Campbell-Walsh-Wein
HANDBOOK *of*
urology

Campbell-Walsh-Wein
HANDBOOK of
urology

Alan W. Partin, MD, PhD
Professor and Director
Department of Urology
The Johns Hopkins School of Medicine
Baltimore, Maryland

Louis R. Kavoussi, MD, MBA
Professor and Chair
Department of Urology
Zucker School of Medicine
   at Hofstra/Northwell
Hempstead, New York;
Chairman of Urology
The Arthur Smith Institute for
   Urology
Lake Success, New York

Craig A. Peters, MD
Chief, Pediatric Urology
Children's Health Texas;
Professor of Urology
UT Southwestern
Dallas, Texas

Roger R. Dmochowski, MD, MMHC, FACS
Professor, Urologic Surgery, Surgery
   and Gynecology
Vice Chair for Faculty Affairs
   and Professionalism
Section of Surgical Sciences
Associate Surgeon-in-Chief
Vanderbilt University Medical Center
Nashville, Tennessee

Associate Editors

Christopher S. Cooper, MD, FAAP, FACS
Professor and Vice Chairman of Urology
Department of Urology
University of Iowa;
Senior Associate Dean of Medical
   Education
University of Iowa Carver College
   of Medicine
Iowa City, Iowa

Kirsten L. Greene, MD, MAS, FACS
Professor and Chair
Department of Urology
University of Virginia
Charlottesville, Virginia

Alexander Gomelsky, MD
B.E. Trichel Professor and Chairman
Department of Urology
Louisiana State University
   Health Shreveport
Shreveport, Louisiana

Robert M. Sweet, MD, FACS
Professor, Department of Urology
   and Surgery (Joint)
Adjunct Professor, Bioengineering
Chief, Division of Healthcare
   Simulation Science
University of Washington
Seattle, Washington

ELSEVIER

Elsevier
1600 John F. Kennedy Blvd.
Ste 1600
Philadelphia, PA 19103-2899

CAMPBELL-WALSH-WEIN HANDBOOK   ISBN: 978-0-323-82747-8
OF UROLOGY

Library of Congress Control Number: 2021948424

Senior Content Strategist: Belinda Kuhn
Content Development Specialist: Denise Roslonski/Laurie Gower
Publishing Services Manager: Deepthi Unni
Project Manager: Beula Christopher
Design Direction: Amy Buxton

Printed in India

Last digit is the print number: 9 8 7 6 5 4 3 2

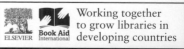

Preface

"Learning is a treasure that will follow its owner everywhere."

Chinese proverb

Access to all forms of **information** has become increasingly easy and exceedingly rapid, whereas access to **knowledge** does not always follow. Our age of information overload has become a blessing and a challenge that we must manage with care. As we edited the *Campbell's Urology* textbook over the past decade, it became evident that our colleagues' demand for practical knowledge had evolved, and with this handbook, we have attempted to address this evolving need. Using the wealth of experience and knowledge of the authors of the Campbell's textbook distilled into a clinically oriented and succinct presentation of the key elements of urology, we have attempted to meet the needs of the clinical urologic student, resident, fellow, or early career provider in an easy access format. We also recognize the need for information review in an efficient format to assist in preparation for exams and other required routine knowledge assessments. This book attempts to provide the basic information and cognitive framework needed by urology providers to both care for patients and assist in examination preparation. We hope the knowledge obtained from using this text will translate into improved care and health for all urologic patients.

From the Editors

Contributors

Gregory M. Amend, MD
Fellow
Department of Urology
University of California San
    Francisco
San Francisco, California

James Anaissie, MD, BSE
Resident
Scott Department of Urology
Baylor College of Medicine
Houston, Texas

Angela M. Arlen, MD
Associate Professor
Department of Urology
Yale University School of
    Medicine
New Haven, Connecticut

**Ramasamy Bakthavatsalam,
    MS, FRCS (G)**
Professor
Department of Surgery and
    Urology
University of Washington
Seattle, Washington

Michael S. Borofsky, MD
Assistant Professor
Department of Urology
University of Minnesota
Minneapolis, Minnesota

Robert E. Brannigan, MD
*Professor, Director of
    Andrology Fellowship*
Department of Urology
Northwestern University,
    Feinberg School of Medicine
Chicago, Illinois

Benjamin N Breyer, MD, MAS
*Professor of Urology and
    Epidemiology and
    Biostatistics*
Department of Urology
University of California San
    Francisco
San Francisco, California

Michael C. Chen, MD
Resident Physician
Department of Urology
Kaiser Permanente Southern
    California
Los Angeles Medical Center
Los Angeles, California

Caitlin T. Coco, MD
Fellow
Children's Health Texas
Department of Urology
University of Texas
    Southwestern
Dallas, Texas

**Christopher S. Cooper, MD,
    FAAP, FACS**
*Professor and Vice Chairman
    of Urology*
Department of Urology
University of Iowa;
*Senior Associate Dean of
    Medical Education*
University of Iowa Carver
    College of Medicine
Iowa City, Iowa

Nicholas G. Cost, MD
Associate Professor
Department of Surgery,
  Division of Urology
University of Colorado School
  of Medicine
Aurora, Colorado

Jessica C. Dai, MD
Assistant Instructor
UT Southwestern Medical
  Center
Dallas, Texas

Atreya Dash, MD
Associate Professor
Department of Urology
University of Washington
Seattle, Washington

Richard J. Fantus, MD
Andrology Fellow
Department of Urology
Northwestern University,
  Feinberg School of Medicine
Chicago, Illinois

Alexander Gomelsky, MD
*B.E. Trichel Professor and
  Chairman*
Department of Urology
Louisiana State University
  Health Shreveport
Shreveport, Louisiana

**Kirsten L. Greene, MD,
  MAS, FACS**
Professor and Chair
Department of Urology
University of Virginia
Charlottesville, Virginia

Sumit Isharwal, MD
Assistant Professor
Department of Urology
University of Virginia
Charlottesville, Virginia

Emily F. Kelly, MD
Resident
Department of Urology
Louisiana State University
  Health Shreveport
Shreveport, Louisiana

**Mohit Khera, MD, MBA,
  MPH**
Professor of Urology
Scott Department of Urology
Baylor College of Medicine
Houston, Texas

Aaron Krug, MD
Resident Physician
Department of Urology
Kaiser Permanente Southern
  California
Los Angeles Medical Center
Los Angeles, California

David A. Leavitt, MD
Assistant Professor
Department of Urology
Vattikuti Urology Institute,
  Henry Ford Health System
Detroit, Michigan

**Gina M. Lockwood, MD,
  MS, FAAP**
Assistant Professor
Department of Urology
University of Iowa
Iowa City, Iowa

Alan W. Partin, MD, PhD
Professor and Director
Department of Urology
The Johns Hopkins School
  of Medicine
Baltimore, Maryland

Craig A. Peters, MD
Chief, Pediatric Urology
Children's Health Texas;
Professor of Urology
UT Southwestern
Dallas, Texas

**Lauren H. Poniatowski,
  MD, MS**
Urology Resident
Department of Urology
University of Washington
Seattle, Washington

Polina Reyblat, MD
Chief of Service
Department of Urology
Kaiser Permanente Southern
  California
Los Angeles Medical Center
Los Angeles, California

**W. Stuart Reynolds, MD,
  MPH**
Associate Professor
Department of Urology
Vanderbilt University Medical
  Center
Nashville, Tennessee

Elizabeth Rourke, DO, MPH
*Female Pelvic Medicine
  and Reconstructive Surgery
  Fellow*
Department of Urology
Vanderbilt University Medical
  Center
Nashville, Tennessee

Bogdana Schmidt, MD, MPH
Assistant Professor
Division of Urology
University of Utah
Salt Lake City, Utah

Bradley F. Schwartz, DO, FACS
Professor and Chairman
Department of Urology
Southern Illinois University
  School of Medicine
Springfield, Illinois

Elisabeth Sebesta, MD
*Female Pelvic Medicine and
  Reconstructive Surgery
  Fellow*
Department of Urology
Vanderbilt University Medical
  Center
Nashville, Tennessee

Douglas W. Storm, MD
Associate Professor
Department of Urology
University of Iowa Hospitals
  and Clinics
Iowa City, Iowa

Peter Sunaryo, MD
Fellow
Department of Urology
University of Washington
Seattle, Washington

Robert M. Sweet, MD, FACS
Professor
Department of Urology and Surgery (Joint)
Adjunct Professor
Bioengineering
Chief
Division of Healthcare Simulation Science
University of Washington
Seattle, Washington

Matthew D. Timberlake, MD
Assistant Professor
Urology and Pediatrics
Texas Tech University Health Sciences Center
Lubbock, Texas

Ernest Tong, MD
Resident
Department of Urology
Louisiana State University Health Shreveport
Shreveport, Louisiana

Samuel Washington III, MD
Assistant Professor
Department of Urology
University of California, San Francisco
San Francisco, California

Dana A. Weiss, MD
Assistant Professor
Department of Urology
University of Pennsylvania;
Attending Physician
Department of Urology
The Children's Hospital of Philadelphia
Philadelphia, Pennsylvania

Jonathan T. Wingate, MD
Assistant Professor
Uniformed Services University of the Health Sciences
Madigan Army Medical Center
Tacoma, Washington

Contents

Evaluation of the Urologic Patient: History, Physical Examination, Laboratory Tests, Imaging, and Hematuria Workup

LAUREN H. PONIATOWSKI, JONATHAN T. WINGATE
AND ROBERT M. SWEET

CONTRIBUTORS OF CAMPBELL-WALSH-WEIN, 12TH EDITION

Sammy E. Elsamra, Erik P. Castle, Christopher E. Wolter, Michael E. Woods, Jay T. Bishoff, Ardeshir R. Rastinehad, Bruce R. Gilbert, Pat F. Fulgham, Michael A. Gorin, and Steven P. Rowe

PATIENT HISTORY AND PHYSICAL EXAMINATION

A proper history and physical examination is essential in evaluating the urologic patient. Completing this assessment reliably and comprehensibly allows for gathering information essential for diagnosis, counseling, treatment, and next steps.

CLINIC VISIT SET-UP

The clinic visit should be comforting and nonthreatening to the patient. The patient room or telehealth visit set-up should include ideal provider-patient positioning and ability to make proper eye contact.

PATIENT HISTORY

Chief Complaint (CC)

The CC is the reason why a patient is seeking urologic care and is the focus of the visit.

History of Present Illness (HPI)

The HPI covers multiple factors related to the CC with the purpose of developing a differential diagnosis.

Constitutional Symptoms. These symptoms include fever, chills, night sweats, anorexia, weight loss, fatigue, and/or lethargy.

Pain. Elicit pain location, radiation, palliative factors, provocative factors, severity (1-10 scale), and timing (including onset and change over time).

- Renal pain (flank pain) – Renal pain is located at the ipsilateral costovertebral angle (CVA) lateral to the spine and inferior to the 12th rib and often radiates toward the abdomen or scrotum/labia.
- Ureteral pain – This is often due to ureteral obstruction and may be present in the ipsilateral abdominal lower quadrant. The pain is often acute in onset and intermittent and may be referred to the scrotum/penis.
- Bladder pain – This type of pain may be due to inflammation (cystitis) or bladder distension (urinary retention). Suprapubic in location with possible improvement after voiding.
- Prostatic pain – This is a deep pelvic pain that may be confused with rectal pain. There are often associated irritative voiding symptoms (urinary frequency, urgency, dysuria).
- Penile pain – Penile pain has a variable presentation with wide differential, including paraphimosis, penile lesions, referred pain, Peyronie's disease, or priapism.
- Scrotal pain – This type of pain may be superficial (skin) or involve the scrotal contents. Testicular torsion is a urologic emergency.

Hematuria. Hematuria is defined as presence of blood in the urine and is divided into categories of gross (visible) versus microscopic (>3 RBC/HPF on microscopic examination) versus pseudohematuria (redness in urine of non-urologic origin). Obtain the presence or absence of associated voiding symptoms, smoking history, chemical exposure history, trauma, urinary tract infections, or recent urologic procedures. Please refer Hematuria section below for more details.

Lower Urinary Tract Symptoms (LUTS). LUTS may be obstructive or irritative in nature. Obstructive symptoms include urinary frequency, intermittency, incomplete emptying, weak stream, hesitancy, and straining with voiding. Irritative symptoms include urinary frequency, urgency, dysuria, or nocturia and may be caused by chronic bladder outlet obstruction, overactive bladder, cystitis, prostatitis, bladder stones, or bladder cancer. The International Prostate Symptom Score (IPSS) is the AUA symptom score with the addition of a quality-of-life score and is a useful tool for assessing LUTS (Table 1.1) (see Chapter 21).

Urinary Incontinence

- Stress incontinence – Involuntary passage of urine with activities that increases intra-abdominal pressure including Valsalva, cough, sneeze, laugh, and/or heavy lifting.
- Urge incontinence – Involuntary passage of urine associated with sudden urge to void. This is often associated with overactive bladder, cystitis, neurogenic bladder, or poorly compliant bladder.
- Mixed incontinence – When a patient experiences both stress and urge incontinence.
- Continuous incontinence – Constant leakage of urine independent of urination patterns or intraabdominal pressure. This is often due to congenital cause or urinary fistula.
- Pseudoincontinence – Incontinence-like symptoms due to non-urologic cause such as vaginal discharge or labial fusions causing retention of urine.
- Overflow incontinence – Leakage of urine due to volume of urine exceeding bladder capacity. This is common in bladder outlet obstruction.
- Functional incontinence – Leakage of urine due to patient immobility or inadequate access to facilities. Patients otherwise have normal urologic anatomy/physiology. See Chapter 16.

Erectile Dysfunction (ED). ED is defined as the inability to attain/maintain penile erection sufficient for satisfactory sexual intercourse. It is important to obtain history related to timing and situational factors of erections. Validated questionnaires for characterizing ED includes the International Index of Erectile Function (IIEF) and the abbreviated IIEF-6 or Sexual Health Index for Men (SHIM). See Chapter 14.

Other Urologic Conditions. Additional topics often covered in a urologic-based HPI include loss of libido, abnormal ejaculation, anorgasmia, hematospermia, pneumaturia, and/or urethral discharge.

Table 1.1 International Prostate Symptom Score

SYMPTOM	NOT AT ALL	<1 TIME IN 5	LESS THAN HALF THE TIME	ABOUT HALF THE TIME	MORE THAN HALF THE TIME	ALMOST ALWAYS	YOUR SCORE
1. Incomplete Emptying							
Over the past month, how often have you had a sensation of not emptying your bladder completely after you finished urinating?	0	1	2	3	4	5	
2. Frequency							
Over the past month, how often have you had to urinate again less than 2 hours after you finished urinating?	0	1	2	3	4	5	
3. Intermittency							
Over the past month, how often have you found you stopped and started again several times when you urinated?	0	1	2	3	4	5	

4. Urgency

Over the past month, how often have you found it difficult to postpone urination?

0   1   2   3   4   5

5. Weak Stream

Over the past month, how often have you had a weak urinary stream?

0   1   2   3   4   5

6. Straining

Over the past month, how often have you had to push or strain to begin urination?

0   1   2   3   4   5

	NONE	1 TIME	2 TIMES	3 TIMES	4 TIMES	≥5 TIMES
7. Nocturia Over the past month, how many times did you most typically get up to urinate from the time you went to bed at night until the time you got up in the morning?	0	1	2	3	4	5

Continued

Table 1.1 International Prostate Symptom Score—cont'd

SYMPTOM	NOT AT ALL	<1 TIME IN 5	LESS THAN HALF THE TIME	ABOUT HALF THE TIME	MORE THAN HALF THE TIME	ALMOST ALWAYS	YOUR SCORE
TOTAL INTERNATIONAL PROSTATE SYMPTOM SCORE							
QUALITY OF LIFE DUE TO URINARY SYMPTOMS	DELIGHTED	PLEASED	MOSTLY SATISFIED	MIXED—ABOUT EQUALLY SATISFIED AND DIS-SATISFIED	MOSTLY DISSATIS-FIED	UNHAPPY	TERRIBLE
If you were to spend the rest of your life with your urinary condition just the way it is now, how would you feel about that?	0	1	2	3	4	5	6

From Cockett A, Aso Y, Denis L. Prostate symptom score and quality of life assessment. In: Cockett ATK, Khoury S, Aso Y, et al., eds. *Proceedings of the Second International Consultation on Benign Prostatic Hyperplasia (BPH); 27-30 June 1993.* Paris, Channel Island: Jersey: Scientific Communication International, 1994:553-555.

Past Medical/Surgical History

It is essential to obtain a complete medical and surgical history (including prior genitourinary or abdominal surgeries). Obtain operative reports when applicable.

Performance Status

Determine the functional ability of patient as a benchmark for his or her tolerance for undergoing challenging or invasive treatments. Assess a patient's ability to perform activities of daily living (ADLs), dressing, eating, toileting, hygiene, preparing meals, shopping, maintaining a house, and interactions with family and community. Grading performance status can be completed using the Eastern Cooperative Oncology Group (ECOG) score or Karnofsky performance status.

Medications

Obtain full medication history including urologic medications and anticoagulants. Also consider medications with urologic side effects (Table 1.2).

Social History

Review where the patient lives, who lives at home with patient, and if there are family/friends in the area. Also obtain occupational history to give insight on socioeconomic status and possible industrial exposures. Review sexual history in a non-accusatory manner such as "Do you partake in sexual relations with men, women, or both? A single partner or multiple?" Obtain drug use history including tobacco, alcohol, illicit drug use. This is important for considering withdrawal or difficulty coping during possible procedures/hospitalizations.

Family History

Ask about urologic conditions/diseases/cancers as well as bleeding disorders, reactions to anesthesia and significant non-urologic conditions/disease/cancers.

Review of Systems

Comprehensive system-based checklist related to other symptoms that may or may not be included in HPI or related to CC.

Table 1.2 Drugs Associated with Urologic Side Effects

UROLOGIC SIDE EFFECTS	CLASS OF DRUGS	SPECIFIC EXAMPLES
Decreased libido Erectile dysfunction	Antihypertensives Psychotropic drugs	Hydrochlorothiazide Propranolol Benzodiazepines
Ejaculatory dysfunction	α-Adrenergic antagonists	Prazosin Tamsulosin α-Methyldopa
	Psychotropic drugs	Phenothiazines Antidepressants
Priapism	Antipsychotics Antidepressants Antihypertensives	Phenothiazines Trazodone Hydralazine Prazosin
Decreased spermatogenesis	Chemotherapeutic agents Drugs with abuse potential Drugs affecting endocrine function	Alkylating agents Marijuana Alcohol Nicotine Antiandrogens Prostaglandins
Incontinence or impaired voiding	Direct smooth muscle stimulants Others Smooth muscle relaxants Striated muscle relaxants	Histamine Vasopressin Furosemide Valproic acid Diazepam Baclofen
Urinary retention or obstructive voiding symptoms	Anticholinergic agents or musculo- tropic relaxants Calcium channel blockers Antiparkinsonian drugs α-Adrenergic agonists Antihistamines	Oxybutynin Diazepam Flavoxate Nifedipine Carbidopa Levodopa Pseudoephedrine Phenylephrine Loratadine Diphenhydramine

Table 1.2 Drugs Associated With Urologic Side Effects—cont'd

UROLOGIC SIDE EFFECTS	CLASS OF DRUGS	SPECIFIC EXAMPLES
Acute renal failure	Antimicrobials	Aminoglycosides
		Penicillins
		Cephalosporins
		Amphotericin
	Chemotherapeutic drugs	Cisplatin
	Others	Nonsteroidal anti-inflammatory drugs
		Phenytoin
Gynecomastia	Antihypertensives	Verapamil
	Cardiac drugs	Digoxin
	Gastrointestinal drugs	Cimetidine
		Metoclopramide
	Psychotropic drugs	Phenothiazines
	Tricyclic antidepressants	Amitriptyline
		Imipramine

PHYSICAL EXAMINATION

Vital Signs

Obtain temperature, heart rate, blood pressure, respiratory rate, and pain rating.

General Appearance

Note level of pain or distress, nutritional status, appearance and self-care, frailty, mobility. Look for stigmata associated with certain disease states.

Kidneys

The kidneys are located in the retroperitoneum and surrounded by the psoas and oblique muscles, peritoneum, and diaphragm. For adults, place the nonexamining hand posteriorly at the costovertebral angle and palpate the kidney with the examining hand through the anterior abdominal wall (Fig. 1.1). Kidneys are typically difficult to palpate and not visible on examination (unless large mass or very thin patient). Assess pain at kidney via percussion by contacting the patient with the closed hand of the examiner at the CVA. Be gentle; a simple tap should elicit a positive sign if present.

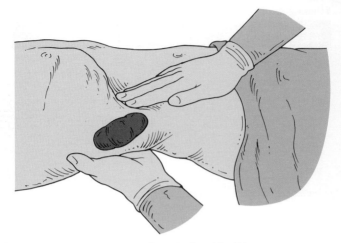

FIG. 1.1 Bimanual examination of the kidney.

Bladder

To examine the bladder, palpate and percuss starting at level of pubic symphysis and ascend toward umbilicus to determine the level of distension. The bladder is palpable when it distends to level above the pubis (~150 cc). The bladder may be visualized when distended at ~500 cc in thin patients. Additionally, A bimanual exam may be performed to assess mobility of the bladder as well as cancer staging.

Penis

Inspect the skin for hair distribution, lesions, presence/absence of foreskin (in adults, retract foreskin to evaluate glans), and Tanner stage. Evaluate the urethral meatus (location, stenosis, presence of urethral discharge). Palpate for any subcutaneous plaques or curvature. Remember to reduce the foreskin at the end of the examination.

Scrotum and Contents

Inspect the scrotal skin for hair distribution, lesions, and infection. Be sure to evaluate the entire scrotum toward the perineum, especially in those with limited mobility or poor self care. Palpate the testicles for size, orientation, pain, or masses. Evaluate for hydrocele, varicocele (patient supine, standing, standing with Valsalva). Palpate the vas deferens. Check for an inguinal hernia by sliding

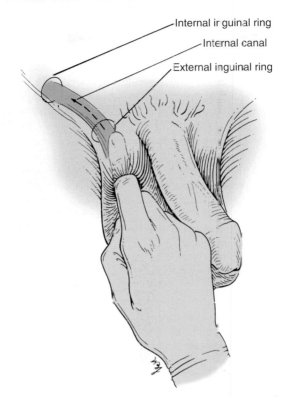

Internal inguinal ring
Internal canal
External inguinal ring

FIG. 1.2 Examination of the inguinal canal. (From Swartz MH. *Textbook of physical diagnosis.* Philadelphia: Saunders, 1939:376.)

the index finger over testis and invaginating the scrotum up toward external ring (Fig. 1.2).

Digital Rectal Examination (DRE)

The DRE is used to assess prostate size and perform screening for prostate cancer. For positioning, the patient should bend 90 degrees at the waist while supporting hand or elbows on the table. Lateral decubitus position with legs flexed at hips is another alternative. The examiner's gloved finger with adequate lubrication then is advanced until the prostate is palpable. A normal prostate is smooth and somewhat soft, whereas nodular firmness is concerning and may warrant biopsy. A bimanual examination (DRE with concurrent lower abdominal exam) is performed in the context of bladder cancer staging.

Pelvic Examination in the Female

The pelvic examination is used to evaluate for pelvic organ prolapse, urinary incontinence, dyspareunia, blood per urethra or vagina, and vaginal masses. Visually inspect external genitalia and introitus (atrophic changes, erosions, ulcers, discharge, lesions). The labia minora should be separated and the urethral meatus inspected for prolapse, caruncle, hyperplasia, or cysts. Use a speculum to visualize vagina and have the patient perform the Valsalva maneuver to evaluate for prolapse. Perform Pelvic Organ Prolapse Quantification (POP-Q) if there is prolapse present. Perform a bimanual examination by placing two of the examiner's fingers of the dominant hand into the vaginal vault and placing the nondominant hand over the lower abdomen and palpating for pelvic mass or tenderness.

LABORATORY TESTS

Urinalysis

The urinalysis (UA) is a fundamental test performed on patients presenting with urinary symptoms. For collection, adults should clean the urethral meatus and surrounding area thoroughly and collect a midstream voided urine sample. Catheterized specimens are preferred for infants and neonates.

UA Evaluation

The evaluation of the UA involves gross examination (Table 1.3), dipstick chemical analysis, and microscopic analysis.

Specific Gravity and Osmolality. Related to patient's hydration or amount of material dissolved in the urine or renal concentrating ability.
- Normal specific gravity 1.001–1.035
- <1.008 = dilute, >1.020 = concentrated
- Normal osmolality 50–1200 mOsm/L

pH. Urinary pH ranges from 4.5–8. Typically reflects serum pH.
- Average urinary pH = 5.5–6.5
- Acidotic urinary pH = 4.5–5.5
- Alkalotic urinary pH = 6.5–8

Table 1.3 Common Causes of Abnormal Urine Color

COLOR	CAUSE
Colorless	Very dilute urine
	Overhydration
Cloudy/milky	Phosphaturia
	Pyuria
	Chyluria
Red	Hematuria
	Hemoglobinuria/myoglobinuria
	Anthocyanin in beets and blackberries
	Chronic lead and mercury poisoning
	Phenolphthalein (in bowel evacuants)
	Phenothiazines (e.g., Compazine)
	Rifampin
Orange	Dehydration
	Phenazopyridine (Pyridium)
	Sulfasalazine (Azulfidine)
Yellow	Normal
	Phenacetin
	Riboflavin
Green-blue	Biliverdin
	Indicanuria (tryptophan indole metabolites)
	Amitriptyline (Elavil)
	Indigo carmine
	Methylene blue
	Phenols (e.g., IV cimetidine [Tagamet], IV promethazine [Phenergan])
	Resorcinol
	Triamterene (Dyrenium)
Brown	Urobilinogen
	Porphyria
	Aloe, fava beans, and rhubarb
	Chloroquine and primaquine
	Furazolidone (Furoxone)
	Metronidazole (Flagyl)
	Nitrofurantoin (Furadantin)
Brown-black	Alcaptonuria (homogentisic acid)
	Hemorrhage
	Melanin
	Tyrosinosis (hydroxyphenylpyruvic acid)
	Cascara, senna (laxatives)
	Methocarbamol (Robaxin)
	Methyldopa (Aldomet)
	Sorbitol

IV, Intravenous.
From Hanno PM, Wein AJ. *A clinical manual of urology.* Norwalk, CT: Appleton-Century-Crofts, 1987:67.

Blood/Hematuria. Normal urine contains less than 3 erythrocytes per HPF. A positive dipstick indicates hematuria, hemoglobinuria, or myoglobinuria. Microscopic examination with greater than 3 RBC/HPF indicates microscopic hematuria. A dipstick result needs to be confirmed with microscopic examination [https://www.aua-net.org/guidelines/asymptomatic-microhematuria-(2012-reviewed-for-currency-2016)]. Hematuria of nephrologic (compared with urologic) source is often associated with casts and significant proteinuria (Table 1.4). Erythrocytes from glomerular disease are typically dysmorphic, whereas tubulointerstitial renal disease and urologic origins have a round shape. Other sources of hematuria include vascular disease like arteriovenous fistulas (AV) fistulas and that is induced by a bought of strenuous exercise. Hematuria in patients on anticoagulants still requires workup. Please refer Hematuria section below for more details.

Leukocyte Esterase (LE) and Nitrite. LE is produced by neutrophils and indicates presence of white blood cells in the urine (false positive indicates specimen contamination). Gram negative bacteria convert nitrates to nitrite and therefore presence of nitrites is strongly suggestive of bacteriuria. If a sample is positive for LE but negative for nitrites, noninfectious causes of inflammation should be considered.

Table 1.4 Glomerular Disorders in Patients With Glomerular Hematuria

DISORDER	PATIENTS
IgA nephropathy (Berger disease)	30
Mesangioproliferative GN	14
Focal segmental proliferative GN	13
Familial nephritis (e.g., Alport syndrome)	11
Membranous GN	7
Mesangiocapillary GN	6
Focal segmental sclerosis	4
Unclassifiable	4
Systemic lupus erythematosus	3
Postinfectious GN	2
Subacute bacterial endocarditis	2
Others	4
Total	100

GN, Glomerulonephritis; *IgA,* immunoglobulin A.
Modified from Fassett RG, Horgan BA, Mathew TH. (1982). Detection of glomerular bleeding by phase-contrast microscopy. *Lancet,* 1(8287):1432-1434.

Bacteria. A fresh uncontaminated urine specimen should not contain bacteria. Presence of bacteria is indicative of a UTI.

Yeast. Funguria is more commonly seen in patients with diabetes mellitus or vaginal candidiasis and typically *Candida albicans*.

Protein. Proteinuria increases suspicion for underlying medical renal disease or overflow of abnormal proteins in the urine (multiple myeloma). If proteinuria is present, consider nephrology consultation.

Glucose and Ketones. Often used for screening patients for diabetes mellitus. The renal threshold for glucose detection in urine is serum glucose >180 mg/dL. Ketones are found in urine when carbohydrate sources in the body are depleted and body fat utilization occurs.

Bilirubin and Urobilinogen. Normal urine contains no bilirubin and only small amounts of urobilinogen.

Urine Cytology

Ordered when urologic malignancy is suspected. Do not order as a screening tool or during initial workup for gross/microscopic hematuria. This test is highly specific for high-grade urothelial cell carcinoma (UCC).

SERUM STUDIES

Creatinine and Glomerular Filtration Rate (GFR)

Obtained to evaluate baseline or current renal function and can aid in investigating renal compromise in the context of urinary tract obstruction.

Prostate-Specific Antigen (PSA)

Tumor marker for diagnostic evaluation of prostate pathology including cancer, benign prostatic hyperplasia (BPH), and inflammatory conditions of the prostate.

Alpha-Fetoprotein (AFP), Human Chorionic Gonadotropin (HCG), and Lactate Dehydrogenase (LDH)

Serum tumor markers for workup of testicular mass/cancer.

Endocrinologic Studies

Total testosterone, free testosterone, luteinizing hormone (LH), follicle-stimulating hormone (FSH), prolactin (PRL), and thyroxine T4 may be ordered in the workup of the male patient with suspected hypogonadism.

Parathyroid Hormone

Ordered for patients with hypercalcemia and calcium-based nephrolithiasis.

OFFICE DIAGNOSTIC PROCEDURES

Uroflowmetry

Used to assess voiding pattern including workup of suspected bladder outlet obstruction. Information obtained includes flow rates, voided volume, and voiding curve/pattern.

Post Void Residual (PVR)

The PVR is the volume of residual urine in the bladder measured via bladder scan (may be inaccurate in patients with obesity or ascites) or catheterization following voiding. Acceptable volumes are patient dependent; however, volumes <100 cc are generally considered within acceptable range.

Cystometography and Urodynamic Studies

Components of urodynamic studies include cystometrography, electromyography, urethral pressure profile, and pressure flow studies. This study is used for patients requiring a comprehensive workup of urinary storage and evacuation.

Cystourethroscopy

This procedure allows for direct visualization and evaluation of the lower urinary tract using a flexible cystoscope.

Imaging of the Urinary Tract

Imaging plays a critical role in the diagnosis and management of urologic disease.

Plain Abdominal Radiography. Conventional radiography study intended to display the kidneys, ureters, and bladder (KUB). Indications for obtaining a plain film include scout film, assessment of residual contrast from previous imaging procedure, pre- and post-treatment assessment of renal calculus disease, assessment of the position of drains and stents (Fig. 1.3), and/or adjunct to the investigation of blunt or penetrating trauma to the urinary tract.

Retrograde Pyelogram (RPG). The RPG allows for opacification of the ureters and intrarenal collecting system via retrograde injection of contrast media (Fig. 1.4). Cystoscopy is performed, and a

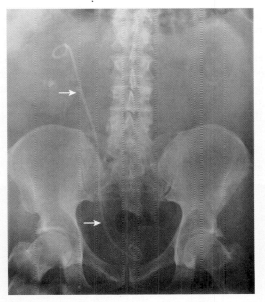

FIG. 1.3 KUB demonstrating residual stone fragments *(arrows)* adjacent to a right ureteral stent 1 week after right extracorporeal shock wave lithotripsy.

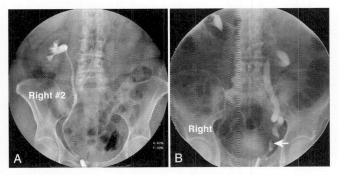

FIG. 1.4 (A) Right retrograde pyelogram performed using an 8-Fr cone-tipped ureteral catheter and dilute contrast material. The ureter and intrarenal collecting system are normal. (B) Left retrograde pyelogram using an 8-Fr cone-tipped ureteral catheter. A filling defect in the left distal ureter *(arrow)* is a low-grade transitional cell carcinoma. The ureter demonstrates dilation, elongation, and tortuosity, the hallmarks of chronic obstruction.

ureteral catheter is used to intubate the desired ureteral orifice. Contrast is injected, and fluoroscopic images are obtained. Indicated to evaluate congenital or acquired ureteral obstruction, elucidation of filling defects and deformities of the ureters or intrarenal collecting systems, opacification or distention of collecting system to facilitate percutaneous access, and evaluation of hematuria, in conjunction with ureteroscopy or stent placement, surveillance of transitional cell carcinoma, and/or evaluation of traumatic or iatrogenic injury to the ureter or collecting system.

Loopography. This is a diagnostic procedure performed in patients having undergone previous urinary diversion (Fig. 1.5). A loopogram

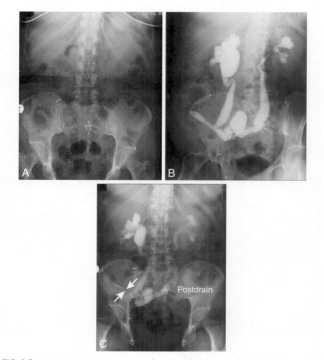

FIG. 1.5 Loopogram in a patient with epispadius/exstrophy and ileal conduit urinary diversion. (A) Plain film prior to contrast administration. (B) After contrast administration via a catheter placed in the ileal conduit, free reflux of both ureterointestinal anastomoses is demonstrated. (C) A postdrain radiograph demonstrates persistent dilation of the proximal loop indicating mechanical obstruction of the conduit *(arrows)*.

performed on an ileal conduit diversion will allow visualization of the ureters and upper collecting systems due to freely refluxing ureterointestinal anastomoses. A small-gauge catheter is inserted via the ostomy and contrast is gently introduced. Plain or fluoroscopic images are obtained. Indications include evaluation of infection, hematuria, renal insufficiency or pain following urinary diversion, surveillance of upper urinary tract for obstruction of urothelial neoplasia and/or evaluation of the integrity of the intestinal segment or reservoir.

Retrograde Urethrography. This is a study to evaluate the anterior and posterior urethra (Fig. 1.6). The patient is positioned obliquely to allow for evaluation of the full length of the urethra. The penis is placed on slight stretch, and contrast is introduced via a catheter inserted into the fossa navicularis. Indications include identifying location and length of urethral stricture, assessment of foreign bodies, evaluation of penile or urethral penetrating trauma, and/or evaluation of traumatic gross hematuria.

Voiding Cystourethrogram (VCUG). This is an imaging study used to the evaluate the anatomy of the bladder and urethra (Fig. 1.7) as

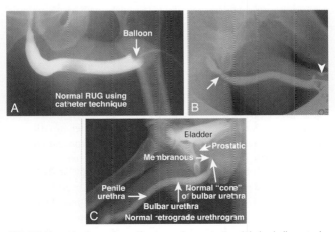

FIG. 1.6 Normal retrograde urethrogram demonstrating (A) the balloon technique for retrograde urethrography, (B) Brodney clamp *(arrowhead)* technique; note the bulbar urethral stricture *(arrow)*, and (C) normal structures of the male urethra.

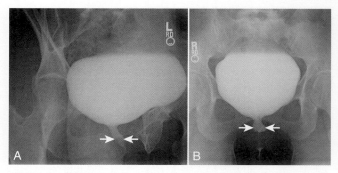

FIG. 1.7 A voiding cystourethrogram performed for the evaluation of recurrent urinary tract infection in this female patient. (A) An oblique film during voiding demonstrates thickening of the midureteral profile *(arrows)*. (B) After interruption of voiding, a ureteral diverticulum is clearly visible extending posteriorly and to the left of the midline *(arrows)*.

well as demonstrating vesicoureteral reflux. The bladder is filled with contrast via catheter (volume varies for children, 200-400 cc for adults). The catheter is removed, and films (AP and oblique) and/or fluoroscopic images are obtained initially, with voiding and post-void. Indications include evaluation of structural and functional bladder outlet obstruction, urethra, and vesicoureteral reflux.

Functional Imaging with Nuclear Scintigraphy

Radionuclide imaging is the procedure of choice to evaluate renal obstruction and function. Common applications for these agents include measurement of renal blood flow, determination of differential renal function, evaluation for the presence and degree of renal obstruction, and assessment of renal scarring.

Technetium ^{99m}–Diethylenetriamine Pentaacetic Acid (^{99m}Tc-DTPA)

- Primarily a glomerular filtration agent useful for evaluation of obstruction and renal function. Upon injection into the bloodstream, ^{99m}Tc-DTPA is extracted by the kidneys entirely through glomerular filtration and is excreted in the urine without being reabsorbed.

- Because of this agent's mechanism of renal clearance, it can be used to calculate GFR.
- This agent is dependent on GFR and less useful in patients with renal failure.

Technetium ^{99m} –Dimercaptosuccinic Acid (^{99m} Tc-DMSA)

- Cleared by glomerular filtration and localizes mostly to the renal cortex.
- Most useful for identifying cortical defects and ectopic kidneys and distinguishing between benign and malignant lesions.
- Because ^{99m} Tc-DMSA is retained by the proximal tubular cells, this imaging agent is ideally suited for imaging cortical processes such as acute pyelonephritis and renal scarring.
- No valuable information on the ureter or collecting system can be obtained with ^{99m} Tc-DMSA.

Technetium ^{99m} -Mercaptoacetyltriglycine (^{99m} Tc-MAG3)

- Cleared mainly by tubular secretion and excreted in the urine.
- Used in diuretic scintigraphy for diagnosis of upper tract obstruction and dynamic renal function (Fig.1.8).

Diuretic Scintigraphy

A renal scan using ^{99m} Tc-MAG3 can provide information regarding differential renal function and obstruction. The patient should be well hydrated the day of the study.

Phamacokinetics. Peak cortical uptake of the ^{99m} Tc-MAG3 radiotracer is typically observed 3 to 5 minutes after intravenous injection, shortly followed by the renal collecting system. By 10 to 15 minutes, the bladder can be visualized as the radiotracer is excreted in the urine.

Phases of Dynamic Renal Imaging. Dynamic renal imaging is performed in the perfusion and functional phases (Fig. 1.9).

- Perfusion phase – Renal plasma blood flow (RPF) to each individual renal unit is measured and compared with flow within the aorta. A curve with a slow rise to peak suggests poor flow to the kidney and likely underlying poor renal function.
- Functional phase – A comparison of the individual renal curves allows for the determination of relative RPF or renal function. A healthy kidney will spontaneously clear the radiotracer within 15 minutes of initial injection. An obstructed renal unit will show retention of radiotracer in the collecting. Some patients

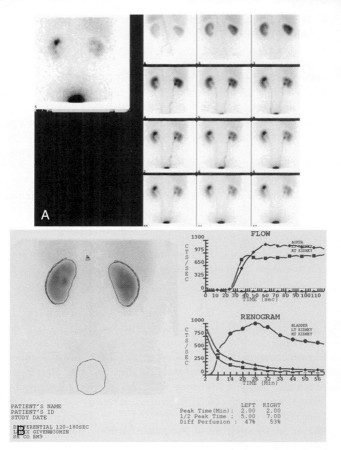

FIG. 1.8 (A) Technetium ^{99m}-mercaptoacetyltriglycine (^{99m}Tc-MAG3) perfusion images demonstrate normal, prompt, symmetric blood flow to both kidneys. (B) Perfusion time-activity curves demonstrating essentially symmetric flow to both kidneys. Note the rising curve typical of ^{99m}Tc-MAG3 flow studies. Dynamic function images demonstrate good uptake of tracer by both kidneys and prompt visualization of the collecting systems. This renogram demonstrates prompt peaking of activity in both kidneys. The downslope represents prompt drainage of activity from the kidneys. Printout of quantitative data shows the differential renal function to be 47% on the left, 53% on the right. The normal half-life for drainage is less than 20 minutes when ^{99m}Tc-MAG3 is used. The half-life is 5 minutes on the left and 7 minutes on the right, consistent with both kidneys being unobstructed.

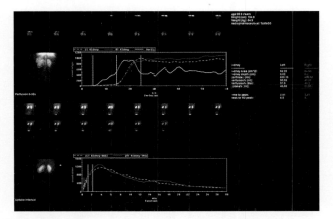

FIG. 1.9 Normal Technetium ^{99m}-mercaptoacetyltriglycine (^{99m}Tc-MAG3) renogram of a patient with history of hydronephrosis being evaluated for obstruction. In the upper portion of the figure, a series of 2-second–per–frame flow images demonstrate the movement of radiotracer from the site of injection, to the heart, aorta/renal arteries, and kidneys. A corresponding time-activity curve is shown. The *white curve* reflects activity in the aorta, and the *purple* and *teal curves* reflect radiotracer activity in the kidneys. Note the sharp upstroke of all three lines and that activity in the aorta precedes activity in the kidneys by several seconds. In the lower half of the figure, a series of 2-minute–per–frame images depicts radiotracer activity within the kidneys as it transitions bilaterally into the collecting systems and then drains down the ureters. In the corresponding time-activity curve, activity within the kidneys peaks at approximately 3 to 4 minutes and then washes out, reaching half-peak approximately 6 to 9 minutes later. The split function of the kidneys is within normal limits, measuring 46% on the left and 54% on the right *(red rectangle)*. No evidence of obstruction is present, and no furosemide is administered.

may experience delayed clearance of radiotracer from the renal pelvis, although they do not have a truly obstructed system (e.g., previously repaired obstructive process such as a ureteropelvic junction obstruction).

- To differentiate these patients from those with obstruction, the diuretic furosemide can be administered when maximum collecting system activity is visualized. The half-time is the time it takes for collecting system activity to decrease by 50% from that at the time of diuretic administration. A post-furosemide half-clearance time of less than 10 minutes is consistent with a patulous nonobstructed system, whereas a half-clearance time of more than 20 minutes is generally consistent with obstruction (Fig. 1.10). A half-clearance time between 10 to 20 minutes is considered indeterminate, and further evaluation is warranted.

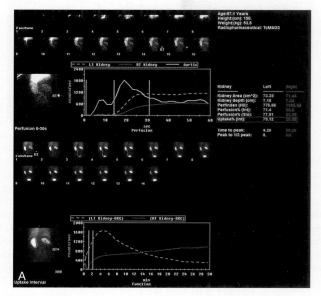

FIG. 1.10 99m Tc-MAG3 renogram of a patient with right-sided renal obstruction. (A) In the 2-second–per–frame flow images at the top of the panel, the left kidney appears much better perfused than the right kidney. This is borne out in the time-activity curve in the upper half of the panel in which the *teal curve* representing the left kidney has a significantly sharper upstroke relative to the *purple curve* of the right kidney. The *white curve* of the aorta is irregular and unreliable because of the abnormal course of the aorta caused by the patient's scoliosis. In the bottom half of the panel, the 2-minute–per–frame images demonstrate normal transit of radiotracer through the left kidney parenchyma and into the collecting system, with drainage to the bladder. This is shown by the *teal curve* of the left kidney on the time-activity curve. The right kidney, which appears smaller and has a central photopenic area corresponding to a dilated renal pelvis, demonstrates increasing uptake throughout the study with very slow transit into the collecting system. This is shown by the *purple curve* of the right kidney in the time-activity curve. A markedly abnormal split function is present, measuring 79% on the left and 21% on the right *(red rectangle)*.

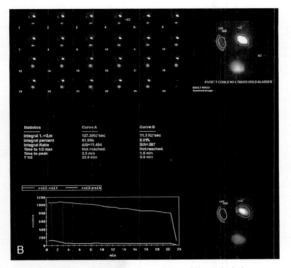

FIG. 1.10, cont'd (B) Given the obstructive pattern of the right kidney, 40 mg of intravenous furosemide was administered. The 1-minute–per–frame images in the upper portion of the panel demonstrate no significant clearing of radiotracer from the left renal collecting system after furosemide administration. This is also seen in the time-activity curve, where the *teal curve* representing the left kidney is nearly horizontal. The lack of response to furosemide is diagnostic of an obstructed collecting system.

Urologic Ultrasonography

Ultrasonography is a versatile and relatively inexpensive imaging modality that utilizes sound waves (Fig. 1.11) to provide real-time evaluation of urologic organs and structures without the need for ionizing radiation.

Renal Ultrasonography. This study is completed using a curved or linear transducer. In adults, the cortex is hypoechoic with respect to the liver (Fig. 1.12). The central band of echoes in the kidney is a hyperechoic area that contains the renal hilar adipose tissue, blood vessels, and collecting system. Renal ultrasonography can be challenging in the context of patient obesity, presence of intestinal gas, or other anatomic abnormalities. Renal ultrasonography has poor sensitivity for renal masses <2 cm.

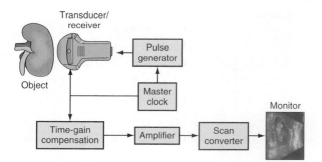

FIG. 1.11 In this simplified schematic diagram of ultrasound imaging, the ultrasound wave is produced by a pulse generator controlled by a master clock. The reflected waves received by the transducer are analyzed for amplitude and transit time within the body. The scan converter produces the familiar picture seen on the monitor. The actual image is a series of vertical lines that are continuously refreshed to produce the familiar real-time, gray-scale image.

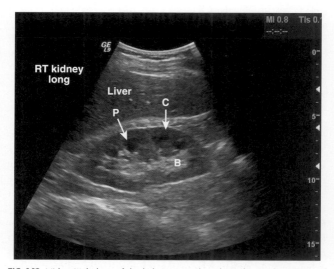

FIG. 1.12 Midsagittal plane of the kidney. Note the relative hypoechogenicity of the renal pyramids *(P)* compared with the cortex *(C)*. The central band of echoes *(B)* is hyperechoic compared with the cortex. The midsagittal plane will have the greatest length measurement pole to pole. A perfectly sagittal plane will result in a horizontal long axis of the kidney.

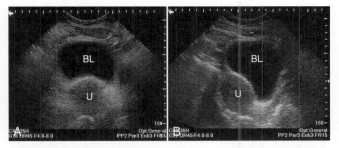

FIG. 1.13 (A) Transverse view of the bladder *(BL)* in this female patient demonstrates the uterus *(U)*. (B) Sagittal view of the bladder shows the uterus posterior to the bladder.

Bladder Ultrasonography. A curved transducer is used, and the patient should have a full bladder to optimize visualization. The bladder is scanned in a sagittal and transverse manner (Fig. 1.13). Evaluation includes the bladder lumen, wall configuration and thickness, presence of lesions/stones/tumors, and emergence of urine from ureteral orifices (ureteral jets).

Scrotal Ultrasonography. Because the scrotum and its contents are superficial, ultrasonography yields excellent and detailed anatomic information including the entire scrotal contents and epididymis. Indications for scrotal ultrasonography include assessment of scrotal and testicular masses, scrotal/testicular pain, scrotal trauma, evaluation of infertility, follow up after scrotal surgery, and evaluation of an empty or abnormal scrotum. Testicular blood flow may be demonstrated with color or power Doppler (Fig. 1.14).

Ultrasonography of the Penis and Male Urethra. Indications include evaluation of penile vascular dysfunction, documentation of fibrosis of the corpora cavernosa, localization of foreign body, evaluation of urethral stricture or diverticulum, or assessment of penile pain or trauma. The most common application of penile ultrasound is in the evaluation of erectile dysfunction (ED) and penile curvature. The proximal portions of the urethra may be evaluated via perineal ultrasonography. Transverse scanning of the

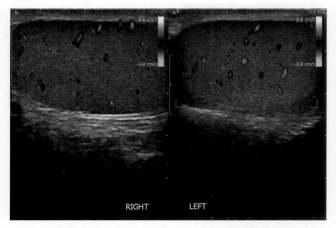

RIGHT   LEFT

FIG. 1.14 Demonstration of normal bilateral intratesticular blood flow by color Doppler.

phallus reveals the two corpora cavernosa dorsally and the urethra ventrally (Fig. 1.15). The sagittal view of the phallus demonstrates the corpora cavernosa with a hyperechoic, double linear structure representing the cavernosal artery. The corpus spongiosum is isoechoic to slightly hypoechoic and contains the coapted urethra.

Transperineal/Translabial Ultrasound. This study allows for visualization of the female bladder, urethra (urethral diverticula, tumors, or foreign bodies), and pelvic floor (Fig. 1.16). This technique can also be used to assess cases of stress urinary incontinence and pelvic organ prolapse in real time and evaluate complications of urethral slings and pelvic reconstruction (sling failure, erosion, de novo voiding dysfunction).

Transrectal Ultrasonography of the Prostate (TRUS). Indications for this study include measurement of prostate volume, abnormal DRE or elevated PSA, ultrasound-guided prostate biopsy, evaluation of cysts, prostatitis, prostate abscess, congenital abnormality, lower urinary tract symptoms, pelvic pain, hematospermia, or

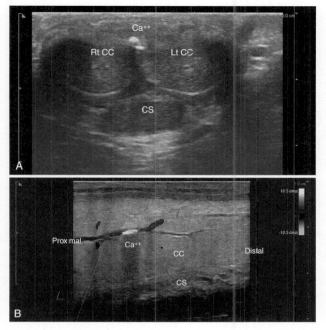

FIG. 1.15 (A) In the transverse plane scanning from the dorsal surface of the midshaft of the penis, the corpora cavernosa (CC) are paired structures seen dorsally, whereas the corpus spongiosum (CS) is seen ventrally in the midline. A calcification (Ca^{++}) is seen between the two CC with posterior shadowing. (B) In the parasagittal plane, the CC is dorsal with the relatively hypoechoic CS seen ventrally. Within the CC, the cavernosal artery is shown with a Ca^{+-} in the wall of the artery and posterior shadowing.

infertility (azoospermia). A digital rectal exam is performed prior to TRUS to evaluate for pain, stricture, mass lesion, or bleeding. The probe is inserted, and a "survey" scan of the prostate is performed from base to apex, including the peripheral zone, transition zone, urethra, seminal vesicles, and rectal wall. Prostate volume is typically calculated using AP, height, and length measurements.

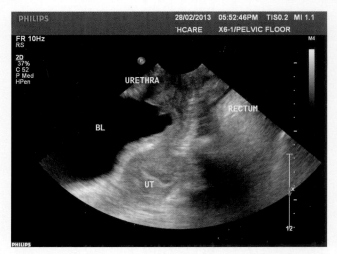

FIG. 1.16 Normal transperineal ultrasound of the female pelvis in the midsagittal plane. The anterior compartment comprises the bladder (BL) and urethra, apical compartment comprises the vagina and uterus (UT), posterior compartment is the rectum. (Image courtesy Lewis Chan, MD.)

Urologic Computed Tomography (CT)

A CT scan produces 3D images of internal structures based on computer reconstruction of cross-sectional images of the body based upon x-ray transmission through thin slices of the body tissue (Fig. 1.17).

Types of CT. CT can be completed with or without intravenous or oral (IV/PO) contrast. IV contrast may be required for better delineation of soft tissue. Oral contrast is not commonly used in urology but may be helpful in certain cases to differentiate bowel from lymph nodes, scar, or tumor. It is important to consider the risks and benefits associated with contrast-enhanced imaging studies.

- **Allergic-like reactions** (mild, moderate, severe) – Consider premedication with corticosteroid/antihistamine.
- **Post-contrast acute kidney injury** – This is defined as deterioration in renal function that occurs within 48 hours following IV iodinated contrast. Avoid iodinated contrast in patients with

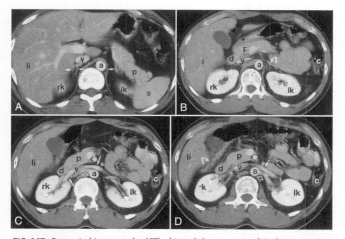

FIG. 1.17 Computed tomography (CT) of the abdomen and pelvis demonstrating normal genitourinary anatomy. (A) The adrenal glands are indicated with *arrows*. The upper pole of the right and left kidneys is indicated with *rk* and *lk*, respectively. *a*, Aorta; *li*, liver; *p*, pancreas; *s*, spleen; *v*, inferior vena cava. (B) Scan through the upper pole of the kidneys. The left adrenal gland is indicated with an *arrow*. *a*, Aorta; *c*, colon; *d*, duodenum; *li*, liver; *k*, left kidney; *p*, pancreas; *rk*, right kidney; *v*, inferior vena cava. (C) Scan through the hilum of the kidneys. The main renal veins are indicated with *solid arrows*, and the right main renal artery is indicated with an *open arrow*. *a*, Aorta; *c*, colon; *d*, duodenum; *li*, liver; *lk*, left kidney; *p*, pancreas; *rk*, right kidney; *v*, inferior vena cava. (D) Scan through the hilum of the kidneys slightly caudal to C. The left main renal vein is indicated with a *solid straight arrow*, and the left main renal artery is indicated with an *open arrow*. The hepatic flexure of the colon is indicated with a *curved arrow*. *a*, Aorta; *c*, colon; *d*, duodenum; *li*, liver; *lk*, left kidney; *p*, pancreas; *rk*, right kidney; *v*, inferior vena cava.

Continued

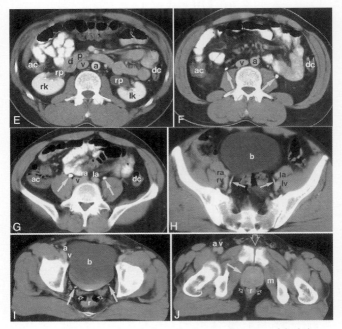

FIG. 1.17, cont'd (E) Scan through the mid to lower polar region of the kidneys. *a*, Aorta; *ac*, ascending colon; *d*, duodenum; *dc*, descending colon; *lk*, left kidney; *p*, pancreas; *rk*, right kidney; *rp*, renal pelvis; *v*, inferior vena cava. (F) CT scan obtained below the kidneys reveals filling of the upper ureters *(arrows)*. The wall of the normal ureter is usually paper thin or not visible on CT. *a*, Aorta; *ac*, ascending colon; *dc*, descending colon; *v*, inferior vena cava. (G) Contrast filling of the midureters *(arrows)* on a scan obtained at the level of the iliac crest and below the aortic bifurcation. *ac*, Ascending colon; *dc*, descending colon; *la*, left common iliac artery; *ra*, right common iliac artery; *v*, inferior vena cava. (H) The distal ureters *(arrows)* course medial to the iliac vessels on a scan obtained below the promontory of the sacrum. *b*, Urinary bladder; *la*, left external iliac artery; *lv*, left external iliac vein; *ra*, right external iliac artery; *rv*, right external iliac vein. (I) Scan through the roof of the acetabulum reveals distal ureters *(solid arrows)* near the ureterovesical junction. The bladder *(b)* is filled with urine and partially opacified with contrast material. The normal seminal vesicle *(open arrows)* usually has a paired bow-tie structure with slightly lobulated contour. *a*, Right external iliac artery; *r*, rectum; *v*, right external iliac vein. (J) Scan at the level of the pubic symphysis *(open arrow)* reveals the prostate gland *(solid arrow)*. *a*, Right external iliac artery; *m*, obturator internus muscle; *r*, rectum; *v*, right external iliac vein.

eFGR <30 mL/min/1.73m². Anuric patients with end-stage renal disease and no functioning transplant kidney may receive IV contrast without risk of additional renal injury. In patients with renal insufficiency on metformin, discontinue metformin the day of iodinated contrast study and hold for 48 hours (risk of developing lactic acidosis).

Hounsfield Units (HU). Unit expressing attenuation values (gray scale of each pixel on a CT depending on the amount of radiation absorbed at that point)

- Air = −1000 HU
- Dense bone = +1000 HU
- Water = 0 HU

Urolithiasis. The standard diagnostic tool for evaluation of kidney stones is noncontrast CT imaging (Fig. 1.18). With the exception of some indinavir stones, all renal and ureteral stones can be detected on CT scan. Stones in the distal ureter can be difficult to differentiate between pelvic calcifications (phleboliths). Low-dose/ultra low-dose unenhanced CT scan should be used when available and is especially important in recurrent stone formers to reduce lifelong radiation exposure.

Cystic and Solid Renal Masses. Renal masses can be characterized as a simple cyst, complex cyst, or solid mass. When the unenhanced CT images of a renal mass are compared with the enhanced images obtained in the cortical medullary or nephrogenic phase, an increase in Hounsfield units (measured in the area of the renal mass) by 15 to 20 HU confirms the presence of a solid enhancing mass, indicating a likely renal cancer. The presence of fat (enhances <10 HU) is diagnostic for angiomyolipoma. A hyperdense cyst shows no change in density between the postcontrast and delayed phase images. Complex cystic masses are characterized by the Bosniak classification system (updated 2019).

Urologic Magnetic Resonance Imaging (MRI)

To obtain an MRI, a patient passes through a magnetic field, and free water protons are oriented along the magnetic field's z-axis. An MR sequence exploits the body's different tissue characteristics and the manner that each type of tissue absorbs and then releases proton energy. Fluid has a low signal intensity and appears dark on T1-weighted MRIs whereas fluid on T2-weighted MRIs has a high

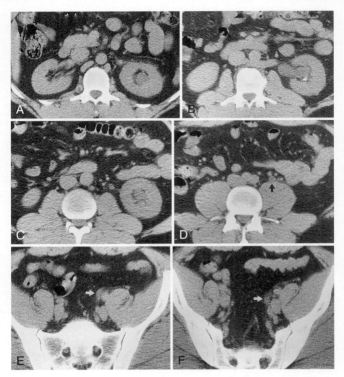

FIG. 1.18 Computed tomography of the abdomen and pelvis in patient with an obstructing ureteral stone at the level of the ureterovesicle junction. (A) Level of the left upper pole. Mild renal enlargement, caliectasis, and perinephric stranding are apparent. (B) Level of the left renal hilum. Left pyelectasis with a dependent stone, mild peripelvic and perinephric stranding, and a retroaortic left renal vein. (C) Level of the left lower pole. Left caliectasis, proximal ureterectasis, and mild periureteral stranding are present. (D) Level of the aortic bifurcation. The dilated left ureter *(arrow)* has lower attenuation than do nearby vessels. (E) Level of the upper portion of the sacrum. A dilated left ureter *(arrow)* crosses anteromedial to the common iliac artery. (F) Level of the midsacrum. A dilated left ureter *(arrow)* is accompanied by periureteral stranding.

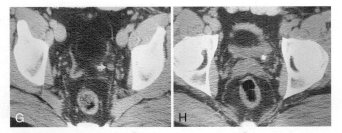

FIG. 1.18, cont'd (G) Level of the top of the acetabulum showing a dilated pelvic portion of the left ureter *(arrow)*. (H) Level of the ureterovesical junction. The impacted stone with a "cuff" or "tissue rim" sign that represents the edematous wall of the ureter. (Reprinted from Talner LB, O'Reilly PH, Wasserman NF. Specific causes of obstruction. In: Pollack HM, et al., eds: *Clinical urography*, 2nd ed. Philadelphia: Saunders, 2000.)

signal intensity and appears bright. Gadolinium contrast should be avoided in patients with eGFR <30 mL/min/1.73m^2 due to risk of nephrogenic systemic fibrosis (NSF). If an MRI is performed in this group, a group II contrast agent should be used. It is not necessary to discontinue metformin for gadolinium contrast studies.

Adrenal MRI. Adrenal lesions are well suited for evaluation with MRI. Benign and malignant lesions are evaluated based on size and lipid content. Pheochromocytoma exhibits a hyperintense "bright" signal intensity on T2-weighted images (Fig. 1.19).

Renal MRI. Benign renal lesions and cysts do not enhance. MRI allows for detecting enhancement of RCC in the wall of complex cysts. Hemorrhage within a cyst results in a high signal on T1-weighted images. MRI allows differentiation of subtypes of RCC using a multiparametric approach (Table 1.5).

Urothelial Cell Carcinoma (Upper and Lower Tract). MR urography can be used in patients in whom other imaging modalities are contraindicated. MR urography uses heavily weighted T2 sequences in which fluid/urine have a high signal intensity or T1-weighted images with gadolinium. Nephrolithiasis or calcification on MRI has no signal characteristics; therefore, it appears as a signal void on imaging. Urothelial tumors, blood clots, gas, or sloughed renal papilla may exhibit a low signal or signal voids on T2-weighted images secondary to the high signal of urine.

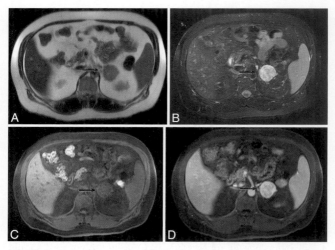

FIG. 1.19 A 50-year-old man with a left side pheochromocytoma and select images from a 1.5T magnetic resonance imaging. (A) Heavily weighted T2 single-shot fast spin echo with an isointense signal (not bright). (B) Moderately weighted T2 fat-suppressed fast recovery fast spin echo with hyperintense signal (bright). (C) T1-weighted precontrast images. (D) T1-weighted postcontrast images with marked early enhancement.

Prostate MRI. Includes anatomic (T1- and T2-weighted imaged) and functional imaging techniques (diffusion-weighted imaging [DWI] with apparent diffusion coefficient [ADC] maps, DCE sequences). Initial T1-weighted sequences are obtained to determine if hemorrhage is present within the prostate and, if present, may limit the diagnostic interpretation of the study. T2-weighted sequences of the prostate provide anatomic information and should include a triplanar (axial, coronal, and sagittal) or comparable sequence (Fig. 1.20). These images provide a detailed anatomic assessment of the gland.

Nuclear Medicine in Urology

Nuclear imaging uses agents labeled with radionuclides to characterize molecular processes within cells. Radiotracers are administered and emit radioactivity that can be detected by an external sensor unit, formatted as an image.

Whole-Body Bone Scan. Skeletal scintigraphy is the most sensitive method for detecting bone metastasis. A "positive" bone scan

Table 1.5 Morphologic and Imaging Characteristics of Incidental Adrenal Lesions (IAL)

IAL	SIZE (cm)	SHAPE	TEXTURE	UNENHANCED CT ATTENUATION (HU)	15-MINUTE CT WASHOUT (%)	MRI SIGNAL CHARACTERISTICS	NUCLEAR MEDICINE CHARACTERISTICS
Adrenal metastasis	Variable	Variable	Heterogeneous when larger	>10	RPW <40	High T2 signal	Positive on PET images
Adrenal cortical carcinoma	>4 cm	Variable	Variable	>10	RPW <40	Intermediate to high T2 signal	Positive on PET images
Pheochromocytoma	Variable	Variable	Variable	>10 rarely <10	RPW <40	High T2 signal	Positive on MIbG
Cyst	Variable	smooth, Round	Smooth	<10	does not enhance	High T2 signal	Negative
Adenoma	1–4 cm	Smooth, round	Homogeneous	<10 in 70%	RPW >40; APW >60	SI dropoff on OP images	Variable on PET images
Myelolipoma	1–5 cm	Smooth, round	Variable with macroscopic fat	<0, often <−50	No data	High T1 signal, India ink, variable SI dropoff on OP images	Negative on PET images
Lymphoma	Variable	Variable	Variable	>10	RPW <40	Intermediate SI	Variable positivity on PET images

Continued

Table 1.5 Morphologic and Imaging Characteristics of Incidental Adrenal Lesions (IAL)—cont'd

IAL	SIZE (cm)	SHAPE	TEXTURE	UNENHANCED CT ATTENUATION (HU)	15-MINUTE CT WASHOUT (%)	MRI SIGNAL CHARACTERISTICS	NUCLEAR MEDICINE CHARACTERISTICS
Hematoma	Variable	Smooth	Variable	>10, sometimes >50	No data	Variable signal	Negative
Neuroblastoma	Variable	Variable	smooth, Round	>10	RPW < 40	Variable if necrotic	Positive
Ganglioneuroroma	Variable	Variable	Variable	>10	No data	Usually intermediate SI	Usually negative
Hemangioma	Variable	Variable	Variable	>10	No data	Usually intermediate SI	Usually negative
Granulomatous	1–5 cm	Smooth	Usually homogeneous	>10	No data	Usually intermediate SI	Positive on PET images if active

APW, Absolute percentage washout; CT, computed tomography; MIBG, m-iodobenzylguanidine; OP, out-of-phase; RPW, relative percentage washout; SI, signal intensity.
From Boland GW, Blake MA. Incidental adrenal lesions: principles, techniques, and algorithms for imaging characterization. Radiology 2008;249(3):756-775; Taffel M, Haji-Momenian S. Adrenal imaging: a comprehensive review. Radiol Clin North Am 2012;50(2):219-243.

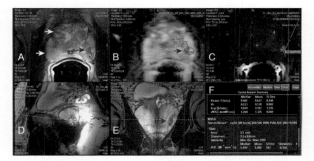

FIG. 1.20 A 66-year-old African American man with a prostate-specific antigen (PSA) of 7.0 and two prior negative biopsies. A 3T mpMRI with an endorectal coil of the prostate was obtained. There were two suspicious areas. (A, D), and (E) are the tri planar axial, sagittal, and coronal plane images, respectively. The peripheral zone *(blue line)* and the central gland *(yellow arrow)* are well visualized. The *red arrow* represents a well-circumscribed heterogeneous benign prostatic hypertrophy nodule (11 mm × 11 mm × 14 mm) within the peripheral zone with no communication to the central gland. (B) The corresponding apparent diffusion coefficient map demonstrates areas of heterogeneous restriction (761 × 10^{-5} mm²/s). (C) The lesion on the dynamic contrast-enhanced (DCE) image exhibits focal type 2 and 3 enhancement curves. (F) The DCE quantitative analysis is listed. The patient underwent a fusion biopsy. The lesion was also appreciated on ultrasonography, and no cancer was detected.

is not specific for cancer and may require plain film radiography, CT, or MRI to confirm as well as correlation with prior history of bone fractures, trauma, surgery, or arthritis.

Positron Emission Tomography (PET). PET/CT and PET/MRI offer diagnostic information based on glucose, choline, or amino acid metabolism depending on the radiotracer used. Molecular imaging of cancer is most commonly performed using PET radiotracer 2-[18F]fluoro-2-deoxy-D-glucose (18F-FDG). It has a well-established role in the detection of residual seminomatous germ cell tumors following chemotherapy (Fig. 1.21).

While it is important to select the study that provides the most useful information, it is also important to consider radiation exposure (Table 1.6) to the patient to be "As Low as reasonably achievable" (ALARA).

HEMATURIA

Hematuria, or presence of blood in the urine, is a concerning urologic sign and it must be thoroughly evaluated because it signals

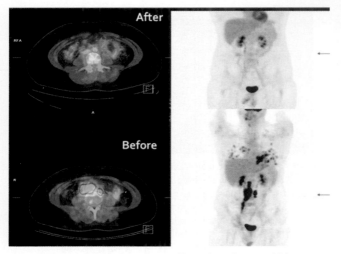

FIG. 1.21 Fluorine-18 fluorodeoxyglucose (^{18}F-FDG) PET/CT is useful for staging and restaging of seminoma in patients treated with chemotherapy. This patient presented with a right-sided seminoma with bulky right-sided retroperitoneal lymph nodes. Positron emission tomography/computed tomography after chemotherapy shows no uptake in the previously positive nodal region.

Table 1.6 Radiation Exposure From Common Urologic Imaging Procedures

RELATIVE RADIATION LEVEL (RRL)	EFFECTIVE DOSE ESTIMATED RANGE	EXAMPLE EXAMINATIONS
None	0	Ultrasound, MRI
Minimal	<0.1 mSv	Chest radiographs
Low	0.1–1.0 mSv	Lumbar spine radiographs, pelvic radiographs
Medium	1–10 mSv	Abdomen CT without contrast, nuclear medicine, bone scan, ^{99m}Tc-DMSA renal scan, IVP, retrograde pyelograms, KUB, chest CT with contrast
High	10–100 mSv	Abdomen CT without and with contrast, whole-body PET

IVP, Intravenous pyelogram; *KUB*, kidney, ureters, bladder
Modified from American College of Radiology: *ACR Appropriateness Criteria Radiation Dose Assessment Introduction.* http://www.acr.org/SecondaryMainMenuCategories/quality_safety/app_criteria/RRLInformation.aspx, 2008.

the presence of a genitourinary (GU) malignancy in up to 25% of patients. Hematuria is classified as gross or microscopic. Gross hematuria (GH) is often alarming to patients, whereas microscopic hematuria (MH) goes unnoticed by the patient until it is detected by urinalysis. Per the American Urological Association (AUA), MH is defined as three or more RBCs/HPF and a single positive urinalysis is sufficient to prompt evaluation.

Causes of Microscopic Hematuria

In most studies, one-thirds to two-thirds of patients evaluated for MH have a demonstrable cause. These include urinary calculus, benign prostatic enlargement (BPH), urethral stricture, and various other conditions (Table 1.7). Malignancy is found in 0.68% to 4.3% of patients being evaluated for MH. The likelihood of identifying malignancy is greater with higher levels of MH (>25 RBCs/HPF), GH, or with risk factors for malignancy (Table 1.8).

Selecting Patients for Evaluation

The AUA guidelines recommend evaluating all adults with asymptomatic MH or GH. A thorough history and exam is required as GH must be distinguished from pigmenturia, which may be due to exogenous sources (e.g., bilirubin, myoglobin), foods (e.g., beets and rhubarb), drugs (e.g., phenazopyridine), and simple dehydration. In women, GH must also be distinguished from vaginal bleeding, which usually can be achieved by obtaining a careful menstrual history.

In order to prevent a misdiagnosis or delay in diagnosis of a more concerning etiology for hematuria, patients who are suspected to have hematuria due to benign causes must have that benign cause substantiated by clinical evidence. They should also be further evaluated once the suspected benign cause has resolved. Patients who develop hematuria in the setting of anticoagulation (e.g., warfarin, enoxaparin, heparin, aspirin, clopidogrel) should still undergo a complete evaluation as the risk of underlying GU malignancy is similar to the patients not on anticoagulation.

Guideline-Based Evaluation of Microscopic and Gross Hematuria

The AUA guidelines has an evaluation algorithm for MH (Fig. 1.22). Again, all patients with gross hematuria should un-

Table 1.7 Differential Diagnosis of Asymptomatic Microhematuria[a]

CATEGORY	EXAMPLES	COMMON CLINICAL PRESENTATION AND RISK FACTORS
Neoplasm	Any	Pelvic irradiation, chronic urinary tract infections, indwelling foreign body
	Bladder cancer	Older age, male predominance, tobacco use, occupational exposures, irritative voiding symptoms
	Ureteral or renal pelvis cancer	Family history of early colon cancers or upper tract tumors, flank pain
	Renal cortical tumor	Family history of early kidney tumors, flank pain, flank mass
	Prostate cancer	Older age, family history, African-American
	Urethral cancer	Obstructive symptoms, pain, bloody discharge
Infection/ inflammation	Any	History of infection
	Cystitis	Female predominance, dysuria
	Pyelonephritis	Fever, flank pain, diabetes, female predominance
	Urethritis	Exposure to sexually transmitted infections, urethral discharge, dysuria
	Tuberculosis	Travel to endemic areas
	Schistosomiasis	Travel to endemic areas
	Hemorrhagic cystitis	Infections, pelvic radiation, certain medications, chemical exposures
Calculus	Any Nephroureterolithiasis	Flank pain, family history, prior stone
	Bladder stones	Bladder outlet obstruction
Benign prostatic enlargement		Male, older age, obstructive symptoms
Medical renal disease[b]	Any	Hypertension, azotemia, dysmorphic erythrocytes, cellular casts, proteinuria
	Nephritis	
	IgA nephropathy	

Table 1.7 Differential Diagnosis of Asymptomatic Microhematuria[a]—cont'd

CATEGORY	EXAMPLES	COMMON CLINICAL PRESENTATION AND RISK FACTORS
Congenital or acquired anatomic abnormality	Polycystic kidney disease	Family history of renal cystic disease
	Ureteropelvic junction obstruction	History of UTI, stone, flank pain
	Ureteral stricture	History of surgery or radiation, flank pain, hydronephrosis; stranguria, spraying urine
	Urethral diverticulum	Discharge dribbling, dyspareunia, history of UTI, female predominance
	Fistula	Pneumaturia, fecaluria, abdominal pain, recurrent UTI, history of diverticulitis or colon cancer
Other	Exercise-induced hematuria[c]	Recent vigorous exercise
	Endometriosis	Cyclic hematuria in a menstruating woman
	Hematologic or thrombotic disease	Family history or personal history of bleeding or thrombosis
	Papillary necrosis	African-American, sickle cell disease, diabetes, analgesic abuse
	Arteriovenous malformation	
	Renal vein thrombosis	
	Interstitial cystitis	Voiding symptoms
	Trauma	History
	Recent genitourinary surgery or instrumentation	History

[a]Differential diagnosis, having ruled out obvious benign causes, such as menstruation, recent instrumentation, uncomplicated cystitis, etc.
[b]Presence of hematologic illness, medical renal illness or use of anticoagulants or antiplatelet agents does not preclude the need for a hematuria evaluation.
[c]Exercise-induced hematuria is a diagnosis of exclusion. Absence of hematuria after abstinence from exercise must be confirmed.
IgA, Immunoglobulin A; *UTI*, urinary tract infection.

Table 1.8 Selected Guidelines for Evaluation of Asymptomatic Microhematuria

GUIDELINE BODY	REFERENCE, YEAR	AGE/SEX	CRITERIA FOR EVALUATION	CYSTOSCOPY	IMAGING	BIOMARKERS
American Urological Association	Davis et al., 2012	Adults	3 or more RBCs/HPF on a single UA	≥35 years old or with risk factors	CT urogram preferred	Not recommended
Canadian Consensus Document	Kassouf et al., 2016	Adults	3 or more RBCs/HPF on 2 out of 3 UAs	≥35 years old	Provider discretion	Not recommended
Kaiser Permanente	Loo et al., 2009	Adults	More than 3 RBCs/HPF on 2 out of 3 UAs	Urologist discretion	CT urogram or IVP + RUS	No consensus on cytology
American College of Obstetricians and Gynecologists and American Urogynecologic Society	Committee Opinion, 2017	Adults Women	Not stated	Avoid in never-smoking women age 35–50; only evaluate if >25 RBCs/HPF	Avoid in never-smoking women age 35–50; only evaluate if >25 RBCs/HPF	Not stated
Japanese	Horie et al., 2014	Adults ≥40 years	5 or more RBCs/HPF on a single UA	≥40 years old, with risk factors	US	+/- Cytology
Dutch	van der Molen and Hovius, 2012	Adults ≥50 years	3 or more RBCs/HPF on 2 out of 3 UAs	>50 years; provider discretion in younger patients	US if >50 years old; provider discretion in younger patients	Cytology recommended in patients with negative evaluation

American College of Physicians	Nielsen and Qaseem, 2016	Adults	3 or more RBCs/HPF on a single UA	Not stated	Not stated	Not recommended
UK National Institute for Health and Care Excellence (NICE)	NICE, 2016; Anderson et al., 2008	Patients over age 60	1+ blood or more on urine dip stick test PLUS Dysuria or elevated leukocytosis	Not stated	Not stated	Not stated

CT, Computed tomography; HPF, high-power field; IVP, intravenous pyelogram; RBC, red blood cell; RUS, renal ultrasound; UA, urinalysis; US, ultrasound.

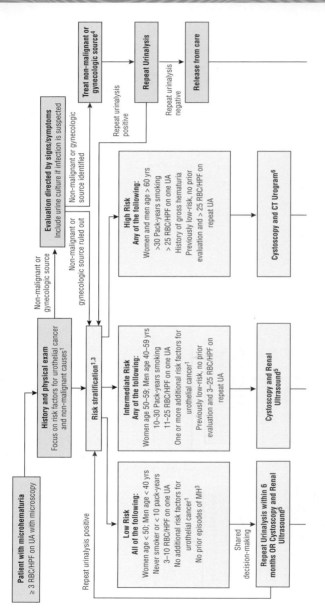

Patient with microhematuria
≥ 3 RBC/HPF on UA with microscopy

History and physical exam
Focus on risk factors for urothelial cancer and non-malignant causes[1]

Evaluation directed by signs/symptoms
Include urine culture if infection is suspected

Non-malignant or gynecologic source identified

Treat non-malignant or gynecologic source[4]

Repeat Urinalysis

Repeat urinalysis negative

Release from care

Repeat urinalysis positive

Non-malignant or gynecologic source ruled out

Non-malignant or gynecologic source

Risk stratification[1,3]

Repeat urinalysis positive

High Risk
Any of the following:
Women and men age > 60 yrs
>30 Pack-years smoking
> 25 RBC/HPF on one UA
History of gross hematuria
Previously low-risk, no prior evaluation and > 25 RBC/HPF on repeat UA

Cystoscopy and CT Urogram[6]

Intermediate Risk
Any of the following:
Women age 50–59; Men age 40–59 yrs
10–30 Pack-years smoking
11–25 RBC/HPF on one UA
One or more additional risk factors for urothelial cancer[1]
Previously low-risk, no prior evaluation and 3–25 RBC/HPF on repeat UA

Cystoscopy and Renal Ultrasound[5]

Low Risk
All of the following:
Women age < 50: Men age < 40 yrs
Never smoker or < 10 pack-years
3–10 RBC/HPF on one UA
No additional risk factors for urothelial cancer[1]
No prior episodes of MH[3]

Shared decision-making

Repeat Urinalysis within 6 months OR Cystoscopy and Renal Ultrasound[5]

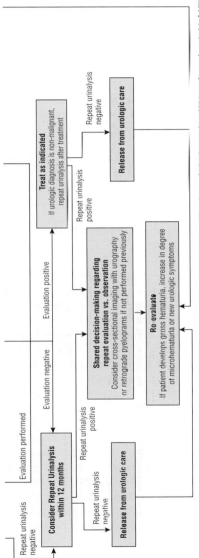

Repeat urinalysis negative

Consider Repeat Urinalysis within 12 months

Evaluation performed

Repeat urinalysis positive

Release from urologic care

Repeat urinalysis negative

Evaluation negative

Evaluation positive

Shared decision-making regarding repeat evaluation vs. observation
Consider cross-sectional imaging with urography or retrograde pyelograms if not performed previously

Treat as indicated
If urologic diagnosis is non-malignant, repeat urinalysis after treatment

Repeat urinalysis positive

Repeat urinalysis negative

Release from urologic care

Re-evaluate
If patient develops gross hematuria, increase in degree of microhematuria or new urologic symptoms

1. Main risk factors for urothelial cancer are those in the AUA risk stratification system (age, male sex, smoking, degree of microhematuria and history of gross hematuria). Additional risk factors for urothelial carcinoma include but are not limited to irritative lower urinary tract voiding symptoms, history of cyclophosphamide or ifosfamide chemotherapy, family history of urothelial carcinoma or Lynch Syndrome, occupational exposures to benzene chemicals or aromatic amines, history of chronic indwelling foreign body in the urinary tract.
2. If medical renal disease is suspected, consider nephrologic evaluation, but pursue concurrent risk-based urological evaluation
3. Patients may be low-risk at first presentation with microhematuria, but may only be considered intermediate- or high-risk if found to have persistent microhematuria
4. There are non-malignant and gynecologic sources of microhematuria that do not require treatment and/or may confound the diagnosis of MH. Clinicians can consider catheterized urine specimen in women with vaginal atrophy or pelvic organ prolapse. Clinicians must use careful judgment and patient engagement to decide whether to pursue MH evaluation in the setting of chronic conditions that do not require treatment, such as the aforementioned gynecologic conditions, non-obstructing stones or BPH.
5. Clinician may perform cross-sectional imaging with urography or retrograde pyelograms if hematuria persists after negative renal ultrasound
6. MR Urogram or Non-contrast imaging plus retrograde pyelograms if contraindications to CT Urogram

FIG. 1.22 Microscopic (MH) Algorithm. https://www.auanet.org/documents/Guidelines/GUI-20-5442%20MH%20Algorithm.pdf.

dergo a complete evaluation of the upper and lower genitourinary tracts. For MH, patients meeting criteria should undergo a risk stratified evaluation, even if one phase of the evaluation shows a suspected cause for the MH. For example, if a patient is found to have nephrolithiasis or a renal tumor on upper tract imaging, they should still undergo cystoscopy for to evaluate for lower tract pathology.

- A thorough history and physical exam should be performed. The goal is to identify causes that may warrant variation from the standard evaluation, such as infection, menstrual bleeding, known medical-renal disease, food/medications, trauma, or recent GU instrumentation. The history should also include an assessment of symptoms, such as GH, voiding symptoms, or flank pain. It should also include risk factors for hematuria. Current medications, including anticoagulants, should be elicited even though it would not preclude an evaluation for hematuria. The history should include questions about tobacco use as it is the number one risk factor for bladder cancer.
- Physical examination should focus on the GU system (e.g., flank tenderness, palpable masses in the flank, abdomen, suprapubic region, urethra; prostate exam, meatal stenosis). If urethral stricture or BPH is suspected, urine flow rate and postvoid residual measurement may be helpful.
- Laboratory testing includes urinalysis (if not performed previously) to assess for hematuria, dysmorphic RBCs, cellular casts, or proteinuria. Urine culture should be performed if the urinalysis is concerning for a urinary tract infection (UTI). Prostate-specific antigen should be checked in the appropriate setting and patient population.
- Urine cytologic examination is highly sensitive and specific for the detection of high-grade urothelial carcinoma. However, current evidence indicates that currently available urinary biomarkers, including cytology, is not sufficiently sensitive to replace cystoscopy or imaging, therefore, it should be not be performed in patients with MH. However, cytologic examination may be considered in patient with a negative initial workup in whom urothelial carcinoma is still suspected, as well as in patients with symptomatic MH or GH.

- If a benign cause of hematuria is found during the initial evaluation (e.g., UTI), that cause should be verified, treated, then the urine should be retested to ensure the hematuria has resolved. If a medical renal cause of hematuria is suspected based on history and laboratory finding, nephrology evaluation is recommended, but the patient should still undergo full urologic hematuria evaluation.

Lower Tract Evaluation

Cystoscopy is the gold standard for lower tract evaluation because it is the most reliable way to evaluate the bladder for the presence of tumors and it allows for evaluation of the urethra. It should be performed in all intermediate and high risk patients. It can be considered in low risk patients rather than a repeat urinalysis (Fig 1.22). Currently, the AUA recommends against the use of blue-light cystoscopy for the evaluation of MH.

Upper Tract Evaluation

Multiphasic computed tomography (CT) urogram (i.e., CT with precontrast, nephrographic, and excretory phases) is the imaging study recommended by the AUA guidelines for the evaluation of high risk patients with hematuria. (Fig. 1.23).

- **First phase** – Unenhanced CT to distinguish between different masses that can be present in the kidney and uncover kidney stones that would later be obscured by the excretion of contrast into the renal collecting system.
- **Second Phase (Corticomedullary Phase)** – 30 to 70 seconds after contrast injection, defines vasculature and perfusion.
- **Third Phase (Nephrogenic Phase)** – 90 to 180 seconds after injection of contrast, allows sensitive detection and characterization of renal masses.
- **Final Phase (Excretory Phase)** – 3 to 5 minutes after injection of contrast. Allows visualization of the collecting system.

It offers complete imaging of the upper GU tract and has the highest sensitivity and specificity for detecting lesions (e.g., nephrolithiasis, renal masses, ureteral masses). In patients whom CT urogram is contraindicated, magnetic resonance (MR) urogram may be used instead. In patients with contraindications for both imaging modalities (e.g. significant renal compromise, contrast

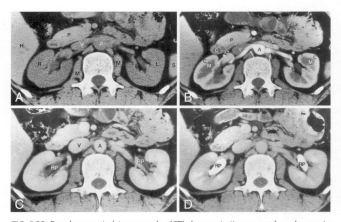

FIG. 1.23 Renal computed tomography (CT) demonstrating normal nephrogenic progression. (A) Unenhanced CT scan obtained at the level of the renal hilum shows right (R) and left (L) kidneys of CT attenuation values slightly less than those of the liver (H) and pancreas (P). *A,* Abdominal aorta; *M,* psoas muscle; *S,* spleen; *V,* inferior vena cava. (B) Enhanced CT scan obtained during a cortical nephrographic phase, generally 25 to 80 seconds after contrast medium injection, reveals increased enhancement of the renal cortex (C) relative to the medulla (M). The main renal artery is indicated with *solid arrows* bilaterally. Main renal veins *(open arrows)* are less opacified with respect to the aorta (A) and arteries. *D,* Duodenum; *P,* pancreas; *V,* inferior vena cava. (C) CT scan obtained during the homogeneous nephrographic phase, generally between 85 and 120 seconds after contrast medium administration, reveals a homogeneous, uniform, increased attenuation of the renal parenchyma. The wall of the normal renal pelvis (RP) is paper thin or not visible on the CT scan. *A,* Abdominal aorta; *V,* inferior vena cava. (D) CT scan obtained during the excretory phase shows contrast medium in the RP bilaterally; this starts to appear approximately 3 minutes after contrast medium administration.

allergies, pacemaker), the upper tracts may be evaluated with non-contrasted CT or ultrasound in conjunction with retrograde pyelography to evaluate the calyces, renal pelvis, and ureters. Ultrasound is also recommended as the primary imaging modality for the low and intermediate risk hematuria patient.

If evaluation reveals nephrolithiasis, renal mass, or bladder tumor, these should be treated per guidelines and will be discussed elsewhere in this handbook. This chapter will discuss treatment of other benign etiologies of hematuria.

Key Points

- A urologist should systematically perform a complete urologic history and physical exam considering a broad differential for the presenting chief complaint.
- It is important to consider all components of a patient's status including social history and performance status as well as special considerations for certain populations including children and the elderly.
- A dipstick urine test alone is inadequate for the diagnosis of microscopic hematuria. AMH must be demonstrated by 3 RBC/HPF on microscopic examination.
- Urine cytology is not recommended during initial workup for AMH, however it is specific for high-grade UCC.
- A CT urogram is sensitive and specific for upper tract urothelial cell carcinoma and is a study used during workup of hematuria.
- A CT noncontrast study of the abdomen and pelvis is key for evaluating urolithiasis with the exception of indinavir stones.
- For a renal mass on MRI, the most important characteristic indicating malignancy is enhancement.

Molecular imaging for urologic malignancies is most often performed using the PET radiotracer 2-deoxy-2-[^{18}F]fluoro-D-glucose (^{18}F-FDG).

Suggested Readings

American College of Radiology (ACR). *Manual on contrast media*. 2020. https://www.acr.org/-/media/ACR/Files/Clinical-Resources/Contrast_Media.pdf.

Barocas DA, Boorjian SA, Alvarez RD, et al. Microhematuria: AUA/SUFU Guideline. *J Urol* 2020;204(4):778-786. https://doi.org/10.1097/JU.0000000000001297.

Barry MJ, Fowler FJ, O'Leary MP, et al. The American urological association symptom index for benign prostatic hyperplasia. *J Urol* 1992;148:1549.

Davis R, Jones JS, Barocas DA, et al. Diagnosis, evaluation and follow-up of asymptomatic microhematuria (AMH) in adults: AUA guideline. *J Urol* 2012;188:2473-2481.

Farwell MD, Pryma DA, Mankoff DA. PET/CT imaging in cancer: current applications and future directions. *Cancer* 2014;120:3433-3445.

Karnofsky DA, Abelmann WH, Craver LF, et al. The use of the nitrogen mustards in the palliative treatment of carcinoma—with particular reference to bronchogenic carcinoma. *Cancer*, 1948;1(4):634-656.

Kriston L, Gunzler C, Harms A, et al. Confirmatory factor analysis of the German version of the international index of erectile function (IIEF): a comparison of four models. *J Sex Med* 2008;5:92.

Oken MM, Creech RH, Tormey DC, et al. Toxicity and response criteria of the Eastern Cooperative Oncology Group. *Am J Clin Oncol* 1982;5(6):649-655.

Silverman SG, Pedrosa I, Ellis JH, et al. Bosniak classification of cystic renal masses, version 2019: an update proposal and needs assessment. *Radiology* 2019;292:475-488.

Steiner H, Bergmeister M, Verdorfer I, et al. Early results of bladder-cancer screening in a high-risk population of heavy smokers. *Br J Urol* 2008;102:291-296.

2

Principles of Urologic Surgery: Perioperative Management

JESSICA C. DAI AND ROBERT M. SWEET

CONTRIBUTORS OF CAMPBELL-WALSH-WEIN, 12TH EDITION

Simpa S. Salami, David Mikhail, Simon J. Hall, Manish A. Vira, Christopher J. Hartman, Casey A. Dauw, Stuart J. Wolf, and Melissa R. Kaufman

PREOPERATIVE EVALUATION

History

A "history and physical" should be completed within 30 days of surgery and updated the day of surgery. Significant comorbidities should be elicited, and any poorly controlled comorbidities should be noted for preoperative optimization.

Physical Exam

A comprehensive physical exam may reveal signs of poorly compensated systemic disease. Body habitus and previous surgical scars should be noted; careful examination of the abdomen, groin, and perineum may help determine the preferred operative approach. The abdomen should also be specifically assessed for potential stoma sites prior to urinary diversion surgery.

Functional Assessment

Preoperative "fitness" is associated with postoperative morbidity and mortality, hospital length of stay, and postoperative return to function. Overall functional status may be assessed through the patient's ability to perform activities of daily living (ADLs) or independent activities of daily living (IADLs), and brief mobility tests (e.g., The Timed up and go test). Frailty may be assessed with standardized instruments (e.g., Fried frailty score). Detailed cognitive assessment (e.g., mini-cog test) may also be performed for those with cognitive impairment or dementia and for geriatric patients.

Preoperative Education

Preoperative education should include discussion regarding the risks, benefits, and alternatives of surgery. Anesthesia type, incision size and location, surgical approach, and postoperative drains or catheters should be addressed. Expectations regarding postoperative recovery, pain management, and anticipated return to activity should be set. Preoperative teaching with a stomal therapist may also benefit patients undergoing urinary diversion.

Risk Stratification Tools

The American Society of Anesthesiologists (ASA) Physical Status Classification is a commonly used framework to risk stratify patients' physical status based on preoperative morbidities. This is an independent predictor of perioperative mortality (Box 2.1). Additional surgical risk calculators such as the American College of Surgeons National Surgical Quality Improvement Program calculator (ACS NSQIP, https://riskcalculator.facs.org/RiskCalculator/PatientInfo.jsp), can also be used to predict a wide range of more individualized postoperative outcomes.

Box 2.1 American Society of Anesthesiologists (ASA) Classification		
1	ASA class I	Normal healthy patient
2	ASA class II	Patient with mild systemic disease
3	ASA class III	Patient with severe systemic disease that limits activity but is not incapacitating
4	ASA class IV	Patient with incapacitating disease that is a constant threat to life
5	ASA class V	Moribund patient not expected to survive 24 hours with or without an operation
6	ASA class VI	A declared brain-dead patient whose organs are being removed for donor purposes
7	ASA class E	In the event of emergency surgery, an E is added after the Roman numeral (in I through V classes)

Preoperative Tests

Routine preoperative laboratory testing for healthy patients undergoing noncardiac surgeries is not mandatory, as this has been shown to be no more cost-effective or predictive of perioperative outcomes than ASA status. However, for select patients, preoperative tests may help guide perioperative management. This may include a complete blood count, basic metabolic panel, prothrombin time (PT), partial thromboplastin time, and internationalized normalized ratio (INR). Urine pregnancy tests should be performed on the day of surgery for all women of childbearing age. Electrocardiograms should be considered for those with cardiac comorbidities or older than 40 years old. Routine chest radiography is not recommended in the absence of preexisting cardiopulmonary disease. For patients with chronic obstructive pulmonary disease (COPD), pulmonary function tests and spirometry may be considered. However, these are not predictive of postoperative pulmonary complications.

OPTIMIZATION OF PREOPERATIVE COMORBIDITIES

Cardiac

Patients with serious preoperative cardiac disorders (e.g., coronary artery disease, heart failure, symptomatic arrhythmias, orthostatic hypotension, and pacemaker or defibrillator dependency) should be identified preoperatively. The American College of Cardiology and American Heart Association task force (2014) has identified three predictors for major adverse cardiac events: clinical markers, functional capacity, and type of surgical procedure. These determine the need for further cardiac evaluation before nonemergent surgeries (Fig. 2.1). Beta-blockers should be continued perioperatively.

Clinical Markers. Major clinical predictors of cardiovascular risk include recent myocardial infarct (<1 month), unstable angina, cardiac ischemia, decompensated heart failure, significant arrhythmias, and severe valvular disease.

Functional Capacity. Metabolic equivalents of the task (MET) refers to the ability to meet the aerobic demands for a specific activity. A 4-MET equivalent is the ability to climb two flights of stairs; a 4-MET capacity generally indicates no further need for invasive cardiac evaluation. The Duke Activity Status Index (Table 2.1) may be used to assess functional capacity.

Type of Surgical Procedure. High-risk procedures include major emergent surgeries and those resulting in long operative times,

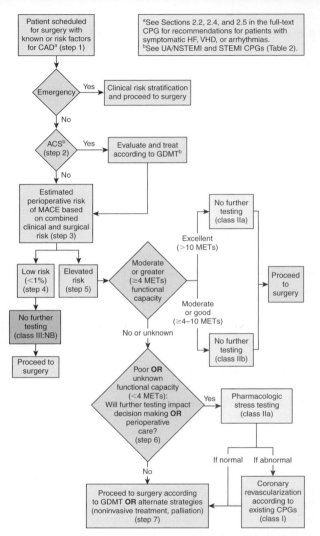

FIG. 2.1 Recommendations for perioperative cardiovascular evaluation and management. From the 2014 American College of Cardiology/American Heart Association guideline recommendations for perioperative cardiovascular evaluation and management of patients undergoing noncardiac surgery. *CAD*, Coronary artery disease; *CPG*, clinical practice guideline; *GDMT*, guideline-directed medical therapy; *MACE*, major adverse cardiac event; *MET*, metabolic equivalents. Reprinted with permission Circulation.2014;130:e278-e333 © 2014 American Heart Association, Inc.

Table 2.1 Duke Activity Status Index[a]

ACTIVITY	YES	NO
Can you take care of yourself such as eating, dressing, bathing, or using the toilet?	2.75	0
Can you walk indoors such as around your house?	1.75	0
Can you walk a block or two on level ground?	2.75	0
Can you climb a flight of stairs or walk up a hill?	5.50	0
Can you run a short distance?	8.00	0
Can you do light work around the house such as dusting or washing dishes?	2.70	0
Can you do moderate work around the house such as vacuuming, sweeping floors, or carrying in groceries?	3.50	0
Can you do heavy work around the house such as scrubbing floors or lifting and moving heavy furniture?	8.00	0
Can you do yardwork such as raking leaves, weeding, or pushing a power mower?	4.50	0
Can you have sexual relations?	5.25	0
Can you participate in moderate recreational activities such as golf, bowling, dancing, doubles tennis, or throwing a baseball or football?	6.00	0
Can you participate in strenuous sports such as swimming, singles tennis, football, basketball, or skiing?	7.50	0

[a]The most widely recognized measure of cardiorespiratory fitness is maximal oxygen consumption (VO_2peak) measured in mL/kg/min. The index score correlates directly with VO_2peak and therefore is an indirect measure of maximal metabolic equivalents (METs).
Duke activity status index (DASI) = Sum of values for all 12 questions.
Estimated peak oxygen uptake (VO_2peak) in mL/min = $(0.43 \times DASI) - 9.6$.
METs = VO_2peak $\times 0.286$ (mL/kg/min)$^{-1}$.
Modified from Hlatky MA, Boineau RE, Higginbotham MB, et al. A brief self-administered questionnaire to determine functional capacity (the Duke Activity Status Index). *Am J Cardiol* 1989;64(10):651-654.

major fluid shifts, or blood loss. Intermediate-risk procedures include minimally invasive surgeries. Low-risk procedures include endoscopic or superficial surgeries and require no further testing. **Cardiac Risk Calculators.** The ACS NSQIP Risk calculator, Gupta Perioperative Risk Myocardial Infarction or Cardiac Arrest Calculator, Goldman's Risk Indices, and Revised Cardiac Risk Index may all be used to more precisely estimate an individual cardiac risk.

Pulmonary

Risk factors for pulmonary complications include age older than 60 years, chronic lung disease, smoking congestive heart failure, obesity, asthma, and obstructive sleep apnea (OSA). Preoperative bronchodilators for COPD patients and corticosteroid inhalers for asthmatic patients should be continued.

Smoking. Smokers have a 4-fold higher risk of perioperative morbidity and 10-fold higher mortality rate. Smoking cessation ≥6 months prior to surgery decreases pulmonary morbidity to nonsmoker rates and cessation ≥4 weeks prior to surgery decreases postoperative wound healing and pulmonary complications. Although it was traditionally believed that smoking cessation within 8 weeks of surgery resulted in greater pulmonary complications, more recent literature does not support this.

Obstructive Sleep Apnea. OSA may be identified preoperatively using validated screening tools (e.g., Berlin Questionnaire, ASA STOP Questionnaire). Perioperative continuous positive airway pressure therapy should be used for these patients.

Hepatobiliary

The Child-Pugh classification estimates perioperative morbidity and mortality for cirrhotic patients using serum markers (e.g., bilirubin, albumin, PT) and clinical signs (e.g., encephalopathy, ascites). Estimated mortality risk is 0% for Child's class A, 30% for Child's class B, and 76%–82% for Child's class C. The Model for End Stage Liver Disease (MELD) score provides even more accurate estimates of perioperative mortality based on serum laboratories (e.g., creatinine, bilirubin, INR) and dialysis status (https://mayoclinic.org/meld/mayomodel9.html). Both provide critical risk assessments for cirrhotic patients.

Endocrine

Careful perioperative management of endocrinopathies are critical to minimize surgical complications.

Diabetes. Perioperative hyperglycemia is associated with impaired wound healing and higher infection rates. Recommended glucose targets are 140–200 mg/dL, depending on illness severity and patient characteristics. Perioperative management of insulin and hypoglycemic agents is summarized in Table 2.2.

Hypothyroidism. A euthyroid state should be achieved prior to elective surgery. Thyroid replacement medication and beta-blockers should be continued perioperatively because hypothyroid patients are at risk for thyrotoxicosis. This may manifest as fevers,

Table 2.2 Management of Perioperative Hypoglycemic Agents

AGENT	DAY PRIOR TO ADMISSION	DAY OF SURGERY
Meglitinides (e.g., repaglinide, nateglinide)	Take as normal	**Surgery in AM:** omit morning dose **Surgery in PM:** give morning dose if eating
Sulphonylurea (e.g., glibenclamide, gliclazide, glipizide)	Take as normal	**Surgery in AM:** omit morning dose **Surgery in PM:** omit morning dose
SGLT-2 inhibitors (e.g., dapagliflozin, canagliflozin)	No dose change	**Surgery in AM:** ½ usual morning dose; check glucose on admission; leave evening meal dose unchanged **Surgery in PM:** ½ usual morning dose; check glucose on admission; leave evening meal dose unchanged NB: also omit day after surgery
Acarbose	Take as normal	**Surgery in AM:** omit morning dose **Surgery in PM:** give morning dose if eating
DPP-IV inhibitors (e.g., sitagliptin, vildagliptin, saxagliptin, alogliptin, linagliptin)	Take as normal	Take as normal
GLP-1 analogues (e.g., exenatide, liraglutide, lixisenatide)	Take as normal	Take as normal
Metformin (procedure not requiring use of contrast media)	Take as normal	Take as normal
Pioglitazone	Take as normal	Take as normal
Basal insulin regimen (e.g., glargine, detemir, NPH)	Take 80% of basal dose	Take 80% of basal dose

DPP-IV, Dipeptidyl peptidase-IV; *GLP-1,* glucagon-like peptide-1; *SGLT-2,* sodium-glucose cotransporter-2.
Adapted from Stoffel JT, Montgomery JS, Suskind AM, Tucci C, Vanni AJ. *Optimizing outcomes in urological surgery: preoperative care for the patient undergoing urologic surgery or procedure.* American Urological Association White Paper, 2018.

tachycardia, confusion, or cardiovascular collapse. Thyroid storm may be managed with iodine and steroids.

Chronic Steroid Use. Stress-dose steroids should be administered for patients with hypothalamic-pituitary axis suppression from chronic high-dose steroid use (daily intake of >20 mg prednisone or equivalents for >3 weeks during the past year). Typically, 50–100 mg intravenous (IV) cortisone is administered prior to induction of anesthesia followed by 25–50 mg hydrocortisone every 8 hours for 24–48 hours. Without supplementation, patients may exhibit signs of adrenal insufficiency, including nausea, vomiting, hypotension, changes in mental status, hyponatremia, or hyperkalemia.

Neurologic

Risk factors for perioperative cerebrovascular accidents include hypertension, diabetes, heart disease, smoking, obesity, age, gender, prior transient ischemic events, brain aneurysms, or arteriovenous malformations. Prior to elective surgery, carotid artery stenting or endarterectomy is indicated for symptomatic, high-grade (>70%) stenosis and should also be considered for asymptomatic patients with >60% stenosis.

PERIOPERATIVE CONSIDERATIONS

Antithrombotic Therapy

Management of antithrombotic therapy requires a careful balance of thrombotic risk and perioperative bleeding risk. The 2014 AUA/International Consultation on Urological Disease (ICUD) White paper provides perioperative recommendations for the management of antiplatelet and anticoagulant agents for commonly performed urologic procedures.

Antiplatelet Agents. Antiplatelet agents (e.g., aspirin, clopidogrel) irreversibly inhibit platelet function and must be stopped 7–10 days before surgery. Dual antiplatelet therapy should be continued for at least 6 weeks following placement of bare-metal cardiac stents and 12 months after drug-eluting stents; elective surgery should be deferred until one or both agents may be stopped. Patients taking antiplatelets for secondary stroke prevention should continue aspirin perioperatively. Low-dose aspirin may be continued perioperatively if significant cardiac risk factors exist. A summary of antiplatelet management is illustrated in Fig. 2.2.

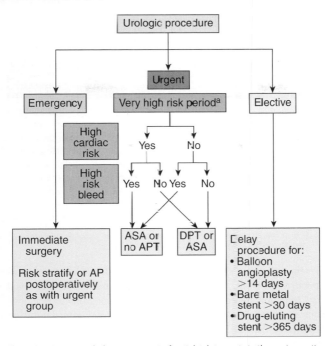

FIG. 2.2 Recommended management of antiplatelet agents in the perioperative period. As published in "Anticoagulation and Antiplatelet Therapy in Urologic Practice: ICUD and AUA Review Paper" 2014. *AP*, Antiplatelet; *APT*, antiplatelet therapy; *ASA*, aspirin; *DPT*, dual antiplatelet therapy.

Anticoagulants. Warfarin should be discontinued 5 days preoperatively (goal INR <1.5). Novel oral anticoagulants require shorter periods of cessation (Table 2.3). Perioperative bridging with therapeutic dose low-molecular-weight heparin (LMWH) or unfractionated heparin (UFH) is recommended for moderate- and high-risk patients (Table 2.4). Anticoagulation should be resumed postoperatively within 12–24 hours if the bleeding risk is acceptable.

Nutrition

Adequate nutrition is critical for wound healing, immune response, return of bowel function, and maintenance of end organ function. Nutritional assessment may include laboratory testing (e.g., lymphocyte count, serum albumin) and validated assessment tools (e.g., Subjective Global Assessment, http://subjectiveglobalassessment.com).

Table 2.3 Suggested Perioperative Management of Novel Oral Anticoagulant Agents for Patients with Normal Renal Clearance

ANTICOAGULANT	TIME TO MAXIMUM EFFECT	LOW BLEEDING RISK SURGERY	HIGH BLEEDING RISK SURGERY
Dabigatran	1.25–3 hours	Last dose 2 days before surgery (skip two doses)	Last dose 3 days before surgery (skip four doses)
Rivaroxaban	2–4 hours	Last dose 2 days before surgery (skip one dose)	Last dose 3 days before surgery (skip two doses)
Apixaban	1–3 hours	Last dose 2 days before surgery (skip two doses)	Last dose 3 days before surgery (skip four doses)

Adapted from Culkin DJ, Exaire EJ, Green D, et al. Anticoagulation and antiplatelet therapy in urological practice: ICUD/AUA review paper. *J Urol* 2014;192(4):1026-1034.

Protein supplements and "immunonutrition" decrease rates of postoperative infection, decrease complications, and length of hospital stay. Malnourished patients may further benefit from preoperative enteral or total parenteral nutrition (TPN) nutrition; enteral nutrition is preferred because it helps maintain the intestinal mucosal barrier. Prior to surgery, solid food, nonhuman milk, and light meals may be consumed up to 6 hours before induction of general anesthesia. Breast milk may be consumed up to 4 hours prior to and clear liquids up to 2 hours prior to surgery.

Bowel Prep

Extrapolating from the general surgery literature, mechanical and oral antibiotic bowel preparations (e.g., neomycin + erythromycin or metronidazole) have traditionally been used prior to major urologic surgery. However, recent meta-analyses have not demonstrated reduced rates of anastomotic leak, wound infection, intra-abdominal abscess, or mortality with the use of mechanical bowel prep. The benefit of antibiotic bowel prep has not been well-studied for urologic surgeries.

INTRAOPERATIVE CONSIDERATIONS

Antibiotic Prophylaxis

Level 1 evidence supports the use of antibiotic prophylaxis to prevent surgical-site infections (SSIs). The most appropriate antibiotic

Table 2.4 Risk Stratification for Arterial or Venous Thromboembolism Events During Perioperative Period in Patients on Chronic Anticoagulant Therapy

	INDICATIONS FOR ANTICOAGULANT THERAPY		
RISK STRATUM	MECHANICAL HEART VALVE	ATRIAL FIBRILLATION	VTE
Low	Bileaflet aortic valve prosthesis without atrial fibrillation and no other risk factors for stroke	CHADS2 score of 0–2 (and no prior stroke or transient ischemic attack)	Single VTE occurred >12 months ago and no other risk factors
Moderate	Bileaflet aortic valve prosthesis plus one or more of the following: atrial fibrillation, prior stroke or transient ischemic attack, hypertension, diabetes, congestive heart failure, age older than 75 years	CHADS2 score of 3–4	VTE within the past 3–12 months Nonsevere thrombophilic conditions (e.g., heterozygous factor V Leiden mutation, heterozygous factor II mutation) Recurrent VTE Active cancer (treated within 6 months or palliative)
High	Any mitral valve prosthesis Any caged-ball or tilting disc aortic valve prosthesis Recent (within 6 months) stroke or transient ischemic attack	CHADS2 score of 5–6 Recent (within 3 months) stroke or transient ischemic attack Rheumatic valvular heart disease	Recent (within 3 months) VTE Severe thrombophilia (e.g., deficiency of protein C, protein S, or antithrombin; presence of antiphospholipid antibodies; multiple abnormalities)

CHADS2, Congestive heart failure, hypertension, age, diabetes, stroke; mo, months; VTE, venous thromboembolism.
Modified from Douketis JD, Spyropoulos AC, Spencer FA, et al. Perioperative management of antithrombotic therapy: Antithrombotic Therapy and Prevention of Thrombosis, 9th ed: American College of Chest Physicians evidence-based clinical practice guidelines. Chest 2012;141(2 suppl):e326S–e350S.

Box 2.2 Patient Factors That Increase the Risk for Infection

- Advanced age
- Anatomic anomalies
- Poor nutritional status
- Smoking
- Chronic corticosteroid use
- Immunodeficiency
- Chronic indwelling hardware
- Infected endogenous or exogenous material
- Distant coexistent infection
- Prolonged hospitalization

Data from Cruse PJ. Surgical wound infection. In: Wonsiewicz MJ, ed. *Infectious disease*. Philadelphia, PA: Saunders, 1992:758-764; Mangram AJ, Horan TC, Pearson ML, et al. Guideline for prevention of surgical site infection, 1999. Hospital Infection Control Practices Advisory Committee. *Infect Control Hosp Epidemiol* 1999;20(4):250-278; quiz 279-280.

agent is determined by patient susceptibility (Box 2.2) and wound class (Box 2.3). The most recent 2019 AUA recommendations for procedure-specific prophylaxis regimens are summarized in Table 2.5 and should be considered in conjunction with local antibiograms. Antimicrobial prophylaxis should be administered 1 hour before incision and continued for <24 hours perioperatively; prolonged use increases the risk of *Clostridium difficile* colitis and antibiotic resistance and increases cost.

Skin Preparation

Hair should be removed when it may interfere with the surgical field. Mechanical clippers or depilatory creams are preferred, though razors may be less traumatic for scrotal skin. Skin preparation may be performed with alcohol, povidone-iodine, or chlorhexidine-based solutions. For clean surgeries, 0.5% chlorhexidine in methylated spirits results in lower rates of SSI than alcohol-based povidone iodine, though insufficient evidence exists to support the superiority of one specific skin prep over others. Although preoperative showering or bathing with antiseptic solution is recommended, there is limited evidence to suggest that this leads to fewer SSIs.

Box 2.3 Surgical Wound Classification

Clean

- Uninfected wound without inflammation or entry into the genital, urinary, or alimentary tract
- Primary wound closure, closed drainage

Clean Contaminated

- Uninfected wound with controlled entry into the genital, urinary, or alimentary tract
- Primary wound closure, closed drainage

Contaminated

- Uninfected wound with major break in sterile technique (gross spillage from gastrointestinal tract or nonpurulent inflammation)
- Open fresh accidental wounds

Dirty Infected

- Wound with preexisting clinical infection or perforated viscera
- Old traumatic wounds with devitalized tissue

Data from Garner JS. CDC guideline for prevention of surgical wound infections, 1985. Supersedes guideline for prevention of surgical wound infections published in 1982. (Originally published in 1985.) Revised. *Infect Control* 1986;7(3):193-200; Simmons BP. Guideline for prevention of surgical wound infections. *Infect Control* 1982;2:185-196.

Positioning

Proper patient positioning is a shared responsibility of the entire operating room team. Careful padding and positioning are critical to avoid positioning-related peripheral neuropathies (Box 2.4). These usually result from excessive stretch, prolonged compression, or ischemia.

Anesthesia

Basic components of anesthesia include hypnosis, amnesia, and analgesia. Appropriate selection of anesthesia depends on patient comorbidities, airway status, procedural complexity, and patient and provider preference.

Regional Anesthesia. Regional anesthesia (e.g. spinal, epidural) is most appropriate for endoscopic or lower abdominal procedures and avoids the cardiopulmonary effects of general anesthesia. Specific complications may include postoperative hypotension due to

Table 2.5 Recommended Antimicrobial Prophylaxis for Urologic Procedures. Duration of Therapy Should be Single Dose and/or ≤24 Hours

PROCEDURE	LIKELY ORGANISMS	WOUND CLASS	ANTIMICROBIAL(S) OF CHOICE	ALTERNATIVE ANTIMICROBIALS
Cystourethroscopy with minor manipulation (e.g., break in mucosal barriers, biopsy, fulguration, etc.)	GNR, rarely enterococci	Clean-contaminated	TMP-SMX, amoxicillin–clavulanate	First- or second- generation cephalosporin + aminoglycoside[a] ± ampicillin
Transurethral cases (e.g., TURP, TURBT, laser enucleation, laser ablation, etc)	GNR, rarely enterococci	Clean-contaminated	Cefazolin, TMP-SMX	Amoxicillin–clavulanate, aminoglycoside[a] ± ampicillin
Prostate brachytherapy, cryotherapy	Staphylococcus aureus, coagulase-negative staphylococci, group A streptococci;	Clean-contaminated	Cefazolin	Clindamycin
Transrectal prostate biopsy	GNR, anaerobes; consider MDR coverage if recent systemic antibiotics (<6 months), international travel, healthcare worker	Contaminated	Fluoroquinolone, first-, second-, or third-generation cephalosporin (ceftriaxone commonly used) + aminoglycoside[a]	Aztreonam May consider infectious disease consultation
Percutaneous renal surgery (e.g., PCNL)	GNR, rarely enterococci, coagulase-negative staphylococci, group A streptococci, S. aureus	Clean-contaminated	First- or second-generation cephalosporin, aminoglycoside[a] + metronidazole,	Ampicillin–sulbactam

Procedure	Organisms	Wound classification		
Ureteroscopy	GNR, rarely enterococci	Clean-contaminated	TMP-SMX, first- or second-generation cephalosporin	Aminoglycoside[a] ± ampicillin, first- or second-generation cephalosporin, amoxicillin–clavulanate
Open, laparoscopic, or robotic surgery without entering urinary tract (e.g., adrenalectomy, pelvic or retroperitoneal lymphadenectomy)	S. aureus, coagulase-negative staphylococci, group A streptococci	Clean	Cefazolin	Clindamycin
Penile surgery (e.g., circumcision, penile biopsy)	S. aureus	Clean-contaminated	N/A	N/A
Urethroplasty (e.g., anterior urethral reconstruction, stricture repair including urethrectomy, controlled entry urinary tract)	GNR, rarely enterococci, S. aureus	Clean, contaminated	Cefazolin	Cefoxitin, cefotetan, ampicillin sulbactam
Involving controlled entry into the urinary tract (e.g., renal surgery, partial or radical nephrectomy, ureterectomy, pyeloplasty, radical prostatectomy, partial cystectomy)	GNR (Escherichia coli), rarely enterococci	Clean-contaminated	Cefazolin, TMP-SMX	Ampicillin–sulbactam, aminoglycoside[a] + metronidazole, or clindamycin

Continued

Table 2.5 Recommended Antimicrobial Prophylaxis for Urologic Procedures. Duration of Therapy Should be Single Dose and/or ≤24 Hours—cont'd

PROCEDURE	WOUND CLASS	LIKELY ORGANISMS	ANTIMICROBIAL(S) OF CHOICE	ALTERNATIVE ANTIMICROBIALS
Involving small bowel (e.g., urinary diversion) cystectomy with small bowel conduit, ureteropelvic junction repair, partial cystectomy	Clean-contaminated	S. aureus, coagulase-negative staphylococci; group A streptococci, GNR, rarely enterococci	Cefazolin	Clindamycin + aminoglycoside[a], cefuroxime (second-generation cephalosporin), aminopenicillin–β-lactamase inhibitor + metronidazole
Involving large bowel, colon conduits	Clean-contaminated	GNR, anaerobes	Cefazolin + metronidazole, cefoxitin, cefotetan, or ceftriaxone + metronidazole, ertapenem[b]	Ampicillin–sulbactam, ticarcillin–clavulanate, piperacillin–tazobactam
Implanted prosthetic devices (e.g., artificial urinary sphincter, inflatable penile prosthesis, sacral neuromodulators)	Clean	GNR, S. aureus; increasing reports of anaerobic + fungal organisms	Aminoglycosid[a] + first- or second-generation cephalosporin or vancomycin	Aminopenicillin–β-lactamase inhibitor (e.g., ampicillin–sulbactam, ticarcillin, tazobactam)

Inguinal and scrotal cases (e.g., radical orchiectomy, vasectomy, vasectomy reversal, varicocelectomy, hydrocelectomy)	GNR, S. aureus	Clean	Cefazolin	Ampicillin–sulbactam
Vaginal surgery, female incontinence (e.g., urethral sling), fistulae repair, urethral diverticulectomy	S. aureus, streptococci, enterococci, vaginal anaerobes, coagulase-negative staphylococci, group A streptococci	Clean-contaminated	Second-generation cephalosporin (cefoxitin, cefotetan) preferred over first-generation cephalosporins because of better anaerobic coverage; cefazolin equivalent for vaginal anaerobic coverage in sling procedures	Ampicillin–sulbactam[a] + aminoglycoside[a] + metronidazole, or clindamycin

[a]Aztreonam may be substituted for aminoglycosides in patients with renal insufficiency.
[b]Intravenous agents used with mechanical bowel preparation and oral antimicrobial (neomycin sulfate + erythromycin base or neomycin sulfate + metronidazole)
GNR, Gram negative rods (commonly include E. coli, Proteus spp., Klebsiella spp. in genitourinary tract); MDR, multidrug resistant; PCNL, percutaneous nephrolithotomy; SSI, surgical site infection; TMP-SMX, trimethoprim–sulfamethoxazole; TURBT, transurethral resection of bladder tumor; TURP, transurethral resection of prostate.
NB: clindamycin, aminoglycoside, + metronidazole or clindamycin are alternatives to penicillin and cephalosporins in patients with penicillin allergy.
Adapted from 2019 AUA Best Practice Statement on Urologic Procedures and Antimicrobial Prophylaxis.

Box 2.4 American Society of Anesthesiologists Task Force Recommendations on the Prevention of Perioperative Peripheral Neuropathies

Preoperative Assessment

- When judged appropriately, it is helpful to ascertain that patients can comfortably tolerate the anticipated operative position.

Upper Extremity Positioning

- Arm abduction should be limited to 90 degrees in supine patients; patients who are positioned prone may comfortably tolerate arm abduction greater than 90 degrees.
- Arms should be positioned to decrease pressure on the postcondylar groove of the humerus (ulnar groove). When arms are tucked at the side, a neutral forearm position is recommended. When arms are abducted on arm boards, either supination or a neutral forearm position is acceptable.
- Prolonged pressure on the radial nerve in the spiral groove of the humerus should be avoided.
- Extension of the elbow beyond a comfortable range may stretch the median nerve.

Lower Extremity Positioning

- Lithotomy positions that stretch the hamstring muscle group beyond a comfortable may stretch the sciatic nerve.
- Prolonged pressure on the peroneal nerve at the fibular head should be avoided.
- Neither extension nor flexion of the hip increases the risk for femoral neuropathy.

Protective Padding

- Padded arm boards may decrease the risk for upper extremity neuropathy.
- The use of chest rolls in laterally positioned patients may decrease the risk for upper extremity neuropathies.
- Padding at the elbow and at the fibular head may decrease the risk for upper and lower extremity neuropathies, respectively.

Equipment

- Properly functioning automated blood pressure cuffs on the upper arms do not affect the risk for upper extremity neuropathies.
- Shoulder braces in steep head-down positions may increase the risk for brachial plexus neuropathies.

Box 2.4 American Society of Anesthesiologists Task Force Recommendations on the Prevention of Perioperative Peripheral Neuropathies—cont'd

Postoperative Assessment

- A simple postoperative assessment of extremity nerve function may lead to early recognition of peripheral neuropathies.

Documentation

- Charting specific positioning actions during the care of patients may result in improvements of care by (1) helping practitioners focus attention on relevant aspects of patient positioning and (2) providing information that continuous improvement processes can use to effect refinements in patient care.

Modified from American Society of Anesthesiologists Task Force on Prevention of Perioperative Peripheral Neuropathies. Practice advisory for the prevention of perioperative peripheral neuropathies: A report by the American Society of Anesthesiologists Task Force on Prevention of Perioperative Peripheral Neuropathies. *Anesthesiology* 2000;92(4):1168-1182.

---

sympathetic blockade (10%–40%), postdural headache (<2%), and serious neurologic deficits (<0.05%).

Monitored Anesthesia Care. Conscious sedation under monitored anesthesia care (MAC) is typically administered using benzodiazepines and IV opioids. MAC requires the same degree of periprocedural monitoring as general anesthesia.

General Anesthesia. General anesthesia is preferred for longer or more complex surgeries. Induction may be attained through inhalational agents (e.g., nitric oxide, isoflurane, sevoflurane, desflurane, halothane) or IV agents (e.g., thiopental, ketamine, propofol, midazolam). These are used in conjunction with opioids and depolarizing or nondepolarizing paralytic agents.

Normothermia

Decreases of even 1–2°C in core body temperature may impair platelet function, clotting, immune function, and tissue perfusion. This results in higher rates of blood loss, transfusion, and SSI. Intraoperatively, peripheral vasodilation and conductive heat loss increase the risk of hypothermia. Normothermia may be maintained using warming blankets, warmed fluids, warm humidified carbon dioxide insufflation, and increased ambient temperature.

Blood Transfusion

Transfusion thresholds must be considered in the context of ongoing or potential surgical bleeding, intravascular volume, comorbidities, and cardiopulmonary reserve. Blood transfusion is recommended for hemoglobin <7 g/dL in hemodynamically stable patients and <8 g/dL for those with underlying cardiovascular disease. Component transfusion of platelets or fresh-frozen plasma is not routinely recommended unless there is severe thrombocytopenia, need for immediate reversal of coagulopathy, or massive transfusion protocol.

Transfusion Reactions. Hemolytic transfusion reactions may present immediately as fevers, chills, chest pain, hypotension, or bleeding diathesis; intravascular hemolysis may present in a delayed fashion. Management includes pausing the transfusion, fluid resuscitation, and urinary alkalinization. Transfusion-related acute lung injury manifests as acute onset noncardiogenic pulmonary edema and accounts for most transfusion-related mortality. Supportive care is the mainstay of treatment.

Infection Risk. In the modern era, there is low risk of bacterial or viral transmission with blood transfusion (1 per 2 million cases for human immunodeficiency virus and hepatitis C; 1 per 200,000 cases for hepatitis B). Platelet transfusion carries the highest risk of bacterial contamination (1/5000 units).

Special Situations. Cell saver, high-dose erythropoietin, or preoperative iron may be considered for patients who do not accept blood products. Those with renal insufficiency or anemia of chronic disease may also benefit from preoperative erythropoietin and iron.

Hemostatic Agents. Hemostatic agents may be useful adjuncts to obtain hemostasis, particularly for oozing from raw tissue surfaces. These include dry matrix agents that provide a substrate for thrombus formation or biologically active agents (Table 2.6).

Radiation Safety

The principle of "as low as reasonably achievable" (ALARA) should be applied to radiation use in all urologic procedures. Low-dose, pulsed fluoroscopy settings may reduce intraoperative radiation exposure by 97%. Use of intermittent fluoroscopy, "last image hold" function, image collimation, C-arm laser beam, and surgeon-controlled foot pedal may additionally decrease exposure. Additional measures include patient shielding and patient placement closest to the C-arm image intensifier.

Table 2.6 Hemostatic Agents for Control of Intraoperative Bleeding

TYPE	PREPARATION	EXAMPLES
Dry matrix agents	Cellulose sheets	Fibrillar, Surgicel, Nu-Knit
	Bovine collagen powder or sheets	Avitene
	Porcine collagen gelatin matrix	Surgifoam, Gelfoam
	Plant starch powder	Arista
Biologically active agents	Thrombin based	Thrombin-JMI, Evithrom, Recothrom, Surgiflo, Floseal
	Fibrin based	Tisseel, Evicel, Evarrest
	Albumin based	BioGlue

INTRAOPERATIVE TECHNICAL DECISIONS

Incisions

The considerations regarding selection and development of midline, Pfannenstiel (Fig. 2.3), Gibson (Fig. 2.4), thoracoabdominal, subcostal and chevron (Figs. 2.5 and 2.6), flank (Fig 2.7), and inguinal (Figs. 2.8 and 2.9) incisions are well-detailed in Campbell-Walsh-Wein Urology, 12th Edition. Midline incisions allow entry

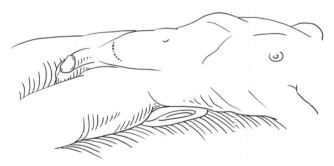

FIG. 2.3 Pfannenstiel incision. A Pfannenstiel is most commonly used by urologists for benign and malignant pelvic organ procedures in pediatric and adult populations. It can also be used for donor nephrectomy and specimen extractions. It heals well cosmetically and has decreased pain postoperatively because it is a muscle-splitting procedure. (From Smith JA Jr, Howards SS, Preminger GM, Dmochowski RR. *Hinman's atlas of urologic surgery*, 4th ed. Philadelphia, PA: Elsevier, 2018; Fig. 69.1.)

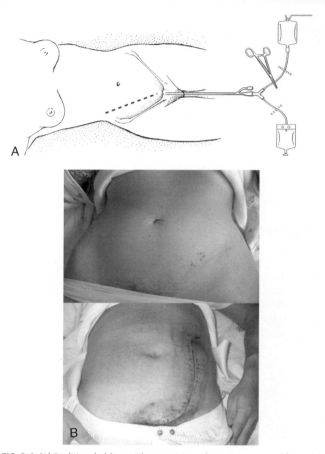

FIG. 2.4 (A) Traditional oblique Gibson incision. This incision is used for renal transplantation and allograft nephrectomy as well as access to the lower ureter and bladder. (B) Traditional oblique Gibson versus "hockey-stick" incision. The modern Gibson incision has become practically more "J-shaped," now also called a "hockey-stick" incision by some. Both incisions serve a similar purpose, with the J-incision able to be extended more superiorly if needed. (A, From Smith JA Jr, Howards SS, Preminger GM, Dmochowski RR. *Hinman's atlas of urologic surgery,* 4th ed. Philadelphia, PA: Elsevier, 2018; B, From Nanni G, Tondolo V, Citterio F, et al. Comparison of oblique versus hockey-stick surgical incision for kidney transplantation. *Transplant Proc.* 2005;37(6): 2479-2481.)

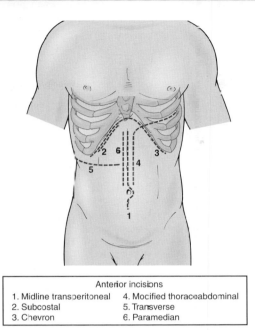

Anterior incisions	
1. Midline transperitoneal	4. Modified thoracoabdominal
2. Subcostal	5. Transverse
3. Chevron	6. Paramedian

FIG. 2.5 Anterior approaches to kidney and retroperitoneum. In a supine position or modified oblique position, there are multiple approaches to the kidney and retroperitoneum anteriorly. These each have different benefits and disadvantages, which are discussed further in Campbell-Walsh-Wein Urology, 12th Edition. (From Smith JA Jr, Howards SS, Preminger GM, Dmochowski RR. *Hinman's atlas of urologic surgery,* 4th ed. Philadelphia, PA: Elsevier, 2018; Fig. 8.4.)

into the abdominal cavity while avoiding major vessels and nerves; pelvic, intraperitoneal, extraperitoneal, and retroperitoneal structures may all be accessed in this manner. The kidney may be approached through anterior or flank incisions; dorsal lumbotomy has also been traditionally used. Inguinal incisions above or below the inguinal ligament may provide access to the spermatic cord, testis, and ilioinguinal lymph nodes.

Suture

Suture selection must be tailored to the tissue characteristics and tensile strength of the wound. A variety of suture materials in monofilament or braided configurations exist, each with distinct tensile strengths, handling qualities, and tissue reactivity (Table 2.7).

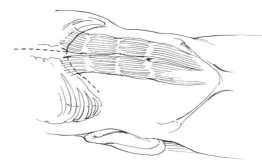

FIG. 2.6 Subcostal incision and extensions. The subcostal incision *(bold black line)* is shown on the left side. It can be used for renal access in the supine or flank position. *Dashed lines* represent possible extension across the midline to a "three-quarters" incision or complete subcostal "chevron" incision. Further extension to include a sternotomy (shown with *dashed lines* as well) is rarely ever used by urologists. (From Smith JA Jr, Howards SS, Preminger GM, Dmochowski RR. *Hinman's atlas of urologic surgery,* 4th ed. Philadelphia, PA: Elsevier, 2018; Fig. 8.8.)

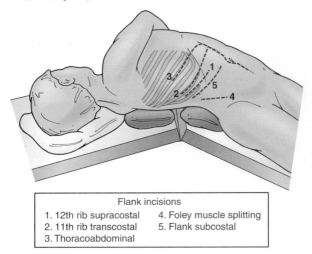

Flank incisions	
1. 12th rib supracostal	4. Foley muscle splitting
2. 11th rib transcostal	5. Flank subcostal
3. Thoracoabdominal	

FIG. 2.7 Flank incisions for renal and retroperitoneal access. Commonly used incisions for renal and retroperitoneal access in the flank position. These incisions can be used for benign and malignant conditions. (From Smith JA Jr, Howards SS, Preminger GM, Dmochowski RR. *Hinman's atlas of urologic surgery,* 4th ed. Philadelphia, PA: Elsevier, 2018; Fig. 8.5.)

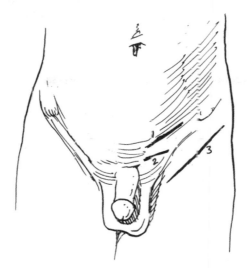

FIG. 2.8 Inguinal incisions. Incision 1: Curvilinear incision for radical orchiectomy and suspected malignancies. Incision 2: Inguinal incision above external inguinal ring for cryptorchidism or inguinal approach to varicocelectomy. Incision 3: Subinguinal incision for inguinal lymphadenectomy for penile cancer. (Modified from Smith JA Jr, Howards SS, Preminger GM, Dmochowski RR. *Hinman's atlas of urologic surgery*, 4th ed. Philadelphia, PA: Elsevier, 2018; Fig 117.1.)

Drains

Passive, open nonsuction drains (e.g., Penrose) may be used to help close potential spaces and prevent fluid accumulation. These should be removed earlier than closed drains because of greater infection risk. Closed nonsuction drains (e.g., pigtail drains) may be used to better quantify or characterize drainage. "Active" closed suction drains (e.g., Jackson Pratt, Blake drains) may be preferred if immediate recognition of small-volume drainage is critical. Suction is typically maintained using a compressible bulb reservoir.

Catheters

Indwelling urinary catheters come in a variety of French (Fr) sizes (1 Fr = 1/3 mm). Although they may be made of many materials (e.g., latex, polyvinyl chloride), silicone may be preferred because of its lack of reactivity, lower risk of bacterial adherence, and safety in patients with latex allergies. Specific designs, such as the curved

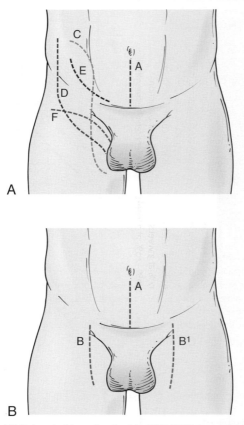

FIG. 2.9 (A) Various incisions described for ILND/PLND in penile cancer. *(A)*, Midline incision for bilateral PLND. *(B)*, Vertical incision allowing for access to superficial and deep ILND. *(C)*, S-shaped incision described for access to complete ILND and ipsilateral pelvic nodes. *(D)*, L-shaped incision for palpable disease, similar access to C. *(E)*, Gibson incision for ipsilateral pelvic node access. *(F)*, Common subinguinal incision for ipsilateral nodes. (B) Another approach for bilateral complete inguinal and pelvic lymphadenectomy. (Modified from Loughlin KR. Surgical atlas. Surgical management of penile carcinoma: the inguinal nodes. *BJU Int* 2006;97(5):1125-1134.)

Table 2.7 Properties of Suture Materials

SUTURE	ORIGIN	TISSUE ABSORPTION	PHYSICAL CONFIGURATION	TENSILE STRENGTH	COMMENTS
Vicryl	Synthetic	Absorbable	Braided	65% at 2 weeks 40% at 4 weeks	Slower loss of function and higher knot-breaking strength than polyglycolic acid (Dexon)
Dexon	Synthetic	Absorbable	Braided	63% at 2 weeks 17% at 3 weeks	Lubricant coating decreases coefficient of friction
Monocryl	Synthetic	Absorbable	Monofilament	30%–40% at 2 weeks (dyed) 25% at 2 weeks (undyed)	Excellent tensile strength allows use of smaller sutures for skin closure
PDS	Synthetic	Delayed absorbable	Monofilament	74% at 2 weeks 50% at 4 weeks 25% at 6 weeks	No absorption until after 90 days; low reactivity; tends to maintain strength in presence of infection; newer barbed version is knotless
Maxon	Synthetic	Delayed absorbable	Monofilament	81% at 2 weeks 59% at 4 weeks 30% at 6 weeks	

Continued

Table 2.7 Properties of Suture Materials—cont'd

SUTURE	ORIGIN	TISSUE ABSORPTION	PHYSICAL CONFIGURATION	TENSILE STRENGTH	COMMENTS
Chromic gut	Natural	Absorbable	Monofilament	0% at 3 weeks	Can also be found as plain gut (untreated) for faster absorption
Nylon	Synthetic	Nonabsorbable	Monofilament	50% at 1–2 years	Very low tissue reactivity
Prolene	Synthetic	Nonabsorbable	Monofilament	No significant loss over time	High plasticity; extremely smooth surface (requires extra knot throws)
Silk	Natural	Nonabsorbable	Braided	Degraded over time	Braided for easier handling; can be prone to infection
Mersilene	Synthetic	Nonabsorbable	Braided or monofilament	No significant loss over time	Braided should not be used in infection

PDS, Polydioxanone suture.

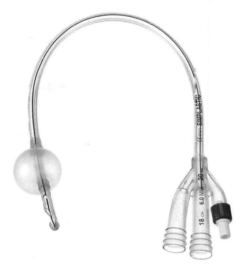

FIG. 2.10 Three-way hematuria catheter. (Image courtesy of Teleflex Incorporated. © 2019 Teleflex Incorporated. All rights reserved.)

coudé tip, Council tip, or reinforced hematuria catheter (Fig. 2.10), may be preferred depending on the specific urologic indication. The duration of drainage must be balanced with urinary tract infection risk from longer catheterization time.

Stents

Ureteral stents typically range 4–7 Fr in diameter and are made from flexible polymers. Self-retaining "double-J" pigtail stents are most commonly used for temporary ureteral drainage. "Single-J" pigtail stents may be used for patients with urinary diversions. Additional stent configurations (e.g., open-ended, spiral-tipped, whistle-tipped) may facilitate ureteral access for drainage or retrograde pyelography. In cases of extrinsic ureteral compression, tandem stents or metal stents may be considered to maintain ureteral patency. The latter require less frequent exchanges, but complication rates exceed 50% (e.g., hyperplastic tissue reactions, encrustation, or tissue ingrowth, uretero-iliac fistula). Indwelling stents may be associated with significant urinary urgency, frequency, and pain. Stent length, but not diameter, is associated with more severe symptoms. Stent discomfort is best treated with alpha-blockers and antimuscarinic

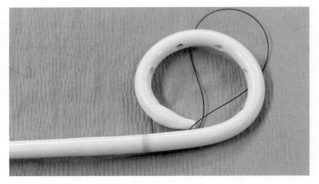

FIG. 2.11 Cope catheter with the retention string loosened for demonstration.

medications. Alternative stent designs to minimize bladder irritation symptoms are also in development.

Nephrostomy Tubes

Nephrostomy tubes range in size from 5 to 32 Fr and are made from a variety of materials such as silicone, polyurethane, or polyethylene. The pigtail tube relies on a curled end for retention within the collecting system. The Cope catheter has a similar design but utilizes a locking internal nylon string to maintain a more secure curled configuration (Fig. 2.11). Nephroureteral stents may be preferred to maintain ureteral access and minimize dislodgement risk. Following PCNL, balloon and malecot catheters have also been used as nephrostomy tubes. A circle catheter may preferred when maintenance of two access tracts is necessary. The Kaye nephrostomy tamponade balloon may be used to maintain control bleeding from a percutaneous access tract.

Fascial Closure

Several fascial closure techniques exist (Figs. 2.12 and 2.13), but no single closure technique has been shown to be superior. Meta-analyses have shown similar incisional hernia rates with continuous or interrupted fascial closures using slowly absorbable or nonabsorbable suture. Additionally, there appears to be no difference in rates of fascial dehiscence or wound infection between interrupted or continuous closure with slowly absorbable suture. Continuous fascial closure should not be performed with rapidly absorbable suture due to increased risk of incisional hernia.

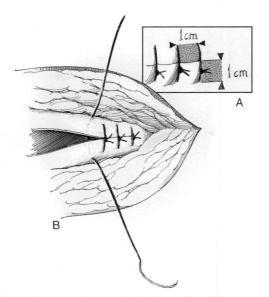

FIG. 2.12 Fascial closure technique. (A and B) Strong fascial closure is important in abdominal incisions. The 2-o nonabsorbable sutures are usually used and should be placed 1 cm from edge and 1 cm apart, as shown here. This can be done in an interrupted fashion (shown here) or running fashion (From Smith JA Jr, Howards SS, Preminger GM, Dmochowski RR. *Hinman's atlas of urologic surgery*, 4th ed. Philadelphia, PA: Elsevier, 2018; Fig. 2.5A3.)

Wound Closure

The specific wound closure technique may be determined by wound type (see Box 2.3). Primary wound closure is appropriate for clean and clean-contaminated wounds. Skin may be closed with absorbable monofilament or staples. Secondary closure is appropriate for heavily contaminated wounds. The fascia is closed primarily, and the skin and subcutaneous tissues are allowed to heal by wound contraction and epithelialization. Delayed primary closure (tertiary closure) is typically reserved for patients with abdominal compartment syndrome or patients requiring planned reoperation, where fascia and skin are closed only after an initial period of observation. Negative-pressure vacuum-assisted closure (VAC) devices may be useful adjuncts for secondary or tertiary closure. These provide enhanced wound debridement and protection from the external

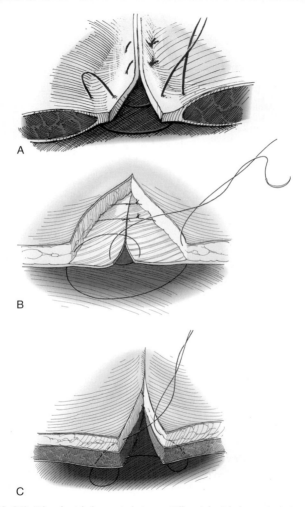

FIG. 2.13 Other fascial closure techniques. Different fascial closure techniques have been described but are less commonly used by urologists. (A) Near-and-far suture for mass closure. (B) Smead-Jones technique in which sutures are 2 cm apart with near and far figure-eight bites. (C) A Gambee stitch or vertical mattress that incorporates both fascial layers. (From Smith JA Jr, Howards SS, Preminger GM, Dmochowski RR. *Hinman's atlas of urologic surgery,* 4th ed. Philadelphia, PA: Elsevier, 2018: Figs. 2.7A–C.)

environment. Open abdominal VAC systems also exist for temporary abdominal closure.

POSTOPERATIVE MANAGEMENT

Venous Thromboembolism (VTE) Prophylaxis

Perioperative thromboprophylaxis must be tailored to the patient's individual risk factors (Box 2.5) and the specific procedure. Patient risk stratification may be performed using a number of different risk assessment models (e.g., Rogers Score, Caprini score). Recommended prophylaxis regimens for different operation classes are shown in Table 2.8. This may include mechanical (e.g., pneumatic compression stockings) or pharmacologic (e.g., LMWH, low-dose UFH) options (Table 2.9). When appropriate, preoperative dosing

---

Box 2.5 Patient-Related Factors Increasing Risk for Venous Thromboembolism

- Surgery
- Trauma (major trauma or lower extremity injury)
- Immobility, lower extremity paresis
- Cancer (active or occult)
- Cancer therapy (hormonal, chemotherapy, angiogenesis inhibitors, radiotherapy)
- Venous compression (tumor hematoma, arterial abnormality)
- Previous venous thromboembolism
- Increasing age
- Pregnancy and the postpartum period
- Estrogen-containing oral contraceptives or hormone replacement therapy
- Selective estrogen receptor modulators
- Erythropoiesis-stimulating agents
- Acute medical illness
- Inflammatory bowel disease
- Nephrotic syndrome
- Myeloproliferative disorders
- Paroxysmal nocturnal hemoglobinuria
- Obesity
- Central venous catheterization
- Inherited or acquired thrombophilia

Modified from Geerts WH, Bergqvist D, Pineo GF, et al. Prevention of venous thromboembolism: American College of Chest Physicians evidence-based clinical practice guidelines (8th edition). *Chest* 2008;133(6 suppl):381S-453S.

Table 2.8 Risk Stratification for Venous Thromboembolism (VTE) and Recommended VTE Prophylaxis for Urologic Procedures

RISK CATEGORY	CLINICAL CHARACTERISTICS	VTE PROPHYLAXIS
Low risk	Minor surgery, younger than 40 years old, no additional risk factors	Early ambulation
Moderate risk	• Minor surgery, additional risk factors • 40–60 years old, no additional risk factors	• Heparin 5000 U SC q12 hours, starting after surgery[a] • Enoxaparin 40 mg (CrCl <30 mL/min = 30 mg) SC daily Pneumatic compression devices if risk of bleeding is high
High risk		• Heparin 5000 U SC q8 hours, starting after surgery[a] • Enoxaparin 40 mg (CrCl <30 mL/min = 30 mg) SC daily Pneumatic compression devices if risk of bleeding is high
Highest risk		• Enoxaparin 40 mg (CrCl <30 mL/min = 30 mg) SC daily AND adjuvant pneumatic compression device Heparin 5000 U SC q8 hours, starting after surgery AND adjuvant pneumatic compression device

[a]American College of Chest Physicians guideline 2012 recommends consideration of preoperative dosing.

CrCl, Creatinine clearance; *q,* every; *SC,* subcutaneous.

Adapted from the American Urological Association Best Practice Statement for the prevention of deep vein thrombosis in patients undergoing urologic surgery (2009).

Table 2.9 Mechanical and Pharmacologic Venous Thromboembolism Prophylaxis

PROPHYLAXIS	DOSE	ADVANTAGES	DISADVANTAGES
Pneumatic compression stockings	N/A	Can be used in patients with high bleeding risk Easily standardized for all patients Studied in multiple patient groups	No standards for size or pressure Individual models not specifically studied Less effective than pharmacologic prophylaxis in high-risk groups
Low-molecular-weight heparin	40 mg SC once daily	Once-daily administration Less risk for heparin-induced thrombocytopenia No blood monitoring necessary	Not reversible High cost Relative contraindication in patients with renal insufficiency
Low-dose unfractionated heparin	5000 units SC q8h	Reversible Can be used safely in patients with renal insufficiency Relatively inexpensive	Needs readministration q8–12h Heparin-induced thrombocytopenia

N/A, Not applicable; *q,* every; *SC,* subcutaneous.

of pharmacologic prophylaxis may be considered. High-level evidence supports the extended use of LMWH prophylaxis for 4 weeks postoperatively to reduce VTE risk among patients undergoing major surgery for abdominal or pelvic malignancy.

Pain Management

Multimodal analgesia is recommended for postoperative pain. This is associated with lower overall opioid requirements and better subjective pain control.

Multimodal Pain Control. Adjunctive medications include acetaminophen, nonsteroidal antiinflammatory drugs (NSAIDs), gabapentin, and pregabalin. These may be augmented by local or neuraxial anesthesia. Additional nonpharmacologic adjuncts include transcutaneous electrical nerve stimulation and acupuncture. Nonopiate pathways for postoperative care have been shown to be feasible and safe for a number of urologic procedures, including ureteroscopy and prostatectomy.

Narcotics. When necessary, oral narcotics are preferred over parenteral administration. When the latter is indicated, patient-controlled analgesia without basal infusion is recommended. Postoperative narcotic use is associated with recovery of bowel function, respiratory depression, sedation, and nausea or vomiting in the postoperative period, as well as long-term addiction potential. To minimize this risk, postoperative narcotic prescriptions should be written at the lowest effective dose for as few doses as necessary to adequately manage postoperative pain.

Gastrointestinal (GI) Recovery

Early refeeding after surgery has been shown to promote nutrition, stimulate bowel motility, and maintain intestinal mucosal integrity; this has been widely adopted across many postoperative enhanced recovery pathways. Recovery of GI function may be optimized by gum chewing or sham feeding. Perioperative use of the μ-opioid receptor antagonist alvimopan (Entereg) has been shown to expedite GI recovery, minimize postoperative ileus episodes, and decrease the length of stay in cystectomy patients. This should be used cautiously in patients with renal dysfunction and is contra-indicated in chronic opiate use. Postoperative wound healing and synthesis of acute phase proteins and immune proteins necessitate greater protein intake. For patients unable to meet their caloric needs within 7–10 days after surgery, supplemental enteral or parenteral nutrition is indicated. When possible, enteral feeding is preferred.

Delirium

Postoperative delirium is an acute change in cognition marked by inattention, fluctuating consciousness levels, and disorganized thinking. This is common in patients older than 65 years old and is associated with longer hospital length of stay, postoperative functional decline, increased care costs, and increased mortality. Preoperative cognitive impairment is a significant predictor of postoperative delirium. Surgical stress, inadequate pain control, electrolyte disorders, polypharmacy, hypoxia, renal insufficiency, sleep deprivation, and urinary catherization exacerbate this risk. Management involves frequent reorientation, maintenance of sleep–wake cycles, and addressing underlying risk factors.

SPECIAL POPULATIONS

Pregnancy

Pregnancy is a unique physiologic state characterized by increased cardiac output, diminished systemic vascular resistance, increased oxygen consumption, chronic respiratory acidosis, expanded plasma volume, hypercoagulability, increased glomerular filtration rate, ureteral collecting system dilation, and alterations in urine chemistry. Additionally, the gravid uterus exerts a mass effect on the vena cava, diaphragm, and uterus. These changes influence the surgical and physiologic management of these patients.

Radiation Exposure. The developing fetus is at highest risk of ionizing radiation exposure from preimplantation to ~15 weeks' gestation. The general principle of ALARA should guide selection of imaging and diagnostic interventions for pregnant patients. Ultrasound and magnetic resonance imaging remain first-line imaging modalities. However, diagnostic imaging studies such as computed tomography should not be withheld from pregnant patients if deemed medically necessary; exposures with standard imaging techniques remain much lower than the doses associated with fetal harm. Iodinated contrast imaging should be avoided.

Surgical Principles. The American College of Obstetricians and Gynecologists recommends that surgery on pregnant women be performed at institutions with neonatal and pediatric services. An obstetric care provider with cesarean delivery privileges should be available, along with qualified individuals to interpret fetal heart rate patterns. Indicated surgeries should not be denied simply because of pregnancy status, but elective surgeries should be postponed until the postpartum period. When possible, nonurgent surgery should be performed during the second trimester, when the risk of teratogenesis and spontaneous abortions is lowest. To date, deleterious effects of anesthetic or sedative agents in human fetuses have not been demonstrated. Appropriate perioperative VTE prophylaxis should be administered given the increased VTE risk during pregnancy. Indwelling stents or nephrostomy tubes placed during pregnancy should be changed every 4–6 weeks because of the risk of rapid encrustation. Asymptomatic bacteriuria should always be treated in this population.

Morbid Obesity

Obesity is defined as body mass index (BMI) >30; morbid obesity is defined as BMI >40, or excess of 100 lb over ideal body weight. Obesity is associated with poor functional capacity and comorbidities such as cardiovascular disease, hypertension, diabetes, and hypoventilation that increase perioperative risk. Additionally, it is a risk factor for postoperative wound infection. Laparoscopic approaches may be preferred to minimize the risk of cardiopulmonary complications for obese patients, and extra-long laparoscopic instruments may be required. Operative times are often longer, putting these patients at greater risk for compartment syndrome or rhabdomyolysis. Additional equipment such as hydraulic tables, side extensions, additional padding, and wide pneumatic compression stockings are also needed to ensure safe intraoperative positioning of obese patients.

Geriatric

Increased age is an independent predictor of perioperative morbidity and mortality. Older patients have diminished physiologic reserve; operative time and intraoperative stress should therefore be minimized for these patients. Additionally, geriatric patients are at high risk of delirium and postoperative complications, and they are more susceptible to medication-associated complications. The 2016 Beers Criteria for Potentially Inappropriate Medication Use in Older Adults provides additional guidance on use of common urology-related medications in this population.

Key Points

- Preoperative risk assessment and optimization of existing comorbidities can reduce perioperative complications and minimize patient morbidity.
- Patient-specific and procedure-specific risks must be carefully considered to determine the appropriate perioperative cardiovascular testing, management of antiplatelet agents and anticoagulants, venous thromboprophylaxis, and optimal antibiotic prophylaxis.
- Surgical site infections can be prevented through several measures: smoking cessation, careful hair removal, thorough preoperative skin preparation, appropriate antimicrobial prophylaxis, maintenance of normothermia, and appropriate wound closure.
- A variety of drains and urinary drainage tubes exist, and use may be tailored to the specific surgery and surgeon preferences.
- Careful fascial closure may minimize the risk of postoperative dehiscence and incisional hernia. Wound closure technique depends on the wound class and degree of contamination.
- Adequate perioperative nutrition is critical for postoperative wound healing. When supplementation is indicated, enteral feeds are preferred over parenteral nutrition.
- Geriatric patients and morbidly obese patients are at high risk for perioperative complications and require additional consideration during surgery.
- Pregnant patients should not be denied indicated diagnostic studies or surgeries. The principle of ALARA should guide diagnostic imaging. Elective surgeries should be deferred until the postpartum period and nonurgent surgeries are ideally performed during the second trimester at a facility with appropriate obstetrics and neonatal expertise.

Suggested Readings

ACS NSQIP Surgical Risk Calculators. https://riskcalculator.facs.org/RiskCalculator/PatientInfo.jsp.

Chrouser K, Foley F, Goldenberg M, et al. *Optimizing outcomes in urologic surgery: Intraoperative considerations.* American Urological Association White Paper, 2018.

Culkin DJ, Exaire EJ, Green D, et al. Anticoagulation and antiplatelet therapy in urological practice: ICUD/AUA Review Paper. *J Urol* 2014;194(4):1026-1034.

Fleisher LA, Fleischmann KE, Auerbach AD, et al. 2014 ACC/AHA guideline on perioperative cardiovascular evaluation and management of patients undergoing noncardiac surgery: a report of the American College of Cardiology/American Heart Association Task Force on practice guidelines. *Circulation* 2014;130:e278-e333.

Forrest JB, Clemens JQ, Finamore P, et al. AUA Best Practice Statement for the prevention of deep vein thrombosis in patients undergoing urologic surgery. *J Urol* 2009;181(3):1170-1177.

Gould MK, Garcia DA, Wren SM, et al. Prevention of VTE in nonorthopedic surgical patients. Antithrombotic Therapy and Prevention of Thrombosis, 9th ed: American College of Chest Physicians Evidence-Based Clinical Practice Guidelines. *Chest* 2012;141(2):e227S-e227S.

Griebling TL, Dineen MK, DuBeau CE, et al. AUA white paper on the Beers criteria for potentially inappropriate medical use in older adults. *Urol Practice* 2016;3(2):102-111.

Lighter DJ, Wymer K, Sanchez J, Kavoussi L. Best practice statement on urologic procedures and antimicrobial prophylaxis. *J Urol* 2020;203(2):351-356.

Smith A, Anders M, Auffenberg G, et al. *Optimizing outcomes in urologic surgery: postoperative.* American Urological Association White Paper, 2018.

Stoffel JT, Montgomery JS, Suskind AM, et al. *Optimizing outcomes in urological surgery: preoperative care for the patient undergoing urologic surgery or procedure.* American Urological Association White Paper, 2018.

White JV, Guenter P, et al. Consensus statement: Academy of Nutrition and Dietetics and American Society for Parenteral and Enteral Nutrition: characteristics recommended for the identification and documentation of adult malnutrition (undernutrition). *J Parenter Enteral Nutr* 2012;36(3):275-283.

3

Principles of Endourology and Fundamentals of Laparoscopic and Robotic Urologic Surgery

PETER SUNARYO AND ROBERT M. SWEET

CONTRIBUTORS OF CAMPBELL-WALSH-WEIN, 12TH EDITION

Brian Duty, Michael Joseph Conlin Roshan M. Patel, Kamaljot S. Kaler, and Jaime Landman

CYSTOSCOPY PREPARATION AND TIPS

Before cystourethroscopy, the skin is prepared with an antiseptic agent. Both chlorhexidine gluconate and alcohol-based solutions can damage mucous membranes and therefore are not recommended for use on the genitalia. Aqueous-based iodophor containing products such as Betadine are safe on all skin surfaces. Plain or lidocaine gel is then injected into the urethra, though meta-analyses have found no difference in procedure tolerance. The most uncomfortable part of the procedure is when the scope passes through the membranous urethra. A randomized trial showed a significant improvement in pain after manual compression of the irrigation bag during passage of the scope. Patients, in particular young men, should be encouraged to relax as much as possible as the scope is advanced through the membranous urethra. Other strategies to decrease pain are allowing patients to observe the monitor or listen to classical music.

URETEROSCOPY TIPS AND KEY POINTS

Basic principles to keep in mind are the importance of access to the upper tract, good visualization, and maintenance of low pressures. In general, semi-rigid ureteroscopy is best below the iliac vessels and flexible ureteroscopy above the vessels. Normal saline should be used as irrigation. Irrigation systems allow visualization, lubrication, and stone manipulation and consist of pressure bags, hand pumps, or foot pumps. The former provides constant flow, and the latter allows for more control. Mobile C-arm fluoroscopy should be used because it provides better image quality and less scatter than fixed units. Before the ureteroscopy proceeds, the bladder is drained to permit accumulation of irrigation fluid during ureteroscopy and minimize buckling of the flexible ureteroscope into the bladder (Fig. 3.1). If a longer rigid

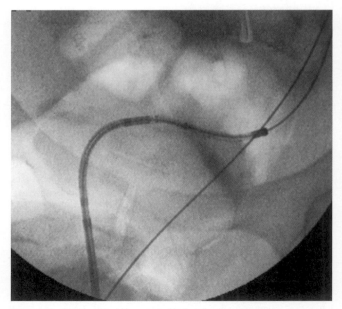

FIG. 3.1 The bladder should be emptied before flexible ureteroscope passage to prevent buckling of the instrument within the bladder if resistance is met at the ureteral orifice.

ureteroscope is being used, the contralateral leg can be elevated to allow for easier introduction of the ureteroscope. A safety guide is critical during rigid ureteroscopy to maintain access and allow placement of a ureteral stent if any problems are encountered. Following the guidewire permits easy identification of the ureteral orifice. By maneuvering the tip of the ureteroscope next to the guidewire posterolaterally, the physician can elevate the wire, thereby propping open the orifice. If necessary, an additional guidewire can be passed and the ureteroscope is then rotated until it is directly between the two wires, which will hold the orifice wide open (Fig. 3.2). When the ureteroscope or access sheath is safely in the intramural ureter, the additional guidewire can be removed.

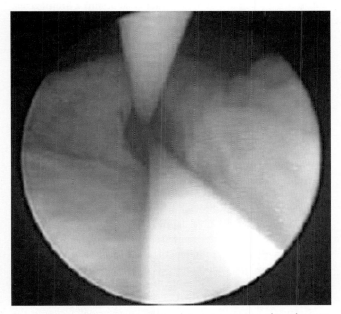

FIG. 3.2 Semirigid ureteroscope passage between two wires. After safety wire placement *(bottom wire)*, a second wire *(top wire)* is passed through the working channel and up the ureter using fluoroscopic guidance to "tent open" the ureteral orifice. The ureteroscope is then gently advanced between the wires until ureteral access is achieved.

Care must be taken when trying to gain access around an impacted stone because of perforation. An angled hydrophilic-coated (tipped or complete) wire, an angled torqueable catheter placed in close proximity to the stone, or both can be helpful. If a guidewire cannot be safely passed beyond the stone, direct inspection of the ureter up to the stone with the rigid ureteroscope may permit passage of the wire under direct vision. If the stone is impacted, it can be helpful to gently manipulate it and/or treat well-exposed areas of the stone with the laser, allowing for improved visibility and safer completion of the lithotripsy. When the proximal ureter is visualized, pass the wire under direct vision prior to completing the lithotripsy.

If there is any suspicion about possible infection above the stone, a urine culture through an open-ended catheter passed antegrade to the obstruction should be sent and a drainage established with a stent or percutaneous nephrostomy. The ureteroscopy should be postponed until the infection has been treated.

A dual-lumen catheter can be advanced over the initial guidewire to gently dilate the ureteral orifice and to introduce a second wire to pass the ureteroscope or a ureteral access sheath over. If the flexible ureteroscope does not pass the orifice, the scope should be rotated 90 to 180 degrees on the guidewire to better position the tip of the ureteroscope. It is important to pass the laser fiber through a straightened flexible ureteroscope to prevent damage to the working channel.

Guidewires – Many are available and offer differing diameters, rigidity, tip design, materials and coating. In general, stiffer wires are better for passing sheaths, dilation systems, and scopes over. Floppy tip, J tip, and double-floppy configurations can be used in certain cases. Guidewires range from 0.018 to 0.038 in size and range from 80 to 260 cm in length. Hydrophilic coated wires are best for establishing challenging access around an obstruction but can easily slide out. New hybrid wires allow for some advantages of both.

Ureteral Access Sheaths – Allow for repeated access to the intrarenal collecting system without having to replace the working guidewire. They have been shown to decrease intrarenal pressure and facilitate fragment retrieval. They come in a range of sizes from 10/12F (inner/outer diameter) up to 14/16F and lengths from 28 cm up to 55 cm. There is a small risk of injury to the ureter from the use of a ureteral access sheath (Table 3.1).

Other Devices – Ureteral dilation, stone retrieval, and antiretropulsion and ureteral biopsy devices are available and useful for ureteroscopic procedures (Table 3.2). New nitinol baskets have provided increased durability and usability.

Table 3.1 Characteristics of Currently Available Ureteral Access Sheaths

MANUFAC-TURER	SHEATH NAME	DILATOR/SHEATH (Fr)	LENGTHS (cm)	UNIQUE FEATURES
Boston Scientific	Navigator	11/13 13/15	28, 36, 46	
	Navigator HD	11/13 12/14 13/15	28, 36, 46	
Applied	Forte (AxP and HD)	10/12–16; 12/14–18; 14/15–18	20, 28, 35, 45 55	
	Forte Plus	10/14	35, 55	Active deflecting mechanism
Bard	Proxis	10/12 12/14	25, 35, 45	
Cook	Flexor	9.5/11; 12/13.7; 14/16	13, 20, 28, 35, 45, 55	
	Flexor DL	9.5/14; 12/16.7	13, 20, 28, 35, 45, 55	Dual-lumen design
	Flexor Parallel	9.5/11; 12/13.7; 14/16	13, 20, 28, 35, 45, 55	Rapid release design for single wire external to sheath
Olympus	UroPass	10/12 11/13 12/14 13/15	24, 38, 46, 54	

Table 3.2 Common Supplies for Ureteroscopy

Ureteroscopes

Rigid
    7 Fr or smaller semirigid ureteroscope
    Larger ureteroscope with straight working channel (optional)
Flexible
    7.5 Fr
    8.6 Fr or larger
    Secondary deflection or exaggerated deflection–capable ureteroscope

Disposable Supplies

Guidewires
    .035 and .038 Angled hydrophilic
    .035 and .038 Straight Teflon coated
    .035 and .038 Nitinol core, polyurethane coated
    .035 and .038 Extra-stiff .035 hybrid
Irrigation
    Hand irrigation device
    Foot irrigation device
    High-pressure working port seal
    Pressure bags
Stone-retrieval devices (3.0 Fr or smaller)
    Helical basket
    Multi-wire basket
    Tipless basket
    Three-prong grasping forceps or equivalent
Catheters
    Dual-lumen catheter
    6- to 12-Fr dilating catheter
    5-Fr Open-ended catheter
    5-Fr Angled-tip torque-able tapered catheter
Dilation devices
    High-pressure ureteral dilating balloons (5–7 mm)
    "Zero-tip" ureteral dilating balloon
Biopsy devices
    3-Fr cup biopsy
    Flat-wire basket
    BIGopsy (optional)
Ureteral stents
    4.7- to 7-Fr, 20- to 28-cm, double-pigtail

Intraluminal Lithotripsy Devices

Holmium laser
Thulium laser
Pneumatic (optional)
Electrohydraulic (optional)

SPECIAL CIRCUMSTANCES

Suprapubic Cystotomy

These individuals are at increased risk of infection, bladder calculi, and bladder cancer. At present there are no level I data showing improved survival in patients with long-term catheters undergoing surveillance cystoscopy. However, in patients with catheters for more than 5 to 10 years, surveillance cystoscopy is a common practice. Every effort should be made to avoid endoscopy through a suprapubic tract until it has had time to mature, which usually takes several weeks from creation. It is advisable to place a wire if endoscopy of an immature tract or an obese patient with a long, tortuous tract is required. Administering intravenous indigo carmine or methylene blue early in the procedure may help visualize the ureteral orifices if there is edema.

Continent Urinary Diversions

Before any endoscopic procedure involving a continent urinary diversion, it is imperative to obtain the operative note. It is important to know the bowel segment used, type and location of the ureteroenteric anastomoses, continence mechanism employed, and whether an afferent limb was created. If a contracture is noted at the urethral anastomosis and the patient does not have outlet obstruction, then it is advisable to use the smallest scope possible rather than dilate or incise the stricture because of the risk of worsening urinary incontinence. Diagnostic procedures on continent cutaneous reservoirs are best accomplished with a flexible cystoscope through the catheterizable channel. Therapeutic procedures should be performed percutaneously into the reservoir, given that continence mechanisms are often fragile. Care must be taken to avoid the vascular pedicle. Begin by irrigating out all of the mucus. Irrigation should then be used judiciously. Too little irrigation will make mucosal folds more prominent and impair visualization, but overdistending the diversion will prevent access to the afferent limb.

FUNDAMENTALS OF LAPAROSCOPIC AND ROBOTIC UROLOGIC SURGERY

Achieving Transperitoneal Access and Establishing Pneumoperitoneum

Closed Technique (Veress Needle). Proper needle function should be ensured before the procedure. The needle is grasped at midshaft and is passed perpendicularly through skin using gentle, steady pressure. Two points of resistance are traversed: the abdominal wall fascia and the peritoneum.

- **Points of Entry** – Insertion is commonly accomplished at the superior border of the umbilicus. Advantages are that the abdominal wall is thinnest, and postoperative cosmesis is excellent. There is potential for injury to a major vessel (e.g., left common iliac vessels, aorta, or vena cava). In nonobese patients, the Veress needle should be passed through the abdominal wall angled toward the pelvis to avoid injury to the bowel and great vessels. In more obese patients, because the umbilicus lies more caudad, less angulation is needed, and the Veress needle should be passed perpendicular. The Palmer point (i.e., subcostal in the midclavicular line on the left side) and at the corresponding site on the right side are other potential sites and preferred when intraabdominal adhesions are suspected. There is the potential to hit the liver on either side or, rarely, the spleen on the left side.

- **Assessing Proper Needle Placement** – First the aspiration-irrigation-aspiration test is performed. A 10-mL syringe containing 5 mL of saline is used to aspirate the needle and check for blood or stool. If negative, then saline is injected. Next, the syringe is again aspirated; no fluid should return. Last, the syringe is detached from the Veress, and any fluid in the hub should fall swiftly (i.e., the "drop" test). Second, the advancement test can be performed. The needle is then advanced 1 cm deeper. Resistance usually means the needle is still in the preperitoneal space and needs to be advanced through the remaining peritoneum. Insufflation is started at 2 L/min with the abdominal pressure set at 10 mm Hg. If free flow of carbon dioxide (CO_2) is noted then after 0.5 L has entered the abdomen, the flow can be increased to maximal capacity and the abdominal pressure set at 15 mm Hg

Open Access Technique: Hasson Technique. Recommended specifically when extensive adhesions are anticipated and involves making a larger incision and increases the chances of port-site gas leakage during the procedure. A semicircular incision is made at the lower edge or slightly below the umbilicus. The fascia and peritoneum are opened individually with a transverse incision, sufficient to accommodate the surgeon's index finger. After visual and digital confirmation of entry into the peritoneal cavity, two 0 silk traction sutures are placed on either edge of the fascia. Next, the Hasson cannula is advanced through the incision with the blunt tip protruding

Hand Port Access. The safest maneuver is to use an open technique and place the hand port into a 6.5- to 7.5-cm open incision in the midline or lower quadrant and then create the pneumoperitoneum through the hand port. Next, a blunt cannula is passed through the hand-assist device, and pneumoperitoneum is established. Additional ports can be placed rapidly with the surgeon's intraabdominal hand being used to guide them. The use of a brown glove on the intraabdominal hand is recommended because they do not reflect the light from the laparoscope and thus reduce glare.

ACHIEVING RETROPERITONEAL ACCESS AND DEVELOPING THE RETROPERITONEAL SPACE

Initial access is obtained through a transverse incision in the midaxillary line, just below the tip of 12th rib. The Hassan technique is then performed. The posterior layer of the lumbodorsal fascia is incised, and muscle fibers are split and the retroperitoneal space is entered by making an incision in the anterior thoracolumbar fascia or by bluntly piercing the fascia. Palpation of the belly of the psoas muscle posteriorly and the Gerota fascia–covered inferior pole of the kidney anteriorly confirms proper entry. Two inflations of the balloon dilator are then done—one directed cephalad and the second directed caudad to fully dilate the retroperitoneal space (Fig. 3.3).

Limitations

Retroperitoneoscopy is associated with limited anatomic landmarks except for the psoas muscle. Retroperitoneal laparoscopy is also associated with a relatively restricted working space compared with transperitoneal laparoscopy. This results in a steeper learning curve with the retroperitoneal approach. Moreover, the fact that a comparatively limited space is available necessitates precise accuracy regarding the strategic placement of ports. Contrary to common conception, the occurrence of an inadvertent peritoneotomy during retroperitoneoscopy does not usually interfere with the subsequent steps of the procedure. However, the occurrence of a peritoneotomy during extraperitoneoscopy may interfere and conversion to a transperitoneal technique may be required. A history of prior retroperitoneal surgery increases the difficulty of reentering the retroperitoneal space.

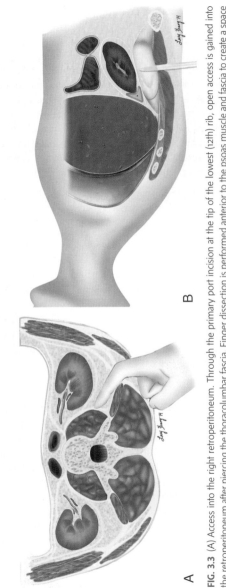

FIG. 3.3 (A) Access into the right retroperitoneum. Through the primary port incision at the tip of the lowest (12th) rib, open access is gained into the retroperitoneum after piercing the thoracolumbar fascia. Finger dissection is performed anterior to the psoas muscle and fascia to create a space for insertion of the balloon dilator. Confirmation that the finger dissection is indeed being performed in the proper plane is obtained by palpating the psoas and erector spinae muscles between the retroperitoneally located index finger and the fingertips of the opposite hand positioned on the patient's back. The fat-covered lower pole of the kidney can be palpated in a cephalad direction by turning the finger clockwise in the retroperitoneum on the right side. (B) Balloon dilation in the posterior pararenal space facilitates the creation of a working space for retroperitoneal laparoscopic nephrectomy (coronal view).

Advantages

Distinct advantages include minimizing inadvertent bowel injury and postoperative ileus, decreased postoperative shoulder tip pain versus transperitoneal laparoscopy, and lower incidence of postoperative trocar site hernias. Another significant benefit is the rapid and direct access to the renal hilum, with the renal artery being the first hilar structure encountered. Furthermore if a partial nephrectomy is planned, it may be more effective to approach a posterior tumor from the retroperitoneal approach.

PHYSIOLOGIC CONSIDERATIONS

CO_2 is the most commonly used insufflant because it is colorless, noncombustible, very soluble in blood, and inexpensive. It is highly soluble in water and easily diffuses in body tissues. However, the characteristic of rapid absorption, which lessens the chance of a gas embolus, may also lead to potential problems e.g., hypercapnia, hypercarbia, arrhythmias). In particular, patients with chronic obstructive pulmonary disease may not be able to compensate for the absorbed CO_2 by increased ventilation Last, CO_2 is also stored in various body compartments and may take hours before the patient has eliminated the extra CO_2 that has accumulated.

Helium is an inert and noncombustible insufflant with no evidence of hypercarbia and is thus useful for patients with pulmonary disease or if hypercarbia develops. However, there is a higher risk of gas embolism because of its lower blood solubility.

The potential for developing hypercarbia exists during both transperitoneal and preperitoneal laparoscopy. A rise in end-tidal CO_2 should prompt the anesthesiologist to adjust the respiratory rate and tidal volume to enhance CO_2 elimination. Simultaneously, the surgeon should decrease the insufflation pressure.

If pneumoperitoneum pressures are increased beyond 20 mm Hg, cardiac output is reduced because of decreasing venous return and hence MAP decreases. Alternatively, in the head-up position, heart rate increases, MAP decreases, systemic vascular resistance increases, and cardiac output decreases. In the head-down position, heart rate drops, MAP rises, systemic vascular resistance falls, and cardiac output increases.

Table 3.3 summarizes the physiologic effects of pneumoperitoneum at various pressures

Table 3.3 Pressure Effects: 5, 10, 20, and 40 mm Hg

EFFECTS	5 mm Hg	10 mm Hg	20 mm Hg	40 mm Hg
Cardiovascular				
Heart rate	↑	↑	↑	↓
Mean arterial pressure	↑	↑	↑	↑
Systemic vascular resistance	↑	↑	↑	↑
Venous return	→/↓	↓↑	↓↑	↓
Cardiac output	→/↓	→/↑	→/↓	↓
Renal				
Glomerular filtration rate	→	↓	↓↓	↓↓
Urine output	→	↓	↓↓	↓↓
Respiratory				
End-tidal CO_2	→	→/↑	→/↑	↑
Pco_2	→	↑	↑	↑
Arterial pH	→	→/↓	↓	↓

CO_2, Carbon dioxide; Pco_2, partial pressure of carbon dioxide.

TROUBLESHOOTING IN LAPAROSCOPIC AND ROBOTIC SURGERY

Preoperative placement of a urethral catheter to drain the bladder is recommended for all major laparoscopic urologic cases. Not only does it largely preclude bladder injury, but it also allows for monitoring urine output. Furthermore, it is helpful to consider having a "hemorrhage" tray available at all times (Box 3.1).

Box 3.1 Contents of Hemorrhage Tray for Laparoscopic Surgery

Laparoscopic Satinsky clamp
10-mm suction-irrigation tip
Endo Stitch device with 4-0 absorbable suture
Lapra-Ty clip applier and a packet of Lapra-Ty clips
6-inch length of 4-0 vascular suture on an SH needle with a Lapra-Ty clip preplaced on the end
Two laparoscopic needle drivers
Topical hemostatic agent of choice

SH, Small half.

Preperitoneal Insufflation. Preperitoneal placement of the Veress needle may preclude successful trocar placement. If the Veress needle is preperitoneal on initial insufflation, pressures are usually higher followed by unequal distention of the abdomen. Second, the Veress needle cannot be easily advanced 1 cm deeper without resistance. If not recognized early, 1 to 2 L of CO_2 may be instilled, and many signs indicative of correct intraperitoneal insufflation may be present, thereby misleading the surgeon. The next step is to evacuate the CO_2 through the sidearm of the trocar and proceed with an open insertion technique. The initial incision can be widened, and the peritoneal surface can be grasped with a pair of Allis clamps and incised. A Hasson cannula is placed, and the peritoneal cavity is insufflated.

Fascial Closure. Incorrect port removal and fascial closure can result in major complications, including herniation, bowel incarceration, and postoperative hemorrhage. Before port removal is initiated, the operative site and the entry sites of each cannula must be carefully inspected with the intraabdominal pressure lowered. Removal of all laparoscopic ports must be under visual control to avoid any possible herniation of intraabdominal contents. Most recommend that on removal of any of the blunt-tipped ports, the fascia does not need to be sutured, except for ports larger than 10 mm placed in the midline. The 5-mm ports are not closed in adults but are closed in pediatric patients. The simplest method is retracting the skin with retractors, grasping the fascia, and suturing it with absorbable 0-0 suture. However, in obese patients, securely accessing the fascia may be difficult. The Carter-Thomason needle-point suture passer consists of a cone that has two integrated, hollow, angled, cylindric passages located 180 degrees opposite each other. With the single-action grasper, the suture is inserted through one of the cylinders thereby traversing muscle, fascia, and peritoneal layers. It is then regrasped and brought out through the other passage.

Suggested Readings

Brackman MR, Finelli FC, et al. Helium pneumoperitoneum ameliorates hypercarbia and acidosis associated with carbon dioxide insufflation during laparoscopic gastric bypass in pigs. *Obes Surg* 2003;13:768-771.

Gill IS, Schweizer D, Hobart MG, et al. Retroperitoneal laparoscopic radical nephrectomy: the Cleveland Clinic experience. *J Urol* 2000;163:1665-1670.

Gunendran T, Briggs RH, Wemyss-Holden GD, et al. Does increasing hydrostatic pressure ("bag squeeze") during flexible cystoscopy improve patient comfort: a randomized, controlled study. *Urology* 2008;72:255-258.

Kavoussi L, Sosa E, Chandhoke P, et al: Complications of laparoscopic pelvic lymph node dissection. *J Urol* 1993;149:322-332.

Meraney A, Gill I. Extraperitoneoscopic pelvic surgery. *AUA Update Ser* 2001;20: 298-303.

Palmer R. Safety in laparoscopy. *J Reprod Med* 1974;13:1-5.

Patel AR, Jones JS, Babineau D. Lidocaine 2% gel versus plain lubricating gel for pain reduction during flexible cystoscopy: a meta-analysis of prospective, randomized, controlled trials. *J Urol* 2008;179:986-990.

Pearle M. *Physiologic effects of pneumoperitoneum*. St. Louis: Quality Medical Publishing, 1996.

Scott D, Julian D. Observations on cardiac arrhythmias during laparoscopy. *BMJ* 1972;1:411-41.

Soomro KQ, Nasir AR, Ather MH. Impact of patient's self-viewing of flexible cystoscopy on pain using a visual analog scale in a randomized controlled trial. *Urology* 2011;77:21-23.

Subramonian K, Cartwright RA, Harnden P, et al. Bladder cancer in patients with spinal cord injuries. *BJU Int* 2004;93:739-743.

Taghizadeh AK, El Madani A, Gard PR, et al. When does it hurt? Pain during flexible cystoscopy in men. *Urol Int* 2006;76: 301-303.

Traxer O, Thomas A. Prospective evaluation and classification of ureteral wall injuries resulting from insertion of a ureteral access sheath during retrograde intrarenal surgery, *J Urol* 189:580-584, 2013.

Wolf JS. Tips and tricks for hand-assisted laparoscopy. *AUA Update Ser* 2005;24:10-15.

Wolf JS, and Stoller M. The physiology of laparoscopy: basic principles, complications and other considerations. *J Urol* 1994;152:294-302.

Yeo JK, Cho DY, Oh MM, et al. Listening to music during cystoscopy decreases anxiety, pain, and dissatisfaction in patients: a pilot randomized controlled trial. *J Endourol* 2013;27:459-46.

4

Urologic Evaluation of the Child

CAITLIN T. COCO AND CRAIG A. PETERS

CONTRIBUTORS OF CAMPBELL-WALSH-WEIN, 12TH EDITION

C.D. Anthony Herndon, Rebecca S. Zee, Rachel Selekman, Hillary L. Copp, and Hans G. Pohl

HISTORY

Evaluating a child with a urologic condition is usually straightforward but can be challenging because of children's anxiety. History and physical examination often reveal the diagnosis and allow development of a treatment plan, yet laboratory studies or imaging may be needed. It is also critical to approach the family members, who are equally anxious, with sensitivity and patience. Open expression of the provider's awareness of their anxiety along with respecting the privacy of older children is important in establishing a trustful relationship.

History often constitutes the most important tool for establishing diagnosis and directing management. The child often provides a more accurate story than the parent. If parents are asking the child about voiding frequency, it is unlikely they know. Children are often oblivious to these issues, but do not underestimate even a younger child's insight.

It is best to ask the historian to report their experience and observations rather than asking for a diagnosis or judgment of "normalcy." For example, ask about frequency and consistency of stool rather than if a child is "constipated."

Engaging the child with a nonthreatening activity or discussion facilitates relaxation during the encounter. Becoming frustrated with an anxious and uncooperative 2-year-old child will result in an unproductive, unpleasant encounter. Sometimes simply returning later helps settle the child.

Children are particularly sensitive to painful touch and temperature; therefore, use clean, warm hands. Examination should be performed at the encounter's end to prevent the guardian from missing out on important clinical details if the child becomes upset.

PHYSICAL EXAMINATION

Examining the Pediatric Patient (Table 4.1)
Testicular Exam

Examination should establish location, size, and texture of the gonads as well as identify pathology of the testicles and scrotum. The patient may be examined supine in frog leg position, with the legs spread apart, sitting, squatting, or standing. The examiner should stand on the contralateral side to area of concern. The nondominant hand is used to gently sweep the testicle toward the internal inguinal ring, sliding from the anterior superior iliac spine to the pubic tubercle. A lubricated glove (with soap and water) may aid the examiner.

Techniques to increase intraabdominal pressure to visualize a bulge include jumping, coughing, laughing, blowing bubbles. If a bulge is not elicited on examination, photographs may be taken by family members. Hydrocele fluid (and neonatal bowel) transilluminates and may appear blue through scrotal skin.

Female Perineal Exam

The female genital examination should visualize the labia, introitus, urethral meatus, clitoris, and anus. The patient should be placed in a frog leg position. The labia majora should be gently pulled laterally and caudally to expose the introitus.

Assessing the Neuromuscular System

The neuromuscular examination can assist with identifying causes of bladder dysfunction. Motor function and balance are assessed by observing the child walk or get on and off the examination table. Strength tests can be performed with cooperative children by having

Table 4.1 Useful Examination Tips

Clearly state area to be examined to guardian/child
Reserve examination for end of encounter
Have guardian bedside for comfort/distraction
Speak in a calm gentle voice throughout examination
Make sure hands are clean and warm

them squeeze fingers or push on provider's hands. Sensation is assessed using cotton swabs and asking the patient to identify the sensation. Newborn and infant motor function can be slightly more challenging. Observation during the encounter includes an assessment of upper and lower extremity mobility. Newborn plantar reflex and palmar grasp reflex should be checked. In older children, knee patellar reflexes and ankle jerk reflexes may be assessed if relevant.

LABORATORY TESTING

Urinalysis

Urinalysis can identify blood, protein, urinary casts, or infectious markers in urine. This includes gross examination for color, turbidity, and debris as well as dipstick and microscopic analyses. Urinary specific gravity usually ranges from 1.001 to 1.035 and can be indicative of hydration status and concentrating ability. Urinary pH can vary from 4.5 to 8 and is reflective of the serum pH. Blood in the urine can be detected on dipstick analysis but may also be positive in the case of myoglobinuria or hemoglobinuria. Microscopic identification of three erythrocytes per high-powered field (HPF) is diagnostic of hematuria. Proteinuria, red blood cell (RBC) casts, and brown-colored urine suggest a nephrogenic origin of hematuria. Leukocyte esterase and nitrite tests suggest bacteriuria.

Urine Culture

Urine culture can indicate infection and identify the responsible organism. Clean-catch urine cultures are notoriously difficult to obtain in children without contamination. A sterile plastic bag with adhesive collar is placed over an infant's genitalia to collect a sample but often is contaminated. If normal, it spares the child from a catheterized urine sample. 100,000 colony-forming units (CFU)/mL of organism plated within 1 hour of collection is necessary to define an infection with clean-catch method. A catheterized or suprapubic aspirate specimen should have a colony count of $\geq$50,000 CFU/mL to constitute an infection.

Urinary Flow Rate

Urinary flow rate in a toilet-trained child is obtained by having the child urinate into a chair or toilet with a flow device synced that records the volume of urine per time. This provides information on voiding patterns and bladder function. Ultrasound measurement of remaining urine defines the postvoid residual (PVR). Flow rates and PVR are useful for monitoring changes in response to therapy. Bell-shaped curves with minimal PVR are considered normal.

Flow-Electromyography studies

Uroflow with electromyography of the pelvic floor (using perineal electrode pads) provides information on bladder pelvic floor coordination. The external urethral sphincter should be quiescent during voiding.

Urodynamics

Video urodynamics assesses continence, bladder stability, capacity, compliance, and sphincteric coordination. Fluoroscopy visualizes anatomy including the bladder outlet during voiding, bladder shape, and reflux into the upper tracts. This is an important study to characterize and trend storage and voiding dynamics in children with structural or neurologic conditions affecting bladder function. It aids in assessment of upper tract injury from high bladder pressures and guides therapeutic interventions. Because this test is invasive requiring catheter placement, knowledgeable and professional staff are paramount to provide a calm, relaxed environment.

IMAGING (Tables 4.2 and 4.3)

Renal and Bladder Ultrasound

Prenatally, sonography visualizes the presence and quality of the renal cortex, laterality of any abnormality, the umbilical cord and anterior abdominal wall anatomy, quantity of amniotic fluid, and urine within the fetal bladder. Many urologic abnormalities are detected on anatomic ultrasound around 20 weeks of gestation. Postnatally, relative to sonography in adults, a newborn kidney's more pronounced corticomedullary differentiation with darker medullary pyramids may be mistaken for hydronephrosis. Hydronephrosis can be underestimated in the several days of the newborn period due to dehydration. Sonography evaluates for hydronephrosis; cortical dysplasia; pelvic and renal cysts (Table 4.4); renal, abdominal, and bladder masses; nephrolithiasis; infection; trauma; posterior urethral valves; ureteroceles; bladder diverticula; and bladder calculi (Fig. 4.1).

Table 4.2 Comparison of Pediatric Urologic Imaging Modalities

	ULTRASOUND	X-RAY/FLUOROSCOPY [a]	COMPUTED TOMOGRAPHY [a]	MAGNETIC RESONANCE IMAGING	NUCLEAR IMAGING [a] RENAL SCINTIGRAPHY MAG3	NUCLEAR IMAGING [a] RENAL SCINTIGRAPHY DMSA
Uses in pediatric urology	• Renal/bladder • Hydronephrosis • Scrotal • Testicular torsion • Prenatal • Spinal • Spinal dysraphism	• Bony abnormalities • Radiopaque stones • Stool burden • Genitogram • Urodynamics • Neurogenic bladder • Voiding cystourethrogram • Vesicoureteral reflux • Posterior urethral valves	• Severe blunt abdominal trauma • Nephrolithiasis • Renal artery disease	• Renal and bladder tumors • Pelvicaliectasis • Genitography • Urogenital sinus	• Renal obstruction	• Pyelonephritis and damage to renal parenchyma • Function of moieties in duplicated systems
Advantages	• Inexpensive • No sedation • Real-time images • No contrast	• Wide range of indications • Real time images	• Available in most settings • Fast • No sedation needed	• Excellent anatomic detail • Urogram phase provides functional info	• Evaluates renal obstruction and function	• Evaluates renal scarring
Disadvantages	• Equipment and operator dependent • Little functional information	• Ionizing radiation	• High doses of ionizing radiation	• Requires sedation in young children • Lack of widely available technology • High cost	• Ionizing radiation	• Ionizing radiation

[a]Utilizes ionizing radiation, which should be minimized in at-risk pediatric population

DMSA, Dimercaptosuccinic acid; *MAG3,* mercaptoacetyltriglycine.

Table 4.3 When to perform imaging for Antenatally detected hydronephrosis

IMAGING PROCEDURE	INITIAL NEONATAL IMAGING	NEONATAL US FINDINGS				
		NORMAL NEONATAL US	ISOLATED MILD (SFU 1-2 OR APRPD <15MM)	MALE WITH MODERATE-SEVERE (SFU 3-4 OR APRPD >15MM) OR ABNORMAL PARENCHYMA, DILATED URETER, BLADDER WALL THICKENING OR DILATED POSTERIOR URETHRA	FEMALE WITH MODERATE-SEVERE (SFU 3-4 OR APRPD >15MM) OR ABNORMAL PARENCHYMA, DILATED URETER, BLADDER WALL THICKENING	MODERATE-SEVERE (SFU 3-4 OR APRPD >15MM) WITH NO EVIDENCE OF VESICOURETERAL REFLUX ON VCUG OR CEVUS
RBUS	✓	✓	✓	✓	✓	✓
VCUG	✗	✗	+/-	✓	✓	Done
ceVUS	✗	✗	+/-	+/-	✓	Done
MAG-3 Renal Scan	✗	✗	✗	✓	✓	✓
RNC	✗	✗	✗	✗	✓	N/A

Abbreviations: RBUS=Renal and bladder ultrasound; APRPD=Anterior-posterior renal pelvic diameter; SFU=Society for Fetal Urology; VCUG=Voiding cystourethrogram; ceVUS=Contrast-enhanced voiding sonourethrogram; RNC=Radionuclide cystogram; MAG-3=mercaptoacetyltriglycine.
Adapted from American College of Radiology Appropriateness Criteria Antenatal Hydronephrosis.

Table 4.4 Imaging Features of Renal Cysts

| MULTICYSTIC DYSPLASTIC KIDNEY | POLYCYSTIC KIDNEY DISEASE | | MULTILOCULAR CYSTIC NEPHROMA[a] | CYSTIC WILMS TUMOR[a] |
	AUTOSOMAL RECESSIVE	AUTOSOMAL DOMINANT		
Unilateral	Bilateral	Bilateral	Unilateral	Unilateral or bilateral
Varying sizes; random distribution	Enlarged and homogeneously hyperechoic parenchyma	Replacement of renal parenchyma by cysts	Noncommunicating cyst of varying sizes but has more parenchymal tissue than MCDK	Noncommunicating cyst of varying sizes but has more parenchymal tissue than MCDK
Bilateral usually lethal	Can be lethal; nonlethal often with liver involvement	Usually later presentation in fourth and fifth decades	Peak incidence 4 years and adolescence	Occurs in children around 2–4 years of age

[a]Although patient age and hallmark sonographic features suggest the diagnosis of renal mass, contrast-enhanced computed tomography of the abdomen should be performed to confirm.

MCDK, Multicystic dysplastic kidney.

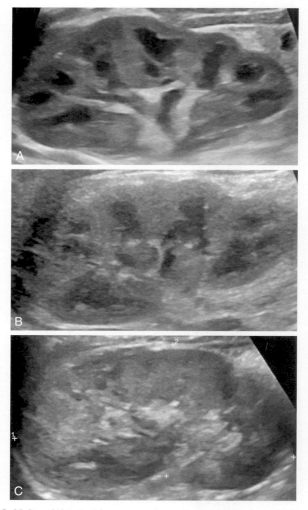

FIG. 4.1 (A and B) Postnatal sonograms demonstrating the high contrast cortico-medullary differentiation typical of a newborn kidney, which might be mistaken for dilated calyces. (C) For comparison, a renal sonogram in an older child.

Testicular Ultrasound

Sonography identifies testicular and paratesticular masses and infectious conditions such as epididymitis. Ultrasound should not be performed for routine cryptorchidism due to poor sensitivity of detecting an undescended testicle. Incidentally discovered testicular microlithiasis does not require further follow-up imaging unless additional risk factors such as infertility with atrophic testis or testis cancer with contralateral microlithiasis exist. Testicular ultrasound may be used to confirm clinical suspicion that an acute scrotum is not caused by torsion by demonstrating testicular blood flow. However, it should not be used to override the clinical impression of testicular torsion because it is not 100% accurate, and these patients may benefit from emergent exploration and detorsion (Table 4.5).

Cystography, Pyelography, and Urogenitography

Ionizing radiation should be used with caution in young children because of their increased sensitivity with subsequent impact on growth and potential for radiation-induced malignancies. Plain abdominal radiography and scout imagery for cystography or pyelography demonstrates bony anatomy of the spine and pelvis, radiopaque stones, and stool burden. Retrograde pyelography requires anesthesia for the injection of contrast into the ureteral orifice to localize obstructive lesions intraoperatively. Urogenitography visualizes urethral and vaginal structures in disorders of sexual differentiation. Voiding cystourethrography (VCUG) assesses anatomy and function of the lower urinary tract and typically does not require sedation. VCUG can evaluate for vesicoureteral reflux and provide excellent anatomic detail of bladder wall and urethral abnormalities like trabeculations, ureteroceles, diverticula, posterior urethral valves, stricture disease, bladder rupture, and foreign bodies

Nuclear Medicine Imaging

Radionuclide Cystography. Direct radionuclide cystography accurately detects vesicoureteral reflux (VUR) with greater sensitive and lower radiation exposure than fluoroscopic VCUG but cannot provide equivalent anatomic detail.

DMSA. Dimercapto-succinic acid (DMSA) is a radioisotope taken up by proximal tubular cells in a renal blood flow dependent pattern. Relative renal function may be determined by the activity in each kidney. Areas of decreased uptake reflect either acute

Table 4.5 Imaging Findings for Scrotal Pathology

TORSION	EPIDIDYMO-ORCHITIS	TESTICULAR OR EPIDIDYMAL APPENDAGE TORSION	TERATOMA	YOLK SAC TUMOR	EPIDERMOID CYST	ADRENAL REST
Color Doppler demonstrates no flow	Hyperemia of the epididymis and/or testicle	Upper pole or epididymal hypoechoic or avascular nodule with surrounding hyperemia	Heterogeneous mass with areas of solid, cystic, and calcified components	Homogeneous well-vascularized mass	Hyperechoic or hypoechoic rings or onion rings with no internal blood flow	Bilateral hypoechoic, hyperemic, heterogenous masses
Whirlpool sign: torsion of spermatic cord on high resolution sonography	May have systemic signs of fever; urine may appear infected	Gradual onset; more early skin changes and scrotal wall edema	Age dependent prognosis; partial orchiectomy considered in prepubertal boys	Most common malignant prepubertal testis tumor	Amenable to testis sparing surgery	Seen in setting of congenital adrenal hyperplasia with improper steroid replacement

inflammatory processes or permanent renal scarring, usually due to infection or congenital maldevelopment.

MAG-3 Diuretic Renography. Mercaptoacetyltriglycine (MAG3) and less commonly used Tc-diethylenetriamine pentaacetic acid (DTPA) are two radioisotopes used in diuretic renography. These studies require a well-hydrated patient, selection of the appropriate region of interest with background subtraction, bladder drainage, and attention to timing of diuretic administration. Differential renal function, washout curves, and washout halftimes can be generated from this protocol, which is helpful to evaluate drainage of the collecting system. Patterns of uptake and drainage should be visually reviewed; simply using the report is often misleading.

Computed Tomography Imaging

Computed tomography (CT) in children should be used judiciously to limit ionizing radiation in developing tissues. Indications when CT scan advantages outweigh risks include blunt abdominal trauma, pediatric renal tumor evaluation, and quantifying stone burden. CT may be required in complex reconstructive situations.

Magnetic Resonance Urography

Magnetic resonance urography (MRU) localizes anatomic abnormalities and assesses differential function and drainage of the urinary tract in a three-phase study. Precontrast T2-weighted (fluid sensitive) fast spin-echo sequences are captured to envisage anatomy. Postcontrast, T1-weighted images assess renal vasculature, parenchymal enhancement, and excretory function. Delayed images detail ureteral anatomy. This protocol takes approximately an hour; therefore, it often requires sedation in children younger than 6 years. MRU characterizes renal masses and cysts, acute inflammatory lesions associated with pyelonephritis, bladder masses such as rhabdomyosarcoma, and other congenital malformations. It is less useful than sonography for the evaluation of stones, acute scrotum, scrotal masses, undescended testicles, and disorders of sexual development.

Incidental and Prenatal Imaging Findings

Kidney

Congenital Malformations. A **solitary kidney** can be visualized on imaging if one kidney failed to develop. As the kidney ascends from the sacral region to its lumbar location, it can arrest at any time, resulting in an abnormally located or **ectopic kidney**. **Horseshoe kidneys** appear as a solitary malrotated kidney on imaging due to the kidneys fusing and becoming entrapped by the inferior mesenteric artery (Fig. 4.2).

Hydronephrosis. Hydronephrosis is typically graded on ultrasound according to the Society for Fetal Urology classification (Fig. 4.3).

Differential Diagnosis – Obstruction (kidney stone, ureteropelvic junction obstruction, ureterovesical junction obstruction), megaureter, vesicoureteral reflux, multicystic dysplastic kidney, cystic nephroma, and nonobstructing nonrefluxing hydronephrosis.

Helpful Imaging Modalities – Ultrasound initially followed by VCUG and/or diuretic renography.

CLINICAL PRESENTATION

Symptoms

Dysuria

Symptoms – Burning or stinging pain with urination

History – The patient and family should be asked about duration, consistency, severity, concomitant hematuria, systemic symptoms like fever, preceding trauma, history of prior infections, weak or deviated urinary stream and voiding patterns–are they "holders"? Is there constipation?

Examination – Meatal caliber should be assessed visually. **Meatal stenosis** can present with a ventral web of tissue below the meatus and usually results in a dorsally defected urinary stream. The presence of erythema in girls or boys suggests local inflammation. The bladder should be palpated to rule out urinary retention. The abdomen can be palpated for the presence of excessive stool.

Labs – A urinalysis can identify possible infection and hematuria. High urinary specific gravity suggests poor hydration. Leukocytes or nitrites on dip stick should prompt a urine culture.

Imaging – Imaging is rarely useful in this setting. A large postvoid residual does suggest significant irritation or an underlying functional issue causing poor emptying.

Differential Diagnosis – The most common cause of dysuria is urinary infection. Nonbacterial viral cystitis presents with significant dysuria and hematuria. Hematuria without infection suggests a foreign body or stone, which can be

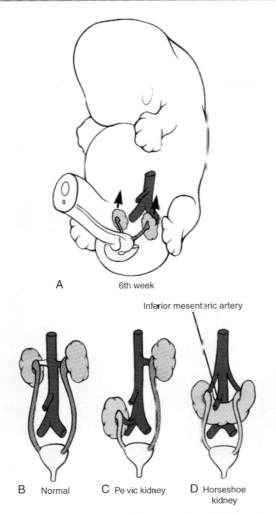

FIG. 4.2 Normal and abnormal ascent of the kidneys. (A and B) The metanephros normally ascends from the sacral region to its definitive lumbar location between the sixth and ninth weeks. (C) Rarely, a kidney may fail to ascend, resulting in a pelvic kidney. (D) If the inferior poles of the kidneys fuse before ascent, the resulting horseshoe kidney does not ascend to a normal position because of entrapment by the inferior mesenteric artery. (Modified from Larsen WJ. *Human embryology*. New York: Churchill Livingstone; 1997.)

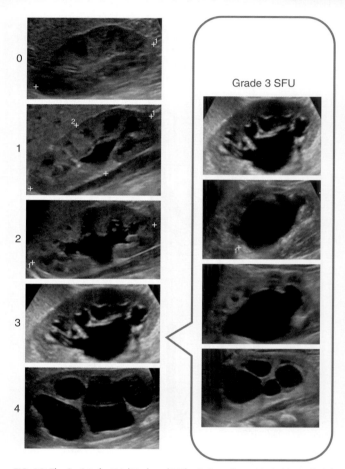

FIG. 4.3 The Society for Fetal Urology (SFU) criteria as demonstrated in postnatal sonograms. Grade 0 shows no central renal dilation. In grade 1, the renal pelvis only is visible; in grade 2, major calices can be identified; in grade 3, major and minor calices can be identified; and grade 4 has features of grade 3 but with parenchymal thinning as well. Within grade 3, there are many different degrees of collecting system dilation that conform to the criteria.

visualized with imaging. Voiding dysfunction is another differential diagnosis to be considered, supported by voiding history, constipation, and possible incontinence. Boys may complain of dysuria and penile pain with voiding dysfunction and voiding postponement. Perineal irritation in girls is common, which may result from vaginal voiding, dysfunctional voiding with postponement, and constipation. Meatal stenosis is common in circumcised boys but does not often cause dysuria.

Treatment – Treatment is directed at the cause. If the cause is unclear, a therapeutic trial of azo-dye medication is useful. Directly treating voiding dysfunction often improves symptoms. Reassurance is important to ensure compliance with voiding improvement programs.

Hematuria

Symptoms – Visible blood in the urine or >3 RBCs per HPF on microscopic examination.

History – Bleeding patterns offer insight into etiology (e.g., terminal bleeding seen with benign urethrorrhagia vs total gross hematuria). Key elements include duration, clot formation or severity of bleeding, difficulty voiding, history of preceding trauma, prior infections, family history of progressive renal disease, and excessive bleeding with prior surgeries. Identifying relevant comorbidities, such as BK virus, provides insight in an immunocompromised child.

Examination – Key findings include blood at the urethral meatus, perineal irritation, flank tenderness, and palpable abdominal masses.

Labs – Urinalysis is obtained to identify infection, proteinuria, and crystalluria. Leukocytes or nitrites should prompt a urine culture. Consider obtaining hemoglobin and hematocrit if concerned for substantial blood loss. Gross hematuria with positive urine dipstick but no RBCs on microscopy suggests myoglobinuria, requiring separate evaluation.

Imaging – Renal sonography can identify masses, hydronephrosis, or an obstructing stone.

Differential Diagnosis – The most common cause of hematuria is urinary tract infection (UTI) followed by perineal irritation, trauma, meatal stenosis with ulceration, coagulation abnormalities, and nephrolithiasis. Less common causes of gross hematuria include sickle cell disease or trait, glomerular disease, malignancies, and benign idiopathic urethrorrhagia.

Treatment – Treatment is severity and etiology specific. Microhematuria can be observed and retested in 6–12 months if urinary crystals, casts, proteinuria, hypertension, and family history of progressive renal disease are absent. Benign idiopathic urethrorrhagia with normal imaging is managed with watchful waiting; 90% of patients have resolution by 2 years. If the cause of gross hematuria is undefined, referral to a pediatric nephrologist is appropriate, particularly with proteinuria. If gross hematuria is substantial enough to require a transfusion or clot retention ensues, admission should be considered. Catheter irrigation in children is limited by urethral size. Cystoscopy with clot evacuation or fulguration, suprapubic tube placement, or urinary diversion may be necessary in order to manage severe gross hematuria.

Incontinence

Symptoms – Leakage of urine. Daytime urinary continence typically occurs by 4 years of age followed by night continence, generally achieved by 5–6 years of age.

History – Inquire about voiding habits cautiously so as not to elicit blanket statements such as "she is always wet." Ask about periods of dryness, worsening with activity, voiding postponement, posturing, drinking habits, bowel habits, neurologic history, and spinal cord injury or surgery. Is this new-onset incontinence or has the child never achieved continence?

Examination – Examination should target the genitalia for signs of irritation or abnormal configuration, the abdomen for stool burden, and the lower extremities for normal gait and feet. A clear history of true continuous incontinence should prompt a search for a perineal ectopic ureteral orifice. Examine the intergluteal cleft for sacral dimpling or hair tufts indicating a possible spinal abnormality.

Labs – A urinalysis can rule out UTIs, which can cause incontinence. Urine culture is indicated if urinalysis is consistent with infection.

Imaging – A postvoid residual bladder ultrasound can rule out overflow incontinence and assess the degree of emptying. Bladder capacity = (age [years] + 2) × 30.

Differential Diagnosis – Bowel and bladder dysfunction, ectopic ureter in girls, UTI, sexual abuse, neurogenic bladder, and epispadias are all in the differential.

Treatment – The most common diagnosis, bowel and bladder dysfunction, typically requires behavioral modification which includes improved hydration, timed voiding every 2–3 hours, and a vigorous bowel regimen. Other etiologies including ectopic ureter and neurogenic bladder necessitate further workup.

Scrotal Pain

Symptoms – Discomfort or tenderness in the scrotal area ± mass and inflammation.

History – Define the duration and onset of pain, preceding trauma, and associated symptoms such as erythema, nausea or vomiting, fevers or chills, or abdominal pain.

Examination – Note testicular lie or position in the scrotum, testicular size, turgor compared with the contralateral side, masses, tenderness, fluctuance, and erythema on examination. Note tenderness in the epididymis in addition to cremasteric reflex. Inguinal region should be palpated for hernia.

Labs – If concerned for a scrotal mass, the following tumor markers should be obtained: human chorionic gonadotropin (bHCG), alpha fetoprotein (AFP), lactate dehydrogenase (LDH). CBC may be helpful if concerned for abscess or infection. A urinalysis or urine culture may support the diagnosis of epididymitis.

Imaging – Testicular ultrasound is useful to assess testicular contour (history of trauma with irregular contour and heterogeneity indicating concern for rupture) and Doppler flow (absence of flow indicates testicular torsion, whereas increased flow to the epididymis indicates inflammation) and to define poorly palpable masses. Renal images should be considered to evaluate for an ectopic ureter causing epididymitis.

Differential Diagnosis – The differential includes testicular torsion, testicular or epididymal appendix torsion, testicular or paratesticular tumor, varicocele, hernia and hydrocele, testicular trauma, epididymo-orchitis, scrotal abscess, cellulitis, and constipation.

Treatment – See Table 4.6.

Table 4.6 Diagnosis and Treatment Options for Various Scrotal Pathology

| DIAGNOSIS | KEY SIGNS AND SYMPTOMS | SCROTAL PATHOLOGY | | | | KEY IMAGING FINDINGS | TREATMENT |
		ERYTHEMA	TENDERNESS	FLUCTUANCE	SWELLING		
Testicular Torsion	Nausea or vomiting Abdominal pain Horizontal lie Hardened testicle Absence of cremasteric reflex	✓	✓		Late finding	Absence of blood flow on Doppler	Emergent bilateral orchiopexy ± orchiectomy
Testicular or paratesticular tumor	Palpable scrotal mass				✓	Mass evident on ultra-sound	Urgent surgical exploration ± radical inguinal orchiectomy
Testicular trauma with rupture	Scrotal ecchymosis		✓		✓	Loss of testicle contour on ultrasound	Urgent surgical exploration
Scrotal abscess [a]	Inflamed, fluctuant scrotum	✓	✓	✓	✓		Consider urgent surgical exploration or debridement

Condition	Physical examination findings	↑ with Valsalva maneuver	↑ with intraabdominal pressure	Tenderness	Ultrasound findings	Management
Varicocele [a]	"Bag of worms"	✓				Consider elective varicocelectomy
Hernia [a]	Inguinoscrotal fullness ± crepitus		✓			Consider repair
Hydrocele [a]	Transilluminates		✓			Consider repair
Testicular or epididymal appendix torsion	Blue-dot sign			Focal	✓	Nonsteroidal antiinflammatory medication
Epididymo-orchitis	Tenderness in epididymal region			✓	Increased blood flow to region on doppler	Antibiotics are indicated with pyuria or positive urine culture
Acute idiopathic scrotitis or cellulitis				✓	"Fountain sign" on ultrasound	Topical steroids, antiinflammatory agents ± antibiotics

[a] Additional clinical information needed to make decision for surgical management

Sources: Gatti JM, Murphy. Current management of the acute scrotum. Semin Plast Surg 2007;16(1):58-63; Lau P, Anderson PA, Giacomantonio JM, Schwarz RD. Acute epididymitis in boys: are antibiotics indicated? Br J Urol 1997;79(5):797-800; and Morey AF, Broghammer JA, Hollowell CMP, et al. Urotrauma Guideline 2020: AUA Guideline. J Urol 2021;205(1):30-35.

Urinary Retention

Symptoms – Inability to spontaneously void with a distended or full bladder relative to expected capacity

History – Time since last void, prior episodes, bowel history, and neurologic disorders should be defined. Pain with urination should be identified as children may hold urine secondary to dysuria. Inquire about recent medication changes and prior urological surgeries.

Examination – Examination includes the urethral meatus and bladder palpation. Neurologic exam is indicated to evaluate for sacral dimpling or tufts and lower extremity motor or sensory deficits.

Labs – Basic metabolic panel (BMP) helps evaluate kidney function with severe retention

Imaging – Bladder ultrasound can quantify urine volume in the bladder and a postvoid residual. Plain film x-ray examination helps determine stool burden and spinal anatomy.

Differential Diagnosis – Differential includes dysfunctional voiding, constipation, neurologic disorders or diagnoses, UTI, adverse drug effect, and locally invading neoplasms. Posterior urethral valves should be considered in a neonate.

Treatment – The first step is identifying the cause of retention. An enema can be administered if constipation or dysfunctional voiding is suspected. Frequently, children void simultaneously with the bowel movement. If other causes are suspected or this management does not resolve the retention, management may necessitate catheterization. Clean intermittent catheterization can be performed and taught to the family as further workup is completed.

Penile Pain

Symptoms – Discomfort or tenderness in the shaft or glans of the penis.

History – Ask about duration, severity, inciting events, erythema, fever, and difficulties with urination and constipation.

Examination – Careful examination of the penis is important. Be sure to explain to the caregiver and child that it is necessary to examine the genitalia. Note foreskin, urethral meatus position and size, penile shaft curvature or torsion, erythema, pubescence, and lesions on the penis because sexually transmitted diseases are prevalent among adolescent boys.

Labs – Urinalysis evaluates for infection. If there is the presence of leukocytes or nitrites on the dip stick, urine culture is appropriate.

Table 4.7 Treatment of Common Penile Conditions

Paraphimosis	Urgent manual reduction
Ischemic priapism	Hydration, oxygenation, alkalization, analgesia. Consider aspiration or irrigation or exchange transfusion (in sickle cell anemia) following failure of above
Balanitis or balanoposthitis	Supportive care, topical antibiotics or antifungals, topical corticosteroids
Penile pain in setting of voiding dysfunction	Voiding improvement program, treatment of constipation, occasional alpha-blockers

Imaging – No imaging is necessary.

Differential Diagnosis – Causes include priapism, paraphimosis, balanitis, urinary retention, constipation, voiding dysfunction, and idiopathic penile edema.

Treatment – See Table 4.7.

Flank Pain or Colic

Symptoms – Discomfort or tenderness on flank may be vague in terms of localization with abdominal pain ("my tummy hurts" may be flank pain).

History – Delve into onset, duration, inciting events, trauma, and associated symptoms such as gross hematuria, dysuria, fevers, and chills. Additional history includes family history of nephrolithiasis, genitourinary (GU) tract structural abnormalities, metabolic conditions associated with stone formation, medications, and prior instances of UTI.

Examination – Examination and careful palpation of the abdomen and flank is important. Localizing pain should be a focus in addition to evaluating for fever.

Labs – A urinalysis evaluates for infection and hematuria. Leukocytes or nitrites on the dip stick should prompt urine culture.

Imaging – If concerned for pyelonephritis or trauma, renal ultrasound is a good first technique to identify hydronephrosis associated with a possible stone, an abscess, or fluid collection. CT is an ideal imaging choice for stone disease, but pediatric radiation exposure is higher risk. CT is reserved for instances in which ultrasound is nondiagnostic with high clinical suspicion.

Differential Diagnosis – Differential diagnosis includes infectious etiology such as pyelonephritis and stone disease. Other differentials include traumatic injury to the area and ureteropelvic junction obstruction.

Treatment – Treatment is etiology specific. Stone management depends on the stability of the patient, stone size, pain control, contralateral kidney function, and indicators of concomitant infection. Infection should prompt urgent decompression with a retrograde ureteral stent or percutaneous nephrostomy tube. Nonacute management options include observation with analgesia, medical expulsive therapy, and surgery. Alpha-blockers are recommended as first-line medical expulsion therapy in children, especially with small, distal stones. Surgical management is like that in adults recommending extracorporeal shock wave lithotripsy and ureteroscopy for smaller stones. Percutaneous nephrolithotomy is reserved for larger renal stone burden. Metabolic evaluation is recommended to identify correctable metabolic abnormalities.

Physical Findings

Male Genitalia
Penis

Swelling and Erythema. Swelling and redness can occur because of many inflammatory conditions. **Paraphimosis** can be distinguished on examination by noting a tight band of tissue behind the erythematous, edematous glans indicating the foreskin was not reduced after retraction. This condition should be addressed immediately with manual reduction. **Balanitis** presents with an irritated, erythematous glans. The preputial skin can be involved (**balanoposthitis**) in uncircumcised children. Penile edema and pruritis in spring or summer with concern for insect bites or outdoor exposure can indicate **summer penile syndrome**, which is typically self-limited and managed conservatively.

Prolonged Erection. **Priapism** is a persistent penile erection, typically affecting only the corpora cavernosa, unrelated to sexual stimulation sustained for >4 hours. Priapism can be ischemic (venoocclusive, low flow), nonischemic (arterial, high flow), and stuttering (intermittent). Completely rigid corpora cavernosa suggests ischemic priapism. Treatment of low-flow priapism resulting from sickle cell disease includes concurrent treatment of the underlying disease with transfusion, alkalization, hydration, and oxygen as well as intracavernous treatment with aspiration (with or without irrigation) or intracavernous injection of sympathomimetics as indicated. Treatment for high-flow priapism is controversial because it may not produce long-term fibrosis.

Meatal Size Abnormalities. The meatus can be abnormally small to the size of a pinpoint after circumcision, indicating **meatal stenosis**, or it can be abnormally large, indicating variants such as **megameatus intact prepuce**.

Lesions. Irregularities of the penile shaft skin can range from mild to severe diaper rash to balanitis xerotica obliterans (BXO).

Abnormal Shape. Nonprogressive, congenital curvature of the penile shaft can occur along the vertical and/or horizontal plane. Surgical correction is indicated with severe angulation because it may interfere with sexual function. Surgical correction with **penile torsion** (rotational deformity) is indicated if rotation is at least 60 degrees.

Urethral Abnormalities. **Hypospadias** has a ventrally displaced urethral meatus typically with ventral curvature and dorsal hooded foreskin, whereas **epispadias** urethral meatus is dorsally displaced with dorsal curvature.

Scrotum

Swelling. A swollen scrotum must be promptly assessed to avoid delayed diagnosis of a testicular torsion or tumor. Most other situations are not acutely dangerous.

Fluid or Solid. Palpation of the affected side helps differentiate a fluid-filled scrotum from a hard mass. Transillumination may help differentiate fluid from solid mass. Fluid is indicative of a **hydrocele**, but this may be reactive fluid with infectious, traumatic, and neoplastic causes. A soft fullness, sometimes with crepitus, can represent a **hernia** with bowel or omentum in the scrotum. If the testis is not able to be palpated, ultrasound imaging is useful.

Tenderness. Scrotal tenderness suggests inflammatory processes, including epididymitis, torsion of a testicular or epididymal appendage causing reactive epididymitis, testicular torsion, hernia, or orchitis. The absence of inflammation with tenderness suggests early torsion or trauma.

Erythema. Scrotal erythema may be caused by cellulitis, an insect bite, or **acute idiopathic scrotitis**. This is an inflammatory process of probable allergic origin that causes significant swelling, erythema and itching. Scrotal ultrasound aids in diagnosis and will show the "fountain sign" or swirling edematous scrotal wall tissues. Topical steroids, antiinflammatory agents, and antibiotics are appropriate if there's suspicion for infection. Rarely, extraintestinal Crohn disease can present with genital swelling.

Undescended Testicles. Unilateral or bilateral absence of the testicles may be true **cryptorchidism** or **retractile testes**. Bilateral nonpalpable testicles without congenital adrenal hyperplasia should have Mullerian inhibiting substance or anti-Mullerian hormone levels drawn. Ultrasound has no role in locating undescended testicles.

Female Genitalia
Interlabial Mass (See Table 4.8)

Urethral Mass. **Urethral prolapse** will demonstrate an erythematous, friable appearing mucosa on vaginal exam. A **prolapsed ureterocele** will be a smooth, congested, mucosa-covered interlabial mass protruding from the urethra and distinct from the vagina. This can be differentiated from urethral prolapse because the ureterocele is not circumferential. Direct reduction can be attempted but is rarely successful. Surgical decompression by incising or puncturing the ureterocele is usually needed.

Paraurethral Mass. A thin-walled golden or whitish cyst anterior to the vagina is typical for a **skene's cyst,** which are commonly self-resolving.

Vaginal Mass. **Botryoid rhabdomyosarcoma** is evident in the vagina as a "cluster of grapes".

Urethral diverticula can present as variably sized, urine-filled periurethral cystic structure protruding through the vaginal opening.

Vaginal Opening Absent

Labial Adhesions. The labia minora are fused in the midline, concealing the vaginal opening. If symptomatic, topical estrogen or steroids can separate the edges, but continued moisturizing ointment will be needed to prevent refusion.

Table 4.8 Diagnosing and Managing Interlabial Masses

	PHOTOGRAPH	DIAGNOSIS	DESCRIPTION	MANAGEMENT
Urethral		Urethral prolapse	Beefy red, friable mucosal covered mass Circumferential Often seen in prepubertal girls with constipation	Topical estrogen or antiinflammatory cream, sitz baths but often surgical manipulation required
		Prolapsed ureterocele	Smooth, congested mucosal covered mass NOT circumferential	Surgical decompression
Para-urethral		Skene's cyst	Golden or white thin-walled cyst anterior to vagina	Often self-resolving
Vaginal		Botryoid rhabdomyosarcomax	"Cluster of grapes"	Possible surgical excision[a]
		Imperforate hymen	Golden or white bulging membrane in introitus May appear blue or purplish in older children	Incision

[a] Clinical picture and staging if indicated are needed for determination of operative management

Source: Rudin JE, Geld VG, Alecseev EB. Prolapse of urethral mucosa in white female children: experience with 58 cases. *J Pediatr Surg* 1997;32(3):423-425.

Imperforate Hymen. Imperforate hymen is usually characterized by a bulging white or yellow membrane in the introitus of an infant or potentially amenorrhea with painful episodes in the older child. Incision for drainage is usually sufficient and dilation is not required.

Cloacal Anomaly. A single perineal opening in a phenotypic female suggests cloacal anomaly where the urethra, vagina, and colon converge. The external appearance is flat with no obvious introitus but may have variable configurations. The bladder may be distended, and the presence of the anomaly may be indicated prenatally. Initial goals are to provide gastrointestinal and urinary drainage. The bladder can be drained with vaginal catheterization or a suprapubic tube, vesicostomy, or even a vaginostomy. A diverting colostomy is usually needed and should be placed relatively high.

Abnormal Clitoris and Pubis

Female Epispadias. A bifid clitoris with a flattened mons pubis and a patulous urethra is characteristic of female epispadias. The vagina appears normally positioned. These girls are nearly always incontinent and require reconstructive surgery.

Ambiguous Genitalia

Examination may not be able to differentiate between phenotypic female versus male. Sensitivity should be paramount when counseling families. Take care not to refer to the child with a specific gender prior to discussions of assigning a sex to rear the child in (using phrases such as "your child" rather than "he/she"). A critical element at initial evaluation is determining the presence of palpable gonads. Palpable gonads indicate that 46, XX congenital adrenal hyperplasia (CAH) is unlikely. Nonpalpable gonads with virilization are concerning for CAH, which requires urgent evaluation for salt wasting. An asymmetric appearance is typical of mixed gonadal dysgenesis.

Major Structural Abnormalities

Epispadias–Exstrophy Complex. A spectrum of conditions ranging from **epispadias** to **classic exstrophy** to the extreme end of **cloacal exstrophy**, with failure of urethral and bladder closure.

Prune Belly Syndrome. Laxity of abdominal musculature, bilateral intraabdominal testes and dimpling of the lateral aspect of the knees can all help identify children with this condition.

Suggested Readings

Barocas DA, Boorjian SA, Alvarez RD, et al. Microhematuria: AUA/SUFU Guideline. J Urol 2020;204(4):778-786.

Bauer R, Kogan BA. Modern technique for penile torsion repair. J Urol 2009;182(1):286-291.

Brandt ML. Pediatric hernias. Surg Clin North Am 2008;88(1):27-43.

Buckley JC, McAninch JW. Use of ultrasonography for the diagnosis of testicular injuries in blunt scrotal trauma. J Urol 2006;175(1):175-178.

Expert Panel on Pediatric Imaging, Brown BP, Simoneaux SF, Dillman JR, et al. ACR Appropriateness Criteria® Antenatal Hydronephrosis—Infant. J Am Coll Radiol 2020;17(11S):S367-S379.

Gatti JM, Murphy P. Current management of the acute scrotum. Semin Pediatr Surg 2007;16(1):58-63.

Geiger J, Epelman M, Darge K. The fountain sign: a novel color doppler sonographic finding for the diagnosis of acute idiopathic scrotal edema. J Ultrasound Med 2010;29(8):1233-1237.

Hoberman A, Wald ER, Reynolds EA, et al. Pyuria and bacteriuria in urine specimens obtained by catheter from young children with fever. J Pediatr 1994;124(4):513-519.

Holm M, Hoei-Hansen CE, Rajpert-De Meyts E, Skakkebaek NE. Increased risk of carcinoma in situ in patients with testicular germ cell cancer with ultrasonic microlithiasis in the contralateral testicle. J Urol 2003;170(4):1163-1167.

Jansson UB, Hanson M, Sillén U, Hellström AL. Voiding pattern and acquisition of bladder control from birth to age 6 years- a longitudinal study. J Urol 2005;174(1):289-293.

Kawaguchi AL, Shaul DB. Inguinal hernias can be accurately diagnosed using the parent's digital photographs when the physical examination is nondiagnostic. J Pediatr Surg 2009;44(12):2327-2329.

Koff SA. Estimating bladder capacity in children. Urology 1983;21(3):248.

Lau P, Anderson PA, Giacomantonio JM, Schwarz RD. Acute epididymitis in boys: are antibiotics indicated? Br J Urol 1997;79(5):797-800.

Majd M, Rushton H. Renal cortical scintigraphy in the diagnosis of acute pyelonephritis. Semin Nucl Med 1992;22(2):98-111.

Montague DK, Jarow J, Broderick GA, et al. American Urological Association guideline on the management of priapism. J Urol 2003;170(4):1318-1324.

Morey AF, Brandes S, Dugi DD 3rd, et al. Urotrauma: AUA guideline. J Urol 2014;192(2):327-335.

Rudin JE, Geldt VG, Alecseev EB. Prolapse of urethral mucosa in white female children: experience with 58 cases. J Pediatr Surg 1997;32(3):423-425.

Sachedina A, Chan K, MacGregor D, et al. More than grapes and bleeding: an updated look at pelvic rhabdomyosarcoma in young women. J Pediatr Adolesc Gynecol 2018;31(5):522-525.

Schulert GS, Gigante J. Summer penile syndrome: an acute hypersensitivity reaction. J Emerg Med 2014;46(1):e21-e22.

Subcommittee on Urinary Tract Infection, Steering Committee on Quality Improvement and Management, Roberts KB. Urinary tract infection clinical practice guideline for the diagnosis and management of the initial UTI in febrile infants and children 2 to 24 months. *Pediatrics* 2011;128:595-610.

Tallen G, Hernáiz Driever P, Degenhardt P, et al. High reliability of scrotal ultrasonography in the management of childhood primary testicular neoplasms. *Klin Padiatr* 2011;223(3):131-137.

Walker BR, Ellison ED, Snow BW, Cartwright PC. The natural history of idiopathic urethrorrhagia in boys. *J Urol* 2001;166(1):231-232.

5

Urinary Tract Infections and Vesicoureteral Reflux

CHRISTOPHER S. COOPER

CONTRIBUTORS OF CAMPBELL-WALSH-WEIN, 12TH EDITION

Christopher S. Cooper, Douglas W. Storm, Antoine E. Khoury, and Elias Wehbi

EVALUATION AND MANAGEMENT OF A CHILD WITH A FEVER

Up to 8% of febrile infections in infants and children are due to urinary tract infection (UTI). Even when another source of fever and infection such as otitis or respiratory infection has been identified, the reduction in risk of a concurrent UTI is only about 50%, so the clinician must consider the possibility of a UTI in any febrile infant. A summary of the evaluation and treatment of a child with a rectal temperature higher than 38°C is provided in Fig. 5.1. A "toxic" appearing febrile child is much more likely to have a serious illness and some symptoms and signs of toxicity include irritability, lethargy, abnormal breathing, tachycardia, and cyanosis.

Definition of a Urinary Tract Infection

What constitutes a "significant" clinical UTI in a child is controversial. The current diagnostic guideline in children 2–24 months from the American Academy of Pediatrics (AAP) requires a urinalysis (UA) with pyuria and/or bacteriuria and at least 50,000 CFU/mL of a uropathogen cultured from a urine specimen obtained through urethral catheterization or suprapubic aspiration. A small proportion of children with a significant UTI may not meet these criteria but do benefit from treatment.

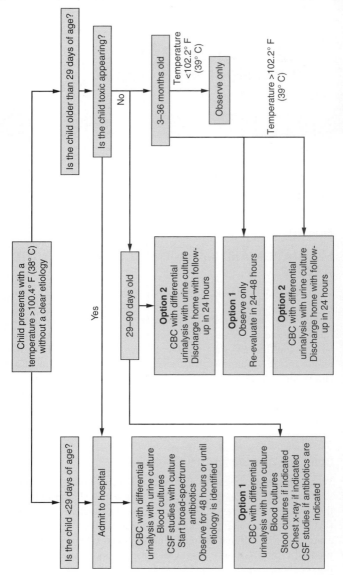

A

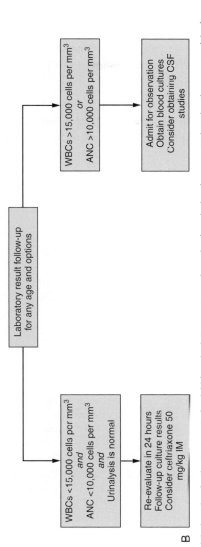

FIG. 5.1 (A) Algorithm for the treatment of a child from birth to age 36 months with a fever higher than 100.4°F (38°C) with no cause of the fever. (B) Continued considerations for the treatment of a child aged 0 to 36 months with a fever higher than 100.4°F (38°C) with no cause of the fever. *ANC,* Absolute neutrophil count; *CBC,* complete blood count; *CSF,* cerebrospinal fluid; *IM,* intramuscular; *WBCs,* white blood cells.

Pathogenesis of UTI Development

Most UTIs begin with periurethral contamination by a uropathogen from the gastrointestinal tract, which is most commonly *Escherichia coli*. These bacteria colonize the urethra, migrate to the bladder, invade the bladder cells, and may then ascend to the kidneys. Kidney colonization results in bacterial toxin production, host tissue damage, and possibly bacteremia (Fig. 5.2).

Risk Factors Leading to Pediatric Urinary Tract Infections

Gender and Age. The only time that UTIs are more prevalent in boys than in girls is at an age younger than 1 year. About 2% of boys and 0.7% of girls experience a UTI during the first year of life; however, 7% of girls and 2% of boys experience a UTI by 6 years of age.

Circumcision. Circumcision reduces UTI development in the first 6 months of life by almost 10-fold.

Anatomic Abnormalities. Anatomic abnormalities predisposing to UTIs include hydronephrosis and hydroureteronephrosis from ureteropelvic junction obstruction (UPJO) or ureterovesical junction obstruction (UVJO), vesicoureteral reflux (VUR), infection stones, infected nonfunctional renal segments or papillae, and urethral obstruction. With the exception of VUR, these abnormalities are often evident on a renal and bladder ultrasound (RBUS), which is currently recommended in young children after their first febrile UTI.

Vesicoureteral Reflux (VUR). VUR occurs in 1%–2% of all newborns, but it is found in 25%–40% of children after their first episode of UTI. The incidence of VUR decreases with increasing age (Table 5.1) VUR facilitates ascent of bacteria from the bladder to the kidney; however, approximately 50%–70% of children with pyelonephritis will not have VUR.

Sexual Activity. Sexual activity increases the risk of UTI.

Bladder and Bowel Dysfunction (BBD). BBD predisposes to UTI, and treatment of BBD reduces recurrent UTIs as well as incontinence and VUR.

Iatrogenic Factors. Catheter-associated UTI (CAUTI) is the most common nosocomial infection, and the risk of UTI increases with the duration of the catheter. Removal of urethral catheters in hospitalized patients is recommended as soon as possible.

Biofilms

Biofilms are communities of microorganisms encapsulated with a self-developed polymeric matrix and adherent to either a living or inert surface. Antibiotics are often unable to eradicate bacteria within a biofilm leading to bacterial persistence.

CLASSIFICATION OF PEDIATRIC URINARY TRACT INFECTIONS

Cystitis and Pyelonephritis

UTIs are classified as cystitis or pyelonephritis based on their symptoms despite a high false-positive rate with this approach. Cystitis is suspected when the child is afebrile and has only lower urinary tract symptoms including urinary urgency, frequency or dysuria, malodorous urine, and/or suprapubic tenderness. Children with a UTI are assumed to have pyelonephritis when they have high fevers, nausea, vomiting, flank pain, or lethargy. Of note, in patients with fever and systemic symptoms, only 50%–66% demonstrated acute inflammatory changes in the kidney on ^{99m}Tc-dimercaptosuccinic acid (DMSA) scans.

Asymptomatic Bacteriuria (ASB)

ASB occurs in 0.8% of preschool girls and is defined as the presence of two consecutive urine specimens yielding positive cultures ($>10^5$ CFU/mL) of the same uropathogen. In school-age girls, spontaneous resolution of ASB occurs in 50%. Children with ASB do not require antibiotics because they do not appear to be at any risk for recurrent symptomatic infections, renal damage, or impaired renal growth. An important exception is that infants with ASB are at risk for developing significant UTIs, and they should be treated with antimicrobial therapy and imaged to evaluate for any congenital abnormalities.

Bacterial Nephritis

Acute bacterial nephritis occurs as the inflammation from bacterial infection spreads throughout the kidney. A localized form of this inflammation is called *acute focal bacterial nephritis* or *lobar nephronia*. Computed tomography (CT) findings include global renal enlargement and inflammatory changes in the perirenal fat and

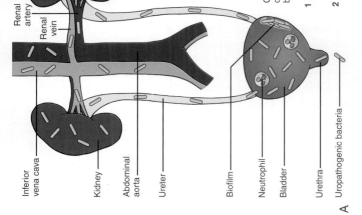

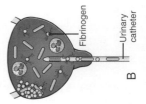

A

Inferior vena cava

Kidney

Abdominal aorta

Ureter

Biofilm

Neutrophil

Bladder

Urethra

Uropathogenic bacteria

Renal artery

Renal vein

11 Bacteremia

10 Host tissue damage by bacterial toxins

9 Colonization of the kidneys

8 Ascension to the kidneys

7 Epithelial damage by bacterial toxins and proteases

6 Biofilm formation

5 Bacterial multiplication and immune system subversion

4 Neutrophil infiltration

3 Inflammation response in the bladder and fibrinogen accumulation in the catheter

Colonization and invasion of the bladder, mediated by pili and adhesins

1 Colonization of the urethra and migration to the bladder

2 Contamination of the periurethral area with a uropathogen from the gut

B

Fibrinogen

Urinary catheter

FIG. 5.2 (A) Uncomplicated urinary tract infections begin when uropathogens that normally reside in the gut colonize the urethra (Step 1). These bacteria then migrate to the bladder (Step 2), where they colonize and invade superficial umbrella cells within the urothelium (Step 3). Innate host inflammatory responses begin to clear bacteria (Step 4). Some bacteria, though, evade the immune system, and these bacteria may then multiply (Step 5) and form a biofilm (Step 6). These bacteria produce toxins and proteases that induce host cell damage (Step 7). They also release nutrients that promote bacterial survival and allow the bacteria to ascend to the kidneys (Step 8). Kidney colonization (Step 9) results in bacterial toxin production and host tissue damage (Step 10). UTIs can ultimately progress to bacteremia if the pathogen crosses the tubular epithelial barrier in the kidneys (Step 11). (B) Uropathogens that cause complicated UTIs follow the same initial steps, including periurethral colonization (Step 1) and migration to the bladder (Step 2). However, for the pathogens to cause infection, the bladder must be compromised. The most common cause of a compromised bladder is an indwelling urinary catheter. There is a robust immune response induced by catheterization (Step 3), resulting in fibrinogen accumulation along the catheter, providing an ideal environment for the attachment of uropathogens that express fibrinogen-binding proteins. This infection induces neutrophil infiltration (Step 4), but after their initial attachment to the fibrinogen-coated catheters, the bacteria multiply (Step 5), form biofilm (Step 6), promote epithelial damage (Step 7), and can seed infection of the kidneys (Steps 8 and 9), where toxin production induces tissue damage (Step 10). These uropathogens can also progress to bacteremia by crossing the tubular epithelial cell barrier (Step 11). (A, From Flores-Mireles AL, Walker JN, Caparon M, et al. Urinary tract infections: epidemiology, mechanisms of infection and treatment options. *Nat Rev Microbiol* 2015;13:269-284.)

Table 5.1 International Classification of Vesicoureteral Reflux

GRADE	DESCRIPTION
1	Into a nondilated ureter
2	Into the pelvis and calyces without dilation
3	Mild to moderate dilation of the ureter, renal pelvis, and calyces with minimal blunting of the fornices
4	Moderate ureteral tortuosity and dilation of the pelvis and calyces
5	Gross dilation of the ureter, pelvis, and calyces; loss of papillary impressions; and ureteral tortuosity

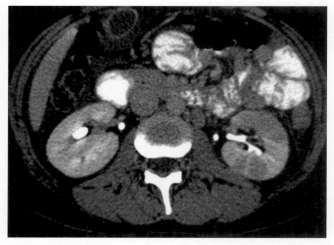

FIG. 5.3 Computed tomography scan demonstrating acute focal pyelonephritis (lobar nephronia).

Gerota fascia. CT with contrast images demonstrate ill-defined, nonhomogeneous areas of decreased parenchymal enhancement that typically are wedge shaped (Fig. 5.3).

Pyonephrosis

Pyonephrosis consists of purulent exudate accumulating in the renal collecting system and is frequently associated with obstructed urinary outflow from the renal pelvis.

Acute Renal Abscess

Symptoms of a renal abscess are similar to pyelonephritis; however, in up to 20% of renal abscess cases, the urine culture result may be negative, which increases the chance that the etiology was via hematogenous seeding of the kidney. CT imaging findings may include (1) a well-defined area of low attenuation or decreased enhancement or (2) a striated, wedge-shaped zone of increased or decreased enhancement.

DIAGNOSING A PEDIATRIC URINARY TRACT INFECTION

Symptoms

The diagnosis of a UTI may be difficult because the symptoms can be nonspecific and require a high degree of suspicion, especially in very young children. Symptoms may include fever, irritability, poor feeding, jaundice, failure to thrive, vomiting, diarrhea, abdominal distention, or foul-smelling urine. In children younger than 2 years of age, the presence of a fever higher than 40°C, history of a previous UTI, suprapubic tenderness, or an uncircumcised penis are the most useful symptoms and signs in predicting a UTI. Older children often present with classic UTI symptoms, including abdominal pain, back pain, dysuria, urinary frequency, and incontinence. The possibility of sexually transmitted diseases in older children and adolescents with symptoms of urethritis must be considered and may be caused by *Neisseria gonorrhoeae*, *Chlamydia trachomatis*, or *Ureaplasma urealyticum*.

Physical Examination

Specific findings on physical examination in young children are rare and may consist of fever or lethargy. An enlarged obstructed bladder or kidney may be palpable as an abdominal or flank mass, respectively. Older children may experience suprapubic, abdominal, or flank tenderness. Costovertebral angle tenderness suggests pyelonephritis. Examination of the external genitalia should be performed to evaluate for signs of trauma, local inflammation, urethral meatal stenosis or discharge, phimosis, foreign body, and anatomic abnormalities in girls such as an ectopic ureteral orifice or urethral mass from a prolapsing ureterocele. Testicular examination may demonstrate tenderness from epididymo-orchitis.

Examination of the back for signs of spina bifida occulta such as a prominent fat pad or asymmetric gluteal cleft or sacral dimple, along with a neurologic examination, may point to underlying neurologic causes predisposing to UTIs.

Urine Collection Methods. The chance of collecting a contaminated urine specimen increases with the decreasing degree of invasive collecting methods. The urine from a collection bag only provides reliable information when the specimen is normal and thereby rules out a UTI. A clean-catch midstream urine sample carries a higher chance of contamination than urine collected via more invasive methods, including catheterization or suprapubic aspiration (SPA). The clean-catch urine is more reliable in an older girl or a circumcised boy. For nontoilet-trained febrile children younger than 2 years of age, the AAP guidelines recommend SPA or catheterization.

Successful catheterization in girls often requires a two-person technique. The labia majora should each be placed on gentle traction outward from the body and slightly lateral to expose the vaginal and urethral openings and facilitate the correct location for catheter insertion. This method, as opposed to using a single hand and fingers spreading the labia laterally, more routinely exposes the normally recessed urethral opening and surrounding anatomic landmarks.

Urine Dipstick Tests. Leukocyte esterase is released from white cells broken down in the urine and serves as a marker for pyuria. False positives result from other causes of inflammation. Urinary nitrite is reduced from nitrates by gram-negative enteric bacteria and requires several hours to occur; thus, a first-morning urine has the best sensitivity with this dipstick test. Frequent urination may not permit enough time for the conversion of nitrates to nitrites and results in a false-negative nitrite test. A dilute urine may also generate a false-negative test or infection with gram-positive organisms that do not reduce nitrates.

The sensitivity of leukocyte esterase for detecting UTI is estimated at 80% with specificity ranging from 64%–92%. The sensitivity of the nitrite test is 50%; however, the specificity is very high at 98%, meaning a positive nitrite test likely reflects a true UTI.

Urine Culture. A positive urine culture is essential for the diagnosis of a UTI; however, the definition of what constitutes a true positive culture based on the number of colony-forming units (CFU) per milliliter of urine is variable between guidelines. The AAP guidelines require 50,000 CFU/mL along with a positive UA for pyuria in a catheterized specimen.

Radiographic Imaging

Controversies with Imaging Strategies. Despite prevalence rates of VUR of up to 40%, the revised AAP guidelines recommended routinely obtaining a renal ultrasound in all children less than 2 years of age with a febrile UTI but not a voiding cystourethrogram (VCUG) if the ultrasound is normal. The Section of Urology of the AAP recommends that a VCUG remain an accepted option following a first febrile UTI. Most agree with obtaining a VCUG in children with recurrent febrile UTIs or if an RBUS demonstrates structural renal anomalies, asymmetry in renal size, ureteral dilation, or bladder anomalies.

Ultrasound. 1%–2% of children with a history of UTI exhibit an abnormality on RBUS requiring additional evaluation. The RBUS is used to follow renal growth in children with a history of UTIs or VUR with kidney size referenced to standard renal growth curves. Of note, the RBUS has a very low sensitivity for the detection of VUR, even in children with high grades of VUR.

Voiding Cystourethrogram. When performed with contrast, the VCUG remains the gold standard imaging technique for the detection and grading of VUR. Because of the improved anatomic resolution, many prefer to use a contrast VCUG as the initial method of evaluation and reserve a radionuclide cystogram (RNC) for follow-up imaging (Fig. 5.4). Recently, in order to eliminate radiation exposure, there is increasing interest and use of contrast-enhanced voiding urosonography in place of VCUG or RNC. In general, the timing of obtaining a VCUG is delayed at least 1 week after treating a UTI to allow for recovery from the infection but may be performed earlier once the urine is sterile and the child has clinically improved. Techniques employed to decrease the child's anxiety and discomfort associated with a VCUG include the use of topical urethral anesthetic, child-life distraction, sedation, and hypnosis.

Five grades of reflux are used to depict the appearance of the ureter, renal pelvis, and calyces as seen on the radiographic contrast images generated by a VCUG (Fig. 5.5).

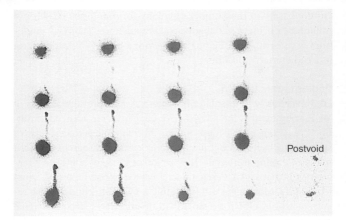

FIG. 5.4 Radionuclide cystogram showing right-sided reflux that worsens with bladder filling. The upper collecting system drains fully with voiding.

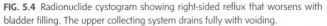

I II III IV V

GRADES OF REFLUX

FIG. 5.5 International classification of vesicoureteral reflux.

Despite the widespread use of the grading system, there is often significant interobserver variability. In addition, the expected concordance between ureteral and calyceal dilation does not always occur (Fig. 5.6). The bladder volume when reflux is first seen during the VCUG should be routinely reported as onset of reflux at lower

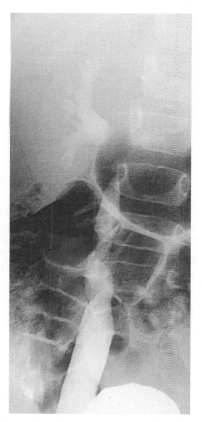

FIG. 5.6 A refluxing ureter with significant dilation of the lower segment but no distortion of the collecting system may be different from the typical system with grade II reflux.

bladder volumes is associated with a lower chance of VUR resolution and a higher chance of recurrent UTIs, independent of the grade of VUR.

99mTc-Dimercaptosuccinic Acid (DMSA) Scan. Cortical renal scan with DMSA, especially when combined with single-photon emission computed tomography (SPECT), is the gold standard for identification of lesions in the renal parenchyma. The uptake of DMSA provides a good proportional representation of glomerular filtration. The timing of DMSA for detection of kidney involvement with a UTI significantly affects its sensitivity. An abnormal scan occurs in 49%–79% of patients within the first 10 days of acute pyelonephritis (APN) but decreases to 30% after 1 month. About 15% of children with these lesions ultimately develop evidence of permanent renal scarring. After the acute inflammatory phase, the ultimate scar involves a loss of tissue that is reflected on radiographic imaging as thinning of the parenchyma over the calyces (Fig. 5.7). Assessment of irreversible renal damage and scar should not be performed earlier than 6 months after APN. VUR, particularly higher grades, is associated with renal maldevelopment/congenital dysplasia that often appears identical to acquired postinfection pyelonephritic scars (Table 5.2).

Computed Tomography (CT). CT provides detailed anatomic imaging; however, the high degree of radiation severely limits any benefit of CT as a routine imaging modality in a child with a UTI. Typical findings associated with renal infection and inflammation include cortical regions of hypoattenuation, wedge-shaped defects, a loss of the corticomedullary differentiation, and striations (Fig. 5.3).

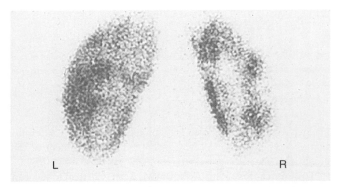

FIG. 5.7 Dimercaptosuccinic acid renal scintigraphy. Pinhole images show a normal left kidney and a right kidney with multiple cortical defects.

Table 5.2 Details of Common Antibiotic Dosing

	DOSE	COMMON SIDE EFFECTS	COMMENTS
Oral Agents			
Amoxicillin-clavulanate	20–40 mg/kg/day in 3 doses	Diarrhea, nausea/vomiting, rash	
TMP-SMX	6–12 mg/kg/day of TMP in 2 doses	Diarrhea, nausea/vomiting, photosensitivity, rash	Contraindicated <6 wk of age
Cefixime	8 mg/kg/day in 1 dose	Abdominal pain, diarrhea, flatulence, rash	
Cefpodoxime	10 mg/kg/day in 2 doses	Abdominal pain, diarrhea, nausea, rash	
Cefprozil	30 mg/kg/day in 2 doses	Abdominal pain, diarrhea, elevated LFTs, nausea	
Cephalexin	50–100 mg/kg/day in 4 doses	Diarrhea, headache, nausea/vomiting, rash	
Nitrofurantoin	3–5 mg/kg in 2 doses	Nausea/vomiting, bad taste	Contraindicated <3 mo of age or when GFR is <50% or in children with G6PD deficiency
Parenteral Agents			
Ceftriaxone	75 mg/kg/day in 1 dose		Single daily dosing acceptable
Cefotaxime	150 mg/kg/day divided q6–8h		
Ceftazidime	100–150 mg/kg/day divided q8h		
Gentamicin	7.5 mg/kg/day divided q8h		Single daily dosing acceptable alternative

Continued

Table 5.2 Details of Common Antibiotic Dosing—cont'd

	DOSE	COMMON SIDE EFFECTS	COMMENTS
Tobramycin	5 mg/kg/day divided q8h		
Piperacillin	300 mg/kg/day divided q6–8h		

G6PD, Glucose-6-phosphate dehydrogenase; GFR, glomerular filtration rate; LFTs, liver function tests; TMP-SMX, trimethoprim-sulfamethoxazole.

MANAGEMENT OF PEDIATRIC URINARY TRACT INFECTION

Antibiotic Treatment

Early antibiotic treatment of febrile UTI limits renal involvement and subsequent scarring. Therefore, the clinician must maintain a high index of suspicion for UTI and routinely begin antibiotics empirically. The incidence of acute scintigraphic renal lesions increased in one series from 22%–59% when the start of antibiotics went from 2 to 3 days after the onset of symptoms. The rate of ultimate scar formation also increased from 11%–76.5% when the start of antibiotics went from 2 to 6 days, respectively.

Inpatient Versus Outpatient Management

Infants older than 2 months and nontoxic children with suspected pyelonephritis can be treated as outpatients if compliance with and tolerance to oral antibiotics is not an issue. Since a febrile UTI in newborns and young infants (less than 2 months) proceeds more frequently to urosepsis and electrolyte abnormalities, this age group requires hospitalization and parenteral antibiotics. Other indications for hospitalization include toxic presentation or dehydration, poor oral intake, questionable compliance with antibiotics and, some suggest, infants under 6 months of age. Within 48 hours of the start of therapy, 90% of children have a normal body temperature, but if a child is not improving after 48 hours, RBUS should be considered.

Antibiotic Duration

With less severe UTI, such as afebrile acute cystitis, a 2- to 4-day course of antibiotics is sufficient. In children with a febrile UTI, antibiotic treatment lasting 7 to 14 days is recommended because shorter courses have been proven inferior. A patient with focal pyelonephritis (previously termed acute lobar nephronia) requires a longer course of antibiotics of at least 3 weeks. A renal abscess may often be adequately treated with antibiotics alone; however, a lack of clinical response or resolution may require percutaneous drainage.

Antibiotic Selection

Trimethoprim-sulfamethoxazole (TMP-SMX) and amoxicillin are used in approximately 50% of outpatient UTI visits but these may be poor empirical choices because of high resistance rates of *E. coli*. Nitrofurantoin or a first-generation cephalosporin is an appropriate narrow-spectrum antibiotic choice for many children with a UTI. Empirical treatment should be based on local/regional antibiograms that are revised and published on an annual basis since uropathogen prevalence and resistance patterns will vary regionally and will change with time. Table 5.2 lists common oral and parenteral antibiotics used for treatment of UTI along with common dosing and side effects.

In addition to *E. coli*, other common gram-negative bacterial uropathogens include *Klebsiella*, *Proteus*, *Enterobacter*, and *Citrobacter*. Gram-positive bacterial uropathogens include *Staphylococcus saprophyticus*, *Enterococcus* and, rarely, *Staphylococcus aureus* (Table 5.3). Neonates and young infants should be covered for

Table 5.3 Commonly Used Prophylactic Antibiotics and Their Dosages

ANTIBACTERIAL AGENT	DOSAGE	CAUTION IN AGE GROUP	ADVERSE EFFECTS[a]
Amoxicillin	5–10 mg/kg/day	None	Diarrhea
Sulfisoxazole (sulfafurazole)	20–30 mg/kg/day	<2 months	Kernicterus
Trimethoprim	2 mg/kg/day	<3 months	Hyponatremia
Trimethoprim/ sulfamethoxazole (cotrimoxazole)	Trimethoprim 1–2 mg/kg/day	<2 months	Kernicterus
Nitrofurantoin	2–3 mg/kg/day	<1 month	Hemolysis in G6PD deficiency
Cefalexin	10 mg/kg/day	None	

[a]The most important adverse effect for each treatment is listed.
G6PD, Glucose-6-phosphate dehydrogenase.

Enterococcus species when choosing empiric antibiotics since the incidence of infections with this uropathogen is higher in early infancy than at a later age. A combination of ampicillin and a third-generation cephalosporin or aminoglycoside is considered a safe empiric choice for neonates and young infants receiving parenteral therapy.

Nitrofurantoin has poor tissue penetration and should not be used for febrile UTI/pyelonephritis. Nitrofurantoin has also been associated with increased risk of hemolytic anemia in infants less than 3 months of age and should not be used in this population. Similarly, TMP is contraindicated in premature infants and newborns less than 6 weeks of age.

MANAGEMENT AFTER URINARY TRACT INFECTION

Routinely repeating a urine culture in children treated with an antibiotic based on previous urine culture susceptibilities is not necessary. Approximately 10%–30% of children develop at least one recurrent UTI, and the recurrence rate is highest within the first 3 to 6 months after a UTI. Identification of the risk factors for a UTI noted at the beginning of this chapter helps direct management aimed at treating or eliminating these risk factors. Renal scarring increases with an increasing number of febrile UTIs and with delayed treatment; therefore, parents should be counseled regarding the high risk of recurrent UTI and seek prompt evaluation for subsequent febrile illnesses in their child. Children who had a febrile UTI should routinely have their height, weight, and blood pressure monitored by their primary care provider. Children with significant bilateral renal scars or a reduction of renal function warrant long-term follow-up for the assessment of hypertension, renal function, and proteinuria.

Chronic Prophylactic Antibiotics (CAPs)

CAP, which may lead to antibiotic resistance and other potential side effects, are not routinely recommended for all children following a febrile UTI. However, the benefits of prophylactic antibiotics in reducing UTIs are more easily demonstrated when used in specific populations at high risk for recurrent UTIs including children with BBD, a history of febrile UTIs, or higher grades of VUR. Common prophylactic antibiotics include TMP-SMX, TMP, nitrofurantoin, and first-generation cephalosporins.

Bladder and Bowel Dysfunction (BBD)

Assessment of underlying BBD as predisposing factors should occur with any pediatric UTI since management of BBD significantly decreases the chance of recurrent UTI in these children. Treatment of constipation alone reduces recurrent UTIs significantly and improves bladder function Children with VUR and bowel and/or bladder dysfunction are at high risk for developing recurrent pyelonephritis and are more likely to benefit from CAP. Recurrent UTI is estimated to occur in about 45% of these children with VUR as opposed to 15% without BBD.

Vesicoureteral Reflux

Several key points regarding VUR are summarized as follows and help guide management of the child with VUR:

1. Antibiotic prophylaxis appears to provide little benefit for those with grade II or lower VUR, particularly in the absence of BBD.
2. Antibiotic prophylaxis does appear to be beneficial for those with grade III or higher VUR, at least among girls.
3. Approximately 15% of children with VUR will have a recurrent febrile UTI within 2 years, and about 15% of these children will develop a renal scar.
4. BBD is a major risk factor for recurrent UTIs on or off antibiotics, which will occur in about 45% of children with BBD as opposed to 15% of those without BBD.
5. A higher grade of VUR is associated with an increased risk for both pyelonephritis and new renal damage.
6. The effect of age on the risk for renal damage is not well defined, although many believe that younger children are more susceptible to renal damage from pyelonephritis.

Etiology of VUR. Reflux is considered primary if it is caused by a deficiency in the ureterovesical junction (UVJ) and secondary if it is caused by abnormally high bladder pressures that overcome an otherwise normal UVJ. Bladder dysfunction is often a major contributor to the presence and persistence of secondary reflux.

The AUA guidelines suggest that BBD is one of the most critical and modifiable variables affecting VUR resolution and UTIs; therefore, symptoms of BBD such as urgency, incontinence, constipation, or encopresis should be recognized and treated.

Spontaneous Resolution. Most cases of low-grade reflux (grade I and II) will spontaneously resolve, whereas grade 3 reflux resolves in approximately 50% of cases, and very few cases of higher-grade reflux (grades 4 and 5, and bilateral grade 3) will resolve. VUR occurring at older age as well as VUR that begins at lower bladder volumes is associated with decreased resolution rates independent of grade (Fig. 5.8).

Principles of Management. Key points in reflux management include:

1. Spontaneous resolution is very common and facilitated by correction of BBD.
2. Higher grades of reflux are less likely to resolve spontaneously, especially in older children.
3. Sterile reflux is unlikely to cause renal damage and, therefore, prevention of UTI is more important than VUR resolution.
4. The use of prophylactic antibiotics is beneficial, particularly in patients at higher risk for UTI such as those with higher-grade VUR, BBD, or a history of recurrent febrile UTIs.
5. There is a role for medical management for most forms of reflux.

Medical Management

Medical management is aimed at decreasing UTI risk factors to prevent infection and maintaining urinary sterility through single daily low-dose CAP. CAP given at night may permit longer duration of antibiotics in the bladder. For children younger than 2 months of age, the most commonly used medication CAP is amoxicillin.

After 2 months of age, the antibiotic of choice often becomes TMP-SMX (Septra, Bactrim). The other drug most commonly used is nitrofurantoin (Macrodantin). Nitrofurantoin may minimize the development of resistance to fecal organisms; however, oral tolerance is lower than that with TMP-SMX because of taste and worse gastrointestinal symptoms.

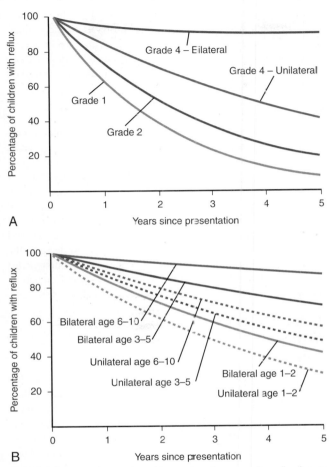

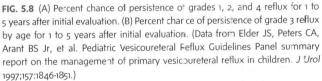

FIG. 5.8 (A) Percent chance of persistence of grades 1, 2, and 4 reflux for 1 to 5 years after initial evaluation. (B) Percent chance of persistence of grade 3 reflux by age for 1 to 5 years after initial evaluation. (Data from Elder JS, Peters CA, Arant BS Jr, et al. Pediatric Vesicoureteral Reflux Guidelines Panel summary report on the management of primary vesicoureteral reflux in children. *J Urol* 1997;157:1846-1851.)

In addition to CAP, timely bladder-emptying habits, healthy dietary and bowel measures to prevent constipation, and evaluating family compliance and access to prompt care are important components of medical management. If a patient has done well on CAP and the risk factors for UTI have been diminished, a trial off of CAP may be warranted.

Surgical Management

Breakthrough febrile UTIs or pyelonephritis while on antibiotic prophylaxis, despite appropriate bladder and bowel habits, are generally considered an indication for surgical correction of the reflux. Other indications may include a failure to resolve higher grades of VUR or a desire to limit antibiotic usage. Surgical options include open ureteral reimplantation for VUR through an intravesical or extravesical approach, which is successful in resolving VUR in more than 98% of cases. Robotic-assisted laparoscopic surgery may also be considered as an approach to ureteral reimplantation in order to decrease the morbidity of an open incision (Fig. 5.9). Endoscopic subureteric injection of bulking agents may be performed in a brief outpatient operation with long-term VUR resolution rates of about 70%.

ASSOCIATED ANOMALIES AND CONDITIONS WITH VUR

Ureteropelvic Junction Obstruction (UPJO)

Up to 3% of children with VUR may have or develop a UPJO, which occurs more frequently in those with high-grade reflux. Three radiologic signs suggest a UPJO in the setting of reflux: if the pelvis shows little or no filling while the ureter is dilated by contrast, if contrast that enters the pelvis is poorly visualized because of dilution, or if a large pelvis fails to drain promptly and retains contrast after voiding (Fig. 5.10). If scintigraphy with catheter drainage confirms a UPJO, correction of the obstruction takes precedence over surgical repair of VUR. However, endoscopic VUR correction at the time of pyeloplasty is a reasonable option.

Ureteral Duplication

VUR is the most common abnormality associated with complete ureteral duplications. Reflux with duplication occurs most commonly into the lower pole of the kidney because of the more lateral and

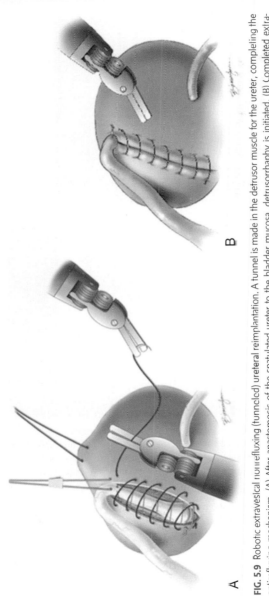

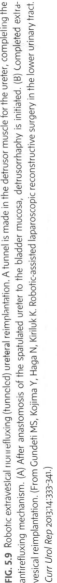

FIG. 5.9 Robotic extravesical nonrefluxing (tunneled) ureteral reimplantation. A tunnel is made in the detrusor muscle for the ureter, completing the antirefluxing mechanism. (A) After anastomosis of the spatulated ureter to the bladder mucosa, detrusorrhaphy is initiated. (B) Completed extravesical reimplantation. (From Gundeti MS, Kojima Y, Haga N, Kiriluk K. Robotic-assisted laparoscopic reconstructive surgery in the lower urinary tract. *Curr Urol Rep* 2013;14:333-341.)

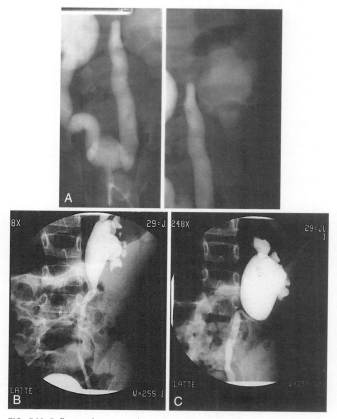

FIG. 5.10 Reflux and ureteropelvic junction (UPJ) obstruction. (A) Significant reflux fills the left ureter to the level of the UPJ. Minimal filling of the pelvis can be a sign of obstruction at this level. (B) In a different patient, reflux is seen as the bladder fills. (C) Significant kinking of the UPJ occurs with voiding.

proximal insertion of its ureter into the bladder with a shorter intramural ureter (Fig. 5.11).

Bladder Diverticula

Some paraureteral diverticulae compromise the antireflux configuration of the UVJ and cause persistent reflux, but in other cases VUR resolves similar to primary reflux (Fig. 5.12)

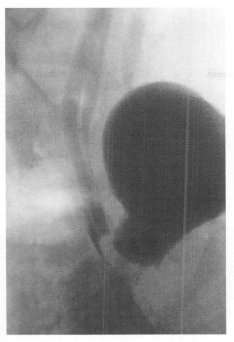

FIG. 5.11 Reflux into both ureters of a complete duplication, as shown here, is less common than reflux into the lower pole ureter alone.

Renal Anomalies

Significant renal anomalies associated with reflux include the multicystic dysplastic kidney (MCDK) and renal agenesis. MCDK has a prevalence of contralateral reflux of approximately 25% with half of these being low grade (1 to 2) VUR. Renal agenesis is also associated with VUR in about 25% of patients.

Megacystis-Megaureter Association

Massive bilateral VUR can cause a gradual remodeling of the entire upper urinary tract resulting in the *megacystis-megaureter association* or syndrome. The large residual urine volume in these patients presents a significant risk factor for recurrent UTI. Vesicostomy may temporize this situation until ureteral reimplantation can be performed.

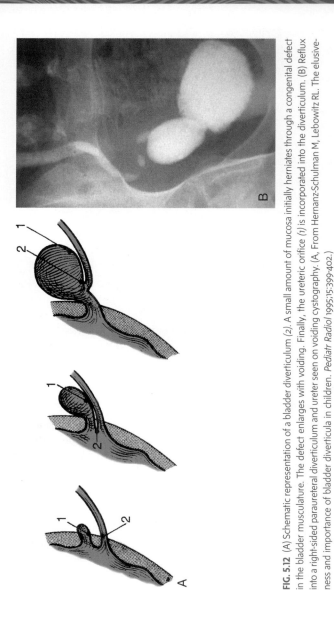

FIG. 5.12 (A) Schematic representation of a bladder diverticulum (2). A small amount of mucosa initially herniates through a congenital defect in the bladder musculature. The defect enlarges with voiding. Finally, the ureteric orifice (1) is incorporated into the diverticulum. (B) Reflux into a right-sided paraureteral diverticulum and ureter seen on voiding cystography. (A, From Hernanz-Schulman M, Lebowitz RL. The elusiveness and importance of bladder diverticula in children. *Pediatr Radiol* 1995;15:399-402.)

Pregnancy and Reflux

Women with a history of reflux have increased morbidity during pregnancy because of UTI-related complications, whether reflux has been corrected or not. In addition, women with hypertension and moderate renal impairment are at risk for preterm birth. Because of the strongly inherited nature of VUR, over 40% of these women's children will also have VUR, which should alert the clinician to the possible need for additional evaluation of the child.

Renal Scars

VUR is associated with a threefold increased risk for detecting renal cortical abnormalities after infection. VUR is less likely to resolve in children with significant renal scars. More severe reflux nephropathy in children increases their risk of developing hypertension, although it remains unclear whether it is the postinfection scarring, congenital dysplasia, or a combination of both that predisposes to hypertension. The medical renal disease that accompanies severe renal scarring can include hyperfiltration, concentrating defects, proteinuria, microalbuminuria (Lama et al., 1997), renal tubular acidosis (Guizar et al., 1996), and chronic renal insufficiency. In addition, many children with VUR fall below the normal age-adjusted growth curve, particularly in patients with bilateral reflux and some degree of renal damage.

Suggested Readings

Cooper CS. Individualizing management of vesicoureteral reflux. *Nephrourol Mon* 2012;4(3):530-534.

Craig JC, Williams GJ, Jones M, et al. The accuracy of clinical symptoms and signs for the diagnosis of serious bacterial infection in young febrile children: prospective cohort study of 15,781 febrile illnesses. *BMJ* 2010;340:c1594.

Elder JS, Diaz M. Vesicoureteral reflux—the role of bladder and bowel dysfunction. *Nat Rev Urol* 2013;10(11):640-648.

Hoberman A, Wald ER, Hickey RW, et al. Oral versus initial intravenous therapy for urinary tract infections in young febrile children. *Pediatrics* 1999;104:79-86.

Koff SA, Wagner TT, Jayanthi VR. The relationship among dysfunctional elimination syndromes, primary vesicoureteral reflux and urinary tract infections in children. *J Urol* 1998;160(3 Pt 2) 1019-1022.

Peters CA, Skoog SJ, Arant BS Jr, et al. Summary of the AUA guideline on management of primary vesicoureteral reflux in children. *J Urol* 2010;184:1134-1144.

Shaikh N, Hoberman A, Keren R, et al. Recurrent urinary tract infections in children with bladder and bowel dysfunction. *Pediatrics* 2016;137(1):e20152982.

Shaikh N, Morone NE, Lopez J, et al. Does this child have a urinary tract infection? *JAMA* 2007;298(24):2895-2904.

Subcommittee on Urinary Tract Infection, Steering Committee on Quality Improvement and Management, Roberts KB. Urinary tract infection: clinical practice guideline for the diagnosis and management of the initial UTI in febrile infants and children 2 to 24 months. *Pediatrics* 2011;128(3):595-610.

6

Lower Urinary Tract Dysfunction and Anomalies in Children

ANGELA M. ARLEN AND CHRISTOPHER S. COOPER

CONTRIBUTORS OF CAMPBELL-WALSH-WEIN, 12TH EDITION

Duncan T. Wilcox, Kyle O. Rove, Aaron D. Martin, Christopher C. Roth, John P. Gearhart, Heather N. Di Carlo, Francisco Tibor Dénes, Roberto Iglesias Lopes, Aseem Ravindra Shukla, Arun K. Srinivasan, Carlos R. Estrada, Stuart B. Bauer, Paul F. Austin, Abhishek Seth, Martin A. Koyle, Armando J Lorenzo, John C. Thomas, Douglass B. Clayton, and Mark C. Adams

LOWER URINARY TRACT AND BOWEL DYSFUNCTION IN CHILDREN

Epidemiology and Pathophysiology

Functional disorders of the lower urinary tract (LUT) encompass abnormalities in bladder filling and include a broad spectrum of clinical entities. Anomalies of bowel and urinary tract frequently coexist, whether functional, anatomic, and/or neuropathic. Constipation may adversely affect bladder function, leading to low functional capacity, incontinence, urinary tract infection (UTI), and triggering or exacerbating vesicoureteral reflux (VUR). LUT dysfunction accounts for up to 40% of pediatric urology clinic visits. Daytime incontinence varies with both age and gender in school-age children and seems to be more common in girls. The most common urinary symptoms include holding maneuvers and urgency. Enuresis stems from a maturational delay in the ultimate development of bladder control, with three organ systems implicated in its pathogenesis: the bladder, kidney, and brain. Approximately 15% of children will have some degree of nighttime wetting at 5 years of age, with a spontaneous resolution rate of approximately 15% per year, so 15 years of age only 1% to 2% of teenagers will still wet the bed.

Clinical Presentation

LUT conditions resulting in urinary stasis are associated with UTI. There is a known association between LUT and VUR, and VUR may be secondary to bladder dysfunction. Clinicians should also be cognizant of association with neuropsychiatric disorders such as attention-deficit/hyperactivity disorder (ADHD) in children with daytime wetting, as these comorbidities may interfere with treatment success. Relationship between abnormal bowel and bladder activity is termed *bowel-bladder dysfunction (BBD)*, and, if present, clear identification and management of any concomitant bowel dysfunction is paramount for successful treatment of voiding symptoms.

Diagnosis and Testing

Evaluation of incontinence, voiding dysfunction, or known LUT pathology begins with thorough history and physical exam. History includes evaluation of urinary symptoms and infections (UTI), diet, bowel function, and developmental milestones, including toilet training. Clinicians should also be cognizant of association with neuropsychiatric conditions such as ADHD in children with daytime wetting because this is likely to interfere with treatment success. Examination should include inspection of the back spine for signs of occult spinal dysraphism or tethered cord such as lipoma, mass, or hair tuft. Constipation/bowel function should be assessed; the Bristol stool scale is often a useful guide (Fig. 6.1). The Rome IV criteria are recommended for diagnosis of functional constipation in children (Table 6.1). If constipation and fecal impaction are obvious on history and physical examination, management based on clinical grounds without imaging studies is recommended. A 7-day bowel and bladder diary and 48-hour frequency volume charts are invaluable in diagnosing simple and complex LUT voiding dysfunction

Noninvasive testing may include urinalysis +/- culture if irritative voiding symptoms (dysuria, urgency, or frequency) are present. Ultrasonography should include prevoid and postvoid

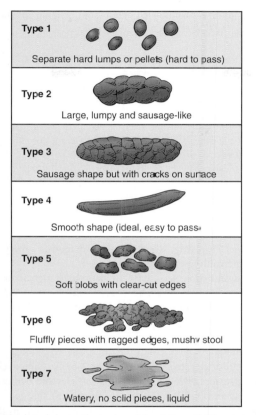

FIG. 6.1 Bristol stool chart with visuals and descriptions of different stool types. This scale provides a helpful, objective reference for documenting stool consistency when talking to patients about bowel function. (Modified from Lewis SJ, Heaton KW. Stool form scale as a useful guide to intestinal transit time. *Scand J Gastroenterol* 1997;32(9):920-924.)

bladder volumes, bladder wall thickness, rectal diameter, and presence of debris. Uroflowmetry provides information regarding flow characteristics during urination, including shape or pattern. Addition of electromyography (EMG) allows for appreciation of coordination between pelvic floor musculature, sphincteric relaxation,

Table 6.1 Rome IV Diagnostic Criteria for Functional Constipation

Must include 1 month of at least two of the following in infants up to 4 years of age:

1. Two or fewer defecations per week
2. History of excessive stool retention
3. History of painful or hard bowel movements
4. History of large-diameter stools
5. Presence of a large fecal mass in the rectum
   In toilet-trained children, the following additional criteria may be used:
6. At least one episode/week of incontinence after the acquisition of toileting skills
7. History of large-diameter stools that may obstruct the toilet

From Benninga MA, Faure C, Hyman PE, et al. Childhood functional gastrointestinal disorders: neonate/toddler. *Gastroenterology* 2016;150(6):1443-1455.E2. https://doi.org/10.1053/j.gastro.2016.02.016.

and bladder emptying, which can help diagnosis synergistic or dyssynergic voiding patterns.

LUT dysfunction secondary to neurologic deficit or severe obstructive uropathy should be assessed with formal urodynamic studies establish bladder pressures. Urodynamic findings that increase concern for upper urinary tract injury include: (1) impaired compliance (>20 mL per cm H_2O is normal); (2) detrusor sphincter dyssynergia (DSD) coupled with poor emptying, inability to void, and/or elevated voiding pressures; (3) sustained, elevated detrusor pressure (Pdet) during filling; (4) elevated detrusor leak point pressure (DLPP) (>40 cm H_2O); and (5) elevated voiding pressures in the setting of poor flow. Routine invasive urodynamics in pediatric patients with LUT symptoms in the absence of neuropathy rarely change management and should be limited.

Treatment

Conservative measures are exhausted before initiating pharmacotherapy, physical therapy, biofeedback, neuromodulation, and/or surgical intervention. The ultimate goal of any structured behavior modification program is to return the child to normal micturition habits. If evidence of bowel dysfunction is present, a regimen that includes high fiber (daily fiber intake is age in years $+15$–20 = total grams to be ingested) and increased fluid intake is initiated, as well as timed voiding every 2 hours. If increased fiber is not feasible or successful, polyethylene glycol can be titrated such that children are eventually having daily Bristol type 4 stools.

Biofeedback uses electronic or mechanical instruments to relay perceptual evidence to assist a child in controlling bladder function. Pharmacologic intervention for LUT dysfunction encompasses anticholinergic agents and α-adrenergic receptor antagonists (i.e., α-blockers) to enhance bladder filling and emptying, respectively. Oxybutynin was among the first generation of modern antimuscarinic medications available for treating incontinence in children. The main side effects include constipation, dry mouth, blurred vision, reduced sweating, flushing, and altered behavior and cognition. Electrical nerve stimulation, also known as *neuromodulation*, has been used to treat refractory nonneurogenic LUTD in children. In neuromodulation, electrical stimuli are exerted in a noninvasive manner to alter the existent neural transmission pattern and modulate detrusor activity.

Initial approach in children with nonmonosymptomatic nocturnal enuresis is as detailed above for LUT dysfunction. Conventional therapies for nocturnal enuresis include behavior modification, the enuresis moisture alarm, and pharmacologic therapy (e.g., desmopressin, anticholinergics, imipramine).

As with bladder management, bowel management algorithms favor conservative measures (Fig. 6.2). Surgical management of defecation disorders includes antegrade enemas, delivered through a catheterizable channel (Malone antegrade continence enema [MACE]) or a cecostomy tube. Retrograde (transanal) washouts with a balloon catheter in the rectum represent a viable and less invasive alternative. Patient selection is critical, and candidates should have failed maximal conventional measures before proceeding to invasive options.

Prognosis

Addressing concomitant bowel dysfunction and ruling out underlying medical disease (such as posterior urethral valves, spinal dysraphism, diabetes mellitus) is key to symptomatic improvement.

PEDIATRIC BLADDER ANOMALIES

Prenatal bladder anomalies may be detected as early as the 10th week of gestation. Bladder agenesis is very rare and compatible with life only if the ureters drain ectopically, resulting in hypoplasia

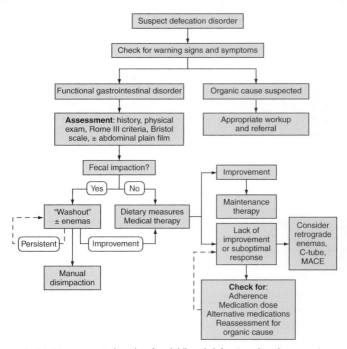

FIG. 6.2 Management algorithm for childhood defecation disorders seen in a pediatric urology practice. Lack of improvement or intractable constipation should be diagnosed based on worsening or absence of suboptimal response to adequate medical treatment for at least 3 months. *MACE,* Malone antegrade continence enema.

due to inadequate filling or storing of urine during development. An enlarged bladder, or "megacystis" with oligohydramnios raises concern for LUT obstruction; however, megacystis resolving before delivery may have no postnatal sequela. Postnatally, megacystis in association with abdominal distention, vomiting, and failure to pass meconium raises suspicion for the megacystis microcolon intestinal hypoperistalsis syndrome.

Bladder diverticula are usually discovered postnatally and may be associated with infection, hematuria, incontinence, or obstruction. Children with generalized connective tissue diseases, such as Ehlers-Danlos, Williams, or Menkes syndrome, are at risk for development of multiple and/or very large posterolateral bladder wall diverticula. Paraureteral diverticula may be acquired/secondary to infravesical obstruction.

Urachal anomalies (Fig. 6.3) may present in the immediate postnatal period with umbilical drainage. Urachal anomalies must be distinguished from omphalitis, which typically presents as a superficial cellulitis and a patent omphalomesenteric duct remnant, which can present with feculent umbilical drainage. Management of an infected urachal cyst or sinus with abscess includes initial drainage and antibiotics followed by complete excision of the patent urachus with a bladder cuff.

Nephrogenic adenoma is a rare benign inflammatory bladder tumor associated with a reaction to infection or trauma. Treatment involves resection although up to 80% may recur.

Hemorrhagic cystitis in children is often related to chemotherapy with cyclophosphamide or ifosfamide as well as BK virus, cytomegalovirus, and adenovirus in immunocompromised children.

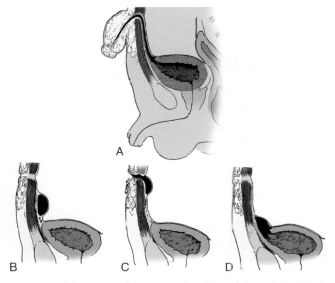

FIG. 6.3 Urachal anomalies. (A) Patent urachus. (B) Urachal cyst. (C) Umbilical-urachus sinus. (D) Vesicourachal diverticulum.

Mesna is given with cyclophosphamide therapy to help prevent hemorrhagic cystitis

POSTERIOR URETHRAL VALVES

Epidemiology and Pathophysiology

PUV are the most common cause of LUT obstruction (LUTO) in boys with an incidence of 1.6–2.1 per 10,000 births. Most valves appear as leaflets arising from the verumontanum that fuse anteriorly (Fig. 6.4). PUV during fetal development results in detrusor hypertrophy with high storage and voiding pressures. PUV may lead to dilation of the posterior urethra, bladder neck hypertrophy, bladder wall thickening, vesicoureteral reflux, upper tract dilation, and—in one third of affected patients—end-stage renal disease.

Clinical Presentation

Neonatal Presentation. Many infants are detected due to prenatal hydronephrosis, oligohydramnios, and/or a thick-walled bladder.

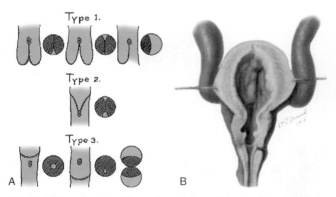

FIG. 6.4 (A) Young's original figures from his 1919 article describing three types of posterior urethral valves. (B) William P. Didusch illustrates the pathognomonic findings associated with posterior urethral valves: the thickened bladder with elevated bladder neck, dilated prostatic urethra, and the valve leaflets commonly ascribed to type 1 valves. The ureters are shown to be dilated. (From Young HH, Frontz WA, Baldwin JC. Congenital obstruction of the posterior urethra. *J Urol* 1919;3:289.)

Initial postnatal course is dictated by the severity of comorbidities such as pulmonary hypoplasia and renal failure.

Delayed Presentation. Despite widespread prenatal sonography, two thirds of children with PUV present after birth; therefore, a high degree of suspicion is warranted in boys presenting with LUT symptoms such as recurrent infections, overflow incontinence, gross hematuria and/or renal dysfunction.

Diagnosis and Testing

Prenatal Diagnosis. Thickened dilated bladder, upper tract dilation, and oligohydramnios have a high sensitivity for PUV on prenatal ultrasonography; a dilated posterior urethra results in the "keyhole sign". Severity of obstruction is indicated by amniotic fluid volume, renal dysplasia, and fetal urinary makers.

Postnatal Diagnosis. Much like the antenatal period, classic ultrasound findings include distended bladder with thickened wall and dilated posterior urethra. Voiding cystourethrogram (VCUG) remains the definitive study to confirm PUV. The bladder often appears thickened and trabeculated with multiple diverticuli, and high-grade VUR is seen in approximately 50% of boys (Fig. 6.5). Postnatal biochemical evaluation of renal function includes electrolytes and creatinine.

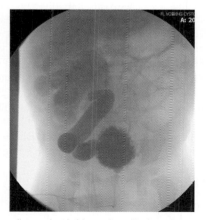

FIG. 6.5 Note small, irregular bladder, unilateral high grade vesicoureteral reflux and posterior urethral filling defect consistent with posterior urethral valves.

Treatment

Prenatal Management. Favorable fetal urine sample obtained after 20 weeks' gestation is suggested by urinary sodium <100 mEq/L, chloride <90 mEq/L, osmolarity <200 mEq/L, and β_2 microglobulin <6 mg/L. Fetal intervention with vesicoamniotic shunting should be selective and undertaken with caution.

Postnatal Management. A 5- or 8-Fr feeding tube should be inserted. Placement may be impeded by the hypertrophied and elevated bladder neck resulting in curling of the catheter within the dilated posterior urethra. Placement of a finger in the rectum may aid in pushing the catheter anteriorly. Alternatively, a coudé tip catheter may facilitate catheter placement. Inflation of a balloon catheter is avoided.

Cystoscopy with PUV ablation is the surgical intervention of choice. A 7.5- or 9-Fr cystoscope with offset lens facilitates passage of various ablating devices. Vesicostomy is reserved for very low birth weight infants whose urethras cannot accommodate the scope and or those with continued impaired renal function, high residuals, and upper tract deterioration. Upper urinary tract diversion is rarely indicated. Circumcision should be encouraged.

Prognosis

Renal dysfunction, VUR, and voiding dysfunction is mediated by bladder dysfunction. Lifetime prevalence of end-stage renal disease is between 20% and 50%. Nadir creatinine value <0.8 mg/dL appears to indicate lower risk while >1.2 mg/dL at 1 year predicts higher risk for renal failure.

The valve bladder evolves through three distinct patterns: (1) detrusor hyperreflexia in infancy and early childhood, (2) decreasing intravesical pressures and improved compliance in childhood, and (3) increased capacity bladder with hypocontractility and atony in adolescence. The focus of VUR management is centered on improving bladder function, and ureteral reimplantation is rarely offered.

BLADDER EXSTROPHY

Epidemiology and Pathophysiology

The exstrophy-epispadias complex is a rare congenital malformation with lower abdominal wall defect exposing an open bladder and urethra, wide diastasis of pubic symphysis, anorectal anomalies, and epispadiac urethral opening.

Clinical Presentation

At birth, bladder mucosa usually appears normal. It should be frequently irrigated with saline and protected with protective dressing. Size and distensibility of exstrophied bladder, as well as size of the fascial defect, affects timing and operative management.

In girls, the vagina is short but of normal caliber. The orifice is frequently stenotic and displaced anteriorly; the labia, mons pubis, and clitoris are divergent (Fig.6.6A). The male genital defect is severe (Fig. 6.6B). The penis is short due to diastasis of the pubic symphysis and marked deficiency of anterior corporeal tissue.

Indirect inguinal hernias are common. The perineum is short and broad with the anus anteriorly displaced and situated directly behind the urogenital diaphragm. Three-dimensional imaging demonstrates extensive pelvic bony defects including pubic diastasis and shortened anterior pubic segment (Fig. 6.7).

Diagnosis and Testing

Prenatal Diagnosis. Only 25% of cases are diagnosed prenatally. Diagnostic criteria on prenatal ultrasound include absence of

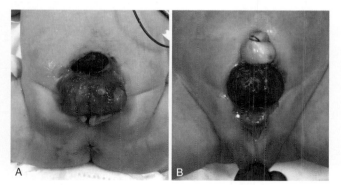

FIG. 6.6 (A) Newborn female with classic bladder exstrophy: note the bifid clitoral halves, divergent labia and mons, as well as the anteriorly displaced anus and diastasis of pubic symphysis. (B) Newborn male: note the short, exposed urethral plate with dorsal curvature.

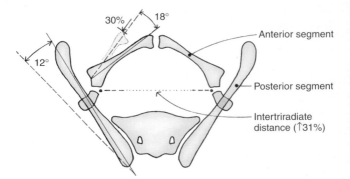

FIG. 6.7 Pelvic bone abnormalities noted in classic bladder exstrophy. The posterior bone segment is externally rotated (12 degrees mean on each side), but the length is unchanged. The anterior segment is externally rotated (18 degrees mean on each side) and shortened by 30%. The distance between the triradiate cartilage is increased by 31%.

bladder filling, low-set umbilicus, widening pubic rami, diminutive genitalia and lower abdominal mass that increases in size as pregnancy progresses (Fig. 6.8). Fetal magnetic resonance imaging (MRI) has been utilized to confirm the diagnosis.

Postnatal Testing. Detailed examination is performed to determine the size and quality of bladder template and urethral plate as well as penile length in males. Pelvic and hip plain films are obtained.

Treatment

Postnatal Management. At birth, the umbilical cord should be tied with 2-0 silk close to the abdominal wall. A hydrated gel dressing or plastic wrap is used to protect the bladder. Preoperative antibiotic prophylaxis is rarely required.

Surgical Repair. Goals of repair are to close bladder and urethra, reconstruct genitalia, and create functional organs for continence, voiding and sexual function. Delayed closure has equal continence rates and no difference in ultimate bladder capacity compared to neonatal closure.

Modern staged repair of bladder exstrophy (MSRE) consists of converting bladder exstrophy into complete epispadias to allow time for bladder to cycle and grow. Complete primary repair of

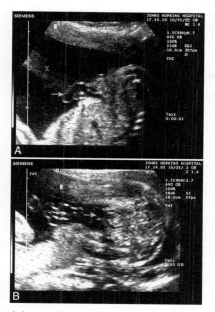

FIG. 6.8 Prenatal ultrasound scan demonstrating bladder exstrophy. (A) Longitudinal view showing the low-set umbilicus *(cyan arrow,* lack of intraabdominal bladder, and lower abdominal mass *(red arrow)* (B) Transverse view through the plane *(X)* in A shows presence of the umbilicus *(cyan arrow)* and the upper edge of the bladder plate that appears hyperechoic *(red arrow).*

bladder exstrophy (CPRE) includes combination of bladder closure, bladder neck reconstruction, urethral elongation, and epispadias repair in a single operation. Pelvic osteotomy is often performed to prevent tension on closure (Fig. 6.9). Penile reconstruction is aimed at (1) correction of dorsal chordee, (2) urethral reconstruction, (3) glanular reconstruction, and (4) skin closure.

Prognosis

Outcomes after exstrophy repair vary widely. Published continence rates vary from 37% to 90%. Erectile function, sensation, and libido are intact for most males. Antegrade ejaculation occurs in 63%; however, sperm quality and quantity are often diminished. Long-term studies have found a minority of men are able to conceive without assisted

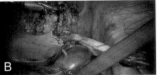
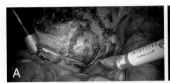
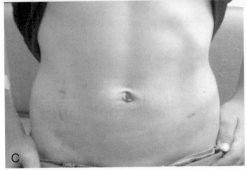

FIG. 6.9 Robot-assisted laparoscopic appendicovesicostomy in a child with valve bladder syndrome and a history of posterior urethral valves. (A) The detrusor muscle is incised in the posterior bladder wall to allow tunneled anastomosis of the appendix. (B) Anastomosis of the appendix to the bladder with a feeding tube traversing the appendix into a cystotomy along the posterior wall of the bladder. (C) Postoperative appearance with appendicovesicostomy stoma visible just inside the umbilicus.

reproductive techniques. For females, sexual intercourse is possible, and may be normal or complicated by dyspareunia. Fertility is unimpaired, however, prolapse occurs more commonly because of lack of pelvic floor support.

PRUNE BELLY SYNDROME

Epidemiology and Pathophysiology

Prune belly syndrome (PBS), also eponymously referred to as Eagle-Barrett syndrome, is characterized by deficient or absent abdominal wall musculature, bilateral intraabdominal cryptorchidism, and urinary tract anomalies, including megalourethra, megacystis, hydroureteronephrosis, and renal dysplasia. By strict definition, which includes cryptorchidism, PBS affects boys, with a contemporary incidence of 1 in 29,000–40,000 live births. Disease severity varies widely, and many patients have cardiopulmonary, gastrointestinal, and musculoskeletal anomalies.

Clinical Presentation

Neonatal abdominal wall appearance immediately suggests PBS (Fig. 6.10). As with PUV, initial postnatal course is dictated by severity of pulmonary hypoplasia.

Diagnosis and Testing

Prenatal Diagnosis. Prenatal findings may appear similar to bladder outlet obstruction; however, the classic findings of hydroureteronephrosis, distended bladder, and irregular abdominal circumference are not consistently seen even at 30 weeks of gestation (Fig. 6.11).

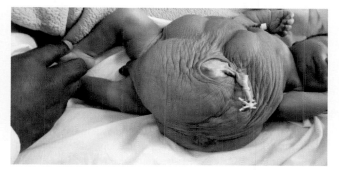

FIG. 6.10 Appearance of a newborn with prune belly syndrome: wrinkled, redundant skin with bulging at the flanks due to deficient of abdominal wall musculature and massively distended bladder.

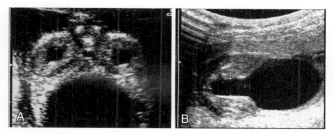

FIG. 6.11 (A) Fetus with prune belly syndrome demonstrating distended bladder with hydronephrotic echogenic kidneys. (B) Distended bladder with dilated prostatic urethra indicative of outlet obstruction from urethral atresia. (Courtesy E. Ruiz.)

Table 6.2 Spectrum of Prune Belly Syndrome

CATEGORY	CHARACTERISTICS
I	Renal dysplasia
	Oligohydramnios
	Pulmonary hypoplasia
	Potter features
	Urethral atresia
II	Full triad features
	Minimal or unilateral renal dysplasia
	No pulmonary hypoplasia
	May progress to renal failure
III	Incomplete or mild triad features
	Mild to moderate uropathy
	No renal dysplasia
	Stable renal function
	No pulmonary hypoplasia

Spectrum of Disease. There are three major categories of neonatal presentation (Table 6.2). Category I includes pronounced oligohydramnios with severe pulmonary hypoplasia and skeletal abnormalities. Boys in category II experience moderate renal insufficiency and moderate-severe hydroureteronephrosis. Category III consists of mild features; renal function is typically normal or mildly impaired and no pulmonary insufficiency.

Postnatal Testing. Baseline assessment of renal function should include ultrasound, blood urea nitrogen (BUN), creatinine, and electrolytes. Unnecessary catheterization should be avoided, however VCUG to assess bladder outlet and emptying is warranted.

Treatment

Postnatal Management. Low-pressure urinary tract dilation is the hallmark of PBS. Bladder is typically enlarged and hypotonic, with elevated compliance and low-pressure VUR in approximately 75%. These bladders are competent at storage, but often demonstrate incomplete emptying with reduced detrusor contractility. UTI avoidance is key. Prophylactic antibiotic therapy is recommended, especially before instrumentation. Circumcision is advisable.

Surgical Repair. Transabdominal or laparoscopic bilateral orchidopexy around 6 months of age is recommended.

Extent and timing of urinary tract reconstruction is tailored to a given child's bladder dynamics while taking into consideration respiratory status. Ureteral reconstruction is considered with repeated UTIs or progressive anatomic or functional upper tract deterioration (Fig. 6.12). Likewise, reduction cystoplasty may be considered in cases of large urachal diverticulum or as part of a more extensive reconstruction, including an

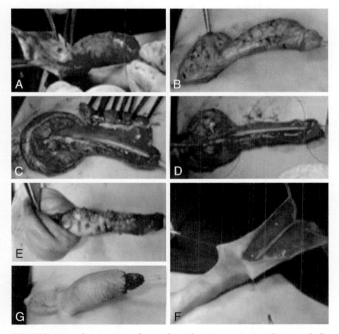

FIG. 6.12 Surgical correction of megalourethra in a patient with prune belly syndrome. (A) Penile deglovement. (B) Exposure of the scaphoid megalourethra. (C and D) Tailoring of the dilated urethral segment. (E) Completed urethroplasty. (F) Presentation of excessive preputial skin. (G) Completed procedure after urethroplasty and circumcision (note the empty scrotum).

appendicovesicostomy to afford better long-term bladder emptying.

Abdominal wall reconstruction, besides obvious cosmetic and psychosocial benefits, has demonstrated improved bladder emptying, more effective cough, and improved defecation. Monfort and Ehrlich abdominoplasties both describe correction of lateral redundancy along with strengthening of abdominal wall by vertical overlapping of the fascia (Fig. 6.13).

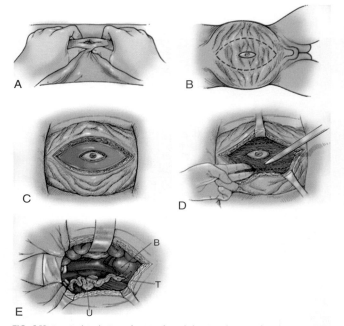

FIG. 6.13 Surgical technique for Monfort abdominoplasty and concomitant reconstruction of prune belly uropathy. (A) Delineation of redundancy by tenting up abdominal wall. (B) Skin incisions are outlined with a separate circumscribing incision to isolate the umbilicus. (C) Skin (epidermis and dermis only) is excised with electrocautery. (D) Abdominal wall central plate is incised at the lateral border of the rectus muscle on either side, from the superior epigastric to the inferior epigastric vessels, creating a central musculofascial plate. (E) Adequate exposure is provided for concomitant transperitoneal genitourinary procedures. *B,* Bladder; *T,* testis; *U,* ureter.

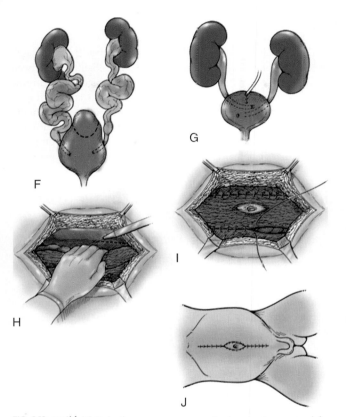

FIG. 6.13, cont'd (F) Only the more normal proximal ureter is preserved for vesicoureteral reimplantation, and the urachal diverticulum is excised. (G) Transtrigonal ureteral reimplantation is performed with or without ureteral tapering as needed. The bladder is closed in two layers, and ureteral stents (not shown) and a cystostomy tube are used. (H) Completion of abdominoplasty by scoring of the parietal peritoneum overlying the lateral abdominal wall musculature with electrocautery. (I) The edges of the central plate are sutured to the lateral abdominal wall musculature along the scored line. (J) Lateral flaps are brought together in the midline, with closed suction drains placed between the lateral flaps and the central plate. Skin is brought together in the midline, enveloping the previously isolated umbilicus. (From Woodard JR, Perez LM. Prune-belly syndrome. In: Marshall FF, ed. *Operative urology*. Philadelphia, PA: Saunders, 1996.)

Prognosis

In the perinatal period secondary to severe pulmonary hypoplasia, 20% of newborns die. Significant pulmonary difficulties have been reported in 55% of PBS survivors. Up to one-third develop chronic renal insufficiency. Nadir creatinine value less than 0.7 mg/dL during infancy portends stable renal function during childhood. Adequate bladder emptying helps reduce risk of UTIs and upper tract deterioration. A normal pattern of sexual development is expected after orchidopexies, although no spontaneous paternity has been reported.

NEUROMUSCULAR DYSFUNCTION OF THE LOWER URINARY TRACT IN CHILDREN

Epidemiology and Pathophysiology

Neural tube defects (NTDs) are the most common congenital cause of neurogenic bladder with meningomyelocele being the most prevalent. Women with low levels of folic acid during early pregnancy are at increased risk for a fetus with an NTD. Neurologic lesions vary depending on the involvement of the neural elements and cannot be reliably predicted based only on the vertebral defect (Table 6.3). Almost all infants with spina bifida have Arnold-Chiari malformation, which is associated with hydrocephalus and developmental brain abnormalities.

Clinical Presentation

Infants who did not undergo prenatal intervention, typically undergo laminectomy with closure within 24 hours of delivery.

Table 6.3 Spinal Level of Myelomeningocele

LOCATION	INCIDENCE (%)
Cervical–high thoracic	2
Low thoracic	5
Lumbar	26
Lumbosacral	47
Sacral	20

Diagnosis and Testing

Prenatal Diagnosis. The majority of infants are diagnosed prenatally. Antenatal ultrasonography suggests the insult to central and peripheral nervous systems is progressive, such that lower limb movement may be lost, and hindbrain herniation and hydrocephalus may worsen during gestation.

Postnatal Testing. Renal-bladder ultrasound is performed as early as possible after birth. Baseline urodynamics and serum creatinine are obtained at 3 months. Three categories of LUT dynamics may be detected: synergic (26%), dyssynergic with and without poor detrusor compliance (37%), and complete denervation (36%).

Infants at risk for urinary tract deterioration as a result of a poorly compliant or overactive detrusor or outflow obstruction from DSD need to be identified.

Treatment

Prenatal Management. Prenatal closure before 26 weeks of gestation improves neuromotor function and decreases need for ventriculo-peritoneal shunting; however, bowel and bladder function do not appear to be improved. There is a significant risk of fetal demise, maternal morbidity, and preterm labor with prenatal intervention.

Postnatal Management. The primary goal of management is preservation of renal function by maintaining low bladder pressures and actively managing symptomatic UTI/VUR. Clean intermittent catheterization (CIC) is implemented if postvoid residuals are elevated. Early intervention with CIC and antimuscarinics to keep filling pressures less than 30 cm H_2O improves the rate of UTI, VUR, and upper urinary tract deterioration, as well as the incidence of chronic kidney disease (CKD) (Fig. 6.14).

Prognosis

Risk factors for renal dysfunction include DSD, high detrusor pressures, detrusor overactivity, febrile UTI, and VUR. Management of neurogenic bowel may also improve bladder function. Up to 70% of males with spina bifida are able to obtain erections, and 40%–75% report ability to ejaculate. Reports suggest that 70%–80% of women with spina bifida are able have an uneventful pregnancy and delivery.

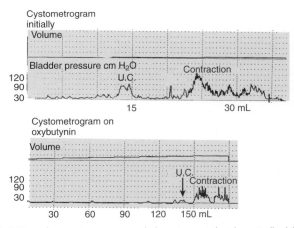

FIG. 6.14 Oxybutynin is a potent anticholinergic agent that dramatically delays detrusor contractions and lowers contraction pressure, as demonstrated on these two graphs. *U.C.*, Uninhibited contraction.

LOWER URINARY TRACT RECONSTRUCTION IN CHILDREN

Most pediatric lower tract reconstructive procedures follow a failure of medical management in correcting a hostile LUT condition. Preoperative urodynamic evaluation, often combined with fluoroscopy, is critical to understand LUT dysfunction and anatomy. Most children require CIC to empty the bladder after LUT reconstruction and they or their family must be willing and capable of performing it on a reliable basis for the lifetime of the patient.

Ureteral reimplantation into native bladder is preferable when an antireflux procedure is necessary. One of the greatest technical challenges regarding bladder reconstruction is reliably providing adequate outflow resistance to achieve continence. Bladder neck repair or slings have variable continence results and may also unmask or result in new bladder hostility; therefore, careful follow-up is mandatory.

Bladder volume achieved through reconstruction must accommodate urinary output for an acceptable period of time, usually 4 hours. Any gastrointestinal segment used for augmentation should be detubularized and reconfigured and widely anastomosed

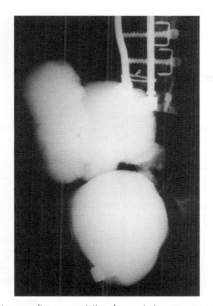

FIG. 6.15 Cystogram after augmentation demonstrates a narrow anastomosis of the bowel segment to bladder. The segment behaves like a diverticulum.

to the bladder to maximize capacity and compliance. Reconfiguration into a spheric shape maximizes the volume achieved and blunts bowel contractions. The native bladder is typically preserved and is widely bivalved to prevent a narrow-mouthed anastomosis which can result in the augmentation segment behaving as a diverticulum (Fig. 6.15). When ileum is used, a segment at least 15 cm proximal to the ileocecal valve is selected.

Unfortunately, long-term complications following bladder augmentation requiring additional procedures are relatively common. Ammonium resorption can cause metabolic acidosis, particularly among patients with renal insufficiency, and increase the risk of kidney stones. Intestinal segments continue to produce mucus and daily bladder irrigations to prevent mucus buildup helps decrease the risk of UTIs and bladder stones. Bacteriuria is common after cystoplasty and does not routinely require treatment. Bladder perforations within the bowel segment may present with vague abdominal symptoms requiring a high index of suspicion. Diagnosis is made by cystogram, computed tomography cystogram, or emergent surgical exploration. Patients with a neurogenic bladder, including those with an augmentation, have an increased risk of bladder cancer.

Suggested Readings

Ashley RA, Inman BA, Routh JC, et al. Urachal anomalies: A longitudinal study of urachal remnants in children and adults. *J Urol* 2007;178:1615-1618.

Austin PF, Bauer SB, Bower W, et al. The standardization of terminology of lower urinary tract function in children and adolescents: update report from the standardization committee of the International Children's Continence Society. *Neurourol Urodyn* 2016 Apr;35(4):471-481.

Burgers RE, Mugie SM, Chase J, et al. Management of functional constipation in children with lower urinary tract symptoms: report from the Standardization Committee of the International Children's Continence Society. *J Urol* 2013;190(1):29-36.

Inouye BM, Massanyi EZ, Di Carlo H, et al. Modern management of bladder exstrophy repair. *Curr Urol Rep* 2013;14:359-365.

Koff SA, Mutabagani KH, Jayanthi VR. The valve bladder syndrome: pathophysiology and treatment with nocturnal bladder emptying. *J Urol* 2002;167(1):291-297.

Lopes RI, Tavares A, Srougi M, et al. 27 years of experience with the comprehensive surgical treatment of prune belly syndrome. *J Pediatr Urol* 2015;11(5):276.e1-276.e7.

Sandler AD. Children with spina bifida: key clinical issues. *Pediatr Clin North Am* 2010;57:879-892.

7

Congenital Anomalies of the Upper Urinary Tract: UPJ Obstruction, Duplication Anomalies, Ectopic Ureter, Ureterocele, and Ureteral Anomalies

MATTHEW D. TIMBERLAKE AND CRAIG A. PETERS

CONTRIBUTORS OF CAMPBELL-WALSH-WEIN, 12TH EDITION

Brian A. VanderBrink, Pramod P. Reddy, John C. Pope IV, Craig A. Peters, Kirstan K. Meldrum, Irina Stanasel, L. Henning Olsen, and Yazan F.H. Rawashdeh

CONGENITAL RENAL ANOMALIES

Renal Agenesis

Renal agenesis (RA) represents congenital absence of one or both kidneys, caused by developmental failures of the ureteral bud and metanephric mesenchyme. Bilateral RA is fatal due to oligohydramnios and pulmonary hypoplasia. Unilateral RA is frequently associated with contralateral ureteral abnormalities, including ureteropelvic junction (UPJ) obstruction (11%), ureterovesical junction (UVJ) obstruction (7%), and vesicoureteral reflux (VUR) (30%). In unilateral RA, consider voiding cystourethrogram (VCUG) because of the high coincidence of VUR, particularly if hydronephrosis or hydroureter is present in the solitary kidney.

Ipsilateral genital duct abnormalities are present in 10%–15% of boys and 25%–50% of girls with unilateral RA. Boys may have

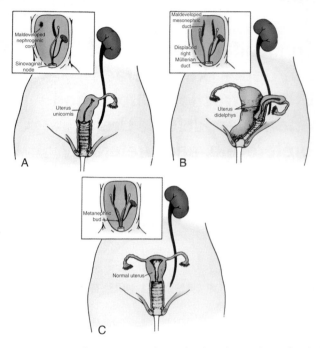

FIG. 7.1 A proposed categorization of genital and renal anomalies in females. See text for details. (From Magee MC, Lucey DT, Fried FA. A new embryologic classification for urogynecologic malformations: the syndromes of mesonephric duct induced Müllerian deformities. *J Urol* 1979;121:265-267.)

ipsilateral vasal agenesis. Girls may have a unicornuate or bicornuate uterus with absent or underdeveloped ipsilateral uterine horn and fallopian tube. Zinner syndrome in boys and obstructed hemivagina ipsilateral renal agenesis syndrome in girls are analogous conditions in which an ectopic ureteral insertion into the genital duct system results in ipsilateral renal agenesis (Fig. 7.1).

Horseshoe Kidney

Horseshoe kidney is the most common renal fusion anomaly with an estimated incidence of 1 in 400 births. Anatomically, horseshoe kidneys have a parenchymatous isthmus connecting the right and left renal moieties, typically at the L3–L4 level, and crossed by the inferior mesenteric artery. Calyces point posteriorly and the ureter inserts in a relatively nondependent and lateral location on the renal pelvis. Approximately 30% of patients with horseshoe kidney have other congenital anomalies, notably Turner syndrome, hypospadias or undescended testis (5%), mullerian abnormalities (5%), VUR (50%), and UPJ obstruction (UPJO). Unobstructed dilation caused by nondependent ureteral insertion is common. Because of relative stasis, children with horseshoe kidney are at increased risk for stones and upper tract infection.

Cross-Fused Ectopic Kidney

Crossed ectopia refers to a kidney positioned contralateral to its ureteral insertion in the bladder. Ninety percent of crossed ectopic kidneys are fused to the opposite renal moiety. Most commonly, the ectopic kidney crosses from left to right, and the ectopic moiety is positioned inferior to the normal moiety. In all types, ureteral orifices are normal and orthotopic. Crossed ectopic kidneys are usually asymptomatic and discovered incidentally, but a minority of patients present with urinary tract infections (UTIs), stones, or hematuria (Fig. 7.2).

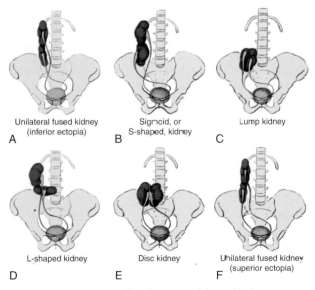

A Unilateral fused kidney (inferior ectopia)

B Sigmoid, or S-shaped, kidney

C Lump kidney

D L-shaped kidney

E Disc kidney

F Unilateral fused kidney (superior ectopia)

FIG. 7.2 Crossed renal ectopia with fusion (A–F).

Renal Duplication Anomalies

Branching of a single ureteral bud results in incomplete pyeloureteral duplication, characterized by a single ipsilateral orifice and bifid renal pelvis or Y-shaped ureter. Incomplete duplication is seldom associated with clinical pathology. By contrast, takeoff of two separate ureteral buds from the same mesonephric duct results in complete ureteral duplication, wherein a relatively cephalad and laterally positioned orifice drains the lower moiety (LM) and a more caudal and medial orifice drains the upper moiety (UM). The UM ureter is more prone to distal obstruction and may be associated with a ureterocele or ectopic ureteral insertion. The LM ureter is more prone to vesicoureteral reflux via a shortened intramural tunnel length.

RENAL OBSTRUCTION: KEY PRINCIPLES

Congenital obstructive uropathy (COU) is distinct from postnatal acquired obstruction in that it alters the growth and differentiation of the developing kidney. Pathophysiological mechanisms remain to be precisely defined but likely reflect alterations of key developmental pathways. Key pathological patterns include fibrosis and altered morphogenesis and ultimately dysplasia in severe cases. Postnatal correction of obstruction does not usually permit normalization but may limit progression. Progression may, however, continue because of altered function and ongoing pathophysiological processes. This can be seen in bilateral obstruction or in solitary obstructed kidneys. Biopsy studies have shown that even with normal uptake on nuclear imaging, affected kidneys may have significant histologic. It has also been shown that early insults to normal kidney development are associated with later progression to renal insufficiency. Few useful biomarkers of obstructive uropathy are currently available to define the need for intervention.

UPJ OBSTRUCTION

Definition

Ureteropelvic junction is the most common form of pediatric upper urinary tract obstruction and is seen in a spectrum of severity with both symptomatic and asymptomatic presentation. The underlying etiology is variable, and spontaneous resolution in many infants is common. Some obstructions are caused by intrinsically abnormal proximal ureteral development and in others extrinsic obstruction is a common cause presenting with flank pain and hydronephrosis. This extrinsic obstruction is often caused by a lower pole vessel of the kidney that creates a kinking of the ureter.

Presentation

Clinical presentation of UPJ obstruction is most commonly through prenatal detection of hydronephrosis but also with symptomatic presentation of abdominal or flank pain. At 20 weeks' gestation, an anatomic screening ultrasound is generally performed. If hydronephrosis is detected, the anteroposterior (AP) diameter of the dilation is followed with serial ultrasonography. Postnatal follow-up is warranted when AP diameter of the dilated pelvis is ≥ 7 mm during the third trimester.

Later presentation with abdominal or flank pain may be mistaken for gastroenterologic problems, and in some children, the appropriate diagnosis is missed for long periods of time. Abrupt onset of severe pain, frequently with nausea and vomiting that is colicky in nature, is the typical pattern and is termed Deitl's crisis. These episodes can last several hours but then typically clear completely with no residual discomfort. They may be often confused for cyclic vomiting syndrome or abdominal migraine. If the child is not having symptoms, imaging may not reveal significant hydronephrosis, but imaging during the acute phase will usually show increased dilation from a baseline study. Providing the family with a standing order for an immediate ultrasound during an episode of pain may provide for a definitive diagnosis. Symptoms may be triggered during a diuretic renogram, although this is inconsistent. There can be a delayed nephrogram for up to 48 hours after an episode of pain on a MAG-3 renal scan.

Following prenatal detection, postnatal evaluation with ultrasonography and selection of further functional imaging in the first weeks of life is typical. Controversy remains over the indications for functional imaging as well as the interpretation of diuretic renography. It is also controversial whether to obtain a VCUG, and some recent reports suggest deferring this unless there is associated ureteral dilation, a duplication anomaly, or a dysmorphic kidney. There will still be an incidence, albeit low, of significant reflux that may be missed.

Evaluation

Key factors to be evaluated using diuretic renography (MAG-3 scan) include the relative function of the affected kidney compared with the contralateral as well as the washout time following Lasix administration. Traditional thresholds for obstruction include washout half-time > 20 minutes, but this is not universally agreed upon in pediatric practice. The actual definition of obstruction remains controversial, with some practitioners considering a system to be significantly obstructed only when there is documented decline in relative renal function over time. For others, reduced function at presentation with a delayed drainage curve suggests the need for surgical intervention.

Management

There are no universally agreed-upon criteria for surgery with congenital hydronephrosis. Most series demonstrate that approximately 25% of children with significant unilateral dilation ultimately undergo operative repair because of decreasing relative renal function or increasing hydronephrosis.

Conservative Management. A practical observation plan would include follow-up ultrasonography every 3 months during the first year of life and then increased to every 6–12 months going forward depending on the severity of the hydronephrosis. Periodic repeat of the nuclear medicine studies to assess function can be performed every 6–12 months or if increasing hydronephrosis is detected. Parental preferences need to be incorporated into the management plan because continued testing can be burdensome.

Clear indications for surgery include markedly increased hydronephrosis, > 10% decrease in relative uptake on renography, and symptoms such as pain or UTI. Persistence of hydronephrosis with no improvement over time may also be an indication for intervention.

Surgical Management. The gold standard for correcting UPJ obstruction is a dismembered pyeloplasty. This can be performed at any age. Retrograde pyelography prior to incision is optional and may be combined with stent placement. The standard approach is a subcostal extraperitoneal incision with mobilization of the renal pelvis and excision of the UPJ segment and part of the renal pelvis. The ureter is spatulated laterally, and an anastomosis with fine absorbable suture is performed. A dorsal lumbotomy approach is another option in children. With open surgery, stenting is optional, as well as wound drain.

More recently laparoscopic and robotic techniques have been employed with equal success rates. These are typically done with a transperitoneal exposure utilizing a running sutured anastomosis. Frequently, a ureteral stent is left in place. This can be done with an extraction string to avoid a later cystoscopy. Wound drains are not typically used.

If an extrinsic obstruction is present, the ureter is dismembered and is transposed anteriorly to the vessel, and a typical spatulated anastomosis is performed. A vascular hitch procedure has been described to fix the renal pelvis inferior to the vessel without any ureteral dismemberment; however, the results with this technique have been inconsistent.

Typical postoperative evaluation includes a renal ultrasound 4–8 weeks after surgery. Continued monitoring is reasonable. Some groups perform a diuretic renogram at 3 months and if this drains well, discontinue further follow-up. However, ongoing monitoring of hydronephrosis for 2–5 years is prudent.

Surgical success rates are typically very high, well above 95% in most series. Complications include urinary leakage, and development of a urinoma may require drainage. Postoperative infection is common, and prophylactic antibiotics may be appropriate. Persisting obstruction, although uncommon, is possible and may require replacement of a ureteral stent, balloon dilation, or reoperative pyeloplasty (Figs. 7.3 and 7.4).

URETEROVESICAL JUNCTION OBSTRUCTION

Definition

Ureterovesical junction obstruction (UVJO), also referred to as primary obstructed megaureter, results from a narrow, a peristaltic segment of intramural ureter, causing a variable degree of upper tract obstruction.

The term "megaureter" is used to describe hydroureter of ≥ 7 mm, regardless of etiology. A megaureter may be associated with UVJO, reflux, or both. Ureteral dilation can be nonpathologic, representing a balanced state of stable dilation.

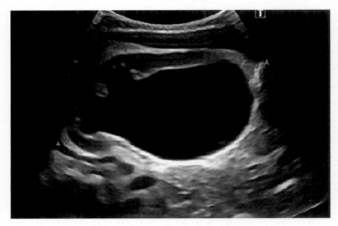

FIG. 7.3 Ultrasound appearance of UPJO.

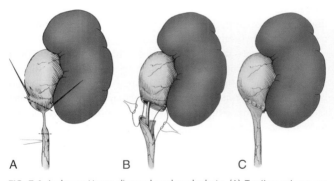

A   B   C

FIG. 7.4 Anderson-Hynes dismembered pyeloplasty. (A) Traction sutures are placed on the medial and lateral aspects of the dependent portion of the renal pelvis in preparation for dismembered pyeloplasty. A traction suture is also placed on the lateral aspect of the proximal ureter below the level of the obstruction. This suture will help maintain proper orientation for the subsequent repair. (B) The ureteropelvic junction is excised. The proximal ureter is spatulated on its lateral aspect. The apex of this lateral, spatulated aspect of the ureter is then brought to the inferior border of the pelvis while the medial side of the ureter is brought to the superior edge of the pelvis. (C) The anastomosis is performed with fine interrupted or running absorbable sutures placed full thickness through the ureteral and renal pelvic walls in a watertight fashion.

Presentation

UVJO is most commonly recognized prenatally. Infants or children may present with febrile UTI, sepsis, pain, stones, or microscopic hematuria. UVJO is more common in boys and more common on the left. The natural history of UVJO tend strongly toward spontaneous resolution in the first years of life.

Evaluation

Prenatally detected hydroureteronephrosis generally prompts ultrasonography and VCUG as initial studies. Patients with UVJO often have significant hydroureteronephrosis without VUR. MAG-3 renogram is obtained around 6 weeks of age to evaluate function and drainage. Washout curves and half times are often considerably delayed but generally do not guide management. Endoscopic evaluation or magnetic resonance urography (MRU) is occasionally needed to differentiate UVJO from ectopic ureter.

Management

Conservative Management. Even in the setting of delayed excretion on renogram, observation is the preferred management approach for children with UVJO who have no infections or functional loss. Infants are typically placed on antibiotic prophylaxis given concern for UTI within a relatively static, dilated system. Serial ultrasounds are obtained frequently during year 1 and every 6–12 months thereafter. A renogram may be repeated less often to confirm functional stability and improved drainage.

Temporizing Management. Infants with UVJO and profound dilation, functional loss, or sepsis may require temporizing diversion as a bridge to definitive reconstruction. Options include end or loop cutaneous ureterostomy or refluxing anastomosis of the pelvic ureter to the lateral wall of the bladder.

Definitive Management. Indications for definitive reconstruction include recurrent or severe infection, ipsilateral function under 40%, and significant or sequential functional decline. Stone formation, pain, or progressive, unremitting dilation may prompt surgery in some patients. UVJO is repaired via excision of the narrow adynamic segment and ureteral reimplantation. Intravesical or extravesical approaches may be utilized. Ureteral tailoring, either by plication or excisional tapering, is usually required (Fig. 7.5).

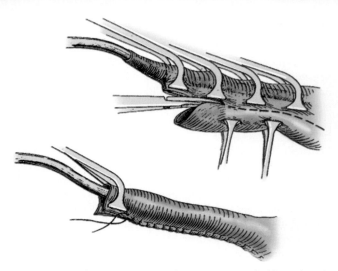

FIG. 7.5 Excisional tapering. Tapering is done over an 8-Fr red rubber catheter in infants or a 10-Fr catheter in older children and adults. After vascularity is defined, special atraumatic clamps are placed over the catheter. Baby Allis clamps help retract the portion of ureter to be resected, which is usually lateral. It is important not to resect too much ureter. Running 5-0 monofilament resorbable sutures are used to reapproximate the proximal two-thirds of the ureter. Its distal third is closed with interrupted sutures to allow for shortening.

Endoscopic management with manual or balloon dilation of the UVJ followed by temporary ureteral stent placement has been described as a minimally invasive alternative to tapered ureteral reimplant.

URETEROCELE

Definition

A ureterocele is a cystic dilation of the distal ureter within the bladder, often associated with upper tract obstruction. Ureteroceles may be associated with single or duplex systems. In the setting of complete duplication, the ureterocele is associated with the UM ureter, while reflux is common in the LM ureter. Ureteroceles are classified according to their location and configuration (Box 7.1).

Box 7.1 Ureterocele Terminology

SINGLE-SYSTEM INTRAVESICAL URETEROCELE
- Entirely within bladder and above bladder neck
- May prolapse into the urethra during voiding

ECTOPIC URETEROCELE
- Some portion of the ureterocele situated permanently at bladder neck or urethra, but orifice is within bladder

CECOURETEROCELE
- Orifice extends beyond bladder neck into urethra
- May not be recognized preoperatively; complexity creates surgical challenges with endoscopic incision

URETEROCELE DISPROPORTION
- Duplex system ureterocele with small (often not visible) associated upper moiety
- Ureterocele visualized in bladder; ipsilateral lower moiety appears unremarkable
- Affected ureter not dilated beyond the bladder

PSEUDOURETEROCELE
- Large ectopic ureter impinges on bladder wall and appears as an intravesical structure on ultrasound
- VCUG shows apparent filling defect, as large ectopic ureter pushes inward on posterolateral bladder

VCUG, Voiding cystourethrogram.

Presentation

Ureteroceles are often identified during evaluation for prenatal hydronephrosis or may present clinically with febrile UTI. Infections may be severe, with bacteremia and sepsis. Infant girls occasionally present with an interlabial mass, representing prolapse of the ureterocele through the urethra. Large ureteroceles can distort trigonal and urethral anatomy and affect the continence mechanism.

Evaluation

Initial evaluation typically consists of renal bladder ultrasound and VCUG. A ureterocele may be differentiated from an ectopic ureter based on ultrasound appearance (Fig. 7.6A, B). The presence of bilateral hydronephrosis may suggest obstruction of the contralateral ureteral orifice or bladder neck. On VCUG, a ureterocele appears as a circular filling defect, best appreciated during early filling (Fig. 7.6C, D). During voiding, ureterocele eversion mimics the appearance of a bladder diverticulum and may indicate a weak trigonal floor. Identification of reflux into the ipsilateral lower pole as well as in the contralateral system is important and will affect management. Nuclear scan can be used to evaluate for obstruction

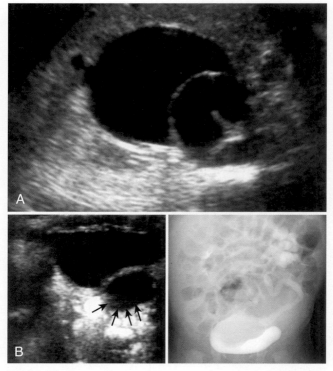

FIG. 7.6 (A) Ultrasound image of an intravesical ureterocele at the bladder level. (B) Ultrasound image of a bladder in a child with an ectopic ureter extending into the bladder. The wall of the ureter is thicker than the ureterocele, and the lumen of the ureter extends well outside the bladder lumen, indicating that this is an ectopic ureter rather than a ureterocele.

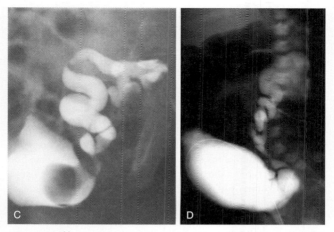

FIG. 7.6, cont'd (C) Voiding cystourethrogram in a child with a ureterocele appearing as a filling defect within the bladder and massive ipsilateral lower pole reflux. (D) Voiding cystourethrogram in a child with a ureterocele and evidence of ureterocele eversion with voiding. The apparent diverticulum is the ureterocele extending outside the bladder wall with increased intravesical pressure. This pattern may be seen with the ureterocele everting or intussuscepting into its dilated ureter. There is lower pole reflux as well.

and relative function of the associated renal unit, though not reliable in the first weeks of life. In the absence of functional loss, the UM of a duplex system should contribute one-third of ipsilateral function, and the lower moiety should contribute two-thirds.

Management

Management goals include preservation of functional renal parenchyma (via correction of obstruction and prevention of VUR), elimination or prevention of infection, maintenance of continence, and minimization of procedural morbidity.

Conservative Management. Infants with improving mild to moderate unilateral hydronephrosis and small intravesical ureteroceles are often managed conservatively. Infants are typically placed on antibiotic prophylaxis and followed with serial ultrasounds. Families are educated on the signs and symptoms of UTI. Nuclear renogram at 6–12 weeks of age may be useful. Factors associated with a more benign clinical course include absent or low-grade ipsilateral VUR and absent function of the associated renal unit (multicystic dysplastic kidney [MCDK], nonfunctioning UM).

Surgical Management. Indications for surgical intervention include infection, severe or worsening ipsilateral hydronephrosis, and bilateral hydronephrosis (secondary to obstruction of bladder outlet or contralateral ureteral orifice). Children with systemic infection or sepsis who do not immediately respond to antibiotics require emergent surgical decompression.

Decompression is accomplished via transurethral incision or puncture of the ureterocele. A cold knife, angled-tip hot wire, Bugbee, laser, or Collins knife is used to achieve a transverse full-thickness incision in the ureterocele. The ureterocele is best visualized endoscopically at low filling volumes. The incision is ideally positioned distally, medially, and close to the bladder floor. Adequacy of the decompression is confirmed visually by escape of urine or distal ureteroscopy in the ureterocele.

The primary risk of endoscopic treatment is ipsilateral de novo reflux via the surgically created defect. Risk is technique-dependent but is thought to be higher for extravesical ureteroceles (70%) compared to intravesical ureteroceles (25%).

In many cases, transurethral incision serves to alleviate obstruction until infants are old enough for definitive reconstruction, often planned between 1 and 2 years of age. Surgical options and considerations for definitive treatment are summarized in Table 7.1.

ECTOPIC URETER

Definition

An ectopic ureter inserts caudal to the normal orthotopic position on the trigone, resulting from an abnormally cephalad ureteral budding from the mesonephric duct. Like ureteroceles, ectopic ureters may be associated with a single system kidney or the UM of a duplex system. Ectopic ureters most commonly insert into the bladder neck or proximal urethra but may also terminate in the genital tract (Fig. 7.7).

Presentation

Prenatal detection is common, often with severe dilation. Infants and children may present with dramatic systemic infection or

Table 7.1 Options for Definitive Surgical Management of Ureterocele

PROCEDURE	IDEAL INDICATIONS	ADVANTAGES	LIMITATIONS
Transurethral incision	• Small infant • Large ureterocele with VUR	• Outpatient procedure[a] • Effective decompression • Occasionally definitive	• De novo reflux into ureterocele segment necessitating subsequent lower tract reconstruction
Upper pole nephrectomy	• **No lower moiety VUR** • Nonfunctioning upper moiety	• May be definitive • Removes pathology • Avoids bladder surgery	• May still require lower tract reconstruction • Risk to lower moiety • Leaves ureterocele in bladder • May develop VUR
UU or ureteropyelostomy	• **No lower moiety VUR** • Functional upper moiety	• Drains obstructed segment with little risk for obstruction or UTI	
Common sheath reimplant with ureterocele excision	• **Associated lower moiety VUR** • Functional upper moiety without significant dilation	• Eliminates obstruction and VUR • Removes ureterocele • No renal risk	• Complex surgery • Risk to vagina and BN • May require ureteral tapering

[a]Unless patient is an infant requiring admission for oxygen monitoring.

BN, Bladder neck; *UTI*, urinary tract infection; *UU*, ureteroureterostomy; *VUR*, vesicoureteral reflux

Female

Male

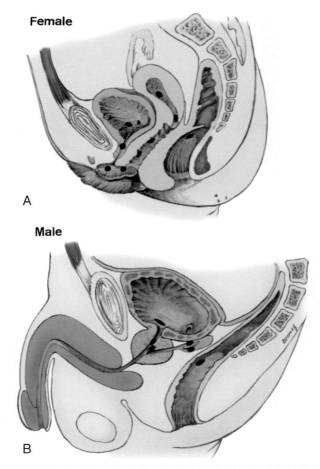

FIG. 7.7 Sites of ectopic ureteral orifices in the a female (A) and male (B) patient.

more subacutely with chronic low-grade fevers yet negative urine culture results. An ectopic ureter should be considered in girls with continuous urinary leakage because insertion into the genital tract bypasses the external sphincter. In contrast, boys never present with incontinence because the ectopic insertion is proximal to the external sphincter. However, when an ectopic ureter inserts into Wolffian duct structures, boys may present with epididymo-orchitis at an unusually early age.

Evaluation

Perineal examination in girls may reveal a dilated Gartner's duct cyst in the vagina, and urine may be expressed from a vaginally inserting orifice. Initial imaging includes renal ultrasound (RUSD), VCUG, and nuclear scan. An ectopic ureter may be differentiated from a ureterocele based on a relatively thicker partition between bladder and ureter on ultrasound and a lumen that extends well outside of the bladder lumen. Reflux into an ectopic ureter may occur if the orifice is positioned near the bladder neck. In a duplex system with ectopic UM ureter, LM reflux is common. Definitive management is guided by nuclear renal scan, which indicates the relative function of the associated kidney or UM. The more remote an ectopic ureteral insertion (i.e., vas deferens, ejaculatory duct, uterus), the higher the risk of dysplasia and reduced function.

MRU may be used when anatomy is complex—massive dilation is present, the location of ectopic insertion is uncertain, or the existence of duplication is unclear. MRU may provide functional information but requires sedation in young children.

Endoscopic evaluation can distinguish an ectopic ureter from a ureterocele, confirm the location of an orifice, or note the presence of duplication. The orifice of the affected ureter is often difficult to visualize within the urethra or vagina.

Management

Surgical intervention is often required to preserve functional renal parenchyma, address infection-related complications, establish continence, or remove a dilated, nonfunctional renal–ureteral unit.

Conservative Management. For infants with dilation and stasis or associated lower moiety VUR, antibiotic prophylaxis is appropriate while awaiting definitive treatment. Children without clinical problems, stable dilation, or a nonfunctioning associated renal unit may be managed with an observational approach.

Temporizing Management. Some infants with ectopic ureter require temporizing diversion with cutaneous ureterostomy as a bridge to definitive reconstruction. Diversion is a consideration in infants with sepsis or massive dilation and uncertain functionality. Loop or end ureterostomy may be used, providing decompression and functional assessment of the affected unit before definitive management. Alternatively, decompression may be achieved via refluxing anastomosis of the lateral bladder wall to the medial aspect of the dilated ectopic ureter. Although the latter option may decrease the risk of UTI and urinary tract colonization, it may also increase the complexity and difficulty of subsequent definitive reconstruction.

Definitive Management. In children with a single-system ectopic ureter and salvageable ipsilateral renal function, ureteral reimplantation with or without tapering is indicated. If the associated kidney is both nonfunctional and problematic, nephrectomy is considered.

For children with a duplex system, definitive reconstruction options mirror those for duplex system ureteroceles, guided by the relative function of the affected moiety and presence or absence of lower moiety VUR.

In general, common sheath ureteral reimplantation is the foremost option for children with UM function and LM VUR because reflux in this setting is unlikely to resolve spontaneously. For those with UM function and no LM VUR, ipsilateral ureteroureterostomy is an excellent option. Last, for children with nonfunctioning UM, heminephrectomy may be considered, with or without LM ureteral reimplantation (Fig. 7.8).

RENAL CYSTIC DISEASE

Multicystic Dysplastic Kidney

MCDK is the most common cause of renal cystic disease in infants and young children and the second most common cause of abdominal mass in newborns (severe hydronephrosis is most common). MCKD may represent an extreme variant of obstructive hydronephrosis or UPJ obstruction, in which all functional parenchyma is compromised. Detection is typically via prenatal ultrasound. Radiographically, MCDK is characterized by haphazard distribution of noncommunicating cysts without a larger central cyst. This is in contrast to severe UPJ obstruction, wherein calyces are organized around and communicate with the central renal pelvis.

Summary of clinical decision making for ectopic ureter

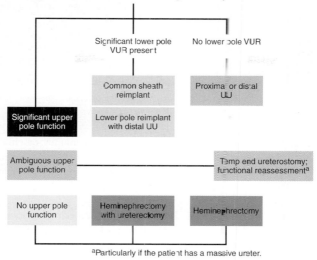

^aParticularly if the patient has a massive ureter.

FIG. 7.8 Algorithm for definitive management.

The natural history of MCDK is benign with a high rate of spontaneous involution. Associated hypertension is rare. Contralateral VUR may be present in 20%–30% of cases. Malignant degeneration is extremely uncommon.

Evaluation includes serial RUSD, generally for the first year of life, to confirm spontaneous involution. VCUG may be obtained to evaluate for contralateral VUR. Nuclear scan is optional to confirm the diagnosis, distinguishing from UPJ obstruction, cystic nephroma, and cystic Wilms tumor. Blood pressure should be carefully followed through childhood.

Nephrectomy is indicated when MCDK causes mass effect with respiratory or gastrointestinal compromise, refractory hypertension, or spontaneous rupture or hemorrhage from trauma (Fig. 7.9).

Polycystic Kidney Disease

Autosomal recessive polycystic kidney disease (ARPKD) results from mutations in the *PKHD1* gene and consequent defects in the fibrocystin protein. In contrast to the more common autosomal

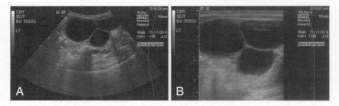

FIG. 7.9 (A and B) Renal ultrasonogram of large left multicystic dysplastic kidney. There are multiple large cysts. No definite renal cortex is seen.

dominant form, ARPKD typically presents in infancy or childhood. Poor renal function may result in oligohydramnios and respiratory distress after delivery secondary to pulmonary hypoplasia. Patients may have flank masses from bilaterally enlarged kidneys.

Radiographically, the kidneys have increased echogenicity because of microcysts. Macrocysts appear with increasing age. All patients have associated congenital hepatic fibrosis and variable degrees of biliary ectasia. For those who survive the neonatal period, hypertension and renal insufficiency are major manifestations. Severely affected patients may require nephrectomy due to mass effect or respiratory or gastrointestinal compromise. Most patients eventually require dialysis and transplantation.

Autosomal dominant polycystic kidney disease typically presents in the third or fourth decade of life. Known autosomal dominant disease in a parent may prompt radiographic screening or genetic testing in childhood, resulting in early detection (Fig. 7.10).

Juvenile Nephronophthisis or Medullary Cystic Kidney Disease

Juvenile nephronophthisis (JN) is an autosomal recessive disorder representing the most common genetic cause of end-stage renal disease in childhood and adolescence. Patients present with polyuria, polydipsia, and small stature. Polyuria is secondary to concentration defect and salt wasting. Blood pressure is typically normal. Anemia and normal urinalysis without proteinuria are common. Patients have small kidneys bilaterally with loss of corticomedullary differentiation and corticomedullary cysts, which may not appear until adolescence or adulthood.

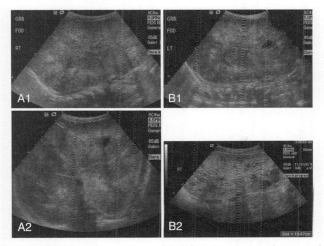

FIG. 7.10 Ultrasonographic appearance of the kidneys in neonates with autosomal recessive polycystic kidney disease (ARPKD) and autosomal dominant polycystic kidney disease (ADPKD) can be similar. (A1 and A2) Newborn with ARPKD. Note the large size and hyperechogenic, homogeneous appearance of the renal parenchyma. A2 is a cross-sectional cut of the baby's abdomen showing both kidneys to be large and occupying a large portion of the abdominal cavity. (B1 and B2) Newborn with ADPKD. Again note the abnormal renal architecture and the hyperechogenic appearance of the kidneys. The parenchyma consists of multiple tiny cysts, with some being slightly larger than others. (Courtesy of Marta Hernanz-Schulman, MD.)

Medullary cystic kidney disease is in an autosomal dominant condition caused by a defect in uromodulin. Presentation and radiographic appearance are nearly identical to JN. However, patients with medullary cystic kidney disease have hypertension and may develop gout during adolescence.

Management for both conditions is supportive, with blood pressure control and sodium replacement in some cases. Dialysis and transplant are often required, and grafts are not susceptible to either disease process (Fig. 7.11).

Von Hippel-Lindau Syndrome

Von Hippel Lindau (VHL) syndrome is characterized by cerebellar hemangioblastoma, retinal angioma, pheochromocytoma, epididymal papillary cystadenoma, renal cysts, and renal cell carcinoma.

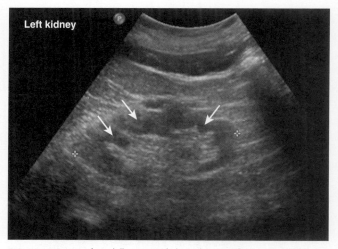

FIG. 7.11 Features of medullary cystic kidney disease. Ultrasonogram demonstrating corticomedullary cysts, some of which are indicated by *arrows*. The hyperechogenicity is secondary to the tubulointerstitial fibrosis. (From Simms RJ, Eley L, Sayer JA. Nephronophthisis. *Eur J Hum Gen* 2009;17:406-416.)

Renal cysts are often the earliest manifestation of the disease, occurring in 80% of patients. Cysts larger than 2 cm are more likely to be malignant. Aggressive imaging surveillance is required in patients with VHL to monitor for development of renal cell carcinoma or pheochromocytoma.

CALYCEAL DIVERTICULUM

A calyceal diverticulum is a cystic cavity lined by transitional epithelium, which communicates with a calyx or renal pelvis through a narrow isthmus. Small diverticula are usually asymptomatic yet may present clinically with pain, infection, milk of calcium, or stone formation.

Ultrasound typically demonstrates a fluid-filled area positioned more centrally than a simple cortical cyst. Computed tomography or magnetic resonance urogram may show pooling of contrast in the diverticulum. Asymptomatic patients do not require treatment. Indications for surgical intervention include febrile UTI, pain, or stone formation. Surgical approach is

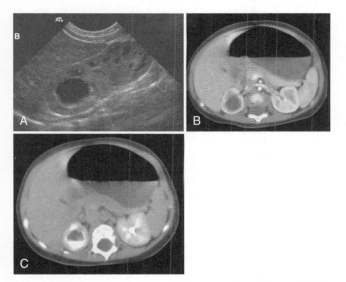

FIG. 7.12 Calyceal diverticulum. (A) Renal ultrasonography reveals a round lesion that could be confused with a renal cyst. Because of the patient's history of recurrent febrile urinary tract infections, contrast-enhanced computed tomography was performed. (B) Early contrast images reveal no enhancement of the lesion; however, delayed imaging (C) reveals contrast layering in a portion of the collecting system, confirming the diagnosis of calyceal diverticulum.

determined by diverticular position and orientation. Posterior diverticula may be approached percutaneously for nephrolithotomy or diverticular ablation. Anteriorly located diverticula may be approached laparoscopically or robotically for marsupialization and epithelial fulguration. Superiorly located diverticula may be approached ureteroscopically with methylene blue localization, diverticular neck dilation, and endoscopic stone extraction (Fig. 7.12).

Suggested Readings

Calderon-Margalit R, Golan E, Twig C, et al. History of childhood kidney disease and risk of adult end-stage renal disease. *N Engl J Med* 2018;378(5):428-438.

Figueroa VH, Chavhan GB, Oudjhane K, Farhat W. Utility of MR urography in children suspected of having ectopic ureter. *Pediatr Radiol* 2014;44(8):956-962.

Han MY, Gibbons MD, Belman AB, et al. Indications for nonoperative management of ureteroceles. *J Urol* 2005;174(4 Pt 2):1652-1655.

Huang WY, Peters CA, Zurakowski D, et al. Renal biopsy in congenital ureteropelvic junction obstruction: evidence for parenchymal maldevelopment. *Kidney Int* 2006;69(1):137-143.

Jawdat J, Rotem S, Kocherov S, et al. Does endoscopic puncture of ureterocele provide not only an initial solution, but also a definitive treatment in all children? Over the 26 years of experience. *Pediatr Surg Int* 2018;34(5):561-565.

Kawal T, Srinivasan AK, Talwar R, et al. Ipsilateral ureteroureterostomy: does function of the obstructed moiety matter? *J Pediatr Urol* 2019;15(1):50.e1-50.e6. doi:10.1016/j.jpurol.2018.08.012.

Sander JC, Bilgutay AN, Stanasel I, et al. Outcomes of endoscopic incision for the treatment of ureterocele in children at a single institution. *J Urol* 2015;193(2):662-666.

Sparks S, Viteri B, Sprague BM, et al. Evaluation of differential renal function and renographic patterns in patients with dietl crisis. *J Urol* 2013;189(2):684-689.

8

Management of Pediatric Kidney Stone Disease

DOUGLAS W. STORM AND CHRISTOPHER S. COOPER

CONTRIBUTORS OF CAMPBELL-WALSH-WEIN, 12TH EDITION

Gregory E. Tasian, and Lawrence A. Copelovitch

EPIDEMIOLOGY OF PEDIATRIC KIDNEY STONE DISEASE

The incidence of nephrolithiasis has increased over the past several decades 5%–10% per year for children. Among all pediatric age groups, the greatest increase is among adolescents, particularly females. Girls have a higher frequency of stones compared with boys. In adults, approximately 75%–80% of stones are calcium oxalate, 5% are calcium phosphate, 10%–20% are struvite, and 5% are pure uric acid. Children have a similar distribution of stones, with calcium phosphate stones being slightly more common and uric acid stones being less common. The notion that most stones that form during childhood are caused by rare genetic causes, inborn errors of metabolism, or infection is not true. Patients who develop kidney stone disease during childhood are at risk for development of comorbidities such as decreased bone mineral density, chronic kidney disease, and heart disease.

EVALUATION

Evaluation of Child with Suspected Nephrolithiasis

Ultrasound is the initial imaging study recommended for children with suspected nephrolithiasis reserving a noncontrast computed tomography (CT) scan for children with a nondiagnostic ultrasound in whom the clinical suspicion for stones remains high. The

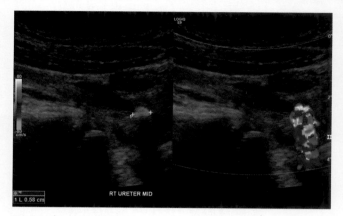

FIG. 8.1 Ultrasonographic appearance of ureteral stone. A stone appears as an echogenic focus on gray-scale with confirmatory "twinkle artifact" on color Doppler. The pulse repetition frequency should be maximized when evaluating with Doppler. Stones smaller than 4 mm typically do not have an associated posterior acoustic shadow using modern ultrasound machines, transducers, and software packages.

criteria for defining a stone on ultrasound are (1) hyperechoic focus in the renal papillae, calyces, or renal pelvis and (2) confirmatory twinkle artifact (Fig. 8.1). Although historically the presence of a posterior acoustic shadow was a necessary diagnostic criterion for a kidney stone, modern harmonic and spatial compounding ultrasound technology does not generate shadows as readily, particularly for stones less than 4 mm. Ultrasound has >70% sensitivity and >95% specificity for detecting urinary tract stones, including stones located in the mid-ureter.

Noncontrast CT has nearly 100% sensitivity and specificity to identify kidney stones. CT, however, delivers ionizing radiation, which is associated with an increased risk for malignancy. Although the attributable risk for cancer from a single CT scan performed for kidney stones is small (0.2%–0.3% above baseline), the cumulative risk is higher for those undergoing repeated studies. When necessary (e.g., stone not visualized on ultrasound but with secondary signs of obstruction such as hydronephrosis), a

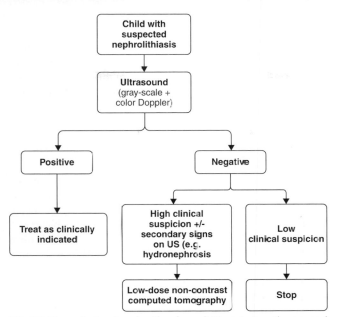

FIG. 8.2 Diagnostic imaging algorithm for pediatric patients with suspected kidney or ureteral stones.

low-dose noncontrast CT of the abdomen and pelvis should be performed (Fig. 8.2).

Medical History

A focused dietary history with special emphasis on fluid and salt intake, vitamin (A, C, D) and mineral supplementation, and special diets (e.g., ketogenic diet) is indicated in every patient. A detailed medication history with special emphasis on corticosteroids, diuretics (furosemide, acetazolamide), protease inhibitors (indinavir), antibiotics and antiepileptics (e.g., topiramate) should also be obtained. Children with a history of prematurity, urinary tract abnormalities, urinary tract infections (UTIs), intestinal malabsorption, and prolonged immobilization are at increased risk for developing stones.

Metabolic Investigation

Children with a metabolic abnormality have a fivefold increased risk for recurrence compared with children with no metabolic disorder. Consequently, some believe all children should undergo a comprehensive metabolic evaluation. The need for such an analysis after a child's first kidney stone has become somewhat controversial, as the composition of pediatric kidney stones have become similar to that seen in adults. An analysis should be performed of a passed or retrieved stone. Further metabolic evaluation could include serum and urine studies in patients in whom stone analysis could not be performed or for those with either calcium or uric acid–based stones. A serum creatinine may be used to evaluate for acute kidney injury or chronic kidney disease. Serum calcium, phosphorous, bicarbonate, magnesium, and uric acid levels are effective in screening for hypercalcemia/hypocalcemia-associated calculi. A 24-hour urine collection will evaluate urinary levels of calcium, oxalate, uric acid, sodium, citrate, cystine, creatinine, as well as urinary volume and pH.

Urine Metabolic Abnormalities

Hypercalciuria is found in 30%–50% of children. The most common cause of hypercalicuria in both children and adults is idiopathic hypercalciuria. Increased urinary oxalate excretion may be caused by an inherited metabolic disorder (primary hyperoxaluria) or, more commonly, as a secondary phenomenon caused by increased oxalate absorption or excessive intake of oxalate precursors. Gastrointestinal absorption varies inversely with dietary calcium intake, and, as a result, calcium-deficient diets may increase oxalate absorption and hyperoxaluria. Cystinuria is an autosomal recessive disorder, resulting in disordered amino acid transport in the proximal tubule. In spite of the higher uric acid excretion observed in children, uric acid nephrolithiasis is rather rare in childhood, accounting for <5% of all renal calculi. Hyperuricosuria in the setting of low urinary pH is the greatest risk factor for uric acid stone formation.

There may be other inborn metabolic diseases that may also lead to pediatric stone formation. A summary of such conditions is included in Table 8.1.

Table 8.1 Inherited Conditions Leading to Nephrolithiasis

CONDITION	INHERITANCE PATTERN/GENETIC CAUSE	PRESENTING SYMPTOMS	MEDIAN PRESENTING AGE	TYPE OF STONE FOUND	MEDICAL TREATMENT
Primary hyperoxaluria	Autosomal recessive; Defect of hepatic AGT enzyme	Renal calculi, nephrocalcinosis, renal impairment, hyperoxaluria, hyperglycoluria	5–6 years; Can be first detected as infant or into adulthood	Calcium oxalate	High fluid intake, potassium or sodium citrate, orthophosphate, pyridoxine, liver/kidney transplantation
Cystinuria	Autosomal recessive	Renal calculi	Second to third decades of life	Cystine	High fluid intake, limited salt intake, urinary alkalinization, low-protein diet, chelators
Phosphoribosyl pyrophosphate (PRPP) synthetase superactivity	X-linked inheritance	Usually young males, gouty arthritis, nephrolithiasis	Childhood	Uric acid	Allopurinol
Hypoxanthine-guanine phosphoribosyl transferase (HGPRT) deficiency Lesch-Nyhan syndrome	X linked inheritance	Neurologic manifestations, self-mutilation, hyperuricemia, hyperuricosuria	Childhood	Uric acid	Allopurinol
Adenine phosphoribosyl transferase (APRT) deficiency	Autosomal recessive	Nephrolithiasis	Early childhood	2,8-Dihydroxyadenine (DHA)	Allopurinol, high fluid intake, dietary purine restriction

Continued

AGT, Alanine-glyoxylate transaminase.

Table 8.1 Inherited Conditions Leading to Nephrolithiasis—cont'd

CONDITION	INHERITANCE PATTERN/GENETIC CAUSE	PRESENTING SYMPTOMS	MEDIAN PRESENTING AGE	TYPE OF STONE FOUND	MEDICAL TREATMENT
Xanthine-oxidase (XOD) deficiency	Mutations of 2p22	Nephrolithiasis, myopathy, low plasma levels of uric acid	5 years	Xanthine	Low purine diet, high fluid intake
Glycogen storage disease Type 1 (GSD-1)	Autosomal recessive	Hepatomegaly, short stature, osteoporosis, hypoglycemia, lactacidemia, hyperlipidemia, hypercalciuria, hypocitraturia, hyperuricemia	Childhood with increasing incidence with age	Calcium	Oral citrate therapy, salt reduction, metabolic control of acidosis
Dent disease	X-linked recessive	Nephrolithiasis, proteinuria, hypercalciuria, rickets, hypotonia, cataracts	Early childhood	Calcium	Thiazides, ACE inhibitors
Familial primary hypomagnesemia with hypercalciuria and nephrocalcinosis (FHHNC)	Autosomal recessive	Nephrolithiasis, polyuria, polydipsia, failure to thrive, seizures, muscular tetany, rickets, severe ocular involvement	1–8 years of age	Calcium	Magnesium supplements, thiazides, renal transplant

ACE, Angiotensin-converting enzyme.

MANAGEMENT OF CHILDREN AND ADOLESCENTS WITH KIDNEY AND URETERAL STONES

Medical Expulsion Therapy

Medical expulsion therapy (MET) is the use of α-blockers or, less commonly, calcium-channel blockers to facilitate passage of a ureteral stone. The mechanism for MET in increasing stone passage is that type 1a and 1d α-receptors are found in high concentrations in the smooth muscle of the distal third of the ureter and at the ureterovesical junction. Spontaneous stone passage without MET is higher among older patients and for smaller (<5 mm) and more distal ureteral stones. The American Urological Association (AUA) and Endourological Society Guideline for the surgical management of urinary stones recommends that pediatric patients with uncomplicated ureteral stones ≤10 mm should be offered "observation with or without MET using α-blockers" (Grade B Level of Evidence).

Surgical Management

Options for Surgical Management. Up to 60% of children with kidney or ureteral stones require surgery. Surgical options for pediatric patients include ureteroscopy (URS), shock wave lithotripsy (SWL), and percutaneous nephrolithotomy (PCNL), all of which require anesthesia and, traditionally, radiation exposure. A recent review reported stone clearance ranging from 70%–97% for PCNL, 85%–88% for URS, and 80%–83% for SWL. The choice of intervention is determined primarily by the size and location of the stone, patient anatomy, and patient (and provider) preference (Table 8.2)

Radiation Risks Associated with Surgical Management. Patients with nephrolithiasis are exposed to radiation during diagnostic evaluation, operative treatment, and for surveillance after surgery. Cumulative radiation exposure is a particularly important consideration for children with nephrolithiasis since they are likely to require future diagnostic imaging and surgical interventions that often use ionizing radiation. Recent techniques utilizing ultrasound for URS, SWL, and PCNL offer decreased radiation exposure in children. Checklists designed to reduce radiation exposure may also reduce fluoroscopy time, improve skin-to-image

Table 8.2 2016 American Urological Association and Endourological Society Recommendations for the Surgical Management of Urinary Stones for Pediatric Patients

RECOMMENDATION	STRENGTH OF RECOMMENDATION	LEVEL OF EVIDENCE
In pediatric patients with uncomplicated ureteral stones <10 mm, clinicians should offer observation with or without medical expulsive therapy using α-blockers	Moderate: net benefit or harm moderate	B: Moderate certainty
Clinicians should offer URS or SWL for pediatric patients with ureteral stones who are unlikely to pass the stones or who failed observation and/or MET, based on patient-specific anatomy and body habitus	Strong: net benefit or harm substantial	B: Moderate certainty
Clinicians should obtain a low-dose CT scan on pediatric patients before performing PCNL	Strong: net benefit or harm substantial	C: Low certainty
In pediatric patients with ureteral stones, clinicians should not routinely place a stent before URS	Panel consensus, based on members' clinical training, experience, knowledge, and judgment for which there is no evidence.	Expert opinion
In pediatric patients with a total renal stone burden ≤20 mm, clinicians may offer SWL or URS as first-line therapy	Moderate: net benefit or harm moderate	C: Low certainty

In pediatric patients with a total renal stone burden >20 mm, both PCNL and SWL are acceptable treatment options. If SWL is utilized, clinicians should place an internalized ureteral stent or nephrostomy tube	Panel consensus, based on members' clinical training, experience, knowledge, and judgment for which there is no evidence	Expert opinion
In pediatric patients, except in cases of coexisting anatomic abnormalities, clinicians should not routinely perform open, laparoscopic, or robotic surgery for upper tract stones	Panel consensus, based on members' clinical training, experience, knowledge, and judgment for which there is no evidence	Expert opinion
In pediatric patients with asymptomatic and nonobstructing renal stones, clinicians may utilize active surveillance with periodic ultrasonography	Panel consensus, based on members' clinical training, experience, knowledge, and judgment for which there is no evidence	Expert opinion

CT, Computed tomography; *MET*, medical expulsive therapy; *PCNL*, percutaneous nephrolithotomy; *SWL*, shock wave lithotripsy; *URS*, ureteroscopy.

intensifier distance, and increase utilization of appropriate dose settings for children undergoing these procedures.

Surgical Antibiotic Prophylaxis. Prophylaxis is indicated in all patients undergoing URS or PCNL and for patients undergoing SWL who are at increased risk for infection. A urine culture should be obtained before all upper tract procedures to determine if the urine is sterile, and culture results are used to guide preoperative antibiotic therapy. Patients undergoing percutaneous procedures, patients with high-grade obstruction, or patients with an indwelling stent are at increased risk of urosepsis highlighting the need for prophylaxis in these patients.

Ureteroscopic Management of Upper Urinary Tract Calculi. Either SWL or URS should be first-line treatment for children with ureteral stones who have failed observation/MET or renal stone burden of ≤20 mm. Because of continued miniaturization and availability of endourologic instrumentation, stone clearance with this technique in children exceeds 85% with complication rates similar to the adult population. Although 25% of children undergoing URS require a staged procedure, routine "prestenting" before URS is not recommended. The complications of URS include ureteral injury, urinary tract infection, and bleeding. Serious complications (> Clavien 3) are uncommon. These include unrecognized ureteral injury, including mucosal flaps and tears, perforation, false passage, and partial to complete ureteral avulsion. Should a ureteral injury occur, the procedure should be aborted, and a ureteral stent should be placed to mitigate shear force injury on the ureter, ischemic damage, and extravasation of irrigant or urine.

Shock Wave Lithotripsy. SWL use in children have reported complication, safety, and stone clearance rates comparable to adult cohorts. Along with URS, SWL is a treatment option for upper tract calculi 15 mm or smaller in children. When used as a primary treatment option for upper tract calculi, SWL efficacy ranges from 68%–84%. However, stone clearance in children with a history of a urologic anomaly or urinary tract reconstruction is low. Depending on body habitus, stone size, and stone location, URS or PCNL may be better treatment options for these children.

Stone size is an important determinant of stone clearance after SWL. Studies report a 91% clearance for mean stone diameter less than 10 mm versus 75% clearance for stone size greater than 10 mm. Although SWL is considered a treatment option for pediatric patients with renal stones greater than 20 mm, the probability of clearance is lower than PCNL and requires multiple treatments.

Stone location is an important determinant of SWL outcomes; however, the most effective management of lower pole calculi has yet to be determined in children. Stone clearance for lower pole stones range from 56% to 61% with retreatment rates of 40%. SWL failure and retreatment rates were associated with increased mean stone burden, increased infundibular length, and an infundibulo-pelvic angle greater than 45 degrees. Stone composition is also an important effect modifier of SWL efficacy. Cystine stones are uniquely challenging because of their hardness and high recurrence rates.

The short-term side effects of SWL include hematuria (up 44%) and subcapsular or perirenal hematoma. In addition, children treated with SWL need to pass stone fragments and are at risk for intermittent renal colic, emergency department visits for pain control, and steinstrasse. There is also concern for an increased risk of developing hypertension following SWL in children although studies to date are not conclusive.

Percutaneous Nephrolithotomy. PCNL is considered first-line therapy for renal stones greater than 20 mm in children, with stone clearances of approximately 90%. The continued miniaturization of access sheaths and nephroscopes and improvements in stone fragmentation technology have allowed use of smaller access tracts, which mitigates the risk for bleeding while maintaining stone-free rates at or above 75%. Despite the AUA guidelines that state both SWL and PCNL are options for children with renal stones greater than 20 mm, PCNL may be a better option for these patients because SWL is less effective than PCNL for large renal stones.

PCNL is technically challenging, and surgeon experience with PCNL is paramount in developing treatment plans to optimize efficacy with minimal morbidity. CT before PCNL is recommended, and the images must be reviewed carefully to determine if stones are amenable to a percutaneous procedure and to determine the optimal calyx to access the stone. Stone size, stone location, and adjacent organs should be considered. In addition, any alteration in renal anatomy caused by scoliosis, lordosis, or kyphosis should also be considered. The risks associated with PCNL include bleeding requiring transfusion, delayed renal hemorrhage requiring angioembolization, sepsis, pneumothorax, hemothorax, urothorax, incomplete stone clearance, and injuries to adjacent organs.

Urinary tract infections should be treated before PCNL. A urine culture and antibiotic sensitivities should be checked 2 to 3 weeks before the procedure. Historically, primary PCNL with adjunctive SWL to clear residual fragments was often performed for children ("sandwich therapy"). However, with efficacy of PCNL around 90% for large stone burdens, miniaturization of nephroscopes, and concerns of potential increased risk of developing hypertension following SWL, the indications for sandwich therapy are limited.

The proportion of children who experience some complication after PCNL ranges from 15% to 39%. Although most of these complications are minor, complications greater than or equal to Clavien 3 occur in 1%–16% (Table 8.3). The probability of operative blood loss requiring transfusion is consistently <10%. Complications included postoperative fever (30%) and need for transfusion (24%). Transfusion was associated with operative time, sheath size, and stone burden. Studies have demonstrated that the most significant determinants affecting complication rates are operative time, sheath size, midcalyceal puncture, and partial staghorn formation. PCNL has not been shown to cause loss of kidney function or scarring.

Should significant bleeding occur, the operation should be aborted, and either a Foley catheter or reentry catheter should be placed in the collecting system through the nephrostomy tract and treated as clinically indicated similar to adult patients. Should a renal pelvis injury occur, the operation should be stopped, and an antegrade ureteral stent should be placed, if feasible. Treatment of known complications of PCNL in children, including hydrothorax, colonic injury, and postoperative bleeding, is similar to adults.

Laparoscopic and Robotic-Assisted Pyelolithotomy. Laparoscopy and robotic-assisted surgery are not indicated for upper tract stones in pediatric patients with normal urinary tract anatomy. The primary exception to this is in children or adolescents with renal or ureteral stones and a coexisting anatomic anomaly, such as ureteropelvic junction (UPJ) obstruction. In these patients, robotic (or laparoscopic) pyeloplasty with concomitant stone removal is indicated.

Table 8.3 Historic and Contemporary Outcomes of Percutaneous Nephrolithotomy for Pediatric Patients

AUTHOR YEAR	YEAR	PATIENTS (n)	MEAN AGE (YEARS)	TRACT SIZE	FRAGMENTA-TION METHOD	STONE CLEAR-ANCE (%)	FEVER	SEPSIS	BLOOD TRANSFU-SION (%)	URINE LEAK	PLEURAL INJURY	DEATH	OVERALL COMPLICA-TIONS	≥ CLAVIAN GRADE 3
Yadav et al.	2017	639	12.2	≤2–4 Fr	Pneumatic Holmium	94	19 (3)	NR	43 (6.5)	5 (1)	0	0	143 (22)	13 (2)
Citamak et al.	2015	346	8.5	14–30 Fr	Pneumatic Holmium	73	NR	4 (0.3)	41 (12)	NR	4 (0.3)	1 (<0.1)	NR	NR
Daw et al.	2015	26	3.7	14 Fr	Holmium	77	4 (15)	0 (0)	1 (4)	2 (8)	0 (0)	0 (0)	8 (31)	3 (11)
Dede et al.	2015	39	5.8	12 Fr	Pneumatic Holmium	82	4 (10)	0 (0)	0 (0)	2 (5)	0 (0)	0 (0)	6 (15)	0 (0)
Goyal et al.	2014	158	10	24–30 Fr	Pneumatic	85	8 (5)	10 (6)	12 (8)	12 (0)	2 (1)	0 (0)	62 (39)	10 (16)
Zeng et al.	2013	331	7.8	14–20 Fr	Pneumatic Holmium	80	23 (7)	13 (4)	10 (3)	NR	2 (1)	0 (0)	51 (16)	5 (1.5)
Ozden et al.	2008	53	9.7	20–30 Fr	Ultrasonic Pneumatic	74	NR	NR	9 (17)	3 (6)	1 (2)	0 (0)	NR	NR
Jackman et al.	1998	11	3.4	11 Fr	Electrohydrau-lic lithotripsy	85	NR	0 (0)	0 (0)	NR	NR	0 (0)	NR	NR

NR, Not recorded.

Medical Management of Pediatric Kidney Stones (Secondary Prevention)

Dietary Measures

1. **Fluid Intake**

   Fluid intake is a critical component of stone prevention by reducing the concentration of lithogenic factors including calcium, oxalate, uric acid, and cystine. Most clinicians recommend intake at least equal to calculated maintenance rates in children and greater than 2–2.5 L in adolescents and adults. Even higher fluid intake levels (1.5–2 L/m^2) may be recommended for children with cystinuria or primary hyperoxaluria. As to fluids other than water, reports suggest that fluids that increase urinary pH and citrate excretion such as orange juice, lemonade, and black currant juice reduce the risk for calcium stone formation. Conversely, grapefruit juice appears to increase the risk for calcium-based stones. Whether or not soft drinks increase lithogenic potential remains controversial.

2. **Sodium**

   There is an association between increased sodium intake, urinary calcium excretion, and calcium stone formation. Increased sodium intake promotes calciuria by competing for reabsorption at the level of the renal tubules. A low-salt diet corresponding to less than 2–3 mEq/kg/day in children or less than 2.4 g/day in adolescents or adults is generally recommended for patients with hypercalciuria or calcium-containing stones. A low-salt diet may also reduce urinary cystine excretion in patients with cystinuria.

3. **Calcium**

   There now is substantial evidence that a higher calcium diet is associated with a reduced risk for stone formation. A potential mechanism explaining this seeming paradox is that higher calcium intake effectively binds dietary oxalate in the gut, thereby reducing intestinal oxalate absorption and eventual urinary oxalate excretion. The current recommendation for stone formers is not to restrict dietary calcium intake.

4. **Animal Protein**

   There is evidence for a role of dietary animal proteins (meat, fish, and poultry) in calcium oxalate stone formation. Vegetable and dairy protein sources do not appear to carry the same lithogenic potential. It is generally recommended that children with calculi should not eat excessive amounts of protein but should aim for 100% of the daily recommended allowance for age.

5. **Oxalate**

The role of dietary oxalate in stone formation is controversial because only approximately 10%–20% of urinary oxalate excretion is derived from the diet. As a precautionary measure, most clinicians recommend limiting dietary oxalate ingestion in calcium oxalate stone formers who demonstrate evidence of hyperoxaluria. High oxalate-containing foods include certain nuts (almonds, peanuts, cashews, walnuts, and pecans), spinach, soybeans, tofu, rhubarb, beets, sweet potatoes, wheat bran, okra, parsley, chives, black raspberries, star fruit, green tea, and chocolate. Vitamin C supplements have been associated with increased risk for calcium oxalate stone formation, and therefore these supplements should be discontinued in calcium oxalate stone formers with hyperoxaluria.

6. **Citrate**

Potassium-rich foods such as fruits and vegetables usually contain large amounts of citrate, which are protective against calcium oxalate stone formation. In many studies, a diet high in potassium is protective against urolithiasis. In addition, a potassium-deficient diet can cause increased urinary calcium excretion, overt hypokalemia, and hypocitraturia. As a result, a diet containing potassium-rich fruits and vegetables can theoretically increase urinary citrate excretion directly because of the citrate content found in these foods and indirectly through the dietary potassium content.

7. **Others**

Magnesium complexes with oxalate and may prevent enteric oxalate absorption and decrease calcium oxalate supersaturation in the urine. In some studies, higher dietary magnesium has been associated with a lower risk for stone formation in men, and supplementation may be helpful in the treatment of children with secondary hyperoxaluria. Carbohydrate ingestion has been associated with hypercalciuria, and sucrose ingestion has been found to be associated with urolithiasis. Phytate, a dietary factor found in many high-fiber foods (e.g., cereals, legumes, vegetables, nuts), appears to bind calcium avidly and may inhibit calcium oxalate stone formation.

Pharmacotherapy

1. **Diuretics**

   A thiazide diuretic is often required for children with hypercalciuria that does not respond to a restricted sodium diet. The usual recommendation is hydrochlorothiazide 1–2 mg/kg per day (adult 25–100 mg/day). Potassium citrate can be added to mitigate the effects of potassium depletion.

2. **Alkali Agents**

   Treatment with either potassium citrate (2–4 mEq/kg/day, adults 30–90 mEq/day) or potassium-magnesium citrate has been shown to reduce the recurrence of calcium oxalate stone formation in patients with low or normal citrate excretion. Treatment is considered safe with only minor gastrointestinal side effects; however, one potential concern is that overtreatment with alkali may increase the risk for calcium phosphate stone formation by increasing the urinary pH >6.5, thereby decreasing the calcium phosphate supersaturation product. Potassium citrate is also used to alkalinize the urine in patients with uric acid lithiasis (goal of urine pH >6.5), cystinuria (goal of urine pH >7), and hyperoxaluria.

3. **Thiol-Containing Agents**

   These agents are used for patients with cystinuria in whom fluid/dietary modifications and urinary alkalinization are ineffective in preventing stone recurrences. The two most common agents are D-penicillamine and α-mercaptopropionylglycine (tiopronin). These agents work by reducing the disulfide bond that bridges two molecules of cysteine. Unfortunately, D-penicillamine has a large number of adverse side effects including febrile reactions, gastrointestinal discomfort, liver dysfunction, impaired taste, bone marrow suppression, trace metal deficiencies, membranous glomerulopathy, myasthenia gravis, and skin eruptions (elastosis perforans serpiginosa). The incidence of adverse effects for α-mercaptopropionylglycine is similar but may be slightly less. Monitoring of liver enzymes, complete blood count, urinalysis, and copper and zinc levels should be performed regularly in patients taking these medications.

4. **Allopurinol**

   The mainstay of therapy for most children with uric acid calculi is a combination of high urine output and urinary alkalinization. Allopurinol (4–10 mg/kg/day, adult maximum 300 mg/day) is indicated in patients with both hyperuricemia and hyperuricosuria. Inhibition of xanthine dehydrogenase by allopurinol may lead to accumulation and urinary excretion of xanthine. Rarely, a secondary xanthinuria with xanthine calculi is observed in children on chronic therapy. Allopurinol may also be the agent of choice for treating hyperuricosuric calcium oxalate urolithiasis if there is no concomitant evidence of hypercalciuria, hyperoxaluria, or hypocitraturia.

5. **Pyridoxine**

   Pyridoxine is an important cofactor of the alanine-glyoxylate transaminase (AGT) enzyme. Approximately 10%–30% of children with PH1 are pyridoxine sensitive (>30% reduction of urinary oxalate excretion). In patients with suspected PH1, treatment should be initiated (2–5 mg/kg/day) and titrated upward (8–10 mg/kg/day) until a diagnosis can be made and response assessed. Large doses of pyridoxine have been known to induce sensory neuropathies. There is currently no evidence to suggest that pyridoxine supplementation is beneficial in the treatment of other forms of hyperoxaluria unless a true pyridoxine deficiency exists.

Suggested Readings

Assimos D, Krambeck A, Miller NL, et al. Surgical management of stones: American Urological Association/Endourological Society Guideline, part I. *J Urol* 2016a; 196(4):1153-1160.

Assimos D, Krambeck A, Miller NL, et al. Surgical management of stones: American Urological Association/Endourological Society Guideline, part II. *J Urol* 2016b; 196(4):1161-1169.

Borghi L, Meschi T, Maggiore U, et al. Dietary therapy in idiopathic nephrolithiasis. *Nutr Rev* 2006;64(7 Pt 1):301-312..

Denburg MR, Jemielita TO, Tasian GE, et al. Assessing the risk of incident hypertension and chronic kidney disease after exposure to shock wave lithotripsy and ureteroscopy. *Kidney Int* 2016;89(1):185-192.

Denburg MR, Leonard MB, Haynes K, et al. Risk of fracture in urolithiasis: a population-based cohort study using the health improvement network. *Clin J Am Soc Nephrol* 2014;9(12):2133-2140.

Kokorowski PJ, Chow JS, Strauss KJ, et al. Prospective systematic intervention to reduce patient exposure to radiation during pediatric ureteroscopy. *J Urol* 2013;190 (4 suppl):1474-1478.

National Research Council. *Health risks from exposure to low levels of ionizing radiation. BEIR VII, Phase 2.* Washington, DC: National Academies Press, 2006.

Routh JC, Graham DA, Nelson CP. Epidemiologic trends in pediatric urolithiasis at United States freestanding pediatric hospitals. *J Urol* 2010a;184(3):1100-1104.

Routh JC, Graham DA, Nelson CP. Trends in imaging and surgical management of pediatric urolithiasis at American pediatric hospitals. *J Urol* 2010b;184(4 suppl):1815-1822.

Tasian GE, Cost NG, Granberg CF, et al. Tamsulosin and spontaneous passage of ureteral stones in children: a multi-institutional cohort study. *J Urol* 2014;192(2):506-511.

9

Conditions of the External Genitalia

DANA A. WEISS and CRAIG A. PETERS

CONTRIBUTORS OF CAMPBELL-WALSH-WEIN, 12TH EDITION

Lane S. Palmer, Jeffrey S. Palmer, Christopher J. Long, Mark R. Zaontz, Douglas A. Canning, Julia Spencer Barthold, Jennifer A. Hagerty, and Martin Kaefer

FEMALE

External

Labial Adhesions

Description – Fusion of labia minor.

Epidemiology – 0.6%–1.8%; usually under age 2 years.

Presentation – Seen on exam or by parent; usually asymptomatic; may cause postvoid dribbling, deviated stream or local irritation.

Treatment – Only if symptomatic; most resolve spontaneously. Topical conjugated estrogen (0.625 mg/g) successful in 90% (side effect: breast budding, skin hyperpigmentation). Manual separation with lubricated probe after lidocaine cream. Recurrence common without continued application of moisturizing ointment.

Urethral Prolapse (Fig. 9.1)

Description – Circumferential eversion of urethral mucosa.

Epidemiology – Prepubertal black girls and postmenopausal women.

Presentation – Bleeding from mucosa causes blood spotting.

Treatment – Observation, sitz baths, topical corticosteroids, conjugated estrogens. Surgical excision of redundant mucosa for recurrence.

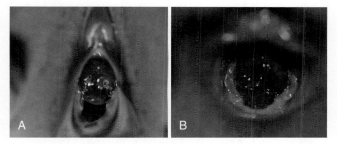

FIG. 9.1 (A and B) Urethral prolapse.

Paraurethral Cyst
Description – Dilation of periurethral glands (Skene's glands) just inside urethral meatus. In neonates, respond to maternal estrogen and secrete mucoid material resulting in cyst formation.

Diagnosis – Displaces urethral meatus and produces deviated urinary stream.

Treatment – Frequently rupture spontaneously. If persistent, can drain by needle puncture.

Gartner's Duct Cyst
Description – Cystic structure representing incomplete regression of the wolffian duct along the anteromedial wall of the vagina. Can be associated with an ectopic ureter entering into the vagina that fails to rupture.

Treatment – Incised to relieve obstruction; can be injected with contrast to delineate anatomy. Ectopic ureter may drain a dysplastic kidney or an upper pole segment which may lead to incontinence.

Vagina

Imperforate Hymen (Fig. 9.2)
Description – Lack of opening in hymenal membrane; can be full of retained vaginal secretions due to maternal estradiol stimulation.

Epidemiology – Most common congenital obstructive anomaly of female reproductive tract.

Diagnosis – Usually at birth, whitish bulge seen; later, identified on exam, or in adolescent with amenorrhea.

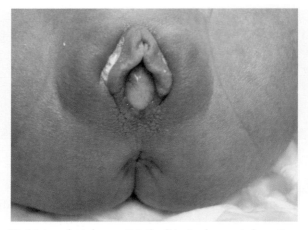

FIG. 9.2 Imperforate hymen. Note the distention from vaginal secretions.

Treatment – In newborns, may be incised transversely at bedside. Needle drainage should not be performed. In older child, incision under anesthesia.

Hymenal Skin Tags

Description – Small excess hymenal tissue, often normal finding.

Treatment – If symptomatic (bleeding, causing tugging), excised and sent for pathology.

Vaginal Septum

Description – Can be at various levels, most frequently in the middle and upper third of the vagina. Usually <1 cm thick, may have small perforations.

Epidemiology – 1 in 70,000 females.

Diagnosis – Present with amenorrhea and distended upper vagina. Imagining: transperineal, transrectal, or abdominal ultrasound, and magnetic resonance imaging (MRI). A high transverse septum must be distinguished from congenital absence of a cervix.

Treatment – Surgery may be delayed with hormonal suppression. Septum can be incised, or completely excised with Z-plasties or vaginal mold to prevent vaginal stenosis.

Vaginal Atresia

Description – Distal vagina fails to form from urogenital sinus; Müllerian structures not affected.

Diagnosis – Distended vagina may be palpable on rectal exam.

Imaging – Ultrasound and/or MRI used to define Müllerian structures.

Treatment – Transverse incision at the hymenal ring with dissection proximally to upper vagina. Pull-through procedure brings vagina to the introitus, sometimes with skin flaps.

Vaginal Agenesis

Description – Congenital absence of proximal vagina in otherwise phenotypically, chromosomally, and hormonally intact female. Component of Mayer-Rokitansky-Kuster-Hauser (MRKH) syndrome. Two forms: type A (typical) – symmetrical uterine remnants and normal fallopian tubes; type B (atypical) – asymmetrical uterine buds and abnormally developed fallopian tubes, with abnormalities in other organ systems.

Epidemiology – 1 in 5000 live female births.

Diagnosis – Present with amenorrhea. Hymenal ring and small distal vaginal pouch present as these derive from the urogenital sinus.

Imaging – Ultrasound and MRI – delineate remnant Müllerian structures, identify if cervix present, and associated renal or skeletal anomalies.

Treatment – Nonoperative – gradual pressure on perineum with dilators creates progressive invagination of the vagina. Operative – skin or intestinal neovagina or buccal mucosal vaginoplasty. Neovagina connected to uterus only if cervix is present.

Complications – Vaginal stenosis – occurs in skin > ileum neovagina > sigmoid neovagina.

Vaginal Rhabdomyosarcoma (Fig. 9.3)

Description – Rhabdomyosarcoma of vagina; best prognosis of female genital tract tumors; primarily embryonal cell type.

Epidemiology – Mean age < 2 years.

Diagnosis – Bleeding or visible mass bulging from introitus, sometimes "grapelike" (botryoid), cluster of tissue.

Imaging – Staging with abdominal/pelvis/chest CT, bone marrow biopsy.

Treatment – Tissue diagnosis by biopsy. Chemotherapy first line, surgery follows for local resection or restaging (see Chapter 11).

Clitoris

Clitoral Hypertrophy

Description – Enlarged clitoral tissue, usually associated with common urogenital sinus.

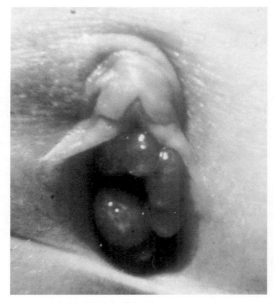

FIG. 9.3 Vaginal rhabdomyosarcoma.

Etiology – Usually enzymatic defect in adrenal steroid synthesis producing excess androgen metabolites. Most common – deficiency of 21-hydroxylase or 11-hydroxylase. Also androgen-producing maternal tumors, local growth factor from neurofibromas.

Evaluation – Serum electrolytes, 17-hydroxyprogesterone level, and karyotype.

Treatment – If congenital adrenal hyperplasia (CAH), replacement of glucocorticoids and mineralocorticoids to prevent production of androgens, further stimulation of the external genitalia.

Prolapsed Ureterocele (Fig. 9.4)

Description – Large ureterocele may prolapse through the urethra.

Diagnosis – Pink or dark purple bulge from urethra; may case urinary retention.

Imaging – Renal and bladder ultrasound (RBUS).

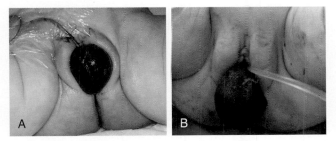

FIG. 9.4 (A and B) Prolapsed Ureterocele.

Treatment – Needle decompression or incision and reduction, placement of urethral catheter.

Urogenital Sinus/Cloacal Anomaly

Description – Confluence of the vagina with the urinary tract; occurs from bladder to the urethral meatus. Persistent cloaca: rectum also joins the vagina posteriorly; single perineal opening.

Epidemiology – Urogenital (UG) sinus usually associated with CAH; incidence 1 in 500 females.

Diagnosis – Single perineal opening; suprapubic mass from distended bladder or hydrometrocolpos.

Imaging – RBUS and pelvic ultrasound; consider MRI.

Treatment – Level of confluence in relation to bladder neck is most critical factor in surgical management; urogenital mobilization to bring urethra and vagina to perineum.

Inguinal Hernia

Description – Patent processus vaginalis extends beyond internal inguinal ring, containing abdominal contents (peritoneal fluid, bowel, omentum, gonads).

Epidemiology – Rarer in girls than boys. May be associated with complete androgen insensitivity syndrome (CAIS).

Diagnosis – Inguinal bulge, occasionally pain.

Treatment – Open or laparoscopic closure of patent processus; ensure phenotypic females are not genetically male: Pelvic ultrasound, vaginoscopy to see cervix, identify ovary and fallopian tube through hernia sac.

MALE

Penis

Phimosis

Description – Physiologic in newborns; pathologic later due to chronic irritation from urine or balanitis (Fig. 9.5A).

Treatment – Spontaneous resolution by 3–4 years in physiologic (due to smegma and erections). If pathologic, treatment with steroid cream first line; circumcision.

Paraphimosis (Fig. 9.5B)

Description – Entrapment of the prepuce behind the glans.

Sequellae – Severe edema of foreskin within hours; ischemia of glans if not reduced.

Treatment – Manual reduction after pressure/icing to reduce edema; dorsal slit procedure.

Smegma

Description – Entrapped sloughed skin cells under unretractable prepuce or under glanular adhesions after circumcision.

Diagnosis – White, round, smooth-walled lesion under skin.

Treatment – Resolution as adhesions open.

Circumcision

Description – Removal of preputial skin.

Risks/Benefits – Benefits: prevention of penile cancer, decreased urinary tract infection (UTI), decrease sexually transmitted diseases. Risks: injury during procedure.

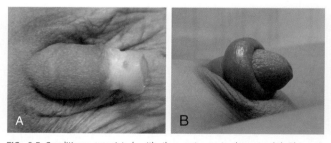

FIG. 9.5 Conditions associated with the uncircumcised penis. (A) Phimosis caused by a preputial ring. (B) Paraphimosis with associated entrapped prepuce behind the glans penis.

- **Procedure** – Neonatal clamp (Gomco, Mogen, Plastibell), local anesthesia (topical and penile block). Later freehand under general anesthesia.
- **Complications** – 0.2%–5% of boys. Bleeding (0.1%) – Usually from frenulum. Wound infection – rare. Skin separation – appears as loss of penile shaft skin. Topical petroleum-based ointment allows closure, usually a normal outcome. Cicatricial scar or secondary phimosis – skin closes over glans. Treat with betamethasone 0.05% or 0.1% (2–3x daily for 21–30 days).

Glanular Adhesions and Penile Skin Bridges

- **Description** – Attachments of inner prepuce to the glans. Adhesions – cell layer thick. Skin bridges – thicker, epithelialized.
- **Epidemiology** – Common in newborns after circumcision, decreasing incidence with age.
- **Treatment** – Lysis or division in office after topical analgesic; under anesthesia with cautery or sutures if broad or thick bridges.

Meatal Stenosis

- **Description** – Narrowing of urethral meatus. Occurs after circumcision.
- **Presentation** – Symptoms: dorsally deflected, narrow urinary stream.
- **Treatment** – Meatotomy – midline ventral incision to enlarge meatus in clinic or in operating room (OR). Meatoplasty – excision of wedge of ventral glans, suture edges of the urethral mucosa to the glans; in OR.

Parameatal Cyst

- **Description** – Small blister or cyst near urethral meatus. Cyst wall is transitional and squamous or columnar epithelium.
- **Treatment** – Complete excision.

Balanitis Xerotica Obliterans (BXO). Lichen Sclerosus Et Atrophicus

- **Description** – Chronic inflammatory, infiltrative dermatosis of glans, meatus, and urethra; can cause phimosis.
- **Presentation** – Tight, scarred phimosis foreskin irritation, discomfort, bleeding; acute urinary retention.
- **Treatment** – For meatus – topical steroids (betamethasone or clobetasol) or systemic tacrolimus. For prepuce: circumcision. After hypospadias repair: excise and replace tissue.
- **Risks** – Recurs in 20%–40%.

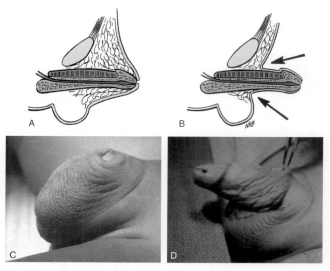

FIG. 9.6 Buried penis (A and C), which may be visualized by retraction of the skin lateral to the penile shaft (B and D).

Inconspicuous Penis, Including Buried/Hidden Penis, Trapped and Webbed Penis (Fig. 9.6)

Description – Penis enclosed in skin, appears small; normal stretched penile length.

Etiology – Congenital – poor penopubic/penoscrotal fixation of skin. Acquired – obesity or trapping from cicatricial scarring.

Surgical correction – Degloving with removal of fibrous bands. Fix subcutaneous tissue to Bucks fascia at penopubic and penoscrotal junctions. Preputial skin used for ventral skin coverage. Alternative for webbing: transverse incision of scrotal web, vertical closure.

Penile Curvature (Chordee)

Description – Usually ventral, associated with skin deficiency; also dorsal or lateral.

Etiology – Usually with hypospadias. Congenital lateral curvature from overgrowth or hypoplasia of corporal body.

Surgical Correction – Deglove penis, excise fibrous tissue superficial to Buck fascia. If resolved – skin coverage. If persists- dorsal plication urethral division and/or corporal grafting (see Hypospadias section). Skin coverage using flaps.

Penile Torsion

Description – Rotational deformity of the penile shaft, usually counterclockwise. Median raphe spirals around the shaft.

Surgical correction – Penis degloved, glans rotated opposite to defect, skin and dartos sutured to coronal collar. For severe torsion, proximal anchoring sutures or rotational dartos flap.

Congenital Hemangioma

Description – Cutaneous/strawberry hemangioma most common. Rapid growth for 3–6 months, then most involute. Subcutaneous/cavernous hemangioma – vascular malformation, tends to enlarge over time.

Workup – Color Doppler ultrasound (CDUS), computed tomography (CT), or MRI to delineate size and depth.

Treatment – For cutaneous – short-term oral corticosteroid or propranolol. For subcutaneous – en bloc resection, preoperative angioembolization may reduce size and risk of bleeding.

Genital Lymphedema

Description – Impaired lymphatic drainage causing progressive penile/scrotal swelling. Anogenital granulomatomosis – associated with Crohn's disease.

Epidemiology – Congenital sporadic (85%), inherited (15%), or acquired. 80% present at puberty.

Treatment – Initially observation. Azathioprine has been used. Surgery if significant or progresses: removal of all involved tissue.

Hypospadias

Description – Classic triad: ectopic, ventrally located urethral meatus; ventral penile curvature; incomplete, dorsally hooded foreskin.

Epidemiology – 1 in 150 to 300 live births. Wide spectrum: intact prepuce with minimal defect (5%), mild, distal variant (70%–85%), severe proximal hypospadias (10%).

Workup – Evaluate for inguinal hernia/hydrocele (9%–16%), cryptorchidism (~7%–10%). If associated with undescended testes, testing for disorder of sexual differentiation (DSD). Routine imaging not recommended.

Surgical correction

Goals – Correction of penile curvature, advancement of urethra. Surgery ideally between 6–12 months old.

Perioperative considerations

Preoperative androgen stimulation – Controversial.

- Benefits: Larger glans to tubularize.
- Concerns: Impaired wound healing, secondary male characteristics.

Urinary diversion – Soft urethral stent facilitates healing; may decrease risk of meatal stenosis and urethrocutaneous fistula.

Antibiotics – Perioperative antibiotics, ± prophylaxis for stent.

Wound care – Petroleum-based ointment.

Postoperative pain control – Combination of acetaminophen and nonsteroidal antiinflammatory drugs (NSAIDs). Ibuprofen safe even in the immediate postoperative period. Minimize narcotics.

Basic Procedure

Assess urethral meatus location, degree of curvature. Circumcising incision, degloving proximal to urethral meatus, reassess curvature. Decision to perform single versus staged repair. Correction of curvature if needed and urethroplasty if single stage, or transfer of skin to ventrum for second stage.

Specific Procedures (Fig. 9.7)

Repairs

Advancement Procedures

- **Urethromeatoplasty** – Single vertical incision between ectopic meatus and distal pit; closed horizontally.
- **Meatal advancement glanuloplasty (MAGPI) and M inverted V glansplasty (MIV)** – For proximal glanular meatus – advance meatus distally by closing the glans underneath, no tubularization of urethra.

Tubularization Procedures

- **Thiersch-Duplay (TD)** – Local tissue distal to meatus tubularized into the neourethra over a catheter; neourethra covered with Dartos flap.
- **Tubularized incised plate (TIP)** – Modification of TD repair – deep incision into the urethral plate to ease tubularization of

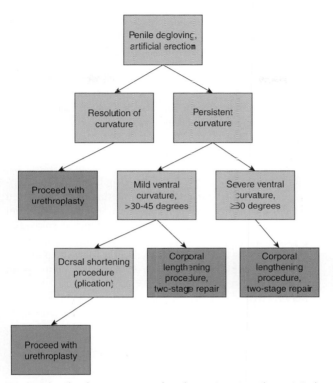

FIG. 9.7 Algorithm for management of penile curvature. Once the penis is degloved, artificial erection is performed. If the curvature is resolved, the urethroplasty can be completed. If there is persistent penile curvature, we use a measurement of 30 degrees as the defining measurement for performing a dorsal plication or a corporal lengthening procedure. If the surgeon is concerned about the quality of the ventral shaft skin in spite of curvature of less than 30 degrees, a corporal lengthening procedure can be considered.

neourethra. Risk of contraction and delayed stricture. Can place dorsal inlay graft (DIG) of inner preputial skin to limit scarring.

- **Onlay island flap (OIF)** – For narrow urethral plate – island flap of dorsal inner preputial skin transposed ventrally, sutured onto urethral plate. Risks: glans dehiscence, urethral diverticulum.

- **Transverse preputial island flap (TPIF)** – Tubularized island flap of inner preputial skin to create entire neourethra in proximal hypospadias if no curvature is present after degloving.

Two-Staged Repairs. Correction of severe penile curvature (plication, division of urethral plate, corporotomy), and tissue transfer (preputial flap or free graft of prepuce or buccal mucosa) in first stage; tubularization of neourethra with U-shaped incision and vascular coverage in second stage.

Complications (Table 9.1)

Epispadias

Description – Mild spectrum of exstrophy-epispadias complex; defect on dorsum of penis, urethra open. Shortened and widened phallus, dorsal chordee. Severity ranges from mild glanular defect to complete penopubic epispadias Associated with abnormal bladder neck, incontinence.

Epidemiology – 1 in 117,000 males, majority complete epispadias.

Workup – RBUS, pelvic x-ray, voiding cystourethrogram (VCUG) to evaluate bladder neck.

Surgical repair – Usually 6–12 months of age. Isolated epispadias repair to separate urethra off corpora and transfer ventrally or combined with bladder neck reconstruction for proximal defect.

Penile and Urethral Abnormal Size or Number

Diphallia

Description – Duplication of penis, usually adjacent. Each phallus may have one or two corporal bodies and urethras.

Epidemiology – 1 in 5 million.

Workup – RBUS and VCUG, penile ultrasound, sometimes MRI. Anal and cardiac anomalies common.

Surgical treatment – Individualized, goal functional and cosmetic result.

Aphallia

Description – Absence of phallus, normally developed scrotum, descended testes; anus anteriorly displaced. Urethra opens at anal verge or in rectum. Karyotype – 46 XY; fertility possible.

Epidemiology – 1 in 10–30 million.

Workup – Karyotype, RBUS, MRI.

Surgical treatment – Neophallus reconstruction with complex local or distant flaps.

Table 9.1 Hypospadias Complications

URETHROPLASTY COMPLICATIONS	SKIN COMPLICATIONS
1. Fistula	1. Skin surplus or deficiency with penile tethering
2. Glans dehiscence	2. Penile torsion >30 degrees
3. Meatal stenosis	3. Lichen sclerosus
4. Urethral stricture	
5. Urethral diverticulum	
6. Recurrent curvature >30 degrees	

Standardized Definitions

- **Fistula**: urethral leak anywhere below the meatus
- **Glans dehiscence**: complete separation of the glans wings resulting in a coronal or more proximal meatus, or complete separation of glans wings with an intervening bridge of skin; objectively: glans fusion measurement <2 mm
- **Meatal stenosis**: obstructive symptoms (straining, prolonged voiding, urinary tract infection, and/or retention) *and* meatal calibration <8 Fr before puberty or <12 Fr after puberty
- **Urethral stricture**: obstructive voiding symptoms (stranguria, prolonged voiding, urinary tract infection, and/or retention) with visual near closure of the urethra on urethroscopy
- **Urethral diverticulum**: visual segmental sacculation of the urethra during voiding
- **Recurrent curvature**: residual ventral, dorsal, or lateral curvature >30 degrees demonstrated on erection (spontaneous or artificial)
- **Skin surplus**: Excess skin ≥2 cm in a circumcised patient when the suprapubic fat pad is retracted
- **Penile torsion**: angle between the normal and true vertical glanular plane >30 degrees from midline (specify clockwise or counterclockwise)
- **Lichen sclerosus**: white cicatrix, preferably with pathology diagnosis

Urethral Duplication

Description – Duplication usually in sagittal plane (94%); ventral urethra usually more normal; dorsal urethra considered accessory. Three types: (Fig. 9.8).

Presentation – Double meatus and double urinary stream visualized. May have incontinence and recurrent UTIs.

Workup – VCUG, direct vision with cystoscopy.

Surgical treatment – Dependent on anatomy; only if symptomatic. Accessory urethra hypoplastic so should not be used as

IA   IB

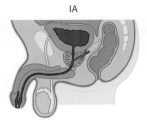   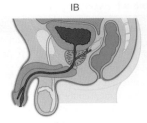

IIA 1   IIA 2

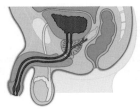   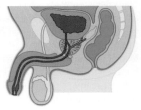

IIA 2 "Y type"   IIB

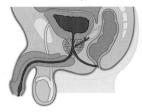   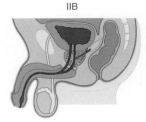

III

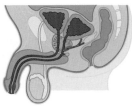

FIG. 9.8 Effman classification.

primary but can be joined to the primary urethra, excised or fulgurated (cautery, sclerosing agents).

Micropenis

Description – Normally formed penis, 2.5 standard deviations below the mean stretched penile length for age (1.9 cm for newborn); testes usually small, frequently cryptorchid. Differentiate buried penis (normal penile shaft but not visualized well) from micropenis. Overweight preteen boys often referred for "micropenis": normal size but appears small due to concealment from prepubic fat pad.

Etiology – Hypogonadotropic hypogonadism, hypergonadotropic hypogonadism (primary testicular failure), and idiopathic.

Priapism

Description – Penile erection > 4 hours without physical or psychological stimulation; usually painful. Four types:

1. Ischemic (venoocclusive, low-flow) – No cavernous blood flow; cavernous blood gas hypoxic, hypercapnic, and acidotic.

Exam – Corpora rigid and painful.

Etiology – Usually homozygous sickle cell disease (predominance of hemoglobin S); Unusual causes: leukemia, other hemoglobinopathies, local malignancy.

Pathophysiology in sickle cell disease – Sickling of red blood cells (RBCs) within sinusoids of corpora during erection → venous stasis → decreased pH, local oxygen tension → more sickling and stasis.

2. Nonischemic (arterial, high-flow) – Unregulated cavernous arterial inflow, usually from vascular fistula. Corpora neither fully rigid nor painful.

Etiology – History of perineal trauma (straddle injury); Fabry disease, sickle cell anemia

3. Stuttering (intermittent) – Recurrent ischemic priapism, short duration with intervening detumescence.

4. Priapism of neonates – Spontaneously resolves.

Etiology – Idiopathic, birth trauma, polycythemia, nitric oxide use.

Treatment of ischemic priapism – Hydration, oxygenation, alkalinization, analgesia; aspiration, irrigation of corpora with α-adrenergic sympathomimetic agent (phenylephrine typically diluted in normal saline to a concentration of 100–200 ug/mL or epinephrine 1:100,000 solution) can follow; exchange transfusion to reduce HbS concentration. To prevent recurrent priapism: pseudoephedrine (α-adrenergic) at bedtime promotes muscle contraction within erectile tissue; phosphodiesterase type 5 (PDE5) inhibitor – PDE5 dysregulation may be involved in priapism.

Testis and Scrotum

Penoscrotal Transposition and Bifid Scrotum

Description – Scrotum extends superiorly to penis or labioscrotal folds completely separated. Usually with proximal hypospadias.

Etiology – Incomplete or failed inferomedial migration of the labioscrotal swellings.

Workup – If complete transposition, RBUS and consider voiding cystourethrography.

Surgical correction – Usually during hypospadias repair. Superior aspects of each half circumscribed and closed ventral to penis.

Risks – Injury to tunica vaginalis and spermatic cord during deeper dissection.

Inguinal Hernia (Fig. 9.9)

Description – Patent processus vaginalis extending beyond internal inguinal ring containing abdominal contents (peritoneal fluid, bowel, omentum, gonads) that pass into the inguinal canal; usually presents as inguinal bulge.

Epidemiology – 1%–5% of children. 5–10x more common in boys; right > left; higher in premature and low birthweight infants.

Imaging – Not required.

Treatment – Surgical repair with high ligation of hernia sac at internal ring; repair soon after diagnosis to prevent incarceration. If incarcerated, urgent exploration. Laparoscopic repair possible.

Complications – Recurrence 0.5%–1%, up to 2% for premature infants; secondary cryptorchidism, testicular atrophy, and vasal injury rare.

Communicating Hydrocele

Description – Patent processus vaginalis containing peritoneal fluid alone, may extend to the tunica vaginalis around testis;

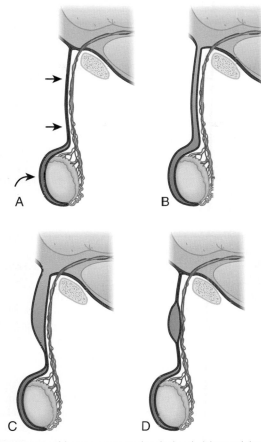

FIG. 9.9 Anatomy of the processus vaginalis in hydrocele. (A) Normal closure of the processus vaginalis; *straight arrows* indicate the funicular process; *curved arrow* is the tunica vaginalis. (B) Communicating hydrocele with complete patency of the processus vaginalis. (C) Funicular hydrocele with distal closure of the processus vaginalis; communication with the peritoneal cavity may also result in hernia. (D) Encysted hydrocele of the spermatic cord. (From Martin LC, Share JC, Peters C, et al. Hydrocele of the spermatic cord: embryology and ultrasonographic appearance. *Pediatr Radiol* 1996;26:523-530.)

fluid flows freely between scrotum and abdomen; may resolve by age 1 year.

Etiology – Increased incidence if abdominal ascites, peritoneal dialysis, or ventriculoperitoneal shunt.

Treatment – See inguinal hernia.

Hydrocele of the Spermatic Cord and Scrotal Hydrocele

Description – Fluid within segment of patent processus vaginalis with obliterated processus distally and proximally (cord) or within tunica vaginalis surrounding the testis without communication proximally (scrotal).

Etiology – ~5% of male infants have scrotal hydrocele; most resolve spontaneously.

Imaging – Not required; may help evaluate testis if not palpable through a tense hydrocele.

Abdominoscrotal Hydrocele

Description – Scrotal hydrocele extending proximally across internal inguinal ring into abdomen, without communication with the peritoneum

Epidemiology – 1.25% of hydroceles, 30% bilateral. Present in infancy, enlarge over time.

Imaging – Ultrasound may show proximal extent.

Treatment – May improve or resolve spontaneously. Primary scrotal approach to drain and excise the enlarged tunica vaginalis with limited dissection decreases inflammation and morbidity from an inguinal dissection. Testes may be undescended; need subsequent orchiopexy.

Cryptorchidism (Fig. 9.10)

Description – One or both testes not located in scrotum; palpable or nonpalpable. Absent testes: lost due to vascular accident or torsion (vanishing), or never formed (agenesis); if never formed, associated with ipsilateral Müllerian duct persistence. Associated with decreased fertility; 2–5x increased risk testicular cancer.

Retractile testes – Scrotal testes that retract out of the scrotum; can be manually pulled to scrotum where they remain temporarily after fatiguing the cremasteric reflex by holding them in place for a minute.

Workup – In case of bilateral nonpalpable testes associated with abnormal penile development, karyotype and hormonal analysis to rule out congenital adrenal hyperplasia.

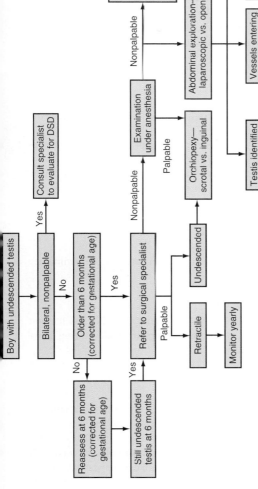

FIG. 9.10 Algorithm for management of the undescended testis. The American Urological Association guideline algorithm for diagnosis and treatment of palpable and nonpalpable testes in patients confirmed to have undescended testis by an experienced examiner. *DSD,* Disorder of sexual differentiation. (From American Urological Association. Evaluation and treatment of cryptorchidism. 2014. http://www.auanet.org/education/guidelines/cryptorchidism.cfm.)

Treatment – Hormonal therapy not recommended. Surgery based on testis location preoperatively. If **palpable**, inguinal approach; if **nonpalpable**, diagnostic laparoscopy defines presence and location of testis in abdomen or if absent (normal vas and vessels entering ring—vanished; blind ending vessels—never formed). Then proceed with laparoscopic orchiopexy, inguinal approach, or scrotal exploration if needed.

Complications – Testicular retraction, atrophy

Follow up – At least 6 months to confirm position of testis. Longer follow-up optional.

Scrotal Pain/Acute Scrotum (Box 9.1)

Torsion of Appendix Testis

Description – Appendix testis (from Müllerian duct) and appendix epididymis (from wolffian duct) can twist, causing pain and swelling.

Epidemiology – Most common cause of scrotal pain in prepubertal boys. Peak age 7–12 years.

Diagnosis – Blue dot sign; focal tenderness at superior pole; preserved symmetric cremasteric reflux; swelling, tenderness, edema (must distinguish from spermatic cord torsion or epididymitis).

Imaging – CDUS – may show abnormal appendage, hyperperfusion of epididymis.

Management – Conservative: ice, oral antiinflammatory agents, limit physical activity.

Testicular Torsion

Extravaginal – infants

Description – Torsion of entire spermatic cord before fixation of tunica vaginalis to dartos; occurs prenatally, during delivery, or postpartum.

Epidemiology – 6.1/100,000 births; increased in high birth weight or difficult delivery; may be bilateral – concurrent or metachronous torsion.

Exam and workup – Testis hard and fixed, scrotum erythematous or dark, may have hydrocele. CDUS.

Treatment – Controversial. If acute change, immediate exploration to attempt salvage, and prevent contralateral torsion. If born with findings, explore immediately to prevent contralateral torsion versus explore electively since unsalvageable

Box 9.1 Differential Diagnosis of Pediatric Adolescent Acute Scrotal Pain

Appendage torsion
    Appendix testis
    Other appendage (epididymis, paradicymis, vas aberrans)
Spermatic cord torsion
    Intravaginal, acute or intermittent
    Extravaginal
Epididymitis
    Infectious
    Urinary tract infection
    Sexually transmitted disease
    Viral
    Sterile or traumatic
Scrotal edema or erythema
    Diaper dermatitis, insect bite, or other skin lesions
    Idiopathic scrotal edema
Orchitis
    Associated with epididymitis with or without abscess
    Vasculitis (e.g., Henoch-Schönlein purpura)
    Viral illness (mumps)
Trauma
    Hematocele or scrotal contusion or testis rupture
Hernia or hydrocele
    Inguinal hernia with or without incarceration
    Communicating hydrocele
    Encysted hydrocele with or without torsion
    Associated with acute abdominal pathology (e.g., appendicitis, peritonitis)
Varicocele
Intrascrotal mass
    Cystic dysplasia or tumor of testis
    Epididymal cyst, spermatocele or tumor
    Other paratesticular tumors
Musculoskeletal pain from inguinal tendonitis or muscle strain
Referred pain (e.g., ureteral calculus or anomaly)

and metachronous torsion rare; concern for increased anesthetic risk in newborn.

Intravaginal

Description – Torsion of spermatic cord within tunica vaginalis; "bell-clapper deformity" and horizontal lie predispose.

Epidemiology – 1/4000 males; left > right; peak ages 12–16 years; familial predisposition.

Evaluation and Workup – Acute severe scrotal pain starting at rest or wakes from sleep; nausea and vomiting. Exam: tender, firm, horizontal orientation, high riding, absent cremasteric reflex, edema and erythema.

Imaging – CDUS – reduced or absent flow compared to contralateral; swirl sign showing twist in cord; heterogeneity of parenchyma.

Treatment – Surgical emergency – viability related to duration of torsion; optimal salvage within 6 hours. Preoperative manual detorsion ("opening the book") – may relieve symptoms exploration still required. Hemiscrotal or midline incision; untwist testis, fasciotomy in tunica albuginea to enhance perfusion an option; fix contralateral testis (three nonabsorbable sutures). If torsed testis viable, pex; if not, orchiectomy. If tunica albuginea incised, use graft of tunica vaginalis to cover.

Intermittent torsion

Description – Intermittent: periodic episodes, self-limited (0.5–2 hours) acute scrotal pain; may precede acute torsion in 30%–50% of patients.

Diagnosis – Often no physical exam or imaging findings by time of evaluation; may have residual swelling.

Imaging – CDUS may show residual edema and hyperemia.

Treatment – Prompt or elective bilateral septopexy.

Epididymitis

Description – Infectious or inflammatory.

Presentation – Insidious onset of pain, sometimes fever and dysuria, nausea rare.

Workup – Diffuse tenderness, scrotal swelling; sometimes pyuria and bacteriuria. Assess history of UTI's, sexual activity, dysfunctional voiding, intermittent catheterization, or urethral anomalies.

Imaging – CDUS – increased epididymal size and blood flow.

Management – Reduce inflammation – ice packs, NSAIDs, scrotal elevation; if infection suspected, antibiotics. Testing and treatment for sexually transmitted infections (STIs) in adolescents.

Varicocele

Description – Abnormal dilation of internal spermatic veins within pampiniform plexus; may be associated with subfertility.

Epidemiology – 8%–16% adolescents, presents after age 10.

Etiology – Increased venous pressure in left renal vein, collateral venous anastomoses, valvular incompetence of the left internal spermatic vein at junction with the left renal vein.

Presentation – Left-sided swelling above testis, found by patient or clinician; sometimes bilateral; rarely – mild pain.

Physical exam – Grading: grade 0 (subclinical): nonpalpable, visualized only on CDUS; grade 1: palpable with Valsalva; grade 2: palpable but not visible; grade 3: easily visible; may be intratesticular in 1%–2%. If veins do not decompress while supine abdominal imaging – to rule out abdominal or pelvic mass. Assess testicular consistency and size. Follow for testicular growth - testes may grow variably throughout puberty.

Workup – Testicular size; semen analysis (no reliable standards for adolescents based on Tanner stage). Controversy regarding correlation between unilateral or total testicular volume and semen parameters; varicocele grade and postoperative catch-up growth do not predict ultimate semen quality.

Treatment – Controversial. Observation for majority. Indications for surgery: size discrepancy (differential or total testicular volume hypotrophy >20%); abnormal semen analysis; pain (rare); intratesticular component of varicocele (not standard indication).

Surgical approaches – inguinal, subinguinal, laparoscopic, or venographic. (Table 9.2).

Epididymal Cyst/Spermatocele

Description – Simple cystic structures on epididymis; similar appearance to spermatocele; spermatocele contain sperm, occur postpubertally.

Epidemiology – ~14% (increasing incidence with age, 35% of boys >15 years)

Table 9.2 Treatment Options for Varicocele

PROCEDURE	COMMENTS	RECURRENCE OR PERSISTENCE	HYDROCELE	TESTICULAR ATROPHY
Open suprainguinal (Palomo)	Mass ligation	2%–4%	0%–30% (10%)[a]	
Laparoscopic:				
Nonlymphatic or artery sparing	Risk of injury to genitofemoral n	0%–9%	11%–32% (7%)[a]	
Artery and/or lymphatic sparing	Risk of injury to genitofemoral n	1%–7%	0%–4%	
Microscopic subinguinal	Artery and lymphatic sparing	0%–10%	0%–6%	Rare
Nonmicroscopic inguinal		7%–33%	8%–14%	
Sclerotherapy		6%–35%	Occasional	Rare

[a]Number in parentheses refers to meta-analysis of Barroso et al., 2009.

       Diagnosis – Palpable by patient or physician; occasionally transient pain; incidental finding on ultrasound.

       Management – May spontaneously resolve; surgical intervention rarely indicated.

Congenital Absence of the Vas Deferens

       Description – Unilateral or bilateral, normal or obstructed contralateral vas; typically infertile.

       Pathophysiology – Associated with less severe mutations of cystic fibrosis gene *CFTR*; associated with persistent mesonephric duct anomaly with renal agenesis or ectopia and partial or complete agenesis of the epididymis and seminal vesicles.

Suggested Readings

American Academy of Pediatrics Task Force on Circumcision: circumcision policy statement. *Pediatrics* 2012;130(3):585-586.

Barthold JS, González R. The epidemiology of congenital cryptorchidism, testicular ascent and orchiopexy. *J Urol* 2003;170(6 Pt 1):2396-2401.

Braga LH, Lorenzo AJ, Bagli DJ, et al. Ventral penile lengthening versus dorsal plication for severe ventral curvature in children with proximal hypospadias. *J Urol* 2008;180(suppl 4):1743-1747 discussion 1747-1748.

Kolon TF, Herndon CD, Baker LA, et al. American Urological Association. Evaluation and treatment of cryptorchidism: AUA guideline. *J Urol* 2014;192(2):337-345.

Montague DK, Jarow J, Broderick GA, et al. American Urological Association guideline on the management of priapism. *J Urol* 2003;170:1318-1324.

10

Disorders of Sexual Development

GINA M. LOCKWOOD AND CHRISTOPHER S. COOPER

CONTRIBUTORS OF CAMPBELL-WALSH-WEIN, 12TH EDITION

Richard Nithiphaisal Yu, David Andrew Diamond, and Richard C. Rink

NORMAL SEXUAL DEVELOPMENT

Normal sexual development can be categorized into three processes: establishment of genotypic (chromosomal) sex, establishment of phenotypic sex, and formation of gender identity. Disruption of any of these interactions is described as a disorder of sexual development (DSD).

During the first 6 weeks of development, the gonadal ridge, germ cells, internal ducts and external genitalia are bipotential in both 46,XY and 46,XX embryos. Multiple genes are thought to determine chromosomal sex. Specifically, **the *SRY* (sex-determining region Y) gene on the Y chromosome is considered the testis-determining factor**. Under this influence, the bipotential gonadal ridges differentiate into testes, and germ cells develop into spermatocytes (Fig. 10.1). In the absence of *SRY*, ovarian organogenesis results (Table 10.1).

The Sertoli cells of the testis secrete anti-Müllerian hormone (AMH) at 7 to 8 weeks of gestation, which promotes Müllerian duct regression. Testosterone secretion by the fetal testis Leydig cells occurs at approximately 9 weeks of gestation. Androgens promote virilization of wolffian duct structures, the urogenital sinus, and the genital tubercle. Testosterone enters target tissues by passive diffusion, and wolffian duct virilization does not occur if local androgens are not present. In some cells, testosterone is converted to dihydrotestosterone (DHT) by intracellular 5α-reductase. Testosterone or DHT then binds to an intracellular

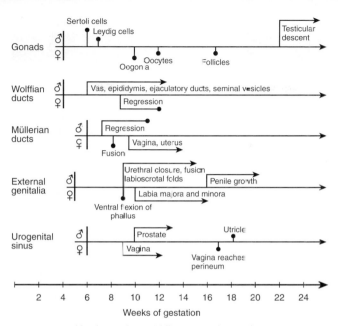

FIG. 10.1 Timetable of normal sexual differentiation. (From White PC, Speiser FW. Congenital adrenal hyperplasia due to 21-hydroxylase deficiency. *Endocr Rev* 2000;21(3):245-291.)

androgen receptor. DHT binds to the receptor with greater affinity and stability than does testosterone. **In tissues equipped with 5α-reductase at the time of sexual differentiation (e.g., prostate, urogenital sinus, external genitalia), DHT is the active androgen.** Masculinization of the external genitalia is complete by 12–13 weeks of gestation (Fig. 10.2). Penile growth and testicular descent occur over the third trimester. In the female fetus, the absence of testosterone maintains the appearance of external genitalia at the 6-week gestational stage (Fig. 10.3).

The wolffian ducts adjacent to the testes form the epididymis, joining with the rete testes. Distally the wolffian ducts join the urogenital sinus to develop into the seminal vesicles. In the female fetus without testosterone, the wolffian ducts regress. Without AMH, the Müllerian ducts develop into the female internal reproductive tract, including the fallopian tubes and uterus. Contact of the ducts with the urogenital sinus ultimately forms the vagina.

Table 10.1 Common Embryologic Origins of Genital Structures.

MALE	EMBRYONIC STRUCTURE	FEMALE
Testis	Indifferent Gonad	Ovary
Seminiferous tubules	Gonadal cortex	Ovarian follicles
Rete testis	Gonadal medullar	Rete ovarii
Gubernaculum testis	Gubernaculum	Ovarian ligament Round ligament of uterus
Efferent ductules of testis Paradidymis	Mesonephric tubules	Epoöphroon Paraoöphoron

Appendix of epididymis
Ductus deferens
Ejaculatory duct and
  seminal vesicle
Ureter, pelvis, calyces,
  collecting tubules
	Wolffian duct
	(mesonephric
	duct)
		Gartner duct
		Ureter, pelvis, calyces,
		  and collecting tubules

Kidney
Nephrons (glomerulus,
  proximal tubule, loop
  of Henle, distal tubule)
	Intermediate mesoderm	Kidney
		Nephrons (glomerulus,
		  proximal tubule, loop
		  of Henle, distal tubule)

Appendix of testis	Müllerian duct (paramesonephric duct)	Paratubal cyst Fallopian tube Uterus Cervix

Bladder and trigone
Urethra
Prostate
Verumontanum
Prostatic utricle
Periurethral glands (Littre)
Bulbourethral glands
  (Cowper's)
	Urogenital sinus	Bladder and trigone
		Urethra
		Vagina, hymen
		Urethral glans (Skene's)
		Greater vestibular glands
		  (Bartholin's)

Penis
Glans penis
Corpora cavernosa of penis
Corpus spongiosum of
  penis
	Genital tubercle	Clitoris
		Glans clitoris
		Corpora cavernosa of
		  clitoris
		Bulb of vestibule

Ventral aspect of penis	Urethral folds/ vestibular folds	Labia minora
Scrotum	Labioscrotal swellings	Labia majora

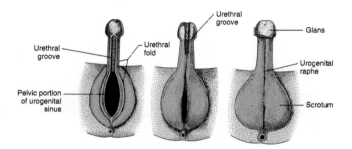

FIG. 10.2 Schematic diagram of differentiation of the male external genitalia. (From Martinez-Mora J. Development of the genital tract. In: Martinez-Mora J, ed. Intersexual states: disorders of sex differentiation. Barcelona: Ediciones Doymer 1994:53.)

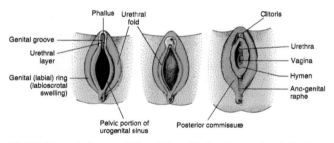

FIG. 10.3 Schematic diagram of differentiation of the female external genitalia. (From Martinez-Mora J. Development of the genital tract In: Martinez-Mora J, ed. *Intersexual states: disorders of sex differentiation.* Barcelona: Ediciones Doymer, 1994:52.)

It is generally accepted that the proximal two thirds of the vagina is formed from the Müllerian ducts and the distal third from the urogenital sinus (Fig. 10.4).

Formation of gender identity is a complex and poorly understood phenomenon. Research suggests that gender identity may be affected not only by chromosomal sex and prenatal hormones but also postnatal environmental factors.

TERMINOLOGY AND DEFINITIONS

The most widely used terminology for the myriad conditions of abnormal sexual differentiation is **disorders of sexual development (DSD)**, or disorders of sexual differentiation. Although there is no clear consensus, individuals affected by DSD may

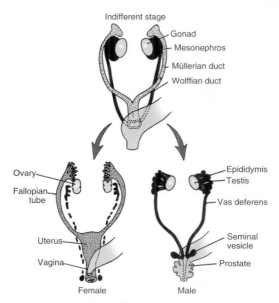

FIG. 10.4 Differentiation of the wolffian and Müllerian duct and urogenital sinus in the male and female. (From Wilson JD. Embryology of the genital tract. In: Harrison HH, Gittes RF, Perlmutter AD, et al., eds. *Campbell's urology.* 4th ed. Philadelphia, PA: WB Saunders, 1979:1473.)

prefer the term difference of sex development, intersex, or more specific terminology to the diagnosis, such as androgen insensitivity syndrome (Table 10.2).

DIAGNOSIS AND MANAGEMENT IN THE NEWBORN WITH AMBIGUOUS GENITALIA

History

Factors to assess include level of prematurity, exposure to exogenous hormones by mother, and prenatal testing such as fetal karyotype or appearance of genitalia on sonogram. Family history should assess neonatal deaths (suggestive of congenital adrenal hyperplasia [CAH]), urologic diagnoses in children or adults, precocious puberty, infertility, amenorrhea, hirsutism, or consanguinity.

Table 10.2 Overview of Nomenclature and Classification for Disorders of Sexual Development

CLASSIFICATION	INCIDENCE	EXAMPLES	PATHOPHYSIOLOGY	PRESENCE OF GONADS
1. Disorders of Gonadal Differentiation and Development				
Klinefelter Syndrome	1/600 (classic)		Classic 47,XXY: meiotic nondisjunction	Bilateral testes
46,XX Male	1/20,000		Translocation of Y chromosome material to X chromosome	Bilateral testes
Gonadal Dysgenesis				
Turner syndrome	1/2500		Classic 45,X; presence of one normal X chromosome and absent/abnormal other chromosome/mosaicism	Bilateral streak (dysgenetic) gonads (primary follicles described in some)
46,XX "pure" gonadal dysgenesis				Bilateral streak (dysgenetic) gonads
Mixed gonadal dysgenesis	Second most common cause of ambiguous genitalia in neonates		Most 45,XU/46,XY	Unilateral testis, contralateral streak gonad

Continued

Table 10.2 Overview of Nomenclature and Classification for Disorders of Sexual Development—cont'd

CLASSIFICATION	INCIDENCE	EXAMPLES	PATHOPHYSIOLOGY	PRESENCE OF GONADS
Partial gonadal dysgenesis			45,X/46,XY or 46,XY	Bilateral dysgenetic testes
46,XY "pure" gonadal dysgenesis (Swyer syndrome)			Complete absence of testis-determining factor; mutations in *SRY* gene in some	Bilateral dysgenetic testes
Embryonic Testicular Regression/Bilateral Vanishing Testes Syndrome			46,XY; loss of testicular tissue during embryogenesis	Bilateral hemosiderin deposition
2. Ovotesticular DSD (True hermaphroditism)			46,XX, 46,XY or mosaicism	Two ovotestes or one ovary/one testis
3. 46,XX DSD (Female pseudohermaphroditism) *Congenital Adrenal Hyperplasia*	1/5000–15,000 (21-hydroxylase)	21-Hydroxylase, 11β-hydroxylase deficiencies	Inborn error of metabolism in one of enzymes involved in cortisol production; increased testosterone production	Bilateral ovaries
Maternal Androgen Excess†			Exogenous androgen effects on fetal development	Bilateral ovaries
4. 46,XY DSD (Male pseudohermaphroditism)				

Leydig Cell Agenesis/Unresponsiveness		Leydig cell aplasia or abnormal LH receptor	Bilateral testes
Disorders of Testosterone Biosynthesis (CAH variants)	StAR deficiency, 3β-hydroxysteroid dehydrogenase deficiency	Defect of enzymes converting cholesterol to testosterone	Bilateral testes
Disorders of Androgen-Dependent Target Tissue			
Syndrome of complete androgen insensitivity	1/20,000–1/60,000	X-linked; androgen resistance secondary to abnormality of androgen receptor	Bilateral testes
Syndrome of partial androgen insensitivity		X-linked; androgen resistance secondary to abnormality of androgen receptor	Bilateral testes
Mild androgen insensitivity syndrome		Androgen resistance secondary to abnormality of androgen receptor	Bilateral testes
5α-Reductase deficiency		Abnormality in type II isoenzyme that converts testosterone to DHT	Bilateral testes
Persistent Müllerian duct syndrome		Abnormality of AMH gene or receptor	Bilateral testes
5. Unclassified DSD **Mayer-Rokitansky-Küster-Hauser Syndrome**	1/4000–5000	46,XX, genetic basis unknown	Bilateral ovaries

AMH, Anti-Müllerian hormone; *CAH*, congenital adrenal hyperplasia; *DHT*, dihydrotestosterone; *DSD*, disorder of sexual development; *LH*, luteinizing hormone.

Physical Examination

The presence of palpable gonads helps narrow the possible diagnoses (see Fig. 10.5). **Because ovaries do not descend, a palpable gonad in the inguinal canal or scrotum is highly suggestive of the presence of a testicle.** Rarely, an ovotestis undergoes descent. **An important tenet is that bilaterally nonpalpable testicles or a unilateral nonpalpable testis in the presence of any degree of hypospadias should be treated as DSD until proven otherwise.** The degree of rugation and pigmentation of the labioscrotal folds should also be assessed.

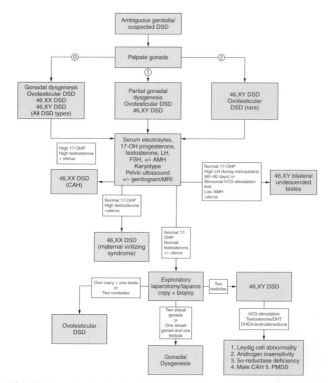

FIG. 10.5 Diagnostic algorithm for DSD based on number of gonads palpated. *17-OHP*, 17-Hydroxyprogesterone; *AMH*, anti-Müllerian hormone; *DHEA*, dehydroepiandrosterone; *DHT*, dihydrotestosterone; *FSH*, follicle-stimulating hormone; *hCG*, human chorionic gonadotropin; *LH*, luteinizing hormone; *MRI*, magnetic resonance imaging.

Phallic examination should include a measure of stretched penile length. Mean stretched penile length in a full-term newborn male in the United States is 3.5 cm (±0.04). The number and location of perineal orifices (three: urethra, vagina and anus or two: urethra and anus) should be documented. The presence of a uterus can sometimes be determined on physical exam by palpation of an anterior midline cordlike structure on rectal examination.

In addition to genital examination, it is important to note other dysmorphic features suggestive of genetic disorders (e.g., short, broad neck associated with Turner syndrome).

Further Evaluation

Immediate serum laboratory evaluation includes karyotype, serum electrolytes, 17-hydroxyprogesterone, testosterone, luteinizing hormone (LH), and follicle-stimulating hormone (FSH). Because karyotyping results can often require several days to return, fluorescence in-situ hybridization (FISH) can act as a rapid alternative to identify X and Y chromosome material.

Serum electrolytes and 17-hydroxyprogesterone are requisite early to rule out a salt-wasting form of CAH.

The presence or absence of testicular tissue can be determined by a human chorionic gonadotropin (hCG) stimulation test, but this test is not needed from 60–90 days of life when there is a natural gonadotropin surge (mini-puberty) and resultant increase in testosterone level. **A failure to respond to hCG in combination with elevated LH and FSH levels or low level of AMH with elevated gonadotropins indicates functional anorchia.**

Imaging is not always required, but pelvic ultrasound or magnetic resonance imaging (MRI) can be helpful to determine the presence of Müllerian structures and/or gonads. A fluoroscopic genitogram can delineate anatomy of a urogenital sinus anomaly before surgical intervention. Sometimes laparotomy or laparoscopy with gonadal biopsy is required if diagnosis with less invasive measures is not sufficient.

Management

DSD in the newborn is most commonly suspected in the setting of ambiguous genitalia and should be treated as both a medical and psychosocial emergency. **Multidisciplinary team management is paramount and if possible should consist of a urologist, endocrinologist, geneticist, and psychiatrist/psychologist/social worker with experience in treating children with DSD.** Initial goals of care should include

1. Medical stabilization
2. Diagnosis
3. Assignment of sex of rearing based on diagnosis, anatomy, and functional potential of the genital and reproductive tract

Sex of rearing in a newborn is mutually agreed on by the parents and medical team based on the best available information, with the understanding that the child may ultimately declare a gender identity different than that assigned.

DIAGNOSIS AND MANAGEMENT FOR THE OLDER CHILD WITH SUSPECTED DSD

Several DSD conditions may go unrecognized until later in childhood, adolescence or even adulthood (Table 10.3). Initial

Table 10.3 Clinical Presentation for Disorders of Sexual Development After the Newborn Period

CLINICAL SCENARIO	DIFFERENTIAL DIAGNOSES
Primary Amenorrhea	
Sexual infantilism + hypergonadotropic hypogonadism	Gonadal dysgenesis, Leydig cell hypoplasia
Normal/partial puberty	CAIS, PAIS, gonadal dysgenesis
Virilization/genital ambiguity at puberty	Disorders of testosterone biosynthesis, 5α-reductase deficiency, Leydig cell hypoplasia, gonadal dysgenesis, nonclassic CAH, PAIS
Incidental Finding	
Absence of uterus in female phenotype	MRKH, CAIS
Atypical gonad given external phenotype	Gonadal dysgenesis, CAIS
Inguinal Hernia in Female Child	CAIS, 5α-reductase deficiency, PAIS, disorders of testosterone biosynthesis
Virilization of Female in Childhood	Nonclassic CAH

CAH, Congenital adrenal hyperplasia; *CAIS,* complete androgen insensitivity syndrome; *MRKH,* Mayer-Rokitansky-Küster-Hauser syndrome; *PAIS,* partial androgen insensitivity syndrome.

evaluation is similar to that in the newborn period including karyotype (or FISH), testosterone, FSH, LH, and pelvic imaging.

PATHOPHYSIOLOGY, PRESENTATION, EVALUATION AND MANAGEMENT OF SPECIFIC DSD

Disorders of Gonadal Differentiation and Development

Klinefelter Syndrome

Definition/Pathophysiology – Klinefelter syndrome is the most common major abnormality of sexual development. Classically associated with a 47,XXY karyotype, the diagnosis requires at least one Y chromosome and at least two X chromosomes.

Presentation – Seminiferous tubules degenerate and are replaced with hyaline resulting in small (less than 3.5 cm in length) and firm testicles. Plasma estradiol levels are high, resulting in gynecomastia, often developing in puberty. Patients are at increased risk for breast carcinoma, as well as extragonadal germ cell tumors and Leydig/Sertoli cell tumors. The majority of patients are infertile with azoospermia.

Evaluation – Karyotype is diagnostic; serum testosterone is low-normal, gonadotropins, and estradiol are elevated.

Management – Androgen supplementation to improve libido, reduction mammoplasty, and assisted reproductive technology to non-mosaic patients are options. **Microdissection testicular sperm extraction results in retrieval rates for sperm in 40%–50%, and intracytoplasmic sperm injection has reported success.**

46,XX Male. This condition is characterized by testicular development in individuals with no Y chromosome. The hypothesized mechanism is translocation of Y chromosome material, including *SRY*, to the X chromosome. Most have normal male external genitalia or hypospadias, but all are infertile. There is a similar endocrinologic profile to Klinefelter syndrome, and hormonal treatment is similar, but because of lack of germ cells, there is no role for sperm retrieval.

Gonadal Dysgenesis. This consists an array of anomalies, all with some degree of abnormal gonad development, ranging from complete gonadal absence to delayed gonadal failure.

Turner Syndrome

Definition/Pathophysiology – This condition is characterized by one normal functioning X chromosome. The other sex chromosome may be absent, abnormal or with mosaicism.

Presentation – Manifestations of 45, X type may include short stature, broad chest, widespread nipples, webbing of the neck, peripheral edema at birth, short fourth metacarpal, hypoplastic nails, multiple pigmented nevi, coarctation of the aorta, bicuspid aortic valve, and renal anomalies. **Sexual infantilism is a hallmark, meaning lack of pubertal development of the external genitalia and lack of development of secondary sex characteristics.** The diagnosis should be considered in any infant with lymphedema or young woman with short stature, lack of secondary sex characteristics, or primary amenorrhea. By birth, gonads are mostly devoid of oocytes, resulting in characteristic streak gonads (Fig. 10.6).

Evaluation/Management – **Determination of Y chromosome material in Turner syndrome is critical because it predisposes to masculinization and gonadoblastoma.** Risk of gonadoblastoma is estimated at 12%–20% and has been reported as early as 5 months of age. Prophylactic gonadectomy in the Y mosaic Turner syndrome patient is advised but not required in the 45,XO patient. Endocrinologic evaluation is needed. Growth hormone or sex hormones may be needed for growth and development. Although spontaneous fertility is rare, pregnancy is a possibility for some patients with spontaneous menses.

46,XX "Pure" Gonadal Dysgenesis

Definition/Pathophysiology/Presentation – These patients have 46,XX karyotype, are characterized by female external genitalia,

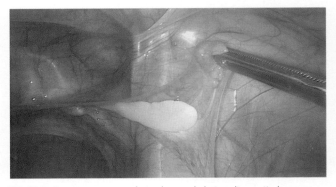

FIG. 10.6 Gross appearance of streak gonad during diagnostic laparoscopy. (Courtesy of D. Diamond, MD.)

normal Müllerian ducts with the absence of wolffian structures, normal height, bilateral streak gonads and sexual infantilism.

Evaluation – Because of streak gonads they have elevated serum gonadotropins.

Management – Estrogen and progesterone replacement are warranted. Because there is no Y chromosome material, gonadectomy is not recommended.

Mixed Gonadal Dysgenesis (MGD)

Definition/Pathophysiology/Presentation – MGD is characterized by a unilateral testis, a contralateral streak gonad, and persistent Müllerian structures associated with varying degrees of masculinization. Most have a 45,XO/46,XY karyotype. There can be phenotypic internal asymmetry, where a dysgenetic or streak gonad on one side will be associated with an ipsilateral uterus and fallopian tube, and a testicle on the contralateral side can be associated with wolffian duct structures (e.g., epididymis, vas deferens). This underscores the effects of local testosterone and AMH secretion. **MGD is the second most common cause of ambiguous genitalia in the neonatal period.**

The risk of gonadoblastoma or dysgerminoma is 15%–35%. **Denys-Drash syndrome and Frasier syndrome are associated with mutations in the Wilms tumor suppressor gene and are associated with mixed gonadal dysgenesis.** Denys-Drash is associated with nephropathy, genital ambiguity, and Wilms tumor. Risk of gonadal tumor in patients with Denys-Drash syndrome is up to 40%. Frasier syndrome is not associated with increased risk of Wilms tumor but a 60% risk of gonadoblastoma in the presence of Y chromosome material (see Table 10.3).

Management – Sex assignment, gonadectomy if indicated, and screening for Wilms tumor are primary considerations. If male gender is selected and the testicle can be brought to the scrotum, physical exam and ultrasound screening for gonadoblastoma must be weighed against prophylactic gonadectomy and androgen replacement.

Partial Gonadal Dysgenesis

Individuals typically have a 45,X/46 XY or 46,XY karyotype, and unlike mixed gonadal dysgenesis, have two dysgenetic testes. There is variability in phenotype depending on AMH and testosterone production. The risk of gonadal malignancy has been estimated to be more than 40% by 40 years of age. Management is similar to mixed gonadal dysgenesis.

46,XY Complete "Pure" Gonadal Dysgenesis (Swyer Syndrome)

Definition/Pathophysiology – There is lack of testis formation despite a Y chromosome, with bilateral streak gonads, normal female genitalia, and well-developed Müllerian structures.

Presentation/Evaluation – The majority present in adolescence with delayed puberty and amenorrhea. There is no genital ambiguity but sexual infantilism. There are high levels of serum gonadotropins, which can lead to elevated androgen levels and clitoromegaly in some.

Management – Risk of germ cell tumors is up to 35% by 30 years of age; therefore, management includes gonadectomy and cyclic hormone replacement.

Embryonic Testicular Regression and Bilateral Vanishing Testes Syndrome

Patients are 46,XY with absent testes but **clear evidence of testicular function (i.e., AMH and/or testosterone production) at some point during embryogenesis.** This is distinguished from gonadal dysgenesis in which testicular function has always been absent. Etiology is postulated to be caused by a genetic mutation, teratogen, or bilateral testicular torsion. Phenotype ranges from typical female to ambiguous to male. Diagnosis can be made with karyotype, castrate levels of testosterone, and elevated gonadotropins during mini-puberty from 2–6 months of age. Treatment is individualized.

Ovotesticular DSD

Definition/Pathophysiology – Ovotesticular DSD describes individuals with both testicular tissue with well-developed seminiferous tubules as well as ovarian tissue with primordial follicles. **Gonads may take the form of one ovary and one testis, or more commonly, one or two ovotestes.** Chromosomal makeup in order of frequency is 46,XX, mosaicism with Y chromosome material, and 46,XY.

Presentation – The differentiation of both the external and internal genitalia is variable and related to the function of the ipsilateral gonad. In most, the genitalia are ambiguous. The ovary, most commonly found on the left side, is usually orthotopic. Testes and ovotestes, more commonly found on the right side, can lie anywhere in the path of testicular descent (Fig. 10.7). Fallopian tubes are consistently present along with the ovary, and vas deferens alongside the testis. Ovotestes can have fallopian tube,

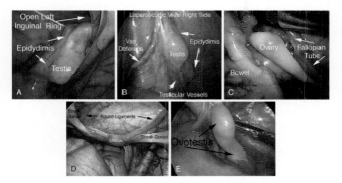

FIG. 10.7 Human intraoperative photographs (A) Intraabdominal testis at internal ring. (B) High intraabdominal testis. (C) Normal ovary. (D) Streak gonads in a patient with XY gonadal dysgenesis. (E) Ovotestis in ovotesticular syndrome.

vas deferens, or both structures. In most patients, a uterus is present. Frequently, the ovarian portion of an ovostestis is normal while the testicular component is dysgenetic.

Management – Although both gonadoblastoma and dysgerminoma have been described, the incidence is low. Gender assignment is based on functional potential of external and internal genitalia. Risks and benefits of gonadectomy versus surveillance should be weighed. There is potential for fertility from an ovarian standpoint if appropriate ductal structures are present.

46,XX DSD

A 46,XX DSD is a phenotypic abnormality of sexual development in which individuals with no chromosomal abnormalities and ovaries have some degree of external masculinization and ambiguous genitalia.

Congenital Adrenal Hyperplasia

Definition/Pathophysiology – CAH is caused by a defect in one of five enzymes involved in the cortisol biosynthetic pathway (see Fig. 10.8). A deficiency in any of the enzymes shown in Table 10.4 may cause CAH. As a result of these defects, production of hydrocortisone is impaired, causing a compensatory increase in secretion of adrenocorticotrophic hormone (ACTH). The increase in ACTH drives formation of additional adrenal steroids proximal to the enzymatic defect and a secondary increase in

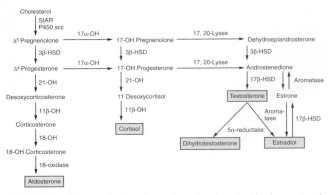

FIG. 10.8 Steroid biosynthetic pathway for mineralocorticoid, glucocorticoid, and sex steroid hormone production.

Table 10.4 Enzyme Deficiencies Involved in Congenital Adrenal Hyperplasia

ENZYME DEFICIENCY	TEST FOR DIAGNOSIS	CLINICAL FEATURES
21-Hydroxylase	Plasma 17-hydroxyprogesterone ↑	Virilization in females, salt wasting with infantile adrenal crisis
11β-Hydroxylase	Plasma 11-Deoxycortisol ↑ 11-Deoxycorticosterone ↑	Virilization (can be late onset), hypertension
3β-Hydroxysteroid dehydrogenase	Plasma 17-hydroxypregnenolone ↑ Plasma dehydroepiandrosterone (DHEA) ↑	Mild clitoromegaly and labial fusion, possible symptoms of aldosterone and cortisol deficiency
17α-Hydroxylase		Nonvirilizing
Cholesterol side chain cleavage enzyme		Nonvirilizing

DHEA, Dehydroepiandrosterone

androgen formation. A deficiency of 21-hydroxylase is responsible for 95% of cases, while a deficiency in 11β-hydroxylase accounts for approximately 5% of cases.

Presentation – CAH is the most common cause of ambiguous genitalia in the newborn. **Patients with 21-hydroxylase**

deficiency exhibit one of three presentations: salt wasting and virilization (concomitant aldosterone insufficiency), simple virilization without salt wasting, and those without evidence of either. In the female with virilization, there is almost always some degree of clitoromegaly and variable labial fusion, as well as a common urogenital sinus (Figs. 10.9 and 10.10). The Prader classification is used to characterize the degree of virilization of the external genitalia in CAH (Fig. 10.11). Müllerian structures are usually normal.

With the salt-losing variant of CAH in both males and females, failure to regain birth weight, weight loss, and dehydration occur in the first few weeks of life. Vomiting can be prominent. In severe cases, adrenal crises occur within the first 10–21 days of life. Death can occur from hyperkalemia, dehydration, and shock without treatment. Presentation of CAH with 11β-hydroxylase deficiency is similar to 21-hydroxylase with the addition of hypertension, thought to be secondary to increased levels of deoxycorticosterone. In males with CAH, there is sexual precocity within the first 2–3 years of life. Unless medical therapy is instituted, there will be short stature and

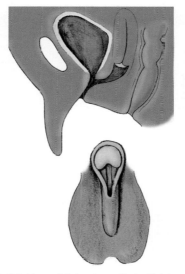

FIG. 10.9 Urogenital sinus in a patient with intersex.

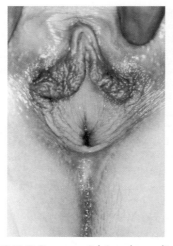

FIG. 10.10 Pure urogenital sinus abnormality.

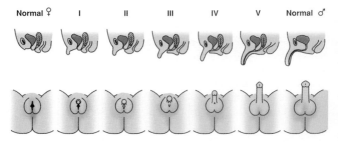

FIG. 10.11 Classification by Prader of the various degrees of masculinization of the external genitalia in females with congenital adrenal hyperplasia that has been applied by some authors to intersexual states in general. (From Prader A. Die Haufigkeit der kongenitalen androgenitalen Syndroms. *Helv Pediatr Acta* 1958;13:426.)

infertility. Testicular adrenal rest tissue (TART) is present in 25%–30% of males, which represents hypertrophy of adrenal rests caused by ACTH stimulation.

Evaluation – See Table 10.4. In classic 21-hydroxylase deficiency, pelvic ultrasound may demonstrate Müllerian structures.

Management – Treatment of CAH consists of hydrocortisone administration in childhood and adolescence. Those with the salt-wasting variant require increased salt intake and mineralocorticoid treatment indefinitely.

Surgical management in CAH patients is controversial. There are three main components: urethroplasty and vaginoplasty to create separate orifices and enlarge the vaginal introitus, clitoroplasty with reduction in size and creation of a clitoral hood, and feminizing vulvoplasty/labioplasty. Long-term fertility in males and feminization and menstruation in females can be anticipated with proper hormonal supplementation.

46,XX DSD Secondary to Increased Maternal Androgens

This diagnosis is now rare, as historically the most common cause of this phenomenon was ingestion of maternal progestins or androgens and more rarely a maternal tumor with virilizing effects on a female fetus. Another possible source is aromatase deficiency in the mother. In any of these cases, a normal hormonal profile should be recognized postnatally, and genital reconstruction, if desired, is the only treatment.

46,XY DSD

This subset of DSD refers to individuals with well-differentiated testicles in whom there are varying degrees of phenotypic feminization.

Leydig Cell Aplasia (Luteinizing Hormone Receptor Abnormality)

A rare autosomal recessive trait in males yields absence of Leydig cells or abnormalities of the LH receptor on Leydig cells. Phenotype varies with bilateral testes. Absent rise of serum testosterone after hCG stimulation is characteristic. Histology of the testicles shows absence of Leydig cells with normal Sertoli cells.

Disorders of Testosterone Biosynthesis

Definition/Pathophysiology – An abnormality in any of the five enzymes required to convert cholesterol to testosterone cause decreased or absent masculinization in a 46 XY fetus. Cholesterol side-chain cleavage enzyme, 3β-hydroxysteroid dehydrogenase, and 17α-hydroxylase are present in both the adrenal glands and testes, thus **these deficiencies not only result in abnormal testosterone production but also impaired production of glucocorticoids and mineralocorticoids**.

Presentation – Syndromes associated with the first two enzyme abnormalities result in nonvirilized genitalia with hyponatremia, hyperkalemia and metabolic acidosis. The syndrome associated with 17α-hydroxylase deficiency causes excess mineralocorticoid activity (water retention, hypertension and hypokalemia) in addition to undervirilization.

The other two enzymes, 17-20 lyase and 17β-hydroxysteroid oxireductase, can be deficient, but only cause abnormal virilization with no effects on glucocorticoid or mineralocorticoids.

Evaluation/Management – Glucocorticoid and mineralocorticoid supplementation as necessary; management of DSD is variable dependent on enzymatic abnormality determined by genetic testing.

Disorders of Androgen-Dependent Target Tissue

These are the most common definable causes of 46,XY DSD and have a range of phenotypes but similar pathophysiology.

Syndrome of Complete Androgen Insensitivity (CAIS)

Definition/Pathophysiology – This X-linked disorder is characterized by 46,XY karyotype, bilateral testes, female-appearing external genitalia, and absence of Müllerian derivatives (due to AMH secretion). A mutation in the gene for the androgen receptor is identified in 95% of cases.

Presentation – Phenotype is typically female. The vagina is short and blind ending. The testes may be identified in the labia, inguinal canal or abdomen. Diagnosis is commonly made in the setting of primary amenorrhea or the finding of a testicle during an inguinal hernia repair. **In phenotypically female patients with inguinal hernias, 1%–2% will have a 46,XY karyotype.**

Evaluation – Endocrine evaluation in the newborn and adolescent reveals normal male levels of testosterone, DHT, and gonadotropins. Pelvic ultrasound and pelvic exam can confirm the diagnosis.

Management – Timing and necessity of gonadectomy should be considered. Many consider leaving testicles in situ beneficial for natural estradiol production. However, there is an increased risk of malignant degeneration of the testes to gonadoblastoma, dysgerminoma, or seminoma. In prepubertal patients, the risk is 0.8%–2%, only slightly more than the cryptorchid testicle. Risk after puberty is unclear, but delayed gonadectomy is thought to be safe in general. Studies support a female gender identity, consistent with androgen resistance of the brain. If orchiectomy is performed, cyclic estrogen/progestin therapy is begun, and short vagina can be treated with dilation.

Syndrome of Partial Androgen Resistance (PAIS)

These are X-linked disorders of incomplete masculinization related to mutations in the androgen receptor gene. Genital ambiguity is variable, but the classic finding is perineoscrotal hypospadias, cryptorchidism, rudimentary wolffian structures, gynecomastia, and infertility. Müllerian structures are absent. Diagnosis can be difficult, but an hCG stimulation test and polymerase chain reaction (PCR) test can confirm diagnosis. The risk for gonadal tumor is slightly less than with complete androgen resistance. Current recommendations are to allow for virilization of the external genitalia to serve as a guide for gender assignment since this may reflect the degree of androgen imprinting of the brain.

Mild Androgen Insensitivity Syndrome (MAIS)

A relatively new designation of androgen receptor gene mutations causing male factor infertility usually presents with male phenotype or mild hypospadias with azoospermia or oligospermia.

5α-Reductase Deficiency

Definition/Pathophysiology – Low DHT is caused by an autosomal recessive mutation in the 5α-reductase type II isoenzyme, which catalyzes conversion of testosterone to DHT. This mutation is expressed at high levels in the prostate and external genitalia.

Presentation – Neonatal phenotypes range from female, to ambiguous genitalia, to penoscrotal hypospadias. A urogenital sinus is present, and the vaginal pouch is short and blind ending. The phallus is usually small. Testes and epididymis are located in the labia, inguinal canals, or abdomen, and vasa terminate in the vaginal pouch. **At puberty, partial masculinization occurs with increase in muscle mass, development of male body habitus, increase in phallic size, and onset of erections.**

Evaluation – Individuals have normal plasma testosterone but low DHT. **After hCG stimulation, the testosterone/DHT ratio increases markedly (20:1).**

Management – This diagnosis is associated with gender reversal at puberty, specifically in a pedigree study from the Dominican Republic, individuals known as *guevedoces* ("testicles at 12," or "penis at 12"). Male gender assignment is usually favored, but studies supporting this were performed in a unique sociologic environment.

Persistent Müllerian Duct Syndrome (PMDS)

Definition/Pathophysiology – PMDS or *hernia uteri inguinale* describes a 46,XY population with normal external male genitalia but the presence of Müllerian structures internally due to gene defects for AMH or AMH receptors.

Presentation – Patients are phenotypic males with unilateral or bilateral undescended testicles, bilateral fallopian tubes, a uterus, and an upper vagina draining into a prostatic utricle (Fig. 10.12). This is encountered most commonly during inguinal hernia repair or orchiopexy.

Management – Patients are usually treated as male with orchiopexies. Management of Müllerian structures is controversial, as the vasa deferentia are in close proximity to the uterus and proximal vagina, and preservation of structures to prevent vas injury has been recommended; however, malignancies have been reported in up to 8% of Müllerian remnants, supporting careful excision.

Unclassified DSD

Mayer Rokitansky Küster Hauser Syndrome (MRKH)

Definition/Pathophysiology – MRKH is associated with congenital absence of the uterus and vagina in a 46,XX individual with female phenotype and normal secondary sexual characteristics. Normal ovaries and fallopian tubes are present, but only uterine remnants remain, along with a shallow vaginal pouch. Upper tract urinary anomalies occur in one third of

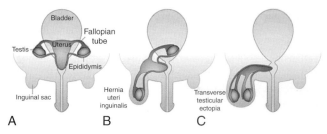

FIG. 10.12 (A to C) Schematic illustration of three presentations of persistent Müllerian duct syndrome. (From Hutson JM, Grover SR, O'Connell M, Pennell SD. Malformation syndromes associated with disorders of sex development. *Nat Rev Endocrinol* 2014;10(8):476-487.)

patients, including renal agenesis, pelvic kidney, and horseshoe kidney.

Presentation – Primary amenorrhea is primary presentation, but it also can present with infertility, cyclic abdominal pain, or dyspareunia.

Evaluation – Abdominal ultrasound or MRI demonstrate an absent uterus. Hormonal profile demonstrates normal female parameters.

Management – Creation of neovagina with dilation or surgery. If present, a hemiuterus should be removed or hormonally suppressed.

Suggested Readings

Bakula DM, Mullins AJ, Sharkey CM, et al. Gender identity outcomes in children with disorders/differences of sex development: predictive factors. *Semin Perinatol* 2017;41(4):214-217.

Bouvattier C. Disorders of sex development: endocrine aspects. In: Gearhart JP, Rink RC, Mouriquand PDE, eds. *Pediatric urology*, 2nd ed. Philadelphia: Saunders Elsevier, 2010.

Cheon CK. Practical approach to steroid 5alpha-reductase type 2 deficiency. *Eur J Pediatr* 2010;170:1-8.

Finney EL, Finlayson C, Rosoklija I, et al. Prenatal detection and evaluation of differences of sex development. *J Pediatr Urol* 2020;16(1):89-96

Heeley JM, Hollander AS, Austin PF, et al. Risk association of congenital anomalies in patients with ambiguous genitalia: a 22-year single-center experience. *J Pediatr Urol* 2018;14(2):153.e1-153.e7.

Hughes IA. Congenital adrenal hyperplasia: a continuum of disorders. *Lancet* 1998;352: 752-754.

Hughes IA. Disorders of sex development: a new definition and classification. *Best Pract Res Clin Endocrinol Metab* 2008;22:119-134.

Kaefer M, Diamond DA, Hendren WH, et al. The incidence of intersexuality in children with cryptorchidism and hypospadias: stratification based on gonadal palpability and meatal position. *J Urol* 1999;162:1003-1007.

Lee PA, Houk CP, Ahmed SF, et al. Consensus statement on management of intersex disorders. International Consensus Conference on Intersex. *Pediatrics* 2006;118: e488-e500.

MacLaughlin DT, Donahoe PK. Sex determination and differentiation. *N Engl J Med* 2004;350:367-378.

Mendonca BB, Domenice S, Arnhold IJ, Costa EM. 46,XY disorders of sex development (DSD). *Clin Endocrinol (Oxf)* 2009;70:173-187.

Saenger P. Turner's syndrome. *N Engl J Med* 1996;335:1749-1754.

11

Pediatric Urologic Oncology
NICHOLAS G. COST AND CRAIG A. PETERS

CONTRIBUTORS OF CAMPBELL-WALSH-WEIN, 12TH EDITION
Michael L. Ritchey, Nicholas G. Cost, Robert C. Shamberger, and Fernando A. Ferrer

ADRENAL TUMORS

Neuroblastoma

Symptoms. Palpable abdominal mass, pain or focal symptoms from metastatic disease (cough, bone pain, neurologic deficits), incidental finding from imaging, hypertension, symptoms of catecholamine excess (tachycardia, anxiety, headaches, seizures), opsoclonus-myoclonus, urinary retention.

History. The patient/family should be asked about duration and acuity of symptoms. Was there any preceding event? The age of the patient is important in prognosis.

Examination. Does the child appear to be overall well or ill appearing? Children with neuroblastoma may be ill appearing or have unstable vital signs (tachycardic, hypotensive, tachypneic) at the time of diagnosis. Thorough examination should assess for any abdominal or pelvic mass as well as any localized areas of tenderness or neurologic deficit. Check for periorbital ecchymosis and any signs of opsoclonus-myoclonus.

Labs. Urinary levels of metabolites of catecholamines, vanillylmandelic acid (VMA) and homovanillic acid (HVA), and also, plasma free metanephrines are important for diagnosis. Check complete metabolic profile and a complete blood count (CBC).

Imaging. Abdominal ultrasound (US) can guide additional cross-sectional imaging. If an abdominal mass is found, the next step is generally a computed tomography (CT) of the chest, abdomen, and

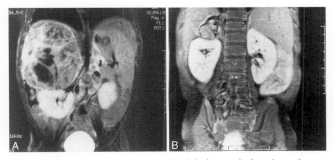

FIG. 11.1 Magnetic resonance imaging (MRI) before and after chemotherapy showing marked reduction in size of right suprarenal neuroblastoma. (A) Before chemotherapy. (B) After chemotherapy.

pelvis. Further specialized imaging such as metaiodobenzylguanidine (MIBG) or positron emission tomography (PET) may be warranted. The classic finding for distinguishing a pediatric abdominal mass as neuroblastoma or nephroblastoma (Wilms tumor) is whether it crosses midline or if it has calcifications. Classically, but not always, neuroblastoma crosses the midline and may have calcifications while nephroblastoma does not generally cross midline or have calcifications (Fig. 11.1)

Differential Diagnosis. The differential diagnosis of an abdominal mass in a child includes malignant tumors of the liver, kidney, adrenal, and bladder. Additionally, findings such as constipation and hydronephrosis may result in a palpable mass.

Treatment. Neuroblastoma generally requires multimodal treatment with surgery, chemotherapy, and radiation. The first step in patient management is stabilization as infants with widely metastatic neuroblastoma may be very ill. In general the next step for a suspected neuroblastoma is biopsy. However, this should only be done after a multidisciplinary discussion with pediatric oncology. Subsequent steps with chemotherapy or surgical resection may require a nuanced analysis of patient and tumor factors.

Prognosis. Highly dependent on risk status, which combines pathologic features, stage and patient age. Low risk has a >95% 5-year overall survival (OS). Intermediate risk = 70%–90% 5-year OS. High risk = 20%–40% 5-year OS.

Pheochromocytoma

Symptoms. Most patients will be symptomatic with hypertension, attacks of hypertension/anxiety, overall symptoms of catecholamine excess (tachycardia, anxiety, headaches, seizures, pallor, tremor, perspiration).

History. Duration and acuity of symptoms and personal or family history of genetic predispositions (von Hippel Lindau, multiple endocrine neoplasia, neurofibromatosis, succinate dehydrogenase mutations).

Examination. Vital signs (heart rate, blood pressure). Thorough investigation for stigmata of hereditary syndromes correlated with pheochromocytoma (Table 11.1).

Labs. Plasma free metanephrines are critical for diagnosis. Check complete metabolic profile and a CBC.

Imaging. If plasma free metanephrines are elevated, the next step is generally a CT or MRI of the abdomen and pelvis (Fig. 11.2).

Table 11.1 Hereditary Syndromes Associated with Pheochromocytoma

SYNDROME	FINDINGS
MEN IIA	Pheochromocytoma, medullary thyroid carcinoma, parathyroid adenoma
MEN IIB (III)	Pheochromocytoma, medullary thyroid carcinoma, ganglioneuromatosis, mucosal neuromas
VHL	Pheochromocytomas, CNS/retinal hemangioblastomas, renal cysts, renal cell carcinoma, endolymphatic sac tumors
NF type I	Neurofibromas and pheochromocytomas

CNS, Central Nervous System; *MEN*, Multiple Endocrine Neoplasia; *NF*, Neurofibromatosis; *VHL*, von Hippel Lindau.

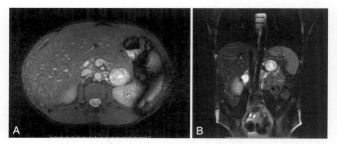

FIG. 11.2 Magnetic resonance imaging (MRI) T2 of left adrenal pheochromocytoma: axial (A) and coronal (B).

Further specialized imaging such as nuclear medicine imaging (MIBG, Dotatate, or PET) may be warranted.

Differential Diagnosis. The differential diagnosis of an adrenal mass with elevated plasma free metanephrines would include an adrenal cortical carcinoma and neuroblastoma.

Treatment. Biopsy is NOT indicated if pheochromocytoma is suspected. Prior to surgery, management with endocrinology for catecholamine blockade. Alpha blockade (phenoxybenzamine or prazosin) should be done first. Beta blockade is only indicated if persistent arrhythmia or tachycardia or hypertension. Increased fluid intake (and increased salt intake) to replete intravascular volume during time of catecholamine blockade. Consultation with anesthesia preoperatively is needed. After a 10- to 14-day blockade, surgery can be done with laparoscopic resection preferred for tumors <8 cm. Early ligation of the adrenal vein will aid in patient stability. Close collaboration with anesthesia is necessary as patients can be very hemodynamically labile during surgery.

Prognosis. 90% of tumors are nonmetastatic and nonmalignant. Complete resection associated with over 80% long-term relapse free survival. Genetic testing should be offered as >10% of patients will have a hereditary predisposition.

RENAL TUMORS (Figs. 11.3 and 11.4) (Table 11.2)

Wilms Tumor (Nephroblastoma)

Symptoms. Palpable abdominal mass, hematuria, fever, anorexia, weight loss, constipation.

History. The patient/family should be asked about duration and acuity of symptoms and personal or family history of genetic predispositions (Table 11.3).

Examination. Does the child appear to be overall well or ill appearing? Children with Wilms tumor are generally well appearing at the time of diagnosis (compared with neuroblastoma). Thorough examination should assess for any abdominal or pelvic mass. Assess for signs of hereditary predisposition (genitourinary anomalies [hypospadias, undescended testis (UDT), ambiguous genitalia], hemihypertrophy, aniridia).

Labs. Complete metabolic profile and a CBC. Assess coagulation profile as 2% of those with Wilms tumor have an acquired von Willebrand factor deficiency.

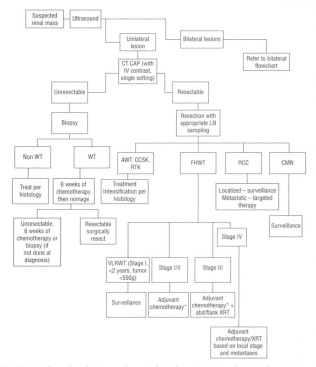

FIG. 11.3 Unilateral pediatric renal mass algorithm. *AWT,* Anaplastic Wilms Tumor; *CAP,* Chest, Abdomen, Pelvis; *CMN,* Congenital Mesoblastic Nephroma; *CT,* Computed Tomography; *FH,* Favorable Histology; *LN,* Lymph Node; *RCC,* Renal Cell Carcinoma; *VLR,* Very Low Risk; *WT,* Wilms Tumor; *XRT,* Radiation Therapy.

Imaging. Abdominal US can help guide additional cross-sectional imaging. If an abdominal mass is found, the next step is generally a CT of the chest, abdomen, and pelvis (Fig. 11.5).

Differential Diagnosis. The differential diagnosis of an abdominal mass in a child includes malignant tumors of the liver, renal, adrenal, and bladder. Additionally, benign findings such as constipation and hydronephrosis may result in a palpable mass. Etiologies of a malignant renal mass in a child include renal cell carcinoma, clear cell sarcoma of the kidney, and rhabdoid tumor. Benign renal lesions include mesoblastic

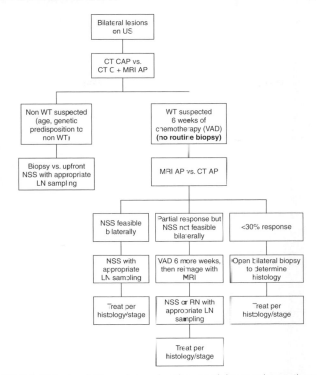

FIG. 11.4 Bilateral pediatric renal mass algorithm. *AP,* Abdomen Pelvis; *C,* Chest; *CAP,* Chest, Abdomen, Pelvis; *CT,* Computed Tomography; *LN,* Lymph Node; *MRI,* Magnetic Resonance Imaging; *NSS,* Nephron Sparing Surgery; *RN,* Radical Nephrectomy US; Ultrasound; *VAD,* Vincristine, Actinomycin, Doxorubicin; *WT,* Wilms Tumor.

nephroma, cystic nephroma, angiomyolipoma, and multicystic dysplastic kidney.

Treatment. Surgery is generally the next step with radical nephrectomy; lymph node sampling is the treatment of choice in most patients with a unilateral, nonsyndromic tumor. Biopsy is generally not indicated outside of extenuating circumstances. Those with bilateral renal tumors or a syndrome-associated unilateral tumor concerning for Wilms should be treated with presurgical chemotherapy followed by attempted partial nephrectomy

Table 11.2 Pediatric Renal Tumor Overview

TUMOR TYPE	EPIDEMIOLOGY	CLINICAL PRESENTATION	IMAGING CHARACTERISTICS	TREATMENT	RISK FOR METASTASES/ RECURRENCE	PROGNOSIS
• Wilms tumor	• Most common pediatric renal tumor • 80% of all pediatric renal tumors (75% favorable histology Wilms tumor, 5% anaplastic Wilms tumor) • Can present at any age but most common at 2–5 years	• Painless abdominal mass, hematuria, hypertension • May be associated with predisposition syndromes	• CT CAP • "Claw sign" of normal kidney around the tumor. The mass typically pushes surrounding structures away rather than invading surrounding organs	• Surgical excision, adjuvant chemotherapy and possibly radiation • Exceptions for the youngest patients (<2 years) with stage I disease – surgery alone. Also, preoperative chemotherapy and partial nephrectomy for bilateral tumors	• About 20% of cases present with metastatic disease • Local recurrence is rare if tumor completely excised • Recurrence increased for those with nodal involvement or tumor rupture	• Prognosis largely impacted by stage and tumor histology • Favorable histology better than Anaplasia • Tumor genetics (LOH at 1p and 16q) can predict outcome as well

• Renal cell carcinoma (RCC)	• Difficult to distinguish from presentation of Wilms tumor • May be associated with predisposition syndrome	• CT CAP • Typically smaller than Wilms tumors but can vary and some are quite large • More likely to have calcifications than Wilms tumors	• Complete surgical excision including removal all involved nodal disease • Clinical trials for those with metastatic disease	• Almost 50% will have advanced stage (stage III–IV) disease • Approximately 1/3 have nodal spread • 25% with metastatic disease at presentation	• Outcome highly dependent on stage. • >85% survival for those with localized disease (even with nodal spread) if completely excised • Poor survival (<25%) for those with metastatic disease
• Second most common renal tumor in patients 0–30 yr (4%–5%) • Most common renal tumor in adolescents (>12 yr) • Most commonly Translocation type RCC (TFE+)					

Continued

Table 11.2 Pediatric Renal Tumor Overview—cont'd

TUMOR TYPE	EPIDEMIOLOGY	CLINICAL PRESENTATION	IMAGING CHARACTERISTICS	TREATMENT	RISK FOR METASTASES/ RECURRENCE	PROGNOSIS
• Congenital mesoplastic nephroma (CMN)	• The most common renal tumor in infants younger than 6 months of age • Patients younger than 6 months with a renal mass are presumed to have CMN	• Classically present as a palpable mass in newborn period • May be detected prenatally, may be associated with polyhydramnios and preterm birth	• Imaging studies (typically US) show this tumor to be confined to the kidney and a full staging work up with CT CAP is indicated	• Radical nephrectomy is both diagnostic and therapeutic • LN sampling is advocated to obtain accurate staging information should this actually be WT	• Traditionally thought of as benign, but recurrent and/or metastatic cases have been rarely reported • Metastases have been reported to occur to the lung, brain, liver, heart, and bone • Risk factors for recurrence include positive surgical margin, cellular subtype	• Prognosis is good, especially if treated in first 6 months of life • There is no established follow up for CMN, but serial abdominal US for the first 2 years is likely prudent

• Clear cell sarcoma of the kidney (CCSK)	• Classically the bone metastasizing tumor with late recurrences • Peak incidence between 1 and 4 years, 2:1 male predominance • No known familial or predisposition syndromes	• Present with a firm palpable mass, with 15%–60% reporting pain due to skeletal metastases	• Imaging studies are similar to that of WT	• Primary radical nephrectomy and LN sampling • Adjuvant therapy includes XRT and multidrug chemotherapy (vincristine, doxorubicin, cyclophosphamide, and etoposide) • With current treatment regimens, brain metastases are becoming more common than the typical bone metastases originally reported • There is a high relapse rate within the first 3 years after treatment, especially in younger patients and those with advanced disease	• 5-year EFS is 75%–85% with 5-year OS 85%–90% • These patients need to be followed closely

Continued

Table 11.2 Pediatric Renal Tumor Overview—cont'd

TUMOR TYPE	EPIDEMIOLOGY	CLINICAL PRESENTATION	IMAGING CHARACTERISTICS	TREATMENT	RISK FOR METASTASES/ RECURRENCE	PROGNOSIS
• Rhabdoid tumor of the kidney (RTK)	• Rare and aggressive • Occasional occurrences of separate CNS primary tumors • 80% of these tumors occur in children younger than 2 years of age with a male predominance (1.5:1) • Median age at diagnosis is 10.6 months • Many patients have a germline mutation that predisposes them to this tumor (incomplete penetrance, possible gonadal mosaicism); consider genetic counseling for families	• Hematuria is the typical presenting complaint, but symptoms associated with metastatic disease (to brain, lung, liver) are present in up to 80% of cases	• Imaging involves CT CAP • Unique to RTK is the need for CNS imaging (brain MRI) given the high risk of metastatic disease to brain; this is more common in patients younger than 1 year at diagnosis	• Early radical nephrectomy with LN dissection is the mainstay of treatment • This tumor is resistant to chemotherapy and XRT	• CNS involvement is almost universally fatal	• 4-year OS is between 20 and 36 months • Lower stage (I/II) patients have a 41.8% OS • Higher stage (III/IV/V) have a 15.9% OS • Age influences OS, with younger patients having worse OS than older patients • Intensive follow up is needed for these tumors

Angiomyolipoma (AML)	• Classically seen in patients with tuberous sclerosis • Made of fat, muscle, and blood vessels and thus prone to bleed	• Retroperitoneal bleeding	• Annual monitoring with US and/or MRI for size stability for the duration of life	• Embolization is the treatment of choice should hematuria become an issue • All attempts at nephron preservation should be made due to the future risk of possible resections	• Higher risk of RCC
Renal medullary carcinoma	• Affects patients with sickle cell trait, thus there is an African American predominance • Very aggressive tumor with almost all cases being fatal	• >90% of patients present with advanced disease	• Imaging with CT CAP	• Treatment revolves around radical nephrectomy • Typically will also receive chemotherapy	• Survival between 4 and 16 months from diagnosis

Continued

Table 11.2 Pediatric Renal Tumor Overview—cont'd

TUMOR TYPE	EPIDEMIOLOGY	CLINICAL PRESENTATION	IMAGING CHARACTERISTICS	TREATMENT	RISK FOR METASTASES/ RECURRENCE	PROGNOSIS
• Multilocular cystic nephroma (MCN)/ cystic partially differentiated nephroblastoma (CPDN)/ cystic Wilms tumor (WT) spectrum	• These usually present in patients before 2 years of age • Males more often than females in children but more common in females in adulthood	• Usually unilateral, presenting with palpable mass • Mimics include multicystic dysplastic kidney, severely obstructed ureteropelvic junction, cellular variant of CMN, CCSK, and cystic RCC	• MCN, CPDN, and cystic WT are indistinguishable on radiologic imaging and require surgical pathologic review • MCN – well circumscribed, cysts and septae • CPDN – poorly differentiated tissue or blastemal cells are found in the septa • Cystic WT – more solid structures between the cysts with stromal/ mesenchymal and/or epithelial components	• Complete resection is considered curative, usually with radical nephrectomy • If using NSS, frozen section to confirm negative margins is mandatory • MCN is a benign lesion, surveillance is all that is needed • Stage I CPDN is followed with surveillance • Stage II CPDN receives chemotherapy • Cystic WT is treated per recommendations for WT		

• Renal cysts	• Rare in children	• Usually incidentally discovered on US	• Bosniak classification system that is well described in adults is not generally applied to children • Modifications to this system have been made, that include US findings as well as Internal flow	• Simple cysts (modified Bosniak I and II) can likely be followed with serial imaging without risk of harboring malignancy • Complex cysts (modified Bosniak III or IV) harbor a risk of intermediate or malignant histology, thus radical nephrectomy is advocated

Continued

Table 11.2 Pediatric Renal Tumor Overview—cont'd

TUMOR TYPE	EPIDEMIOLOGY	CLINICAL PRESENTATION	IMAGING CHARACTERISTICS	TREATMENT	RISK FOR METASTASES/ RECURRENCE	PROGNOSIS
			• Anything beyond a simple cyst should have an MRI with and without intravenous contrast to assess the cyst wall and for solid components			

AML, Angiomyolipoma, CAP, chest, abdomen, pelvis, CCSK, clear cell sarcoma of the kidney, CMN, congenital mesoblastic nephroma, CPDN, cystic partially differentiated nephroblastoma, CT, computed tomography, LN, lymph node, LOH, loss of heterozygosity, MCN, multilocular cystic nephroma, MRI, magnetic resonance imaging, OS, overall survival, RCC, renal cell carcinoma, RTK, rhabdoid tumor of the kidney, US, ultrasound, WT, Wilms tumor, XRT, radiation therapy.

Table 11.3 Hereditary Syndromes Associated with Wilms Tumor

SYNDROME	GENETICS	ASSOCIATED FEATURES
Wilms tumor, Aniridia, Genital abnormalities, Range (WAGR) of mental development	11p13 WT1, PAX6	Wilms Tumor (WT) Aniridia Genital abnormalities Mental retardation
Denys Drash	WT1	WT Genital abnormalities Renal failure/nephropathy (mesangial sclerosis)
Beckwith-Weideman and hemi-hypertrophy	11p15.5 WT2	Pre- and postnatal overgrowth Hem hypertrophy (growth asymmetry) Macroglossia Anterior abdominal wall defects Ear creases/pits
Frasier syndrome	WT1	Nephropathy (FSGS) Genital abnormalities Gonadoblastoma WT

FSGS, Focal segemental glomerulonephritis; *WAGR*, Wilms tumor, Aniridia, Genital abnormalities, Range of mental development; *WT*, Wilms Tumor.

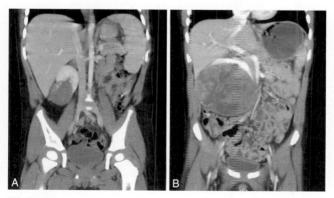

FIG. 11.5 (A) Computed tomography of a Wilms tumor that was pretreated with chemotherapy. (B) After 6 weeks of chemotherapy, the tumor is much smaller in size.

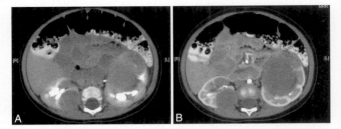

FIG. 11.6 Patient with bilateral tumors who was treated with chemotherapy. (A) Computed tomography (CT) before treatment. (B) CT after 12 weeks of chemotherapy, revealing only minimal decrease in the size of the tumors. Bilateral partial nephrectomies were performed, revealing mature tumor elements with rhabdomyoblastic differentiation.

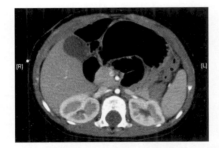

FIG. 11.7 Postoperative image from patient shown in Fig. 11.6. Demonstrates that the kidneys have pretty near normal volume after resection of the bilateral tumors.

(Figs. 11.6 and 11.7). Surgical pathology and imaging will guide stage-specific adjuvant chemotherapy and possibly radiation.

Prognosis. Highly dependent on tumor histology and stage. Five-year OS for favorable histology is >90%. Five-year OS for unfavorable histology range from 30% to 80%, depending on stage.

Renal Cell Carcinoma

Symptoms. Palpable abdominal mass, hematuria, fever, anorexia, weight loss, constipation.

History. The patient/family should be asked about duration and acuity of symptoms. Also, about known personal or family history of genetic predispositions (Table 11.4).

Table 11.4 Hereditary Syndromes Associated with Renal Cell Carcinoma

SYNDROME	GENE	PRESENTATION
Von Hippel Lindau	3p; *VHL* tumor suppressor	Clear cell RCC Retinal and CNS hemangioblastomas Pheochromocytomas Pancreatic cysts/tumors Epididymal cystadenomas
Tuberous sclerosis	*TSC1* or *TSC2*	AMLs Clear cell RCC Seizures Mental retardation Facial angiofibromas Hamartomas
Hereditary papillary RCC	*MET* proto-oncogene	Low-grade type 1 papillary RCC
Birt-Hogg-Dubé	*FLCN* tumor suppressor	Chromophobe RCC Fibrofolliculomas Lung cysts and blebs
Hereditary leiomyomatosis and RCC	*FH* tumor suppressor	High grade type 2 papillary RCC Uterine fibroids at young age
Succinate dehydrogenase deficiency	*SDH*	Different RCCs Paragangliomas pheochromocytomas
Sickle cell disease/trait	HbS	Renal medullary carcinoma

RCC, Renal Cell Carcinoma; *CNS*, Central Nervous System; *AMLs*; Angiomyolipomas

Examination. Thorough examination should assess for any abdominal or pelvic mass. Assess for signs of hereditary predisposition (table above).

Labs. Complete metabolic profile and a CBC.

Imaging. Abdominal US can help guide additional cross-sectional imaging. If an abdominal mass is found, the next step is generally a CT of the chest, abdomen, and pelvis.

Differential Diagnosis. Includes malignant tumors of the liver, renal, adrenal, and bladder. Additionally, benign findings such as constipation and hydronephrosis may result in a palpable mass. Etiologies of a malignant renal mass in a child include Wilms tumor, clear cell sarcoma of the kidney, and rhabdoid tumor. Benign renal lesions include mesoblastic nephroma, cystic nephroma, angiomyolipoma and multicystic dysplastic kidney.

Treatment. Radical nephrectomy with lymph node sampling is the treatment of choice in most patients with a unilateral, non-syndromic tumor. Biopsy is generally not indicated outside of extenuating circumstances. Those with bilateral renal tumors or a syndrome-associated unilateral tumor concerning for renal cell carcinoma should be treated with attempted partial nephrectomy. Complete surgical resection is the treatment of choice, no role for adjuvant therapy in nonmetastatic disease.

Prognosis. Dependent on stage. The majority of renal cell carcinoma in children is translocation type RCC. These generally involve chromosomal translocations in Xp11 (TFE gene). Five-year OS by stage: stages I and II, >90%; stage III, 80%; and stage IV, <25%.

BLADDER AND PROSTATE TUMORS

Rhabdomyosarcoma

Symptoms. Urinary frequency/urgency, stranguria, hematuria, constipation, palpable abdominal mass, fever, anorexia, weight loss.

History. The patient/family should be asked about duration and acuity of symptoms. As about known personal or family history of genetic predispositions (Li-Fraumeni, neurofibromatosis).

Examination. Assess for abdominal or pelvic mass. An exam of the urethral meatus may visualize a prolapsing urethral mass, more commonly appreciated in female patients than male patients. Evaluate for urinary retention.

Labs. Complete metabolic profile and a CBC.

Imaging. Abdominal US can help guide additional cross-sectional imaging. Assess for signs of renal failure prior to any contrasted imaging. If a pelvic mass is found, the next step is generally a CT of the chest, abdomen and pelvis. Staging for rhabdomyosarcoma will also include a PET scan. MRI of the pelvis may be helpful for fine anatomic details (Fig. 11.8).

Differential Diagnosis. The differential diagnosis of a pelvic mass in a child includes bladder, prostate, perirectal/perianal, vaginal/uterine, and ovarian malignancy. Additionally, benign findings such

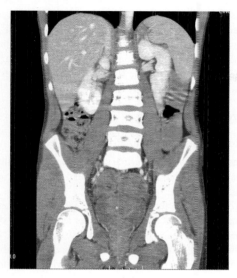

FIG. 11.8 Magnetic resonance imaging of abdomen and pelvis in boy with bladder-prostate rhabdomyosarcoma.

as constipation and urinary retention may result in a palpable mass.

Treatment. The urgent steps in management are to ensure urinary drainage typically with placement of an indwelling urethral catheter. Full staging will require biopsy of the primary tumor and likely a bone marrow biopsy. Biopsy is ideally achieved endoscopically. Depending on the ability to fully resect at diagnosis, surgical excision or chemotherapy are the most likely next steps. This requires a multidisciplinary discussion with pediatric oncology and radiation oncology. In addition to the systemic therapy with chemotherapy, local control is typically achieved with surgery, radiation, or a combination of the two. Major goals of treatment are organ preservation and avoiding the morbidity of complete urinary diversion; therefore, many patients are managed with radiation to preserve the bladder. Final disease staging and grouping (based on imaging, surgical approach, and pathology) will dictate the length of chemotherapy and need for radiation therapy.

Prognosis. Bladder and prostate primary rhabdomyosarcoma are considered an unfavorable site so survival is less than for gynecologic or paratesticular primary tumors. Otherwise, the prognosis is dependent on tumor histology and stage. Three-year OS for embryonal rhabdomyosarcoma is >80%. Three-year OS for alveolar rhabdomyosarcoma is 40%.

GYNECOLOGIC TUMORS

Gynecologic Rhabdomyosarcoma

Symptoms. Vaginal bleeding, urinary frequency/urgency, stranguria, hematuria, constipation, palpable abdominal mass, fever, anorexia, weight loss.

History. The patient/family should be asked about duration and acuity of symptoms. Also, about known personal or family history of genetic predispositions (Li-Fraumeni, neurofibromatosis).

Examination. Thorough examination should assess for any abdominal or pelvic mass. An exam of the introitus may visualize a prolapsing vaginal mass (Fig. 11.9). Evaluate for urinary retention.

Labs. Complete metabolic profile and a CBC.

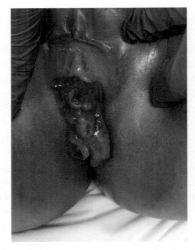

FIG. 11.9 Botryoid vaginal rhabdomyosarcoma emanating from the introitus of a young girl.

Imaging. Abdominal US can help guide additional cross-sectional imaging. Assess for signs of renal failure prior to any contrasted imaging. If a pelvic mass is found, the next step is generally a CT of the chest, abdomen, and pelvis. Staging for rhabdomyosarcoma will also include a PET scan. MRI of the pelvis may be helpful for fine anatomic details.

Differential Diagnosis. The differential diagnosis of a pelvic mass in a child includes bladder, prostate, perirectal/perianal, vaginal/uterine, and ovarian malignancy. Additionally benign findings such as constipation and urinary retention may result in a palpable mass.

Treatment. The urgent steps in management are to evaluate for urinary or bowel obstruction for primary mass. This may involve urinary drainage typically with placement of an indwelling urethral catheter. Full staging will require biopsy of the primary tumor and likely also requires a bone marrow biopsy. Biopsy is ideally achieved endoscopically and/or transvaginally. Depending on the ability to fully resect at diagnosis, surgical excision or chemotherapy is the most likely next step. This requires a multidisc plinary discussion with pediatric oncology and radiation oncology In addition to the systemic therapy with chemotherapy, local control is typically achieved with surgery, radiation, or a combination of the two. Major goals of treatment are organ preservation and avoiding the morbidity of complete pelvic exenteration; therefore, many patients are managed with radiation to preserve the vagina/uterus. Final disease staging and grouping (based on imaging, surgical approach, and pathology) will dictate the length of chemotherapy and need for radiation therapy.

Prognosis. Gynecologic primary sites for rhabdomyosarcoma are considered a favorable site. Otherwise, prognosis depends on patient age and tumor stage. Five-year OS for gynecologic rhabdomyosarcoma is >80% (>90% in those younger than 10 years old and 70% in those older than 10 years old).

TESTICULAR AND PARATESTICULAR TUMORS

Testicular Germ Cell Tumors (GCTs)

Symptoms. Palpable scrotal/testicular mass or swelling, scrotal/testicular pain, dysuria, or focal symptoms from metastatic disease (cough, bone pain, neurologic deficits).

History. Duration and acuity of symptoms, history of cryptorchidism, family history of testicular cancer and genetic syndromes (Klinefelter syndrome, DICER-1, Peutz-Jeghers syndrome, Carney complex, congenital adrenal hyperplasia).

Examination. Evaluate the scrotum, testes, and paratesticular structures and presence or absence of varicocele. Perform an abdominal and pelvic exam to assess for any abdominal masses. Assess for any signs of precocious puberty or gynecomastia.

Labs. Serum tumor markers include alpha fetoprotein (AFP), beta-human chorionic gonadotropin (bHCG), and lactate dehydrogenase (LDH). Note that AFP may be physiologically elevated in the first year of life. If concern for a testicular stromal tumor, also include an inhibin-B, testosterone, and estradiol. Should also check complete metabolic profile and a CBC.

Imaging. Scrotal US can localize the tumor to the testis or paratesticular structures (Fig. 11.10). Evaluate the contralateral testis and also comment on the presence of microlithiasis. Germ cell tumors may be associated with concomitant microlithiasis. Teratoma and epidermoid/dermoid cysts may have a classic appearance of "onion skin lesion" on US. If a mass is found on US concerning for malignancy, the next step in imaging is full staging with CT of the chest, abdomen, and pelvis.

Differential Diagnosis. The differential diagnosis of a scrotal mass in a child includes both benign (teratoma, testicular stromal

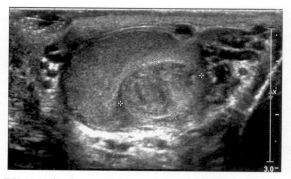

FIG. 11.10 Testicular ultrasound of a pure embryonal carcinoma in a 14-year-old male patient.

tumors) and malignant (germ cell tumor, rhabdomyosarcoma) tumors of the testis or paratesticular structures. Also, entities such as a testicular torsion, hernia, hydrocele, and varicocele may appear as a scrotal mass. Scrotal US can help in distinguishing etiology. Of note a primary tumor may present with a hydrocele so the exam should involve specific evaluation the testis to assess for a mass.

Treatment. Largely dependent on tumor location and the status of the tumor markers and the patient's pubertal status. The following pertains to a primary testicular tumor; for a paratesticular tumor, refer to that separate section later. For prepubertal patients with physiologically normal (remember the physiologic elevation in AFP in the first year of life) serum tumor markers, an inguinal approach to partial orchiectomy (with intraoperative frozen section) is the treatment of choice. Radical inguinal orchiectomy is reserved for prepubertal patients with elevated markers. For pubertal/postpubertal adolescent patients, there is less role for partial orchiectomy because the incidence of a malignant GCT is higher compared with prepubertal patients. However, an inguinal approach to partial orchiectomy (with intraoperative frozen section) can be considered in selected adolescents with normal serum markers and a small (<2 cm) testicular tumor. Postsurgical treatment depends on tumor type and staging work up. For benign tumors, surgical excision (partial or radical orchiectomy) is curative. For malignant GCTs localized, stage I tumors active surveillance is recommended. For those with metastatic disease, adjuvant chemotherapy is indicated. Postchemotherapy residual masses are rare in prepubertal patients. Pubertal/postpubertal adolescents with GCT should be managed in line with adult GCT guidelines, including the need for postchemotherapy retroperitoneal lymph node dissection for those with residual disease.

Prognosis. Dependent on tumor histology and stage but generally excellent prognosis regardless (stage I disease 98%–99% OS; patients with metastatic disease >90% OS).

Testicular Stromal Tumors (Leydig Cell Tumor, Sertoli Cell Tumor, Granulosa Cell Tumors)

Symptoms. Palpable scrotal/testicular mass or swelling, scrotal/testicular pain, dysuria, or focal symptoms from metastatic disease (cough, bone pain, neurologic deficits).

History. Duration and acuity of symptoms, history of cryptorchidism, family history of testicular cancer, and genetic syndromes (Klinefelter syndrome, DICER-1, Peutz-Jeghers syndrome, Carney complex, congenital adrenal hyperplasia).

Examination. Evaluate the scrotum, testes and paratesticular structures, and varicocele. Abdominal and pelvic exam to assess for any abdominal masses. Assess for any signs of precocious puberty or gynecomastia.

Labs. If concern for a testicular stromal tumor, serum tumor markers such as inhibin-B, testosterone, and estradiol should be drawn. To help distinguish from a GCT, AFP, bHCG, and LDH are recommended. Note that AFP may be physiologically elevated in the first year of life. Should also check complete metabolic profile and a CBC.

Imaging. Scrotal US can localize the tumor to the testis or paratesticular structures and may also evaluate the contralateral testis (Fig. 11.11). If pathology is concerning for malignancy, the next step in imaging is full staging with CT of the chest, abdomen, and pelvis.

Differential Diagnosis. The differential diagnosis of a scrotal mass in a child includes both benign (teratoma, testicular stromal tumors) and malignant (germ cell tumor, rhabdomyosarcoma) tumors of the testis or paratesticular structures. Also, entities such as a testicular torsion, hernia, hydrocele, and varicocele may appear as a scrotal mass. Scrotal US can help in distinguishing etiology. Of note, a primary tumor may present with a hydrocele, so the exam should involve specific evaluate on the testis to assess for a mass.

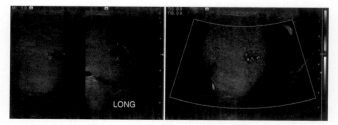

FIG. 11.11 Testicular ultrasound of a Leydig cell tumor in a 15-year-old male patient.

Treatment. Testicular stromal tumors are largely considered benign in prepubertal boys. Thus, for prepubertal patients with physiologically normal (remember the physiologic elevation in AFP in the first year of life) serum tumor markers, an inguinal approach to partial orchiectomy (with intraoperative frozen section) is the treatment of choice (Fig. 11.12). Radical inguinal orchiectomy may be indicated for those with larger masses not amenable to partial orchiectomy. For pubertal/postpubertal adolescent patients, there is less role for partial orchiectomy because the incidence of a malignant GCT is higher compared with prepubertal patients. However, an inguinal approach to partial orchiectomy (with intraoperative frozen section) can be considered in selected adolescents with normal serum markers and a small (<2 cm) testicular tumor. Postsurgical treatment depends on

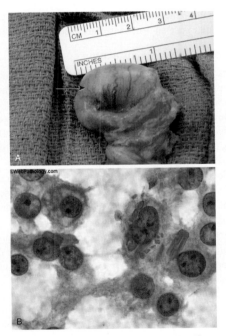

FIG. 11.12 (A) Leydig cell tumor demonstrating characteristic brown appearance related to abundant lipofuscin pigmentation. (B) Reinke crystals. (*A,* Courtesy Fernando Ferrer, MD; *B,* from http://www.webpathology.com.)

pubertal status, tumor type and staging workup. For prepubertal patients with localized stromal tumors (stage I), surgical excision (partial or radical orchiectomy) is curative. Pubertal/postpubertal adolescents with stage I stromal tumors should be followed with surveillance, though an ideal surveillance strategy is not established. Metastatic stromal tumors are rare, and, in such cases, multidisciplinary discussion is needed prior to further therapy. As a separate note, stromal tumors may be associated with DICER-1 mutations, so referral to a genetic counselor is indicated.

Prognosis. Surgical excision with partial or radical inguinal orchiectomy is considered curative in almost all cases of pediatric and adolescent testicular stromal tumors. Unfortunately, there are rare cases of adult patients with metastatic stromal tumors who are typically incurable. Therefore, surveillance is utilized in some cases of pediatric and adolescent stromal tumors as we extrapolate from the adult experience in these rare cases.

Paratesticular Rhabdomyosarcoma

Symptoms. Palpable scrotal/testicular mass or swelling, scrotal/testicular pain, dysuria, or focal symptoms from metastatic disease (cough, bone pain, neurologic deficits).

History. Duration and acuity of symptoms, history of cryptorchidism, family history of testicular cancer, and genetic syndromes (Klinefelter syndrome, DICER-1, Peutz-Jeghers syndrome, Carney complex, congenital adrenal hyperplasia).

Examination. Evaluate the scrotum, testes and paratesticular structures, and varicocele. Abdominal and pelvic exam to assess for any abdominal masses. Assess for any signs of precocious puberty or gynecomastia.

Labs. If concern for a testicular stromal tumor, serum tumor markers such as inhibin-B, testosterone, and estradiol should be drawn. To help distinguish from a GCT, AFP, bHCG, and LDH are recommended. Note that AFP may be physiologically elevated in the first year of life. Should also check complete metabolic profile and a CBC.

Imaging. Scrotal US can localize the tumor to the testis or paratesticular structures and may also evaluate the contralateral testis (Fig. 11.13). If pathologic is concerning for malignancy, the next step in imaging is full staging with CT of the chest, abdomen, and pelvis. Staging for rhabdomyosarcoma will also include a PET scan.

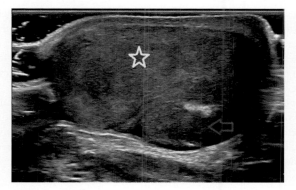

FIG. 11.13 Testicular ultrasound of a paratesticular rhabdomyosarcoma in a 2-year-old male patient. (Yellow star indicates the large paratesticular mass. Red arrow indicates the normal testicle adjacent to the mass.

Differential Diagnosis. The differential diagnosis of a scrotal mass in a child includes both benign (teratoma, testicular stromal tumors) and malignant (germ cell tumor, rhabdomyosarcoma) tumors of the testis or paratesticular structures. Also, entities such as a testicular torsion, hernia, hydrocele, and varicocele may appear as a scrotal mass. Scrotal US can help in distinguishing etiology. Of note, a primary tumor may present with a hydrocele, so the exam should involve specific evaluation on the testis to assess for a mass.

Treatment. Paratesticular rhabdomyosarcoma is initially treated with a radical, inguinal orchiectomy. In cases when the diagnosis is not clear, an inguinal exploration with excisional biopsy and intraoperative frozen section can be considered. However, if the biopsy is inconclusive the preference is for completion radical orchiectomy. Scrotal approaches to orchiectomy or situations in which a prior biopsy is done and the testicle replaced into the scrotum will require hemiscrotectomy if the final pathology is rhabdomyosarcoma.

All patients with paratesticular rhabdomyosarcoma receive adjuvant chemotherapy. Boys younger than 10 years old with no metastatic disease on imaging do not need a staging retroperitoneal lymph node dissection prior to adjuvant chemotherapy. However, those who are 10 years of age or older require a staging ipsilateral retroperitoneal lymph node dissection prior to adjuvant chemotherapy. A bone marrow biopsy may also be indicated depending on the imaging. Final disease staging and grouping (based on imaging, surgical approach, and pathology) will dictate the length of chemotherapy and potential need for radiation therapy.

Prognosis. Paratesticular is considered a favorable site for rhabdomyosarcoma. Prognosis for those without distant (nonnodal) metastatic disease is good with >95% OS. This good survival includes even those with retroperitoneal nodal involvement. However, distant metastatic disease is associated with much lower OS (25%).

Suggested Readings

Caldwell BT, Wilcox DT, Cost NG. Current management for pediatric urologic oncology. *Adv Pediatr* 2017;64(1):191-223.

Dangle PP, Correa A, Tennyson L, Gayed B, et al. Current management of paratesticular rhabdomyosarcoma. *Urol Oncol* 2016;34(2):84-92.

Dome JS, Fernandez CV, Mullen EA, et al. Children's Oncology Group's 2013 blueprint for research: renal tumors. *Pediatr Blood Cancer* 2013;60:994.

England RJ, Haider N, Vujanic GM, et al. Mesoblastic nephroma: a report of the United Kingdom Children's Cancer and Leukaemia Group (CCLG). *Pediatr Blood Cancer* 2011;56(5):744-748.

Geller JI, Cost NG, Chi YY, et al. A prospective study of pediatric and adolescent renal cell carcinoma: a report from the Children's Oncology Group (COG) Study AREN032. *Cancer* 2020;126(23):5156-5164.

Grantham EC, Caldwell BT, Cost NG. Current urologic care for testicular germ cell tumors in pediatric and adolescent patients. *Urol Oncol* 2016;34(2):65-75.

Green DM. The evolution of treatment for Wilms tumor. *J Pediatr Surg* 2013;48(1):14-19.

Kieran K, Ehrlich PF. Current surgical standards of care in Wilms tumor. *Urol Oncol* 2016;34(1):13-23.

Kieran K, Shnorhavorian M. Current standards of care in bladder and prostate rhabdomyosarcoma. *Urol Oncol* 2016;34(2):93-102.

Matthay KK, Maris JM, Schleiermacher G, et al. Neuroblastoma. *Nat Rev Dis Primers* 2016;2:16078.

Nakamura L, Ritchey M. Current management of wilms' tumor. *Curr Urol Rep* 2010;11(1):58-65.

Peard L, Cost NG, Saltzman AF. Pediatric pheochromocytoma: current status of diagnostic imaging and treatment procedures. *Curr Opin Urol* 2019;29(5):493-499.

Ross JH. Prepubertal testicular tumors. *Urology* 2009;74(1):94-99.

Ross JH, Rybicki L, Kay R. Clinical behavior and a contemporary management algorithm for prepubertal testis tumors: a summary of the Prepubertal Testis Tumor Registry. *J Urol* 2002;168(4 Pt 2):1675-1678; discussion 1678-1679.

Rove KO, Maroni PD, Cost CR, et al. Pathologic risk factors in pediatric and adolescent patients with clinical stage I testicular stromal tumors. *J Pediatr Hematol Oncol* 2015;37(8):e441-446.

Saltzman AF, Cost NG. Current treatment of pediatric bladder and prostate rhabdomyosarcoma. *Curr Urol Rep* 2018;19(1):11.

Taskinen S, Fagerholm R, Aronniemi J, et al. Testicular tumors in children and adolescents. *J Pediatr Urol* 2008;4(2):134-137.

12

Infections and Inflammatory Conditions of the Genitourinary System

MICHAEL C. CHEN, AARON KRUG, AND POLINA REYBLAT

CONTRIBUTORS OF CAMPBELL-WALSH-WEIN, 12TH EDITION

Kimberly L Cooper, Gina M. Badalato, Matthew P. Rutman, Kristy Mckiernan Borawski, Alicia H. Chang, Brian G. Blackburn, Michael Hsieh, Robert M Moldwin, Phillip M. Hanno, Michael Pontari, Richard Edward Link, and Nikki Tang

URINARY TRACT INFECTIONS

An **uncomplicated urinary tract infection (UTI)** is an infection in a healthy patient with a structurally and functionally normal urinary tract. Most of these infections resolve with a short course of oral therapy. A **complicated UTI** is associated with factors that increase the chance of acquiring bacteria and decrease the efficacy of therapy (Box 12.1). Here, the urinary tract is structurally or functionally abnormal, the host is compromised, and the bacteria have increased virulence or antimicrobial resistance.

Escherichia coli **is the most common pathogen**, accounting for 85% of community-acquired and 50% of hospital-acquired infections. An important step in the uropathogenisis of *E. coli* is the bacterial adherence with appendages (pili or fimbriae) to the surface urothelium of the host (Fig. 12.1). **Type 1 pili** are **mannose sensitive** because their adhesion ability is inhibited by mannose. **Type P pili** exhibit tropism to the kidney and are found in most strains of *E. coli* that cause pyelonephritis. Type P pili are **mannose resistant** since mannose does not affect their adhesion ability.

Box 12.1 Factors That Suggest a Complicated Urinary Tract Infection

- Functional or anatomic abnormality of the urinary tract
- Male gender
- Pregnancy
- Older adult patient
- Diabetes
- Immunosuppression
- Spinal cord injury
- Childhood urinary tract infection
- Recent antimicrobial agent use
- Indwelling urinary catheter
- Urinary obstruction
- Urinary tract instrumentation
- Hospital-acquired infection
- Symptoms for >7 days at presentation

Cystitis is associated with symptoms of dysuria, frequency, and/or urgency; suprapubic pain; hematuria; and fever. **Acute pyelonephritis** is associated with fever, chills, flank pain, costovertebral-angle tenderness, nausea, vomiting, and malaise. Painless gross hematuria, or microhematuria in the absence of a positive culture, should always raise the suspicion for urologic malignancy, and a hematuria evaluation must be initiated. Imaging studies are not required in most cases of UTI; however, some clinical scenarios may warrant imaging to identify underlying abnormalities requiring procedural intervention or modification of medical management (Boxes 12.2 and 12.3).

Diagnosis of UTI is dependent on a properly collected urine sample (Box 12.4). **Urine dipsticks** are most helpful in ruling out a UTI. Positive nitrites, leukocyte esterase, and blood most accurately diagnose a UTI. Multiple aspects of the **complete urinalysis** may indicate an acute inflammatory response. **Pyuria** is defined as >5 white blood cells (WBCs)/high-power field (HPF). Moderate pyuria (>50 WBCs/HPF) in conjunction with urinary symptoms may indicate a UTI. The mere presence of WBCs in the urine, however, is not diagnostic of a UTI because pyuria can be found in several common urologic conditions. **Leukocyte esterase** is produced by the breakdown of WBCs in urine. Its presence is an indication of pyuria but not bacteria specifically. **Nitrites** are

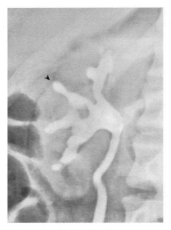

FIG. 12.1 Excretory urogram demonstrates focal, coarse scarring in the right kidney of an 18-year-old girl with a history of many recurrent fevers between 2 months and 2 years of age. A cystogram when the patient was 2 years old established an atrophic left kidney with marked reflux up to the left kidney and slight reflux up to the right kidney. Excretory urography at the age of 6 years established severe atrophy of the left kidney. She had no infections between the ages of 6 and 15 years. Several reinfections occurred at the age of 15 years, and they ceased with prophylactic therapy. Her blood pressure has remained normal, and her serum creatinine level was 0.9 mg/dL at the age of 18 years. At 21 years of age, she stopped antimicrobial prophylaxis for 18 months without infections or introital colonization with Enterobacteriaceae. Note that all calyces are blunted and that one extends to the capsule *(arrowhead)* because of atrophy of the overlying cortex.

Box 12.2 Important Information in Evaluation of Urinary Tract Infections

- Recent infections/antibiotic use
- Recent hospitalizations
- Comorbidities
- History of pediatric voiding dysfunction
- Sexual and reproductive history
- Anatomic urologic abnormalities
- Prior surgery of genitourinary tract, reproductive organs, spine
- Family history
- Current medications

Box 12.3 Indications for Radiologic Investigation in Acute Pyelonephritis

- Potential ureteral obstruction (e.g., caused by stone, ureteral stricture, tumor)
- History of calculi, especially infection (struvite) stones
- Potential papillary necrosis (e.g., patients with sickle cell anemia, severe diabetes mellitus, analgesic abuse)
- History of genitourinary surgery that predisposes to obstruction, such as ureteral reimplantation or ureteral diversion
- Poor response to appropriate antimicrobial agents after 5–6 days of treatment
- Diabetes mellitus
- Polycystic kidneys in patients in dialysis or with severe renal insufficiency
- Neuropathic bladder
- Unusual infecting organisms, such as tuberculosis, fungus, or urea-splitting organisms (e.g., *Proteus*)

Box 12.4 Factors That Affect Ability to Provide Adequate Midstream Clean-Catch Sample

- Increased body mass index
- Vaginal atrophy
- Poor manual dexterity
- Inability to bear weight
- Intravaginal pessary
- Nonsterile collection receptacle

---

present when bacteria reduce dietary nitrates via the bacterial enzyme nitrate reductase. Not all bacteria produce nitrites, so the absence of nitrites does not mean bacteria are not present. All Enterobacteriaceae produce nitrites, including *E. coli, Klebsiella, Enterobacter, Proteus, Citrobacter, Morganella, and Salmonella.* Nonnitrite producing bacteria include all gram positives and pseudomonads (*Pseudomonas and Acinetobacter*) (Fig. 12.2). **Urine culture** is the gold standard for identifying bacteriuria, which supports a diagnosis of UTI in the symptomatic patient. Urine culture results are reported as negative, commensal flora, or positive. Commensal flora includes coagulase-negative

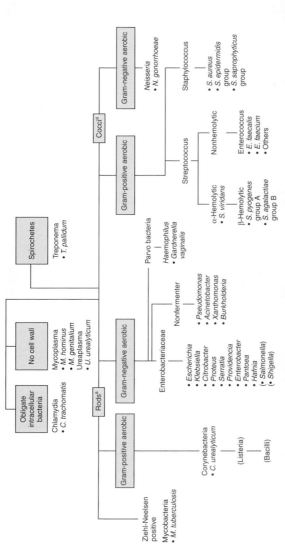

FIG. 12.2 Relevant bacteria for urological infections. [a]Anaerobic bacteria not considered (see Grabe et al., 2015, p. 60 for clarification). (From Grabe M, Bartoletti R, Bjerklund Johansen TE, et al. *Guidelines on urological infections.* 2015. https://uroweb.org/wp-content/uploads/19-Urological-infections_LR2.pdf.)

staphylococci, α- and nonhemolytic streptococci, diphtheroids, nonpathogenic *Neisseria* spp., and yeast. In dysuric patients, an appropriate threshold value for defining significant bacteriuria is 10^2 colony-forming unit (CFU)/mL of a known pathogen.

Asymptomatic Bacteriuria (AB)

AB occurs when a person has no signs or symptoms of UTI, yet bacteria are identified in a urine sample. In women, the term is used when the same bacteria are identified in quantitative counts of ≥100,000 CFUs in two consecutive voided samples that are obtained in a fashion that minimizes contamination. In men, only one positive, clean-catch sample is necessary. **AB should not be treated in most patients,** but treatment is recommended in pregnant women and in patients undergoing procedures in which transmucosal bleeding is anticipated (Box 12.5).

Antimicrobial Therapy. Antimicrobial selection should be influenced by efficacy, safety, cost, and compliance. The choice of agent and duration of therapy are critical in preventing the perpetuation of antimicrobial resistance as well as treatment-related adverse effects. The mechanism of action, reliable coverage, common adverse reactions, precautions, and contraindications for antimicrobial agents used in the treatment of UTIs are summarized in Tables 12.1 to 12.4.

Uncomplicated Cystitis

Uncomplicated cystitis is characterized by an acute onset of dysuria and change in baseline voiding symptoms. Possible first-line antimicrobial therapies include nitrofurantoin, trimethoprim-

---

Box 12.5 Decision to Treat Asymptomatic Bacteriuria

Do not treat: premenopausal women, nonpregnant patients, patients with diabetes, older community dwellers, older adult institutionalized patients, patients with spinal cord injuries; patients with indwelling catheters, and patients with pyuria with asymptomatic bacteriuria

Treat: pregnant women and those undergoing procedures in which transmucosal bleeding is anticipated

Table 12.1 Bacteriostatic Versus Bactericidal Agents

BACTERIOSTATIC	BACTERICIDIAL
Chloramphenicol	Aminoglycosides
Clindamycin	Quinolones
Macrolides	β-Lactams
Sulfonamides	Vancomycin
Tetracycline	
Trimethoprim	

Table 12.2 Mechanism of Action of Common Antimicrobials Used in the Treatment of Urinary Tract Infections

DRUG OR DRUG CLASS	MECHANISM OF ACTION	MECHANISMS OF DRUG RESISTANCE
β-Lactams (penicillins, cephalosporins, aztreonam)	Inhibition of bacterial cell wall synthesis	Production of β-lactamase Penicillin-binding protein altercation Changes in cell wall porin size
Aminoglycosides	Inhibition of ribosomal protein synthesis	Downregulation of bacterial drug uptake Aminoglycoside-modifying enzymes
Quinolones	Inhibition of bacterial DNA gyrase	Mutation in DNA gyrase-binding site Changes in cell wall porin size, active efflux
Fosfomycin	Inhibition of bacterial cell wall synthesis	Novel amino acid substitutions or the loss of function of transporters
Nitrofurantoin	Inhibition of several bacterial enzyme systems	Not fully elucidated
Trimethoprim-sulfamethoxazole	Antagonism of bacterial folate metabolism	Draws folate from environment
Vancomycin	Inhibition of bacterial cell wall synthesis (at β-lactams)	Enzymatic alteration of peptidoglycan

Table 12.3 Reliable Coverage of Antimicrobials Used in the Treatment of Commonly Encountered Pathogens

ANTIMICROBIAL AGENT OR CLASS	GRAM-POSITIVE PATHOGENS	GRAM-NEGATIVE PATHOGENS
Amoxicillin or ampicillin	Streptococcus Enterococci	Proteus mirabilis
Amoxicillin with clavulanate	Streptococcus Enterococci	P. mirabilis, Klebsiella spp.
Ampicillin with sulbactam	Staphylococcus (not MRSA) Enterococci	P. mirabilis, H. influenzae, Klebsiella spp.
Antistaphylococcal penicillins	Streptococcus Staphylococcus (not MRSA)	None
Antipseudomonal penicillins	Streptococcus Enterococci	Most, including Pseudomonas aeruginosa
First-generation cephalosporins	Streptococcus Staphylococcus (not MRSA)	Escherichia coli, P. mirabilis, Klebsiella spp.
Second-generation cephalosporins (cefamandole, cefuroxime, cefaclor)	Streptococcus Staphylococcus (not MRSA)	E. coli, P. mirabilis H. influenzae, Klebsiella spp.
Second-generation cephalosporins (cefoxitin, cefotetan)	Streptococcus	E. coli, Proteus spp. (including indole-positive) H. influenzae, Klebsiella spp.
Third-generation cephalosporins (ceftriaxone)	Streptococcus Staphylococcus (not MRSA)	Most, excluding P. aeruginosa
Third-generation cephalosporins (ceftazidime)	Streptococcus	Most, including P. aeruginosa
Aztreonam	None	Most, including P. aeruginosa
Aminoglycosides	Staphylococcus (urine)	Most, including P. aeruginosa
Fluoroquinolones	Streptococcus[a]	Most, including P. aeruginosa

Continued

Table 12.3 Reliable Coverage of Antimicrobials Used in the Treatment of Commonly Encountered Pathogens—cont'd

ANTIMICROBIAL AGENT OR CLASS	GRAM-POSITIVE PATHOGENS	GRAM-NEGATIVE PATHOGENS
Nitrofurantoin	*Staphylococcus* (not MRSA), enterococci	Many Enterobacteriaceae (not *Providencia*, *Serratia*, *Acinetobacter*) *Klebsiella* spp.
Fosfomycin	Enterococci	Most Enterobacteriaceae (not *P. aeruginosa*)
Pivmecillinam	None	Most, excluding *P. aeruginosa*
Trimethoprim-sulfamethoxazole	*Streptococcus*, *Staphylococcus*	Most Enterobacteriaceae (not *P. aeruginosa*)
Vancomycin	All, including MRSA	None

MRSA, Methicillin-resistant *Staphylococcus aureus*
[a]May be given with an initial one-time intravenous dose of a long-acting parenteral antimicrobial such as 1 g of ceftriaxone or a consolidated 24-hour dose of an aminoglycoside. See IDSA recommendations.

sulfamethoxazole, fosfomycin, and pivmecillinam (Fig. 12.3). Three and 7 days of therapy are preferred in women and men, respectively. Approximately 90% of women are asymptomatic within 72 hours after initiating antimicrobial therapy. A follow-up visit, culture, and further urologic evaluation are not necessary in women who respond to therapy.

Complicated UTIs

Complicated UTIs are those that occur in a patient with a compromised urinary tract or are caused by a very resistant pathogen. These complicating factors may be readily apparent from the severity of the presenting illness or past medical history or may be evident after failure to respond to appropriate therapy. For patients requiring hospitalization, parenteral (intravenous [IV]) antimicrobials should be administered based on the susceptibility patterns of the known uropathogens. Every effort should be made to correct any underlying urinary tract abnormalities. Therapy is usually continued for 10–14 days on culture-specific antibiotics and switched from IV to oral therapy when the patient is afebrile and clinically stable. Repeat urine cultures should be performed if the patient fails to respond to therapy.

Table 12.4 Common Adverse Reactions, Precautions, and Contraindications for Antimicrobial Agents Used in the Treatment of Urinary Tract Infections

DRUG OR DRUG CLASS	COMMON ADVERSE REACTIONS	PRECAUTIONS AND CONTRAINDICATIONS
Amoxicillin or ampicillin Amoxicillin with clavulanic acid Ampicillin with sulbactam	Hypersensitivity (immediate or delayed) Gastrointestinal (GI) upset	Increased risk of rash with concomitant viral disease, allopurinol therapy
Antistaphylococcal penicillins	Same as with amoxicillin/ampicillin Acute interstitial nephritis (especially methicillin)	
Antipseudomonal penicillins	Same as with amoxicillin/ampicillin Hypernatremia (these drugs are given as sodium salt)	Use with caution in patients very sensitive to sodium loading
Cephalosporins	Hypersensitivity GI upset (with oral agents) Positive Coombs test Decreased platelet aggregation	Should not be used in patients with immediate hypersensitivity to penicillins; may use with caution in patients with delayed hypersensitivity reactions
Aztreonam	Hypersensitivity (less than with penicillins)	<1% incidence of cross-reactivity in penicillin or cephalosporin allergic patients
Aminoglycosides	Ototoxicity Nephrotoxicity: nonoliguric azotemia Neuromuscular blockade with high levels	Avoid in pregnant patients and patients with severely impaired renal function, diabetes, or hepatic failure Use with caution in patients with myasthenia gravis Use with caution with other potentially ototoxic and nephrotoxic drugs

Continued

Table 12.4 Common Adverse Reactions, Precautions, and Contraindications for Antimicrobial Agents Used in the Treatment of Urinary Tract Infections—cont'd

DRUG OR DRUG CLASS	COMMON ADVERSE REACTIONS	PRECAUTIONS AND CONTRAINDICATIONS
Fluoroquinolones	Mild GI effects; dizziness, lightheadedness; photosensitivity Central nervous system effects, including dizziness, tremors, confusion, mood disorder, hallucinations Tendon rupture	Avoid in children or pregnant patients Concomitant antacid, iron, zinc, or sucralfate use dramatically decreases oral absorption Can significantly increase theophylline plasma levels; avoid quinolones or monitor theophylline levels closely. Can lower seizure threshold Monitor glucose levels in patients taking antidiabetic agents because hypoglycemia and hyperglycemia have been reported Can enhance warfarin effects; closely monitor coagulation tests
Fosfomycin	Headache, GI upset, vaginitis	Hypersensitivity to fosfomycin
Pivmecillinam	Rash, GI upset	Use with caution in patients with penicillin hypersensitivity

Table 12.4 Common Adverse Reactions, Precautions, and Contraindications for Antimicrobial Agents Used in the Treatment of Urinary Tract Infections—cont'd

DRUG OR DRUG CLASS	COMMON ADVERSE REACTIONS	PRECAUTIONS AND CONTRAINDICATIONS
Nitrofurantoin Peripheral polyneuropathy	GI upset Hemolysis with G6PD deficiency Pulmonary hypersensitivity reactions	Do not use in patients with low creatinine clearance (<50 mL/min) because adequate urine concentrations will not be achieved Monitor long-term patients closely Avoid concomitant probenecid use, which blocks renal excretion of nitrofurantoin Avoid concomitant magnesium or quinolones, which are antagonistic to nitrofurantoin
Trimethoprim-sulfamethoxazole	Hypersensitivity, rash GI upset Photosensitivity Hematologic toxicity (patients with AIDS)	Higher incidence of all adverse reactions occurs in patients with AIDS and in older adults Avoid in pregnant patients Avoid in patients receiving warfarin; concomitant use can significantly elevate prothrombin time
Vancomycin	"Red-man syndrome" Nephrotoxicity and/or ototoxicity when combined with other nephrotoxic and/ ototoxic drugs	Use with caution with other potentially ototoxic and nephrotoxic drugs

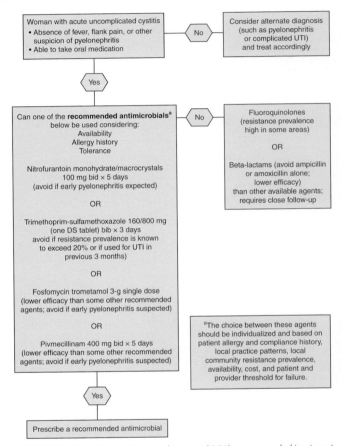

FIG. 12.3 Infectious Diseases Society of America (IDSA)-recommended treatment of acute uncomplicated cystitis

Emphysematous Cystitis (EC). **EC** is a rare and potentially life-threatening form of complicated cystitis that is associated with a high mortality rate. The pathognomonic finding of this disease process is gas noted within the bladder wall on computed tomography (CT) image (Fig. 12.4). EC is typically observed in older women with poorly controlled diabetes. The majority of these patients are treated with medical therapy alone, which consists of IV antibiotics, bladder

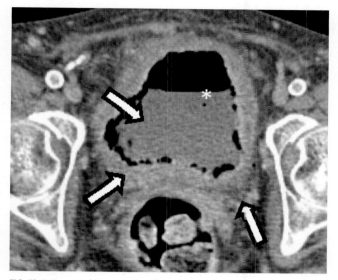

FIG. 12.4 Computed tomography of emphysematous cystitis. *Arrows* indicate intramural gas; there is also air in the bladder lumen *(asterisk).*

drainage, and aggressive treatment of underlying medical conditions. Initial antibiotic treatment regimens must offer broad gram-negative coverage. If initial Gram stain identifies gram-positive cocci, ampicillin or amoxicillin should be added for better enterococcal coverage. Surgical intervention is reserved for those who respond poorly to initial medical management or those who have severe necrotizing infections.

Recurrent UTIs

A **recurrent UTI** is defined as two UTIs in a 6-month period or ≥3 UTIs in a 12-month period. Medical history should detail the prior number of infections and their frequency, culture results, associated symptoms, and identifiable triggers or risk factors (Box 12.6). Suprapubic fullness should be noted, and pelvic examination should be performed. Imaging and cystoscopic evaluation are not warranted in all women with recurrent UTIs however, these should be performed in women with risk factors for a complicated UTI (Box 12.7) (Fig. 12.5).

Box 12.6 Risk Factors for Recurrent Urinary Tract Infections

- Sexual activity
- New sexual partner within past year
- Family history of urinary tract infection (UTI) in first-degree female relative
- Recent antimicrobial use
- Spermicide use
- History of UTI before menopause
- Menopause
- Incontinence, elevated postvoid residual, cystocele

Box 12.7 Indications for Further Investigation of Recurrent Urinary Tract Infections

- Previous urinary tract trauma or surgery
- Previous bladder or renal calculi
- Gross hematuria after resolution of infection
- Obstructive symptoms, high post-void residual (PVR)
- Urea-splitting bacteria on culture
- Previous abdominopelvic malignancy
- Bacterial persistence after sensitive-based treatment
- Diabetes or other immune compromise
- Pneumaturia, fecaluria, anaerobic bacteria, or history of diverticulitis
- Repeated pyelonephritis
- Asymptomatic microhematuria after resolution of infection

Acute Pyelonephritis

Acute pyelonephritis is the inflammation of the kidney as a result of an infection of the renal parenchyma. *E. coli*, which constitutes a unique subgroup that possesses special virulence factors, accounts for 80% of cases. More resistant species, such as *Proteus, Klebsiella, Pseudomonas, Serratia, Enterobacter,* or *Citrobacter,* should be suspected in patients who have recurrent UTIs, are hospitalized, or have indwelling catheters and in those who underwent recent urinary tract instrumentation. Except for *E. faecalis, S. epidermidis,* and *S. aureus,* gram-positive bacteria rarely cause pyelonephritis.

Classic symptoms consist of an **acute onset of fever, chills, and flank pain** and/or costovertebral tenderness. The clinical presentation

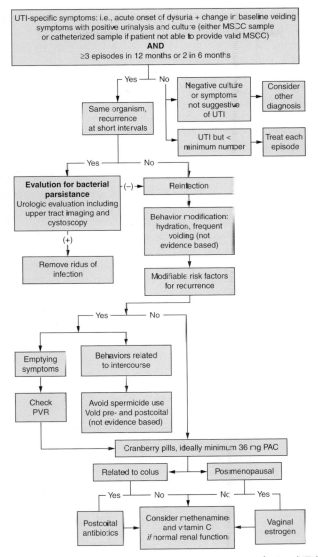

FIG. 12.5 Algorithm for management of recurrent urinary tract infections (UTIs). *MSCC*, Midstream clean-catch sample; *PAC*, proanthocyanidin; *PVR*, post void residual.

is wide-ranging, from gram-negative sepsis to cystitis with mild flank pain. There is often flank tenderness to deep palpation.

Urinalysis (UA) may reveal pyuria, bacteria, and large amounts of granular or leukocyte cast. Blood cultures are positive in ~25% of cases of uncomplicated pyelonephritis in women. The majority replicate the urine culture and do not influence decisions regarding therapy. **Blood cultures** should be obtained in patients with systemic toxicity, those requiring hospitalization, or with risk factors such as pregnancy. Ultrasound (US) may show focal parenchymal swelling and regions of increased or decreased echogenicity (Fig. 12.6). **CT and magnetic resonance imaging (MRI) also may show focal swelling and diminished and/or heterogeneous parenchymal contrast enhancement** (Fig. 12.7). Without contrast, CT may show diminished density of affected areas and MRI may show regions of restricted diffusion.

Acute pyelonephritis infections can be subdivided into (1) uncomplicated infections that do not warrant hospitalization, (2) uncomplicated infections in patients with normal urinary tracts who are ill enough to warrant hospitalization for parenteral therapy, and (3) complicated infections associated with hospitalization, catheterization, urologic surgery, or urinary tract abnormalities (Fig. 12.8, Table 12.5). In patients with a fever lasting longer than 72 hours, CT is most helpful for ruling out obstruction and identifying renal and perirenal infections.

Renal Abscess

Renal abscess is a collection of purulent material confined to the renal parenchyma. Gram-negative organisms are typically implicated.

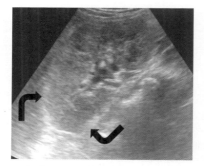

FIG. 12.6 Ultrasound of acute pyelonephritis. *Arrows* show an abnormally echogenic and swollen upper pole.

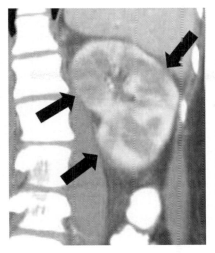

FIG. 12.7 Computed tomography of focal pyelonephritis. *Arrows* show patchy regions of diminished heterogeneous enhancement and swelling.

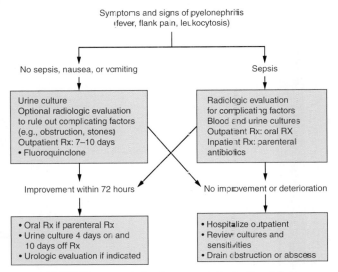

FIG. 12.8 Management of acute pyelonephritis. *Rx,* Prescription.

Table 12.5 Treatment Regimens for Acute Complicated and Uncomplicated Pyelonephritis in Women

CIRCUMSTANCE	ROUTE	DRUG	DOSE[e]	FREQUENCY PER DOSE	DURATION (DAYS)
Outpatient—moderately ill, no nausea or vomiting	Oral[a]	TMP-SMX DS[b]	160–800 mg	q12h	14
		Ciprofloxacin[c]	500 mg	q12h	7
		Ciprofloxacin[c] (extended release)	1000 mg	q24h	7
		Levofloxacin[c]	750 mg	q24h	5
Inpatient—severely ill, possible sepsis	Parenteral[d]	Ampicillin and gentamicin	1–2 g 1–1.5 mg/kg	q6h q8h	10–14
		Levofloxacin[c]	500–750 mg	q24h	10–14
		Ceftriaxone	1 g	q24h	10–14
		Carbapenem	(dose varies)		10–14
Pregnant	Parenteral[d]	Ampicillin and gentamicin	1–2 g 1–1.5 mg/kg	q6h q8h	10–14
	Oral	Aztreonam	1 g	q8h	10–14
		Cephalexin	500 mg	q6h	

DS, Double strength; q, every; TMP-SMX, trimethoprim-sulfamethoxazole.
[a]May be given with an initial one-time intravenous dose of a long-acting parenteral antimicrobial such as 1 g of ceftriaxone or a consolidated 24-hour dose of an aminoglycoside. See IDSA recommendations.
[b]Appropriate choice if uropathogen is known to be susceptible. If susceptibility is unknown, an initial dose of long-acting parenteral antimicrobial such as 1 g of ceftriaxone or a consolidated 24-hour dose of an aminoglycoside is recommended.
[c]May be used in areas where the prevalence of resistance of community uropathogens to fluoroquinolones is not known to exceed 10%.
[d]For parenteral agents, take until afebrile then transition to oral agents according to sensitivities.
[e]All dosages should be adjusted for renal function.

Ascending infection associated with tubular obstruction from prior infections or calculi appears to be the primary pathway. Gram-positive infections may occur via hematogenous seeding in patients with multiple skin carbuncles or in IV drug users.

Patients may present with **fever, chills, abdominal or flank pain**, and, occasionally, weight loss and malaise. The diagnosis of renal abscess is often preceded by urinary tract symptoms consistent with UTI or pyelonephritis.

Patients typically have marked **leukocytosis**. Pyuria and bacteriuria may not be evident unless the abscess communicates with the collecting system. Bacteremia may be present. Urine cultures may show no growth or a microorganism different from that isolated from the abscess. US may show a low-echodensity lesion with increased transmission. **CT is the diagnostic procedure of choice** and will characteristically show abscesses as well-defined lesions with decreased attenuation (Fig. 12.9).

Patients should be immediately started on **IV antibiotics**. Conservative management with antibiotics and careful observation may be employed in clinically stable patients with small abscesses (<3–5 cm in diameter). The size of the abscess may be assessed radiographically for improvement. Image-guided needle aspiration may be necessary to differentiate abscess from tumor. **Percutaneous**

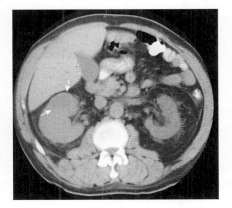

FIG. 12.9 Acute renal abscess. Nonenhanced computed tomography scan through the midpole of the right kidney demonstrates right renal enlargement and an area of decreased attenuation *(arrows)*. After antimicrobial therapy, a follow-up scan showed complete regression of these findings.

drainage remains the first-line procedure of choice for most renal abscesses >5 cm in diameter.

Perinephric Abscess

A **perinephric abscess extends beyond the renal capsule but is contained by Gerota's fascia**. It usually results from rupture of an acute cortical abscess into the perinephric space, extravasated infected urine from obstruction or trauma, infection of a perinephric hematoma, or hematogenous seeding.

Patients may present **similar to a renal abscess**. An abdominal or flank mass can be felt in approximately half of the cases. Laboratory features include leukocytosis, elevated serum creatinine, and pyuria. Blood and urine culture may or may not be positive. CT is valuable for demonstrating the primary abscess (Fig. 12.10).

All patients should be **immediately started on IV antibiotic therapy**. Small abscesses may be treated with antibiotics alone in clinically stable and immune competent patients. **Unlike renal abscesses, early percutaneous drainage of abscesses >3 cm in diameter is recommended.** Nephrectomy may be necessary if the kidney is nonfunctioning or severely infected.

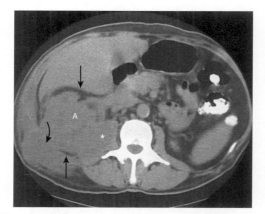

FIG. 12.10 Nonenhanced computed tomography scan through the lower pole of the right kidney (previous left nephrectomy) shows extensive perinephric abscess. Extensive abscess (*A*) distorts and enlarges the renal contour, infiltrates perinephric fat *(straight arrows)*, and extends into the psoas muscle *(asterisk)* and the soft tissues of the flank *(curved arrow)*. Also note that normal renal collecting system fat has been obliterated by the process.

Xanthogranulomatous Pyelonephritis (XGP)

XGP is a rare, severe, chronic renal infection typically resulting in diffuse renal destruction. The primary factors involved in the pathogenesis are nephrolithiasis, obstruction, and infection. XGP is characterized by accumulation of lipid-laden, foamy macrophages. It begins within the pelvis and calyces and subsequently extends into and destroys renal parenchymal and adjacent tissues.

XGP should be suspected in patients with UTIs and a **unilateral, enlarged, nonfunctioning, or poorly functioning kidney with a stone or a mass lesion** indistinguishable from malignancy. Patients with XGP commonly experience flank pain, fever, chills, and persistent bacteriuria. *Proteus* is the most common organism involved, followed by *E. coli*. Blood tests often reveal anemia and, possibly, hepatic dysfunction. Azotemia or frank renal failure is rare. CT classically shows unilateral renal enlargement with little or no function and a large calculus in the renal pelvis. Renal parenchyma is replaced by multiple water density masses representing dilated calyces and abscesses. Tc-99m DMSA (2,3 dimercaptosuccinic acid), a technetium renal scan may be used to confirm and quantify the differential lack of function in the involved kidney (Fig. 12.11).

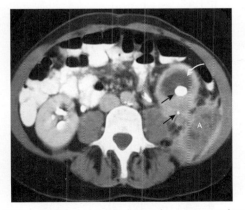

FIG. 12.11 Xanthogranulomatous pyelonephritis. Enhanced computed tomography scan shows collecting system and parenchymal calculi *(straight black arrows)* with lower pole pyonephrosis *(curved white arrow)* and an irregular, predominantly low-density perinephric abscess *(A)* extending into the soft tissues of the flank.

XGP is treated by **surgical excision** of the infected kidney and all surrounding inflammatory tissue. Antimicrobial therapy may be necessary to stabilize the patient preoperatively. The surrounding inflammatory reaction may make surgery difficult. Intraoperative frozen section is unreliable because the lipid-laden macrophages associated with XGP closely resemble clear cell adenocarcinoma. Incision and drainage or **percutaneous drainage is not curative**.

Emphysematous Pyelonephritis (EP)

EP is a urologic emergency characterized by an **acute necrotizing parenchymal and perirenal infection caused by gas-forming uropathogens**. The condition usually occurs in patients with diabetes and in the setting of urinary tract obstruction, papillary necrosis, and significant renal impairment.

The **usual presentation is severe acute pyelonephritis with the classic triad of fever, vomiting, and flank pain**. Hypoalbuminemia, shock at initial presentation, bacteremia, hemodialysis requirement, thrombocytopenia, altered mental status, and polymicrobial infection are associated with a poor prognosis and increased mortality. Urine culture is invariably positive, most commonly with *E. coli*. *Proteus* and *Klebsiella* are less common. CT will demonstrate mottled gas distributed in the renal parenchyma (Fig. 12.12).

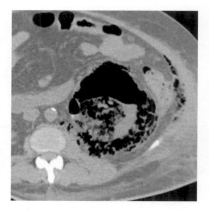

FIG. 12.12 Computed tomography of emphysematous pyelonephritis. There is air within and surrounding the left kidney.

EP is a **urologic emergency**. Most patients are septic and require intensive care. Fluid resuscitation, glucose and electrolyte management, and broad-spectrum antimicrobial therapy are essential. Patients may **initially be managed via placement of a ureteral stent or percutaneous nephrostomy** tube. Nephrectomy is advised in cases where patients do not respond to conservative management or if there is extensive and diffuse gas with renal destruction.

Acute Orchitis and Epididymitis

Acute orchitis and epididymitis involve pain, swelling, and inflammation of the testicle and epididymis, respectively. *E. coli* and *Pseudomonas* are common causative microorganisms. Examination of the scrotum usually reveals a tender testis and spermatic cord. Urine culture should be obtained in all patients. Sexually transmitted infection (STI) testing should be performed, if indicated. Imaging with scrotal US can help to distinguish testicular torsion from orchitis and identify testicular tumors and abscesses. In patients with signs of infectious orchitis, antibiotics to treat gram-negative uropathogens should be started and treatment adjusted based on the result of urine culture. A patient suspected of having a STI should have appropriate treatment started. Patients with orchitis, especially those whose symptoms do not resolve, need follow up to rule out missed torsion or testicular tumor.

Fournier Gangrene

Fournier gangrene (FG) is a **potentially life-threatening** progressive infection of the perineum and genitalia. Risk factors for developing FG include alcoholism, diabetes, recent urogenital or colorectal instrumentation or trauma, and preexisting peripheral vascular disease. Infection may spread along fascial planes. The diagnosis of FG is a surgical emergency as the soft tissue infection can spread very rapidly. Treatment involves a combination of broad-spectrum antibiotics and extensive surgical debridement to margins of healthy bleeding tissue. (https://www.cdc.gov/std/default.htm)

GONOCOCCAL URETHRITIS

Symptoms in men may include urethritis, epididymitis, prostatitis, and proctitis. Women are usually asymptomatic and may present with sequelae of the disease (e.g., pelvic inflammatory disease, tubal scarring, infertility, ectopic pregnancy, and chronic pelvic pain).

Nucleic-acid amplification tests (NAATs) are the preferred method for detecting both N. gonorrhoeae **and** C. trachomatis. In symptomatic men, a positive Gram stain of a male urethral specimen that demonstrates polymorphonuclear leukocytes with intracellular gram-negative diplococci can also be considered diagnostic. Because of its low sensitivity, a negative Gram stain does not rule out N. gonorrhoeae infection.

Treatment involves a single dose of both ceftriaxone 250 mg intramuscularly and azithromycin 1 g orally. Alternative regimens are single oral doses of cefixime 500 mg plus azithromycin 1 g. Patients with allergies to cephalosporins should be treated with azithromycin 2 g orally and, either oral gemifloxacin 320 mg or intramuscular gentamicin 340 mg. Additionally, **all patients diagnosed with gonorrhea should be tested for other STIs**.

NONGONOCOCCAL URETHRITIS (Fig. 12.13)

Chlamydial Urethritis

Chlamydia, caused by C. trachomatis, is the **most frequently reported infectious disease** in the United States. Ascending chlamydial infections in women can lead to scarring of the fallopian tubes, pelvic inflammatory disease, pelvic pain, and infertility. NAAT using first-catch urine is the most sensitive test for detecting C. trachomatis infections in men. The recommended treatment is single-dose, oral azithromycin 1 g or oral doxycycline 100 mg twice daily for 7 days. Concurrent testing for gonorrhea, human immunodeficiency virus (HIV), and syphilis should be performed. As with gonorrhea, **all sex partners within the 60 days preceding the onset of symptoms** should be referred for evaluation.

Mycoplasma Genitalium

M. genitalium is responsible for 15%–20% of nongonococcal urethritis (NGU) cases, 20%–25% of nonchlamydial urethritis cases, and ~30% of persistent or recurrent urethritis cases. Transmission is primarily by direct genital-genital mucosal contact. Because of the lack of approved diagnostic tests, M. genitalium should be suspected in cases of persistent or recurrent urethritis. There have been reports

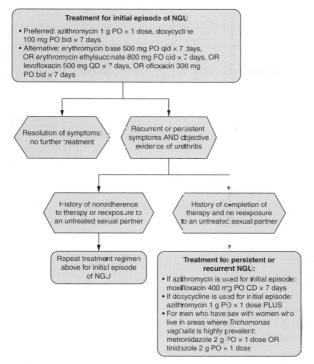

Treatment for initial episode of NGU

- Preferred: azithromycin 1 g PO × 1 dose, doxycycline 100 mg PO bid × 7 days
- Alternative: erythromycin base 500 mg PO qid × 7 days, OR erythromycin ethylsuccinate 800 mg PO qid × 7 days, OR levofloxacin 500 mg QD × 7 days, OR ofloxacin 300 mg PO bid × 7 days

Resolution of symptoms: no further treatment

Recurrent or persistent symptoms AND objective evidence of urethritis

History of nonadherence to therapy or reexposure to an untreated sexual partner

History of completion of therapy and no reexposure to an untreated sexual partner

Repeat treatment regimen above for initial episode of NGU

Treatment for persistent or recurrent NGU:

- If azithromycin is used for initial episode: moxifloxacin 400 mg PO QD × 7 days
- If doxycycline is used for initial episode: azithromycin 1 g PO × 1 dose PLUS
- For men who have sex with women who live in areas where *Trichomonas vaginalis* is highly prevalent: metronidazole 2 g PO × 1 dose OR tinidazole 2 g PO × 1 dose

FIG. 12.13 Treatment algorithm for nongonococcal urethritis (NGU).

of treatment failure due to increasing antibiotic resistance. The Centers for Disease Control and Prevention (CDC) currently recommends a single dose of 1 g azithromycin as first-line therapy.

Trichomonas vaginalis

T. vaginalis is a flagellated parasite that preferentially infects the urethra in men and the urethra, vagina, and vulva in women. NAATs or wet mounts of cultures are used for diagnosis. The low prevalence of *T. vaginalis* in NGU does not warrant using these tests in the initial workup, although they should be considered for male sexual partners of women with trichomoniasis and for other male populations in high-prevalence areas. The recommended treatment is a single dose of oral metronidazole 2 g or tinidazole 2 g.

Anogenital Warts (Condyloma Acuminatum)

Human papillomaviruses (HPVs) are a small group of nonenveloped, double-stranded DNA viruses. **HSV 6 and 11 are nononcogenic and are responsible for ~90% of anogenital warts.** High-risk mucosal HPV types, predominantly 16, 18, 31, 33, and 35, have been associated with most cervical, penile, vulvar, vaginal, anal, and oropharyngeal cancers and precancers. **HPV 16 and 18 are the most common high-risk types and are responsible for >70% of all cervical cancer cases.** The diagnosis is made by clinical examination. Biopsy may be indicated in cases of uncertainty or lack of response to treatment. Patient-applied topical therapies include imiquimod cream (3.75% and 5%), podofilox 0.5% solution, and sinecatechins 5% ointment. Procedural treatments include cryotherapy, surgical excision, and trichloroacetic acid or bichloracetic acid application. **The CDC recommends routine vaccination against HPV at 11 or 12 years of age.**

GENITOURINARY TUBERCULOSIS (TB)

A group of closely related acid-fast bacteria called the *Mycobacterium tuberculosis* complex (MTBC) causes TB. MTBC initially enters the host via inhalation of cough-generated infectious aerosols. TB may infect the genitourinary (GU) tract via seeding through ascending infection or hematogenous seeding. When left untreated, GU TB can lead to irreparable tissue damage with serious consequences such as renal failure and infertility.

The **typical TB constitutional symptoms** are fever, weight loss, night sweats, and malaise. GU-specific symptoms may include dysuria, storage symptoms, hematuria and flank pain. Sterile pyuria and hematuria are typical. The **kidneys are the most common site** of GU TB. Renal infection is progressive and highly destructive over time. Granulomas form in the renal parenchyma and coalesce, forming caseating cavities with necrotic material. These can result in abscesses, chronic pyelonephritis, and parenchymal and papillary necrosis. As infection advances, the calyces become inflamed and eventually calcify, resulting in calyceal distortion, dilation, and stenosis.

Ureteral involvement occurs via descent of infection from the kidneys. "Pan-ureteral" strictures may result in a **"beaded corkscrew"** appearance. Obstruction and urinary reflux may develop (Figs. 12.14 and 12.15). Bladder ulcerations may develop in areas

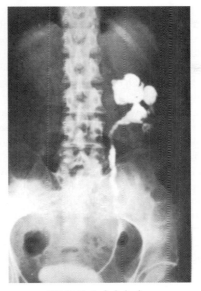

FIG. 12.14 Occluded calyx.

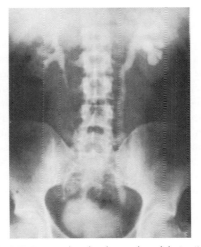

FIG. 12.15 Severe calyceal and parenchymal destruction.

where large granulomas coalesce, with the bladder dome most commonly affected. Bladder contractures develop after approximately 1 year of chronic inflammation and mucosal scarring, which leads to urinary frequency, urgency, pain, and dysuria. The epididymis is the second most common GU site of hematogenous seeding after the kidney. Epididymal TB can extend into the testes and may cause infertility.

GU TB is **diagnosed** with urine acid-fast bacilli culture. **Three to five first-void urine samples obtained on consecutive days** should be collected for maximum yield. Abdominopelvic radiography frequently demonstrates calcifications caused by TB. CT with urography is the most frequently used modality for imaging TB in developed countries, where it has largely replaced IV urography.

Treatment should start with the administration of antituberculosis medications. **Prompt drainage of upper tract obstruction** with percutaneous nephrostomy tube or ureteral stent is warranted in cases of uremia or sepsis. Open ureteral reconstruction may be necessary if obstruction persists after successful medical treatment of TB. Nephrectomy is considered in patients with a nonfunctional kidney and recalcitrant or recurrent TB despite optimal medical therapy or in cases of medically resistant hypertension. Augmentation cystoplasty and bladder substitution are options in the management of the tuberculous contracted bladder.

INTERSTITIAL CYSTITIS

Interstitial cystitis/bladder pain syndrome (IC/BPS) is defined clinically as a **sensation of pain, pressure, and discomfort, perceived to be related to the urinary bladder, associated with lower urinary tract symptoms of** >6 weeks' duration, in the absence of infection or other identifiable causes. Pelvic pain and discomfort are the central symptoms of IC/BPS and the most frequent reason for seeking health care. Urinary frequency is also commonly described. Patients with IC/BPS often describe a compelling need to void centered on mounting pain, pressure, or pelvic discomfort that occurs with filling. Typically, patients with IC/BPS void to avoid or relieve pain. Symptoms tend to fluctuate, and flares are commonly experienced for several days. Triggers for flares vary widely.

The **diagnosis of IC/BPS is challenging** due to the heterogeneity of symptoms and the presence of many medical conditions

Box 12.8 Medical History for Patients with Interstitial Cystitis/
Bladder Pain Syndrome

1. Location of pelvic pain and relationship to bladder filling and emptying
2. Presence or absence of initiating event for pain
3. Duration, quality, and radiation of pain
4. Presence or absence of regional pain (i.e., penile, urethral, vulvar, perineal, perianal, testicular, inguinal, coccygeal)
5. Presence or absence of voiding and/or bowel dysfunction
6. Relationship of pain to menstrual cycle
7. Presence or absence of sexual pain
8. Factors that trigger or decrease pain
9. Response to previous therapies
10. History of urologic/gastroenterological, gynecologic/neurologic/rheumatic disease
11. Previous bladder/pelvic surgery
12. Previous urinary tract infection
13. Previous pelvic irradiation
14. Autoimmune diseases
15. Associated syndromes (irritable bowel, fibromyalgia, chronic fatigue)

with similar symptoms. The initial assessment should include a thorough history, with particular focus on the location and quality of pain symptoms, triggers, and other identifiable causes (Box 12.8). Voiding symptoms may also be evaluated with a voiding diary and pain symptoms quantified with scale or symptom score.

Abdominal examination should focus on documenting abdominal wall tenderness, hernias, abdominal distension, bladder distension, and suprapubic tenderness. A vaginal examination should be performed with inspection for abnormal discharge, musical atrophy, lichen sclerosis, and vaginal and pelvic floor tenderness. A digital rectal examination with complete scrotal and penile examination should be performed in men.

Urine **cytology** should be ordered in patients with gross hematuria and those in high-risk groups for malignancy. Although cystoscopy is not mandatory for diagnosis, a flexible office cystoscopy may be considered early in the course of care to exclude the presence of Hunner's lesions. Urodynamics are not necessary for making the diagnosis in uncomplicated presentations and are usually

Box 12.9 Tiered Therapy for Interstitial Cystitis/Bladder Pain Syndrome per American Urological Association Guidelines

FIRST-LINE TREATMENTS

- General relaxation/stress management
- Patient education
- Self-care/behavior modification
- Pain management

SECOND-LINE TREATMENTS

- Specialized manual physical therapy
- Oral agents: amitriptyline, hydroxyzine, cimetidine, pentosan polysulfate sodium (PPS)
- Intravesical therapy: dimethyl sulphoxide (DMSO), heparin, lidocaine
- Pain management

THIRD-LINE TREATMENTS

- Cystoscopy under anesthesia with hydrodistention
- Treatment of Hunner lesions, if found
- Pain management

FOURTH-LINE TREATMENTS

- Intradetrusor onabotulinumtoxinA
- Neuromodulation
- Pain management

FIFTH-LINE TREATMENTS

- Cyclosporine A
- Pain management

SIXTH-LINE TREATMENTS

- Urinary diversion (with or without cystectomy)
- Substitution cystoplasty
- Pain management

reserved for complex cases. An in-office bladder filling examination may allow an assessment of bladder capacity and reproduction of pain with bladder filling.

Treatment is aimed at ameliorating symptoms and proceeds from least invasive to most invasive options. The 2014 American Urological Association (AUA) guidelines on IC/BPS regarding treatment algorithm are shown in Box 12.9.

Suggested Readings

AUA Core Curriculum Topics
Adult Urinary Tract Infection
Prostatitis
Sexually Transmitted Infection
Interstitial Cystitis

AUA Guidelines
Diagnosis and Treatment Interstitial Cystitis/Bladder Pain Syndrome (2014). https://www.auanet.org/guidelines/interstitial-cystitis-(ic/bps)-guideline.

Recurrent Uncomplicated Urinary Tract Infections in Women: AUA/CUA/SUFU Guideline (2019). https://www.auanet.org/guidelines/recurrent-uti.

13

Male Infertility

RICHARD J. FANTUS AND ROBERT E. BRANNIGAN

CONTRIBUTORS OF CAMPBELL-WALSH-WEIN, 12TH EDITION

Craig S. Niederberger, Samuel J. Ohlander, Rodrigo L. Pagani, and Marc Goldstein

EPIDEMIOLOGY

Infertility affects nearly one in six couples worldwide. **Maternal age is the most important predictive factor of a couple's fertility**. Systematic reporting of in vitro fertilization (IVF) outcomes has led to a better understanding of female factor infertility, but this is not the case for **male factor infertility, which is estimated to contribute to 50% of all cases of infertility**. Furthermore, up to 27% of men in infertile couples are not being evaluated. While the need to workup male factor infertility is sometimes obviated by the existence of IVF, it is important to recognize that the goal of the male workup is for more than procreation. The goals of work up include

- Diagnose and treat reversible causes of infertility.
- Diagnose irreversible causes of infertility amenable to assisted reproductive technology (ART).
- Identify comorbidities that contribute to infertility or harm patient.
- Identify genetic mutations, when appropriate, that may harm patient or offspring.

The **failure to conceive after 12 months of properly timed, unprotected intercourse** remains the standard definition for infertility. Of couples that become pregnant by natural means, nearly 88% achieve pregnancy by 6 months. Thus, initiating workup sooner than 12 months is sometimes reasonable, especially in higher risk couples (i.e., advanced maternal age family history of infertility). While the workup often begins with the woman, early simultaneous evaluation of the male partner could expedite the processes, potentially offer different treatment modalities, and identify undiagnosed comorbid conditions in the man.

PATHOPHYSIOLOGY

Male reproductive physiology requires the coordinated release of hormones from the hypothalamic-pituitary-gonadal (HPG) axis, normal testis histology, a nonobstructed excurrent ductal system, an intact somatic and autonomic nervous system, and functioning external genitalia. Disorders in one or more of these domains can result in pathology ranging from decreased semen quality to the inability producing sperm.

The HPG axis at the simplest level requires gonadotropin-releasing hormone (GnRH) from the hypothalamus to act on the anterior pituitary to release follicle-stimulating hormone (FSH) and luteinizing hormone (LH). FSH acts on the Sertoli cells to stimulate spermatogenesis, and LH acts on Leydig cells to produce testosterone, which is also required for normal spermatogenesis. This axis can be interrupted at any level. Prolactinomas can inhibit GnRH release via negative feedback while other pituitary lesions, like craniopharyngiomas, can disrupt the production of LH and FSH. Likewise, disturbances of androgen synthesis in the testicle can completely disrupt sperm production.

Intratesticular testosterone is necessary for sperm production and serum levels of <300 ng/dL are found in up to 45% of azoospermic men. Testosterone levels are highly susceptible to a number of host conditions, including medications or exposure to toxic metabolites, inflammatory or infectious conditions, childhood disease, and even overall health status. Estrogen levels are also important, as testosterone is aromatized to estrogen in adipose cells and can lead to decreased serum testosterone through negative feedback at the hypothalamic and pituitary levels. Furthermore, the balance of testosterone to estrogen (optimally >10:1) has also been shown to affect male fertility.

Similar to the HPG axis, the testicular microenvironment is tightly regulated, and even small perturbations can cause disruption of spermatogenesis. Spermatagonial stem cells (SSCs) undergo meiosis to ultimately become spermatids through the process of spermatogenesis. This process is exquisitely susceptible to the effects of toxins (environmental, chemotherapy), temperature (varicoceles, cryptorchidism), and radiation. This may result in changes ranging from decreased sperm count to the complete depletion of SSCs.

Spermatids undergo spermiogenesis to become mature spermatozoa, which are ushered into the epididymis. In the epididymis, the spermatozoa gain motility and are stored for reproduction. The autonomic and somatic nervous systems allow for sperm transport from the epididymis to the tip of the urethra during ejaculation, and injuries to either the nerves or pelvic floor musculature (from retroperitoneal lymph node dissection, low-anterior resection, abdominal perineal resection, and so on) can disrupt this process. Furthermore, at the corpus of the epididymis, the numerous efferent ductules condense into a single epididymal tubular structure, and interruptions to this tubular structure at any point can significantly affect semen parameters. Unilateral or bilateral blockages can occur in the epididymis and the vas deferens, and disruptions can occur in the ejaculatory duct and urethra.

Finally, genetic mutations, ranging from syndromes to isolated issues with sperm production, affect male fertility. The most common genetic cause of impaired fertility is Klinefelter syndrome (1:500 to 1:1000 male live births), resulting in hypergonadotropic hypogonadism and typically azoospermia. Complete microdeletions on the long arm of the Y chromosome in AZFa and AZFb result in azoospermia, while men with deletions in AZFc regions can still harbor sperm on microscopic testicular sperm extraction (mTESE). Mutations in the cystic fibrosis transmembrane regulator (CFTR) gene can affect fertility due to segmental hypoplasia/aplasia of the excurrent ductal system. Heterozygous mutations in this gene are relatively common with an incidence of ~1 in 25 non-Hispanic, white men.

CLINICAL MANIFESTATIONS

Men presenting for infertility vary widely in phenotype, making diagnosis based solely on history and physical impossible. The cornerstone for determining the etiology is evaluating for laboratory abnormalities in either semen parameters or hormonal workup. Table 13.1 shows normal semen parameters based on the World Health Organization references ranges, and Table 13.2 shows normal

Table 13.1 World Health Organization V Semen Parameter Reference Ranges

PARAMETER	5TH PERCENTILE OF FERTILE MEN	50TH PERCENTILE OF FERTILE MEN	95TH PERCENTILE OF FERTILE MEN
Volume (mL)	1.5	3.7	6.8
Concentration (M/mL)	15	73	213
Motility (%)	40	61	78
Morphology (%)	4	9	44

Table 13.2 Suggested Laboratory Values[a]

PARAMETER	SUGGESTED VALUES
FSH	<7.6 mIU/mL
LH	<9 MIU/mL
Estradiol	<57 pg/mL
Testosterone	>300 ng/dL
T:E ratio	>10:1
Prolactin	<13

[a]Although reference ranges vary by lab, these reference values for follicle-stimulating hormone (FSH) and testosterone (T) are the commonly accepted levels and are important clinical indicators.
E, Estradiol; *LH,* luteinizing hormone.

laboratory parameters (normal ranges of gonadotropins, estrogen, and prolactin may vary by laboratory).

DIAGNOSIS AND TESTING

The first step in evaluation should always be a **complete history and focused physical exam** (Fig. 13.1). In addition to asking about potential toxic exposures (chemotherapy, radiation), previous infections (systemic, genitourinary, sexually transmitted infections [STIs]), childhood disease, and surgeries (orchidopexy, hernia repair, vasectomy, pelvic surgery), the clinician should take a detailed sexual history. This includes ascertaining facts about erectile dysfunction and ejaculatory disorders as well as into the frequency of intercourse and the potential inadvertent use of spermicidal lubricants.

Additionally, it important to determine if the complaint of infertility is primary (patient has never fathered a child) or secondary (patient has had previous paternity). Likewise, understanding the

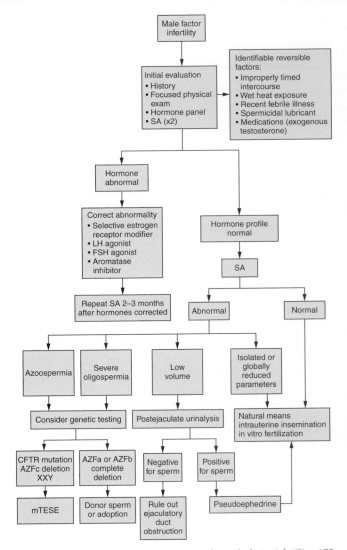

FIG. 13.1 Overview of treatment management for male factor infertility. *AZF,* Azoospermic factor; *FSH,* follicle-stimulating hormone; *LH,* luteinizing hormone; *mTESE,* microsurgical testicular sperm extraction; *SA,* Semen Analysis.

partner's age, menstrual cycle, previous fertility testing, and previous fertility status is important because it may alter the man's clinical course.

A comprehensive assessment of comorbid conditions and medications is also vital. The clinician can potentially identify conditions associated with infertility (i.e., cystic fibrosis, primary ciliary dyskinesia, Klinefelter syndrome). Identifying gonadotoxic medications (e.g., exogenous testosterone) that can cause impairments in semen parameters and even azoospermia is necessary.

The physical exam should focus on the overall appearance of the patient, secondary sexual characteristics, and the genitourinary exam. Signs of decreased body hair or the presence of gynecomastia could indicate a potential testosterone deficiency and/or estrogen excess. The phallus should be expected for plaques, urethral position, and presence of nonretractile foreskin, all of which could interfere with semen deposition. Scrotal contents should be inspected, namely the size, constancy, location, and presence of the testicles. A supine examination of the spermatic cord may reveal the presence or absence of the vas deferens, and a standing examination can lead to a diagnosis of a varicocele. Digital rectal exam may reveal dilated seminal vesicles (seen in ejaculatory duct obstruction [EDO]) or prostate hypoplasia.

Laboratory evaluations as discussed earlier remain the cornerstone of evaluating potentially infertile patients. While there are heterogeneities in clinical practice, a **baseline morning total testosterone level and FSH are necessary**. Additional tests, such as LH and prolactin (for low testosterone), estrogen, and free testosterone, can be included depending on the clinical situation. Semen analysis (SA) should consist of **at least two samples preceded by 2–5 days of abstinence and 2–3 weeks apart**. It is important to identify potential reproductive insults prior to patients producing a sample (e.g., wet heat exposure, febrile illness) to ensure they have an accurate collection (ideally >72 days after the exposure). Additional analysis of semen parameters such as DNA fragmentation can be used in the setting of recurrent miscarriages; however, this should not be solely relied on as a predictive pregnancy metric. Additional tests of sperm function are infrequently utilized and have varying clinical significance.

Imaging such as **scrotal ultrasonography is often not necessary** because most abnormalities may be identified with physical exam alone. Adjunct imaging tests such as transrectal ultrasound (TRUS) or magnetic resonance imaging (MRI) may be useful in cases of ejaculatory duct obstruction. MRI for prolactinoma or pituitary pathology should only be considered if prolactin is reproducibly twice the upper limit of normal. Perhaps the most important imaging test to consider is a **renal ultrasound in the setting of unilateral or bilateral absence of the vas deferens**, as this may identify renal aplasia.

FSH levels and testicular size are intimately associated with azoospermia and **diagnostic testis biopsy is rarely needed**. If FSH is ≤7.6 and testis long axis is >4.6 cm, then there is a 96% chance that the patient has obstructive azoospermia. Conversely, if the FSH is >7.6 and testis long axis is ≤4.6 cm, then there is an 89% chance that the patient has nonobstructive azoospermia.

Genetic testing is not routinely recommended to all men who initially present with infertility. In men with severe oligospermia (≤5 million sperm per mL) and azoospermia, a clinician can consider obtaining germline karyotype to assess for aneuploidy and chromosomal translocations and Y chromosome microdeletion testing. Men with **complete deletion of the AZFa or AZFb regions of the long arm of Y chromosome** are missing requisite genes necessary for spermatogenesis and thus **should not be offered mTESE**, whereas men with deletions of AZFc can have sperm found up to 50% of the time on mTESE. **Men with congenital bilateral (or unilateral) absence of the vas deferens should undergo CFTR testing, as should their partners**.

TREATMENT

The goal of the urologist is to medically and surgically optimize the male's chances of conception in a cost effective and minimally invasive way. Some easily identifiable and potentially reversible risk factors can be gleaned from the history alone. Recent febrile illness, wet heat exposure, use of spermicidal lubricants, improperly timed intercourse, and potential female factors should all be investigated prior to more invasive treatments.

Hormone abnormalities occur in up to 20% of men presenting for infertility. Testosterone enhancement (goal of >300 ng/dL) using clomiphene citrate, human chorionic gonadotropin (hCG), an aromatase inhibitor, and/or a combination of these agents should be pursued in hypogonadal men. Men with decreased testosterone to estrogen ratios (<10:1) or signs of hyperestrogenemia

Table 13.3 Medications Commonly Used in the Treatment of Male Infertility

SELECTIVE ESTROGEN RECEPTOR MODIFIER	AVAILABLE FORMULATION	RECOMMENDED DAILY DOSE
Clomiphene Citrate	50-mg capsule	25–50 mg every other day to daily
Tamoxifen	20-mg capsule	Daily
Toremifene	60-mg capsule	Daily
Raloxifene	60-mg capsule	Daily
Aromatase Inhibitors		
Anastrozole	1-mg capsule	Daily
Letrozole	2.5-mg capsule	Daily
Gonadotropin Agonists		
hCG	SC injection	1000–3000 IU × 2–3 times per week
FSH	SC injection	75–150 IU × 2–3 times per week
hMG	SC injection	75 IU × 2–3 times per week

FSH, Follicle-stimulating hormone; hCG, human chorionic gonadotropin; hMG, human menopausal gonadotropin; SC, subcutaneous.

can be treated with aromatase inhibitors to optimize the testicular hormonal milieu. In general, these medications are well tolerated with minimal adverse effects (Table 13.3).

While erectile issues are addressed elsewhere (Fig. 13.1), potential ejaculatory issues can also sometimes be identified on SA. Men with **low volume azoospermia or severe oligoasthenospermia may have a component of retrograde ejaculation, anejaculation, or EDO**. Retrograde ejaculation can be managed with sympathomimetic agents such as **pseudoephedrine** administered 1 hour prior to ejaculation, with return of sperm in the ejaculate up to 25% of the time. If this fails, the urine can be alkalinized or drained and replaced with a sperm-friendly wash media prior to ejaculation. The subsequent postejaculate urine sample is then collected and processed for use in intrauterine insemination (IUI) or IVF.

Anejaculation requires a similar retrieval protocol but additional stimulation. Penile vibratory stimulation and electroejaculation can both be used to stimulate emission. In patients with spinal cord injury, it is important to know the level of injury because men with lesions at T6 or higher may require pretreatment with sublingual nifedipine to prevent autonomic dysreflexia. Sperm can be recovered in up to 90% of men using these techniques.

EDO is typically diagnosed by low volume azoospermia or severe oligoasthenospermia and dilated seminal vesicles (anteroposterior diameter >12–15 mm) on ultrasound. Transurethral resection of the ejaculatory ducts (**TURED**) at the lateral aspect of the verumontanum can result in increased semen volume in up to 66% of patients and the presence of sperm in up to 50% of previously azoospermic patients. Resulting reflux of urine into the ejaculatory ducts is a possible complication and can result in an abnormally acidic semen sample and/or necrospermia, and retrograde flow of urine can lead to epididymitis, both of which can damage sperm.

Similarly, the increased temperature in the scrotum due to varicoceles can cause testicular alterations, including diminished sperm concentration, motility, and morphology, and even Leydig cell function dysfunction. Varicoceles can be repaired via a retroperitoneal, radiographic, laparoscopic, inguinal, or subinguinal approach with or without the use of operative magnification. **Complications include testicular artery injury (with the potential for testicular atrophy), hydrocele, and varicocele recurrence** (see Table 13.1). The repair of larger varicoceles often yields more improvements in semen parameters than correction of smaller varicoceles. In subfertile men with varicoceles, up to 44% of men achieved pregnancy within 1 year of surgical correction, and up to 50% of men with azoospermia saw the return of sperm to their ejaculate.

Men with obstructive azoospermia due to a **vasal or epididymal obstruction** can either undergo **surgical reconstruction or sperm extraction**, depending on the etiology. Injury to the vas deferens during hernia repair or vasectomy can be surgically repaired. It is imperative that the surgeon recognizes the most proximal site of obstruction, which is not always the site of the initial insult. The surgeon can test fluid from the testicular end of the vas deferens (proximal to the suspected obstruction) to determine patency of the excurrent ductal system from that point to the level of the testicle. The **character and quality of the fluid will determine whether a vasovasostomy (VV) or a vasoepididymostomy (VE) is indicated**. Similarly, the abdominal end of the vas deferens will need to be assessed for patency because multiple vasal injuries or inadequate vasal length may preclude microsurgical reconstruction. **VV, and the more technically challenging VE, should be performed by urologist trained in microsurgical techniques to maximize success rates**. Reported success rates of return of sperm to the ejaculate are over 90% for VVs and range from 70% to 90% for VEs when performed in the correct setting by trained microsurgeons. The most common complication is delayed stenosis of the surgical repair ranging from 5% to 12% for VV and 10% to 25% for VE. Other complications such as hematoma and infection are exceedingly rare.

If the patient's injuries or pathologies are not amenable to reconstruction, the patient does not desire surgical reconstruction, or the patient has nonobstructive azoospermia (NOA) and desires biological paternity, one should proceed with sperm extraction. In the setting of obstructive azoospermia, multiple different procedures can be performed to retrieve sperm. **For NOA, however, microdissection testicular sperm extraction (mTESE) is the gold standard**, as it maximizes sperm retrieval and minimizes inadvertent injury to collateral structures. With this approach, a thorough, meticulous, and methodical search of the testicle is undertaken, searching for dilated or full seminiferous tubules that is sometimes indicative of the presence of active spermatogenesis. These sperm can be extracted and subsequently used in assisted reproductive techniques, namely IVF and intracytoplasmic sperm injection (ICSI).

PROGNOSIS

The unique endpoint of infertility, having a baby, can be achieved through a variety of means. While natural conception is the least expensive and most desirable approach preferred by most couples, a variety of other methods exist. IUI, IVF with or without ICSI, the use of donor sperm, and adoption are also options available to eligible couples (Table 13.4). Means of conception ultimately depends on the quantity and quality of sperm, as well as the site from where sperm are obtained (i.e., testicular sperm cannot be used in IUI or IVF alone; it must be used in the setting of IVF/ICSI).

Table 13.4 Per-Cycle Success Rates of Various Forms of Intervention for the Female Partner and the Associated Multiple Birth Rate Based on 2008 National Data From the Society for Assisted Reproductive Technologies

TECHNIQUE	DELIVERY RATE PER CYCLE (%)	MULTIPLE BIRTH RATE PER PREGNANCY (%)
Timed intercourse	2–3	1
IUI alone	5	1
Clomid alone	5	10
Clomid and IUI	8	10
hMG alone	12–15	15
hMG and IUI	15–18	15
In vitro fertilization	30–32	31

hMG, Human menopausal gonadotropin; IUI, intrauterine insemination.
From Van Voorhis BJ. What to know about the infertile female. In: Niederberger CS, ed. *An introduction to male reproductive medicine.* New York: Cambridge University Press, 2011:134-151.

Suggested Readings

Asafu-Adjei D, Judge C, Deibert CM, et al. Systematic review of the impact of varicocele grade on response to surgical management. *J Urol* 2020;203(1):48-56.

Cooper TG, Noonan E, von Eckardstein S, et al. World Health Organization reference values for human semen characteristics. *Hum Reprod Update* 2010;16(3):231-245.

Dabaja AA, Schlegel PN. Medical treatment of male infertility. *Transl Androl Urol* 2014;3(1):9-16.

Krausz C, Riera-Escamilla A. Genetics of male infertility. *Nat Rev Urol* 2018;15(6):369-384.

Practice Committee of the American Society for Reproductive Medicine. Diagnostic evaluation of the infertile male: a committee opinion. *Fertil Steril* 2015;103(3):e18-25.

Schlegel PN, Sigman M, Collura B, et al. Diagnosis and treatment of infertility in men: AUA/ASRM guideline Part I. *J Urol* 2021;205(1):36-43. doi:10.1097/JU.0000000000001521.

Schlegel PN, Sigman M, Collura B, et al. Diagnosis and treatment of infertility in men: AUA/ASRM guideline Part II. *J Urol* 2021;205(1):44-51. doi:10.1097/JU.0000000000001520

Schoor RA, Elhanbly S, Niederberger CS, Ross LS. The role of testicular biopsy in the modern management of male infertility. *J Urol* 2002;167(1):197-200.

The Optimal Evaluation of the Infertile Male: AUA Best Practice Statement. 2010. https://www.auanet.org/guidelines/male-infertility-optimal-evaluation-best-practice-statement.

14

Evaluation and Management of Sexual Dysfunction in Men and Women

JAMES ANAISSIE AND MOHIT KHERA

CONTRIBUTORS OF CAMPBELL-WALSH-WEIN, 12TH EDITION

Alan W. Shindel, Tom F. Lue, Arthur L. Barnett Ii, Ranjith Ramasamy, Gregory A. Broderick, Chris G. Mcmahon, Matthew J. Mellon, John J. Mulcahy, Allen D. Seftel, Hailiu Yang, Ervin Kocjancic, Valerio Iacovelli, and Omer Acar

ERECTILE DYSFUNCTION

Epidemiology

Erectile dysfunction (ED) is the inability to attain and/or maintain penile erection sufficient for sexual performance or satisfaction. ED affects up to 20% of men worldwide older than 20 years old and worsens with age. Prevalence begins at 1%–10% for men younger than 40 years and approaches 50%–100% for men older than 70 years. Medical comorbidities, such as metabolic syndrome and cardiovascular disease, are associated with ED. Lower education and cigarette smoking are additional predictors for developing ED. The inverse is also true, and ED is now considered a sentinel for future risk of cardiovascular disease. The major risk factors for ED are in Table 14.1.

Pathophysiology

ED and can be broadly separated into psychogenic and organic etiologies (Box 14.1), with most having a functional organic disorder. Organic causes include vasculogenic (most common), neurogenic,

Table 14.1 Major Erectile Dysfunction Risk Factors

CONDITION	MULTIVARIATE ADJUSTED ODDS RATIO
Diabetes mellitus	2.9
Hypertension	1.6
Cardiovascular disease	1.1
Hypercholesterolemia	1.0
Benign prostate enlargement	1.6
Obstructive urinary symptoms	2.2
Increased body mass index ($>$30 kg/m^2)	1.5
Physical inactivity	1.5
Current cigarette smoking	1.6
Antidepressant use	9.1
Antihypertensive use	4.0

Data from Francis ME, Kusek JW, Nyberg LM, Eggers PW. The contribution of common medical conditions and drug exposures to erectile dysfunction in adult males. *J Urol* 2007;178:591-596; and Selvin E, Burnett AL, Platz EA. Prevalence and risk factors for erectile dysfunction in the US. *Am J Med* 2007;120:151-157.

anatomic, and endocrinologic. The metabolic syndrome and its components cause impaired penile perfusion secondary to generalized atherosclerosis, subsequent increased vascular resistance, vascular tone, and fibrosis. These, in turn, lead to a decline in erectile function.

ED can also be secondary to neuronal dysfunction. Because erection is a neurovascular event, any disorder of the brain, spinal cord, or peripheral nerves can negatively impact erectile function. Similarly, iatrogenic damage to the cavernosal nerves and vasculature after radical pelvic surgery or after pelvic fracture may cause ED. Damage to the peripheral nervous system from diabetes mellitus can decrease erectile function. Endocrine disorders such as low serum testosterone, as well as hyperprolactinemia, hyperthyroidism, and hypothyroidism, levels often lead to decreases in erectile function and libido.

Last, ED can be drug induced. Many antihypertensive medications can lead to reversible ED, as seen in Table 14.2. Other drug classes correlated with ED include antipsychotics, antidepressants, recreational drugs, and more. Table 14.3 summarizes many of these medications and suggests possible alternatives.

Clinical Manifestations

ED manifests with marked difficulty in obtaining erections, maintaining them until completion of sexual activity, and/or a

> **Box 14.1** Classification of Male Erectile Dysfunction
>
> **ORGANIC**
>
> I. Vasculogenic
>   A. Arteriogenic
>   B. Cavernosal
>   C. Mixed
> II. Neurogenic
> III. Anatomic
> IV. Endocrinologic
> V. Medication induced
>
> **PSYCHOGENIC**
>
> I. Generalized
>   A. Generalized unresponsiveness
>   1. Primary lack of sexual arousability
>   2. Aging-related decline in sexual arousability
>   B. Generalized inhibition
>   1. Chronic disorder of sexual intimacy
> II. Situational
>   A. Partner related
>   1. Lack of arousability in specific relationship
>   2. Lack of arousability because of sexual object preference
>   3. High central inhibition because of partner conflict or threat
>   B. Performance related
>   1. Associated with other sexual dysfunction (e.g., rapid ejaculation)
>   2. Situational performance anxiety (e.g., fear of failure)
>   C. Psychological distress or adjustment related
>   1. Associated with negative mood state (e.g., depression) or major life stress (e.g., death of partner)

significant decrease in erectile rigidity. Many men have a poor understanding of ED and its symptoms and may confuse ED with decreased libido or disorders of ejaculation.

Diagnosis and Testing

The diagnosis of ED differs from most urologic diagnoses in that extensive diagnostic procedures are generally not required. Therefore, the diagnosis can be made based on the patient's report of consistent inability to attain and/or maintain an erection

Table 14.2 Effect of Antihypertensive Agents on Sexual Function

AGENT	EFFECT	MECHANISM
Diuretics	ED (twice as common as placebo)	Unknown
β-Blocker (nonselective)	ED	Prejunctional α_2-receptor inhibition
α_1-Blocker	Decreases ED rate but may cause alteration of ejaculation	Failure of sympathetic-induced (1) closure of internal sphincter and proximal urethra and (2) failure of seminal emission during ejaculation
α_2-Blocker	ED	Inhibition of central α_2-receptor
Angiotensin-converting enzyme inhibitor	Possible reduction in ED	
Angiotensin II receptor blocker	Possibly reduction in ED	

ED, Erectile dysfunction.

sufficient for satisfactory sexual intercourse. Several well-validated questionnaires, such as the Index of Erectile Function (IIEF), are useful adjuncts to the patient's history. The physical exam should focus on the neurologic, cardiovascular, and genital systems. Obvious physical signs of hypogonadism such as small testes or gynecomastia should be noted. (https://www.auanet.org/guidelines/guidelines/erectile-dysfunction-(ed)-guideline)

Laboratory tests are not mandatory for diagnosis of ED but can help delineate the etiology. **Recommended laboratory tests include serum chemistries, fasting glucose or hemoglobin A1c, complete blood count (CBC), lipid profile, and morning serum total testosterone.** Further diagnostic testing such as intracavernosal injection of erectogenic medications with or without penile duplex ultrasonography (PDU) are used at the clinician's discretion to better characterize the arterial or veno-occlusive mechanisms of ED.

Table 14.3 Drug-Induced Erectile Dysfunction and Suggested Alternatives

CLASS	KNOWN TO CAUSE ERECTILE DYSFUNCTION	SUGGESTED ALTERNATIVES
Antihypertensives	Thiazide diuretics General β-blockers	**Angiotensin-converting enzyme inhibitors** **Angiotensin II receptor antagonists** **Selective** β-blockers α-Blockers Calcium channel blockers
Psychotropics	Antipsychotics Antidepressants Anxiolytics	Newer anxiolytics (bupropion, buspirone)
Antiandrogen	Androgen receptor antagonists Luteinizing hormone–releasing hormone agonists 5α-Reductase inhibitors	N/A
Recreational drugs	Tobacco Alcohol (large volume)	Tobacco cessation Alcohol in moderate

Treatment

The most recent American Urological Association (AUA) guidelines advocate that all therapeutic options for ED be offered, with any being a valid initial therapy. This demonstrates a shift from the traditional escalation from least to most invasive treatments. An algorithm for ED treatment pathways is seen in Fig. 14.1.

Lifestyle modification is a primary treatment for ED. Weight loss, diet, exercise, and decrease in cigarette smoking can lead to meaningful improvements in ED. Switching or ceasing a causative medication can lead to significant improvement. The AUA guidelines also propose a referral to a mental health professional to promote treatment adherence, reduce performance anxiety, and integrate treatments into a sexual relationship

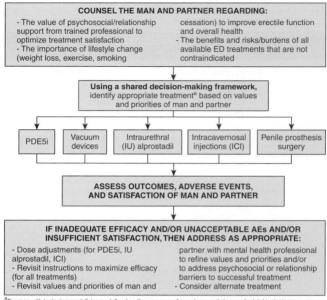

COUNSEL THE MAN AND PARTNER REGARDING:
- The value of psychosocial/relationship support from trained professional to optimize treatment satisfaction
- The importance of lifestyle change (weight loss, exercise, smoking cessation) to improve erectile function and overall health
- The benefits and risks/burdens of all available ED treatments that are not contraindicated

Using a shared decision-making framework, identify appropriate treatment[a] based on values and priorities of man and partner

| PDE5i | Vacuum devices | Intraurethral (IU) alprostadil | Intracavernosal injections (ICI) | Penile prosthesis surgery |

ASSESS OUTCOMES, ADVERSE EVENTS, AND SATISFACTION OF MAN AND PARTNER

IF INADEQUATE EFFICACY AND/OR UNACCEPTABLE AEs AND/OR INSUFFICIENT SATISFACTION, THEN ADDRESS AS APPROPRIATE:
- Dose adjustments (for PDE5i, IU alprostadil, ICI)
- Revisit instructions to maximize efficacy (for all treatments)
- Revisit values and priorities of man and partner with mental health professional to refine values and priorities and/or to address psychosocial or relationship barriers to successful treatment
- Consider alternate treatment

[a]For men with testosterone deficiency, defined as the presence of symptoms and signs and a total testosterone <300 ng/dL, counseling should emphasize that restoration of testosterone levels to therapeutic levels is likely to increase efficacy of ED treatment other than prosthesis surgery.

FIG. 14.1 Algorithm for shared decision making and treatment planning. *ED,* Erectile dysfunction; *PDE5i,* phosphodiesterase type 5.

The most common medications for ED are oral phosphodiesterase type 5 inhibitors (PDE5is). These medications augment (but do not induce) the erectile response. Each PDE5i has similar efficacy but different biochemical properties, and several can be used daily or on demand. These medications result in **successful sexual intercourse rates of approximately 70%**. Success may be lower in patients with DM, previous pelvic surgery, or radiation. **Side effects include headache, dyspepsia, flushing, and visual disturbances**. Dose titration is recommended. The only true contraindication is coadministration with nitrate-containing medications for angina.

Intracavernosal injection (ICI) of alprostadil, papaverine, phentolamine, or a combination is another highly effective pharmacologic therapy. Because of a higher risk of priapism, it is recommended that the first injection be in clinic and to start with a low dose. ICI is contraindicated in men with psychological instability, coagulopathy, unstable cardiovascular disease, reduced manual dexterity, and concurrent use of monoamine oxidase inhibitors. Alprostadil can also be administered as an intraurethral suppository (IUS), albeit with lower success rates (~50%). It is thus often used in combination with PDE5i. IUS should also be tested in the office to avoid the rare case of hypotension. Vacuum erection devices can be an effective alternate but are often considered cumbersome by patients.

In patients with subnormal testosterone values who are considering ED treatment with PDE5is, they can be counseled that testosterone replacement therapy (TRT) can improve the efficacy of PDE5i but should not be used as monotherapy.

One of the most effective methods of ED treatment is the surgical placement of a penile prosthesis. Inflatable penile prostheses (IPPs) are more popular than a malleable variant. IPPs have high patient and partner satisfaction because they can be utilized on demand for as long and as frequently as desired. On the other hand, implantation is associated with the inherent risks of surgery and leads to irreversible ED if removed. Device failure is rare. Loss of penile length is a common complaint but, if present, is minimal. Patients should be extensively counseled about this risk preoperatively.

Many emerging therapies, such as extracorporeal shock wave therapy, ICI of stem cells, and platelet-rich plasma injections, have shown promising preliminary results. However, due to lack of quality data, they are **still considered investigational in the 2018 AUA ED guidelines.**

PRIAPISM

Epidemiology

Priapism is defined as an erection that lasts more than 4 hours after sexual stimulation and orgasm. Its incidence in the United States is 5.34 per 100,000 men per year. The most prominent risk factor for developing priapism is sickle cell disease (SCD). The lifetime probability of a man with SCD developing priapism is 29%–42%, or approximately one third of all priapism cases. Potential etiologies are listed in Box 14.2.

Box 14.2 Causes of Priapism

α-ADRENERGIC RECEPTOR ANTAGONISTS
Prazosin, terazosin, doxazosin, tamsulosin

ANTIANXIETY AGENT
Hydroxyzine

ANTICOAGULANTS
Heparin, warfarin

ANTIDEPRESSANTS AND ANTIPSYCHOTICS
Trazodone, bupropion, fluoxetine, sertraline, lithium, clozapine, risperidone, olanzapine, chlorpromazine, thioridazine, phenothiazines

ANTIHYPERTENSIVES
Hydralazine, guanethidine, propranolol

ATTENTION-DEFICIT/HYPERACTIVITY DISORDER AGENTS
Methylphenidates (Concerta, Daytrana, Focalin, Metadate, Methylin, Quillivant, Ritalin)
Atomoxetine (Strattera)

RECREATIONAL DRUGS
Alcohol, cocaine (intranasal and topical), crack cocaine, marijuana, synthetic cannabinoids

GENITOURINARY CONDITIONS
Straddle injury, coital injury, pelvic trauma, kick to penis or perineum, penile bypass surgery, urinary retention

HEMATOLOGIC DYSCRASIAS
Sickle cell disease, thalassemia, granulocytic leukemia, myeloid leukemia, lymphocytic leukemia, multiple myeloma, hemoglobin Olmsted variant, fat emboli associated with hyperalimentation, hemodialysis, glucose-6-phosphate dehydrogenase deficiency

HORMONES
Gonadotropin-releasing hormone, testosterone

INFECTIOUS (TOXIN-MEDIATED) CAUSES
Scorpion sting, spider bite, rabies, malaria

Box 14.2 Causes of Priapism—cont'd

METABOLIC CONDITIONS

Amyloidosis, Fabry disease, gout

NEOPLASTIC CAUSES (METASTATIC OR REGIONAL INFILTRATION)

Prostate, urethra, testis, bladder, rectum, lung, kidney

NEUROGENIC CONDITIONS

Syphilis, spinal cord injury, cauda equina compression, autonomic neuropathy, lumbar disk herniation, spinal stenosis, cerebral vascular accident, brain tumor, spinal anesthesia cauda equina syndrome

VASOACTIVE ERECTILE AGENTS

Papaverine, phentolamine, prostaglandin E_1, oral phosphodiesterase type 5 inhibitors, combination intracavernous therapy

Modified from Lue TF. Physiology of penile erection and pathophysiology of erectile dysfunction and priapism. In: Walsh PC, Retik AB, Vaughan ED, et al., eds. *Campbell's urology.* Philadelphia: Saunders, 2002:1610-1696.

Pathophysiology

Priapism is typically classified by its etiology: ischemic (low-flow), nonischemic (high-flow), and stuttering. Ischemic priapism accounts for the majority of cases.

Ischemic Priapism. The pathophysiologic process of **ischemic priapism** begins after an erection persists beyond 4 hours. In SCD, sickled erythrocytes obstruct penile venous outflow, leading to stagnant blood in the corpora cavernosa and ischemia. Several other blood dyscrasias or thrombotic states can lead to ischemic priapism. Rarely, metastases to the penis from other sites can lead to venous outflow obstruction and priapism. Ischemic priapism can also be iatrogenic. Up to 5% of men receiving diagnostic ICI of an erectogenic medication subsequently develop ischemic priapism, which can also happen with home use. Oral (PDE5i) monotherapy, on the other hand, rarely causes priapism.

Nonischemic Priapism. This is usually secondary to blunt or penetrating trauma resulting in laceration of the cavernous artery or one of its penile branches. The most common cause is straddle injury, with trauma during sexual intercourse, kicks to the penis or perineum, and pelvic fracture comprising additional mechanisms. Occasionally, treatment of ischemic priapism with multiple injections, aspiration, or shunts, may lead to rapid conversion to high-flow, non-ischemic priapism.

Stuttering Priapism. This is recurrent priapism that may be associated with stuttering nocturnal or early morning erections, dehydration, fever, and exposure to cold. Patients with SCD may experience this from childhood, and any patient who has experienced ischemic priapism in the past is at increased risk of developing stuttering priapism.

Clinical Manifestations

Ischemic and nonischemic priapism differ in their clinical presentation. Patients with ischemic priapism report a fully rigid and painful erection. In nonischemic priapism, the patient is usually less than fully rigid and has a painless erection. In stuttering priapism, patients often awaken with an erection that persists over 4 hours and becomes painful secondary to ischemia. The erection lasts several hours before spontaneous remission. A comparison of the common clinical findings between the types of priapism is in Table 14.4.

Diagnosis and Testing

Diagnosis of priapism is made after an erection lasts longer than 4 hours. Rapid and early detection of priapism is essential because

Table 14.4 Key Findings in Priapism

FINDINGS	ISCHEMIC PRIAPISM	NONISCHEMIC PRIAPISM
Perineal trauma	Seldom	Usually
Hematologic abnormalities	Usually	Seldom
Recent intracorporal injection	Sometimes	Sometimes
Corpora cavernosa fully rigid	Usually	Seldom
Penile pain	Usually	Seldom
Abnormal penile blood gas	Usually	Seldom
Cavernous inflow (on Doppler)	Seldom	Usually

Modified from Montague DK, Jarow J, Broderick GA, et al. American Urological Association guideline on the management of priapism. *J Urol* 2003;170:1318-1324.

Table 14.5 Typical Blood Gas Values

SOURCE	Po$_2$ (mm Hg)	Pco$_2$ (mm Hg)	pH
Normal arterial blood (room air)	>90	<40	7.40
Normal mixed venous blood (room air)	40	50	7.35
Ischemic priapism (first corporal aspirate)	<30	>60	<7.25

Modified from Montague DK, Jarow J, Broderick GA, et al. American Urological Association guideline on the management of priapism. *J Urol* 2003;170:1318-1324.

treatment is time sensitive. Ischemia should be suspected if the patient has penile pain that progresses with duration of erection, has used a known drug associated with priapism, has SCD, or has a known spinal cord condition. If the prolonged erection is not associated with pain or there is known straddle injury, then nonischemic priapism is more likely. Physical examination should include palpation of the penis, with tenderness and full rigidity of corpora, but not glans, suggestive of ischemic priapism, and lack of tenderness and partial erection indicating a nonischemic etiology.

Basic laboratory tests such as CBC and coagulation studies should evaluate for blood dyscrasias, while a sickle cell panel should be performed in African Americans. Urine toxicology can be included if recreational drug use is suspected. A corporal blood gas is recommended and can reliably differentiate ischemic from nonischemic priapism (Table 14.5). (https://www.auanet.org/guidelines/guidelines/priapism-guideline). Imaging is not generally needed for diagnosis, but PDU can demonstrate lack of blood flow in ischemic priapism and high flow for nonischemic cases.

Treatment

The treatment of ischemic priapism is often performed in the emergent setting. A common treatment algorithm is in Fig. 14.2, and, in general, progresses from conservative to invasive interventions, as indicated. Per the AUA guidelines, initial treatment consists of either therapeutic aspiration of the corpora (with or without irrigation of saline), ICI of phenylephrine, or both. The success of corporeal aspiration is improved if combined with phenylephrine injection, which is injected at a concentration of 100–200 µg/mL and administered as 1-mL ICI every 3–5 minutes with a maximum dose of 1 mg in 1 hour.

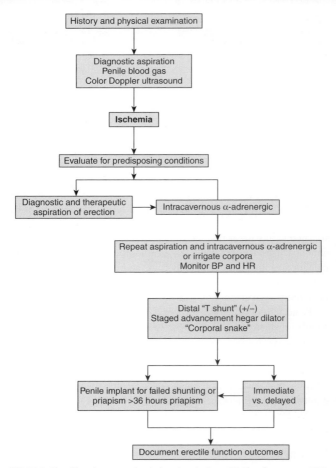

FIG. 14.2 Algorithm for managing ischemic priapism. *BP,* Blood pressure; *ECG,* electrocardiogram; *HR,* heart rate.

Vital signs should be monitored because this can cause hypertension, reflex bradycardia, and cardiac arrhythmias. If the above fails, then the next step is creation of a distal corporoglanular shunt, as seen in Fig. 14.3. These include the Winter (large biopsy needle), Ebbehøj (scalpel), and Al-Ghorab (excision of tunica albuginea at the tip of

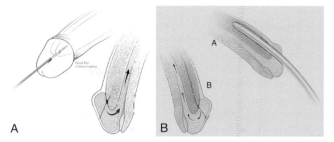

FIG. 14.3 (A) Winter shunt. The distal cavernoglanular shunt procedure is created by transglanular placement of a large-bore needle or angiocatheter into the distal glans and corpus cavernosum. (B) Corporal snake maneuver is a modification of the Al-Ghorab shunt. After excision of a 5-mm circular core of distal tunica albuginea, a 7/8 Hegar dilator is inserted down each corporal body through the tunica window. (B, Copyright Brady Urological Institute. From Burnett AL, Pierorazio PM. Corporal 'snake" maneuver: corporoglanular shunt surgical modification for ischemic priapism. *J Sex Med* 2009;6:1171-1176.)

the corpus cavernosum). Proximal shunting using the Quackels or Grayhack procedures may be warranted if more-distal shunting procedures have failed to relieve the priapism. Underlying SCD or blood dyscrasias should be treated concurrently with intracavernous therapy.

The mainstay of treatment of nonischemic priapism is observation because many resolve spontaneously. Corporal aspiration has only a diagnostic role. Selective arterial embolization is a treatment option if needed. Surgical management of nonischemic priapism is a last resort and should be performed with intraoperative PDU. Treatment of stuttering priapism is focused on prevention. Systemic therapy with α-adrenergic agonists, PDE5i, terbutaline, digoxin, gonadotropin-releasing hormone, and antiandrogens or self-ICI of phenylephrine can be utilized.

DISORDERS OF MALE ORGASM AND EJACULATION

Epidemiology

Ejaculatory dysfunction (EjD) ranges from premature ejaculation (PE), to delayed ejaculation (DE), to a complete inability to ejaculate. The 2020 AUA PE guidelines (https://www.auanet.org/guidelines/guidelines/disorders-of-ejaculation) define lifelong PE as poor ejaculatory control, associated bother, and ejaculation within ~2 minutes of initiation of penetrative sex. Interestingly, although abnormal intravaginal latency times (IVLT) affect only 2.5% of the general male population, a much higher number report having the disorder. The prevalence (20%–30%) varies widely.

The prevalence of DE is less clear, with studies suggesting that up to 40% of men are impacted and worsening with age. Retrograde ejaculation (RE) primarily develops after surgical bladder outlet procedures for lower urinary tract symptoms (LUTS). Another common cause of DE is the use or abrupt cessation of selective serotonin reuptake inhibitors (SSRIs). Five to 15% of men using SSRIs will have sexual dysfunction, sometimes following the first dose.

Other rare disorders of orgasm and ejaculation include orgasmic headache, painful ejaculation, and post orgasmic illness syndrome. Although these are rare, painful ejaculation can occur in up to 25% of men with benign prostatic hypertrophy (BPH)/LUTS.

Pathophysiology

EjD can be acquired or lifelong, with the latter being secondary to neurobiological and genetic variations. Acquired sexual dysfunction is usually secondary to sexual performance anxiety and/or relationship problems. Almost half of all men with ED also complain of PE, likely secondary to "rushing" sex to avoid premature detumescence. DE or absent ejaculation has a wide variety of possible etiologies (Table 14.6).

Clinical Manifestations

EjD has variable presentations. PE is the most common, in which men have a recurrent pattern of ejaculation within 2 minutes of vaginal penetration that is bothersome to the patient and partner. This can either be lifelong or acquired. DE (usually after ~25–30 minutes), anejaculation, and anorgasmia constitute the other end of the spectrum. RE commonly presents after surgical procedures that compromise the bladder neck, such as transurethral resection of the prostate (TURP).

Diagnosis and Testing

Lifelong PE is present since the patient's first sexual experience, whereas, in acquired PE, patients experience IVLT that is markedly reduced from prior sexual encounters. A significant amount of men

Table 14.6 Causes of Retrograde Ejaculation, Delayed Ejaculation, Anejaculation, and Anorgasmia

Aging man	Degeneration of penile afferent nerves
Psychogenic	Inhibited ejaculation
Congenital	Müllerian duct cyst
	Wolffian duct abnormality
	Prune belly syndrome
Anatomic causes	Transurethral resection of prostate
	Bladder neck incision
Neurogenic causes	Diabetic autonomic neuropathy
	Multiple sclerosis
	Spinal cord injury
	Radical prostatectomy
	Proctocolectomy
	Bilateral sympathectomy
	Abdominal aortic aneurysmectomy
	Para-aortic lymphadenectomy
Infective	Urethritis
	Genitourinary tuberculosis
	Schistosomiasis
Endocrine	Hypogonadism
	Hypothyroicism
Medication	α-Methyldopa
	Thiazide diuretics
	Tricyclic and SSRI antidepressants
	Phenothiazine
	Alcohol abuse

SSRI, Selective serotonin reuptake inhibitor.

who self-report PE fail to satisfy these criteria. Standardized questionnaires can be used as an adjunct to a full history in diagnosis, especially to evaluate for the commonly concurrent presence of ED. Physical exam and labs are of limited utility. All other forms of EjD are similarly diagnosed by history and physical exam. RE may be confirmed by obtaining a postejaculation urine sample for presence of sperm. Other testing should be used as clinically indicated but may be of limited utility.

Treatment

All men with PE should receive basic psychosexual education or coaching, which is often used in conjunction with pharmacologic therapy (Fig. 14.4). First-line medical treatment includes

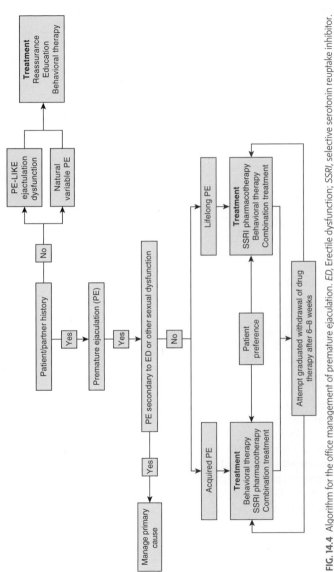

FIG. 14.4 Algorithm for the office management of premature ejaculation. *ED,* Erectile dysfunction; *SSRI,* selective serotonin reuptake inhibitor.

daily SSRIs, on-demand dapoxetine or clomipramine, and topical penile anesthetics. On-demand medications are available but allow for less sexual spontaneity. Tramadol can be recommended if the patient has failed first-line therapy. A full list of possible pharmacologic treatments of PE is in Table 14.7. Lastly, ED is commonly associated with PE and should be treated first. Any surgical options for PE are considered experimental.

Delayed or absent ejaculation is also treated with psychosexual therapy, but pharmacotherapy has very limited success. Table 14.7 in the AUA guidelines on PE lists many medications that may lead to delayed ejaculation and can lead to improvement after cessation. ED should be treated concurrently. Treatment algorithms for DE are in Fig. 14.5. RE has proven difficult to treat, but case reports have shown success with pseudoephedrine and its analogues, tricyclic antidepressants, and bladder neck reconstruction.

PEYRONIE DISEASE

Epidemiology

Peyronie disease (PD), or an abnormal curvature of the penis, is affects 3%–20% of all men. The peak age of onset is in the early 50s. The incidence of symptomatic PD appears to be increasing, likely due to increased awareness and medical visits for ED medications.

Pathophysiology

PD is currently thought to be a wound-healing disorder of the tunica albuginea that results in contractile scar tissue and resultant penile deformity (Fig. 14.6). Unfortunately, the scars in PD do not undergo normal wound healing and thus do not resolve spontaneously.

PD appears to go through an active phase during which the scar can grow, resulting in progressive deformity and pain. However, once PD has stabilized (chronic phase), there is usually no further progression. The exact cause has yet to be fully elucidated, but it is thought it may be due to penile trauma or repeated microtrauma. Genetic predisposition, autoimmune factors, and aberrant wound healing may also contribute.

Table 14.7 Drug Therapy for Premature Ejaculation (PE)

DRUG	DOSE	DOSING INSTRUCTIONS	INDICATION	COMMENTS	LEVEL OF EVIDENCE
Dapoxetine	30–60 mg	On demand, 1–3 hours before intercourse	Lifelong PE Acquired PE	Approved in >50 countries	High
Paroxetine	10–40 mg	Once daily	Lifelong PE Acquired PE		High
Sertraline	50–200 mg	Once daily	Lifelong PE Acquired PE		High
Fluoxetine	20–40 mg	Once daily	Lifelong PE Acquired PE		High
Citalopram	20–40 mg	Once daily	Lifelong PE Acquired PE		High
Clomipramine	12.5–50 µg	Once daily	Lifelong PE Acquired PE		High
	12.5–50 µg	On demand, 3–4 hours before intercourse	Lifelong PE Acquired PE		High
Tramadol	25–50 mg	On demand, 3–4 hours before intercourse	Lifelong PE Acquired PE	Potential risk of opiate addiction	Low
Topical lignocaine/ prilocaine	Patient titrated	On demand, 20–30 minutes before intercourse	Lifelong PE Acquired PE		High

Alprostadil	5–20 mcg	Patient administered intracavernosal injection 5 minutes before intercourse	Lifelong PE Acquired PE	Risk of priapism and corporal fibrosis	Very Low
PDE5 inhibitors	Sildenafil 25–100 mg Tadalafil 10–20 mg Vardenafil 10–20 mg Avanafil 50–200 mg	On demand, 30–50 minutes before intercourse	Lifelong and acquired PE in men with normal erectile function		Low
			Lifelong and acquired PE in men with ED	Improved efficacy if combined with SSRI	Moderate

ED, Erectile dysfunction; *PDE5*, phosphodiesterase type 5; *SSRI*, selective serotonin reuptake inhibitor.

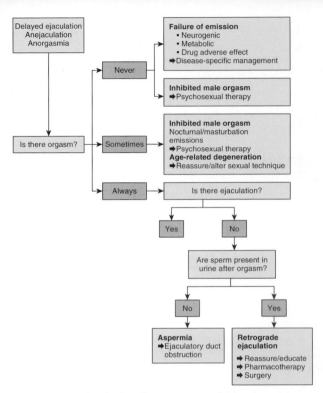

FIG. 14.5 Algorithm for the office management of delayed ejaculation.

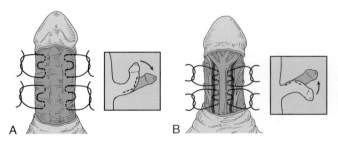

FIG 14.6 The dot procedure employs no incision. The tunica albuginea is plicated with permanent suture using an extended Lembert-type suture placement following four dots per plication. (A) Suture placement for dorsal curve. (B) Suture placement for ventral curve.

Clinical Manifestations

PD usually presents as a gradually worsening penile curvature (typically dorsal), pain with intercourse, and resultant emotional distress. Other common deformities include indentation, hinge effect, or shortening. There is usually an acute phase, lasting 6–18 months with painful erections and worsening deformity, followed by a chronic phase when the plaque stabilizes and pain resolves. Concomitant ED is present in about one third of PD cases.

Diagnosis and Testing

Although a thorough history is essential for the diagnosis of PD, the physical exam is the most crucial component. (https://www.auanet.org/guidelines/guidelines/peyronies-disease-guideline). To assess for PD, the flaccid penis should be evaluated on stretch to document stretched length and presence of a penile plaque. More important is an evaluation of the erect penis. Per the AUA guidelines, physicians should perform an in-office ICI erectogenic test with or without PDU to assess for plaque location, size, and characteristics as well as degree of curvature or deformity prior to consideration of any form of invasive treatment.

Treatment

Treatment of PD is predominantly via intralesional injectable (ILI) or surgical therapy. Many oral and topical therapies have been studied, but none has proven effective, and they are thus not recommended. Risks, benefits, and expectations should be outlined.

The only ILI therapy approved by the Food and Drug Administration (FDA) for PD is collagenase clostridium histolyticum (CCH), which degrades the collagen in aberrant PD plaques. CCH is indicated for patients with stable disease, curvature >30 degrees, and intact erectile function. It is administered as serial treatments and often combined with manual modeling (bending of the penis opposite to the site of curvature). Average reduction in curvature is ~35%. Common adverse events include penile ecchymosis, swelling, and pain, with the rare occurrence of corporal rupture. Off-label ILI medications for PD include interferon α-2b or verapamil. The patient should be counseled on the potential adverse effects of each off-label treatment. ESWT may improve penile pain but not curvature.

Surgical intervention remains the gold standard for the treatment of stable PD. The goal is to make the penis "functionally straight," generally regarded as ≤20 degrees of curvature. Choosing the correct surgical intervention depends on the degree of deformity. In a penis with curvature <70 degrees with intact erectile function, tunical plication is recommended. This involves shortening of the longer (convex) side of the penis to match the shorter side (Fig. 14.6). It often causes penile shortening. A plaque excision with or without grafting is recommended in men with more complex curvatures or curvatures >70 degrees. Of note, both of these therapies require men to have erectile rigidity adequate for coitus. In men with PD and ED refractory to medical therapy, IPP placement is an effective treatment for both. If deformity exists after IPP placement and manual modeling, the practitioner can consider additional plication sutures and/or plaque incision and grafting. Several alternative treatments exist but lack the clinical evidence for recommendation (Table 14.8).

SEXUAL DYSFUNCTION IN FEMALES

Epidemiology

Female sexual dysfunction (FSD) can take many forms (Table 14.9). Although data are limited, 5.8% of women report symptoms consistent with FSD. Prevalence may be higher, with one study demonstrating that >33% of women reported a new sexual disorder within the previous 12 months. Hypoactive sexual desire was the most prevalent sexual complaint (21.4%), followed by problems in arousal (11.4%), satisfaction (10.4%), orgasm (8.8%), and lubrication (8.7%). Decreased sexual desire is 20% in women younger than 25 years of age and approaches 70%–80% in women 55–74 years of age.

Pathophysiology

The pathophysiology of FSD is highly complex and must be considered in a biopsychosocial context. Biologic factors such as common comorbidities and their treatment modalities (e.g., antihypertensives) have been associated with FSD (Table 14.10). Pregnancy, breastfeeding, and a postmenopausal state are often associated with decreased libido. Aging is also known to contribute to FSD because

Table 14.8 External Force Application for Peyronie Disease

TREATMENT	MECHANISM OF ACTION	STUDY OUTCOMES	ADVERSE EFFECTS
Electromotive drug administration	Bypasses hepatic metabolism, increases concentration of drug to target tissues compared with topical application alone	Verapamil alone: no benefit Verapamil + dexamethasone: decreases in plaque volume and penile curvature from 43 to 21 degrees	Temporary erythema at the electrode site
Extracorporeal shock wave therapy	Direct damage to the penile plaque; increases vascularity of the targeted area, inducing an inflammatory reaction, resulting in lysis of the plaque and removal by macrophages	Improvements in pain, IIEF-5 score, and mean QoL score; no curvature reduction	Local petechiae and ecchymoses
Penile traction	Decreases α-smooth muscle actin; increases matrix metalloproteinases involved in collagen degradation	Length increased 0.5–2.0 cm; girth increased 0.5–1.0 cm; curvature mean decrease of 20 degrees; pain decreased, softening or shrinking of plaque; overall satisfaction, 85%	Erythema in the balanopreputial sulcus, discomfort
Vacuum therapy	Unknown; mechanical effects similar to traction have been suggested	Reduction in angle of curvature by 5–25 degrees in 21 of 31 patients	Development of PD, urethral bleeding, skin necrosis, and penile ecchymosis
Radiation therapy	Antiinflammatory effects via functional modulation of the adhesion of white blood cells to activated endothelial cells and modulation of the induction of nitric oxide synthase in activated macrophages	No clinical benefit	Possible malignant change, increased risk for ED in older patients

ED, Erectile dysfunction; IIEF, International Index of Erectile Function; PD, Peyronie disease; QoL, quality of life.

Table 14.9 Definitions of Female Sexual Dysfunction

DSM-IV-TR	DSM-5
Sexual Desire Disorders	**Female Sexual Interest or Arousal Disorder**
Hypoactive sexual desire disorder: Deficiency or absence of sexual fantasies and desire for sexual activity *Sexual aversion disorder:* Aversion to and active avoidance of genital sexual contact with a sexual partner	Lack of or significantly reduced sexual interest or arousal as manifested by three of the following: 1. Absent or reduced interest in sexual activity 2. Absent or reduced sexual or erotic thoughts or fantasies 3. No or reduced initiation of sexual activity and unreceptive to partner's attempts to initiate 4. Absent or reduced sexual excitement or pleasure during sexual activity in almost all or all (75%–100%) sexual encounters 5. Absent or reduced sexual interest or arousal in response to any internal or external sexual or erotic cues (written, verbal, or visual) 6. Absent or reduced genital or nongenital sensations during sexual activity in almost all or all (75%–100%) sexual encounters
Sexual Arousal Disorders	
Female sexual arousal disorder: Persistent or recurrent inability to attain or to maintain until completion of the sexual activity, an adequate lubrication-swelling response, or sexual excitement	
Orgasmic Disorder	**Female Orgasmic Disorder**
Female orgasmic disorder: Persistent or recurrent delay in, or absence of, orgasm after normal sexual excitement	Presence of either of the following on all or almost all (75%–100%) occasions of sexual activity: 1. Marked delay in, marked infrequency of, or absence of orgasm 2. Markedly reduced intensity of orgasmic sensations

Table 14.9 Definitions of Female Sexual Dysfunction—cont'd

DSM-IV-TR	DSM-5
Sexual Pain Disorders	**Genitopelvic Pain or Penetration Disorder**
Dyspareunia: Genital pain that is associated with sexual intercourse *Vaginismus:* Recurrent or persistent involuntary contraction of the perineal muscles surrounding the outer third of the vagina when vaginal penetration with a penis, finger, tampon, or speculum is attempted	Persistent or recurrent difficulties with one or more of the following: 1. Vaginal penetration during intercourse 2. Marked vulvovaginal or pelvic pain during intercourse or penetration attempts 3. Marked fear or anxiety about vulvovaginal or pelvic pain in anticipation of, during, or because of vaginal penetration 4. Marked tensing or tightening of pelvic floor muscles during attempted vaginal penetration

Table 14.10 Medical Conditions That Can Affect Female Sexual Function

MEDICAL CONDITION	POSSIBLE IMPACT ON FEMALE SEXUAL FUNCTION
Coronary artery disease	May affect pelvic perfusion, arousal disorder
Dermatologic conditions (e.g., lichen sclerosus, lichen planus, eczema)	Genital pain, problems with lubrication
Diabetes mellitus	Low desire
Hypertension	Low desire
Hypothyroidism	Problems with lubrication and orgasm
Malignancy and its treatment (breast, anal, colorectal, bladder, gynecologic)	Problems with desire, arousal, orgasm, and genital pain
Neuromuscular disorders, spinal cord injury, multiple sclerosis	Problems with desire, arousal, orgasm, and genital pain
Parkinson disease, dementia	Low desire
Urinary incontinence	Desire, arousal, and pain domains can be affected

Modified from Faubion SS, Rullo JE. Sexual dysfunction in women: a practical approach. *Am Fam Physician* 2015;92(4):281-288.

Table 14.11 Classes and Examples of Medications That Might Be Associated With Low Sexual Desire

Anticonvulsants	Carbamazepine
	Phenytoin
	Primidone
Cardiovascular medications	Angiotensin-converting enzyme inhibitors
	Amiodarone
	β-blockers (atenolol, metoprolol, propranolol)
	Calcium channel blockers
	Clonidine
	Digoxin
	Diuretics (hydrochlorothiazide, spironolactone)
	Lipid-lowering agents
Hormones	Antiandrogens (flutamide)
	Gonadotropin-releasing hormone agonists
	Oral contraceptives
Analgesics	Nonsteroidal antiinflammatory drugs
	Opiates
Psychotropic medications	Antipsychotics
	Anxiolytics (alprazolam, diazepam)
	Selective serotonin reuptake inhibitors
	Serotonin norepinephrine reuptake inhibitors
	Tricyclic antidepressants
Illicit drugs	Amphetamine
	Cocaine
	Heroin
	Marijuana
Others	Histamine receptor antagonists
	Alcohol
	Indomethacin
	Ketoconazole
	Chemotherapeutic agents

Modified from Clayton AH, Kingsberg SA, Goldstein I. Evaluation and management of hypoactive sexual desire disorder. *Sex Med* 2018;6(2):59-74.

levels of estrogen and testosterone decline. Many medications can be associated with FSD (Table 14.11).

From a psychosocial perspective, it is well known that psychiatric disorders and their treatments (e.g., SSRIs) can lead to FSD. Sexual abuse and trauma in childhood, as well as problems with body image, are also common contributors. External factors such as religion, culture, relationship factors, career stress, and financial stress can also worsen FSD.

Clinical Manifestations

The most common manifestation of FSD is low desire, followed by low arousal and orgasmic dysfunction. In female sexual interest-arousal disorder (FSID), women present with absent or decreased desire, fantasizing, excitement, and/or pleasure. With female orgasmic disorders, desire may be present, but the patient has absent, delayed, or weak orgasms. The third classification is genitopelvic pain-penetration disorder, in which there is significant difficulty, distress, and/or pain in achieving or maintaining vaginal penetration.

Diagnosis and Testing

The main barrier to the proper diagnosis of FSD is that <20% of women with sexual issues will seek medical treatment, likely secondary to sociocultural barriers. Assessment is best approached by addressing biologic, psychological, sociocultural, and interpersonal factors (Table 14.12). In addition to a thorough

Table 14.12 Biopsychosocial Model of Assessing Sexual (Dys)Function

Biologic factors	Medications
	Hormonal status
	Neurobiology
	Physical health
	Aging
Psychological factors	Depression
	Anxiety
	Self-image
	Substance abuse
	History of sexual abuse, trauma
Sociocultural factors	Upbringing
	Cultural norms and expectations
	Religious influences
Interpersonal factors	Relationship status or quality
	Partner's sexual function
	Life stressors

Modified from Bitzer J, Giraldi A, Pfaus J. Sexual desire and hypoactive sexual desire disorder in women. Introduction and overview. Standard operating procedure (SOP Part 1). *J Sex Med* 2013;10(1):36-49; Fugl-Meyer KS, Bohm-Starke N, Damsted Petersen C, et al. Standard operating procedures for female genital sexual pain. *J Sex Med* 2013;10(1):83-93; Latif EZ, Diamond MP. Arriving at the diagnosis of female sexual cysfunction. *Fertil Steril* 2013;100(4):898-904.

medical and sexual history, all female patients, regardless of age, should be screened for sexual dysfunction using one of many well-validated questionnaires. Additionally, a history of the sexual partner is often helpful. A thorough physical examination of internal and external pelvic organs must accompany the history. Laboratory testing is rarely indicated.

Treatment

The treatment of FSD is focused on the psychosocial aspect, with medications available as an adjunct. Addressing modifiable factors such as disease states, medications, and relationships can have a large impact.

There are two FDA-approved treatment options for FSID. Flibanserin (Addyi) is taken daily and can increase sexual desire by ~50%. The second option is bremelanotide (Vyleesi), which is administered intramuscularly 45 minutes before sexual intercourse. Estrogen replacement therapy can reduce many of the symptoms associated with sexual dysfunction, and testosterone therapy can increase desire and satisfaction. A treatment algorithm for FSID is in Fig. 14.7.

Female orgasmic disorder (FOD) without sufficient arousal often requires patient and partner psychotherapy with sexual education. Like FSID, FOD is responsive to hormonal therapy with estrogen or testosterone. If patients have sufficient arousal, on-demand oxytocin can improve rates of orgasm.

Female sexual arousal disorder (FSAD) is best treated with hormones, but success has also been noted with the use of PDE5i, prostaglandins, and other medications. Treatment of female persistent genital arousal disorder with duloxetine, pregabalin, and varenicline has limited success. Genitopelvic pain and penetration disorder treatments include biofeedback, vaginal dilation, and, in refractory cases, vestibulectomy. Last, almost half of women with LUTS and/or prolapse report some form of sexual dysfunction, and treatment of the underlying disease can lead to significant sexual improvement.

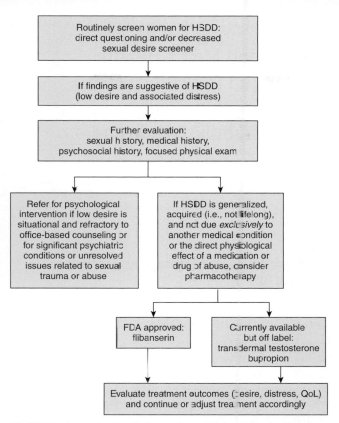

FIG. 14.7 Treatment algorithm for hypoactive sexual desire disorder. (Data from Clayton AH, Kingsberg SA, Goldstein I. Evaluation and management of hypoactive sexual desire disorder. *Sex Med* 2018b;6[2]:59-74.)

15

Integrated Men's Health: Androgen Deficiency, Cardiovascular Risk, and Metabolic Syndrome

ERNEST TONG AND ALEXANDER GOMELSKY

CONTRIBUTORS OF CAMPBELL-WALSH-WEIN, 12TH EDITION

Neil Fleshner, Miran Kenk, and Steven Kaplan

OVERVIEW OF THE PROBLEM

In almost every country, health outcomes among males are significantly inferior to those of females. Efforts to reduce gender inequality in health require a substantial adjustment in multiple facets of life. Human longevity continues to increase on a global scale with advances in medicine. **On average, men throughout the world live shorter lives than women** (Fig. 15.1). Men also fall ill at younger ages and are more prone to chronic diseases (Table 15.1). **Six of the 10 most common causes of death among Americans, including heart disease, cancer, and diabetes, are more prevalent among males.**

EXPLANATION OF THE POORER HEALTH OF MEN

Several factors place men at higher risk of death and disease. Men have **increased exposure to physical and environmental harm in the workplace**, and up to 97% of all risk fatalities are in males. Men have a **propensity for risk-taking behaviors**, such as alcohol use, smoking, and risky sexual practices. In addition, males experience relatively **more social pressure to endorse**

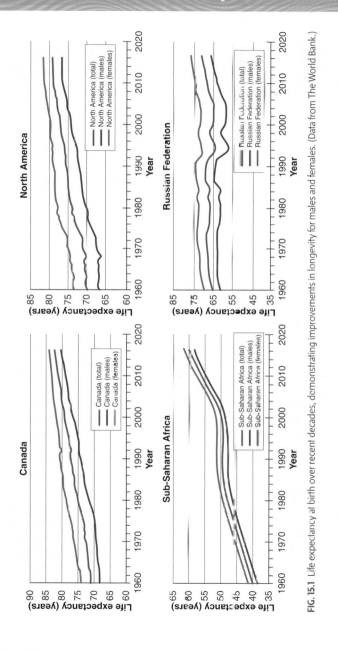

FIG. 15.1 Life expectancy at birth over recent decades, demonstrating improvements in longevity for males and females. (Data from The World Bank.)

Table 15.1 Major Causes of Death, United States, 2016

CAUSE OF DEATH	ANNUAL NO. OF DEATHS	MALE-TO-FEMALE INCIDENCE RATIO
Heart disease	633,842	1.12
Cancer	595,930	1.11
Chronic obstructive lung disease	155,041	0.88
Accidents	146,571	1.73
Stroke	140,323	0.71
Dementia	110,561	0.44
Diabetes	79,535	1.18
Influenza or pneumonia	57,062	0.89
Nephrological conditions	49,959	1.03
Suicide	44,193	3.33

From Centre for Disease Control and Prevention/National Center for Health Statistics (CDC/NCHS). *National vital statistics system, mortality 2017.* Atlanta: US Department of Health and Human Services, 2017.

gender stereotypes, such as independence and toughness, and may postpone or dismiss their health care needs.

METABOLIC SYNDROME AND MEN'S HEALTH

Metabolic syndrome is defined as a series of biochemical, physiologic, metabolic, and clinical factors that increase the individual's risk of type 2 diabetes mellitus (T2DM), heart disease, and early mortality. Depending on the definition and population studied, the prevalence of metabolic syndrome ranges between 10% and 84% of the population. Risk factors include sedentary lifestyle, excess caloric intake, and higher socioeconomic status. Several definitions are available (Fig. 15.2; Table 15.2).

PHYSIOLOGY OF METABOLIC SYNDROME

The physiologic alterations associated with metabolic syndrome have not been fully elucidated, but it is believed that **genetic risk factors interact with lifestyle exposure (physical inactivity, smoking, caloric excess, psychological stress) to create a positive energy imbalance.** This leads to alterations in fatty acid metabolism, endothelial dysfunction, atherogenesis, insulin resistance, and inflammation (Fig. 15.3).

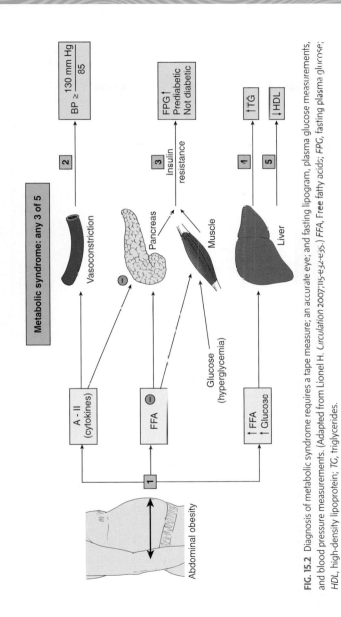

FIG. 15.2 Diagnosis of metabolic syndrome requires a tape measure; an accurate eye; and fasting lipogram, plasma glucose measurements, and blood pressure measurements. (Adapted from Lionel H. *Circulation 2007;115:e32-e35.*) *FFA,* Free fatty acids; *FPG,* fasting plasma glucose; *HDL,* high-density lipoprotein; *TG,* triglycerides.

Table 15.2 Metabolic Syndrome Definitions and Criteria

CLINICAL PARAMETER	WHO (1999)	EGIR (Balkau and Charles, 1999)	ATP III (NCEP, 2001)	AACE (Einhorn et al., 2003)	IDF (Alberti et al., 2005)
Obesity/body fat distribution	Waist/hip ratio >0.90 in men, >0.85 in women or BMI >30 kg/m²	Waist circumference ≥94 cm in men, ≥80 cm in women	Waist circumference >102 cm in men, >88 cm in women	BMI ≥25 kg/m²	Waist circumference ≥94 cm in men, ≥80 cm in women
Insulin resistance/hyperglycemia	IGT, IFG, T2DM, or other evidence of insulin resistance	Hyperinsulinemia (plasma insulin >75th percentile)	Fasting glucose ≥110 mg/dL	Fasting glucose ≥110 mg/dL	Fasting glucose ≥100 mg/dL, T2DM
Triglyceridemia	≥150 mg/dL	≥177 mg/dL	≥150 mg/dL	>150 mg/dL	>150 mg/dL or on treatment
Cholesterol	HDL-C <35 mg/dL in men or <39 mg/dL in women	HDL-C <39 mg/dL	HDL-C <40 mg/dL in men; <50 mg/dL in women	HDL-C <40 mg/dL in men; <50 mg/dL in women	HDL-C <40 mg/dL in men; <50 mg/dL in women; or on treatment
Blood pressure	≥140/90 mm Hg	≥140/90 mm Hg or on treatment	>130/85 mm Hg	≥130/85 mm Hg	>130/85 mm Hg or on treatment
Other	Microalbuminuria[a]			Other features of insulin resistance[b]	

AACE, American Association of Clinical Endocrinologists; ATP III, National Cholesterol Education Program Adult Treatment Panel III Report; BMI, body mass index; EGIR, European Group for the Study of Insulin Resistance; HDL-C, high-density lipoprotein cholesterol; IDF, International Diabetes Federation; IFG, impaired fasting glucose; IGT, impaired glucose tolerance; T2DM, type 2 diabetes mellitus; WHO, World Health Organization.

[a]Microalbuminuria defined as urinary albumin excretion ≥20 μg/min or albumin/creatine ratio ≥30 mg/g.

[b]Family history of T2DM, hypertension, or CVD; polycystic ovary syndrome; sedentary lifestyle; advancing age; ethnic groups having high risk for T2DM or CVD.

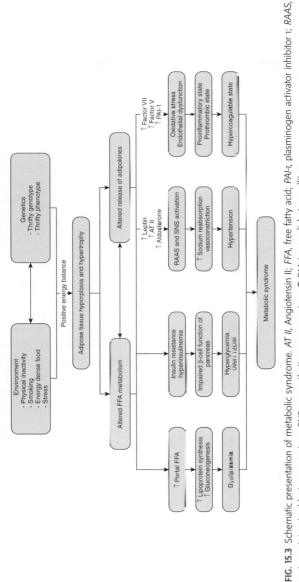

FIG. 15.3 Schematic presentation of metabolic syndrome. *AT II,* Angiotensin II; *FFA,* free fatty acid; *PAI-1,* plasminogen activator inhibitor 1; *RAAS,* renin-angiotensin-aldosterone system; *SNS,* sympathetic nervous system; *T2DM,* type 2 diabetes mellitus.

INDIVIDUAL FACTORS

Obesity, especially abdominal, is driven by excess caloric intake and diminished physical activity. With progressive adipocyte enlargement, adipocyte hypoxia ensues, leading to inflammation and atherosclerosis. **Insulin resistance** occurs when normal insulin concentration fails to induce normal responses in target tissues. Pancreatic beta cells fail to produce sufficient insulin to correct the worsening insulin resistance, which leads to T2DM. **Dyslipidemia** is characterized by lipid anomalies and activity of atherogenic lipoproteins and cholesterol. These anomalies are closely associated with increased oxidative stress and endothelial dysfunction, characterizing the inflammatory nature of atherosclerotic disease. Studies suggest that hyperglycemia and hyperinsulinemia activate the renin-angiotensin system (RAS), which increases renal sodium reabsorption and causes vasoconstriction, resulting in **hypertension**.

Genetics may play a major role, potentially explaining why certain populations are at highest risk for metabolic syndrome. Metabolic syndrome is also characterized by impaired **endothelium-dependent vasodilation**, accelerated atherosclerosis, and a proinflammatory state with **anomalies in procoagulant factors**. **Diets high in fat** and processed foods are associated with generation of reactive oxygen species and a proinflammatory state. Chronic **cortisol hypersecretion** may lead to increased visceral fat and sarcopenia, which lead to dyslipidemia, hypertension, and T2DM. Finally, the increased degree of sleep-disordered breathing seen in **obstructive sleep apnea (OSA)** is associated with metabolic syndrome components.

METABOLIC SYNDROME AND UROLOGIC DISORDERS

Although metabolic syndrome is classically associated with cardiovascular disease, diabetes, and stroke, **urologic conditions are highly prevalent among those with metabolic syndrome.**

RENAL CONDITIONS

Metabolic syndrome and T2DM have a significant impact on renal physiology. Three major renal conditions associated are renal insufficiency, urolithiasis, and renal cell carcinoma (RCC). Renal disorders are a major cause of death and disability. Patients with **renal insufficiency** have accelerated rates of death largely from impending cardiovascular disease. These processes are consequences of metabolic syndrome. **Urolithiasis** is more frequent in patients with metabolic syndrome. Calcium oxalate and uric acid stones were more prevalent among patients with obesity and antihypertensive medications may predispose for stone formation. In addition, there is an association between metabolic syndrome and RCC, with some studies showing a 26% increase in risk of RCC in men with T2DM.

BLADDER CONDITIONS

Metabolic syndrome was associated with a significantly increased risk of **bladder cancer** in men but not in women. Obese patients experienced worse outcomes with an increased risk of disease recurrence, progression, cancer-specific mortality, and any cause of mortality. As metabolic syndrome fosters endothelial dysfunction it may lead to ischemic damage during bladder distention. Many studies examining the linkage between metabolic syndrome and **OAB** were positive. Data suggest that **lower urinary tract symptoms** may be associated with metabolic syndrome and inflammation. The degree of inflammation directly correlates with prostatic volume and International Prostate Symptom Score (IPSS).

PROSTATE CANCER

Men with metabolic syndrome are **more likely to have cancer and to exhibit high-risk features** among a cohort of men presenting for prostate biopsy. Obese men who undergo active surveillance were also found to be at higher risk for disease progression.

LOW TESTOSTERONE AND ERECTILE DYSFUNCTION

Low testosterone is associated with the development of central obesity and metabolic syndrome. Castration therapy among older men with prostate cancer induces metabolic syndrome and elevated risk of cardiovascular disease and T2DM.

TARGETING METABOLIC SYNDROME AS A NOVEL STRATEGY IN UROLOGIC DISEASE

Although the extent to which reversing metabolic syndrome can alter the natural history of the disease remains debatable, evidence shows that both behavioral and medical therapy can have a positive impact. Testosterone and cortisol increase after exercise, with testosterone levels increasing immediately after exercise, while the cortisol response tends to be delayed. **Statins** are approved for the management of hypercholesterolemia and prevention of secondary cardiac events. Although significant epidemiologic literature suggests that **statins may provide protection from the progression of prostate cancer, the only evidence has come from association studies.** **Metformin** is a biguanide drug that has been used to treat T2DM and elicits its metabolism-modifying effects by energetic stress in the liver. Studies suggest that men with diabetes treated with metformin have **lower risk of incidence and death from a number of cancers, including prostate and, potentially, bladder carcinoma.** Because metabolic syndrome is associated with low testosterone levels, treatment with **exogenous testosterone** may partially reverse individual aspects of metabolic syndrome.

Obesity has been associated with dyslipidemia, T2DM, hypertension, cardiovascular disease, stroke, and many urologic conditions. There are several modifiable risk factors, such as **diet and physical fitness, that may affect incidence and outcomes in men with prostate cancer**. Radical prostatectomy is more challenging in obese patients. **Obesity is related to increased risk and biochemical recurrence**. Exercise is associated with improved sexual function in men who had received external beam radiation therapy but does not improve ED after prostatectomy. It is important to **promote long-term strategies for every type of patient, creating individualized approaches and improving men's health overall.**

TESTOSTERONE THERAPY AND CARDIOVASCULAR RISK: ADVANCES AND CONTROVERSIES

Impact of Testosterone Supplementation

Despite the lack of clinical data, testosterone supplementation has increased, with most of the supplementation in men without frank hypogonadism. In the trial by Snyder et al. (2016), testosterone replacement therapy was associated with significantly improved sexual performance and erectile function. There was modest impact on physical functioning. Testosterone replacement elicited no significant benefit with respect to vitality but was associated with small, but significant, benefits to mood, depression symptoms, and energy.

CARDIOVASCULAR RISK

The trial by Basaria et al. (2010) showed fivefold higher incidence of cardiovascular events among testosterone-using men, while Xu et al., 2013 estimated a 54% increase in the risk of cardiovascular events in men on testosterone therapy. The results of many trials led Food and Drug Administration to issue a warning regarding the potential association between cardiac events and testosterone supplementation. Guidelines from The Endocrine Society recommend that clinicians (1) limit the diagnosis of testosterone deficiency to symptomatic males with low testosterone levels, (2) recommend against testosterone replacement therapy in men with relative contraindications (e.g., planning fertility in the near term, those with breast or prostate cancer, and cardiovascular risk factors), and (3) discuss risks of replacement therapy.

ASSOCIATION BETWEEN CARDIOVASCULAR DISEASE AND ERECTILE DYSFUNCTION

There are a host of predisposing risk factors and underlying pathophysiologic processes for cardiovascular disease (CVD) and ED, including dyslipidemia, smoking, hypertension, and T2DM. ED is a risk factor for CVD. **The temporal relationship between ED and subclinical CVD progression is less clear; however, ED may be the single warning of the elevated risk of sudden CVD events**. It is prudent to tease out subclinical CVD before and after the onset of ED.

MENTAL HEALTH AND OPIOID ABUSE IN MEN

Mental illnesses, including anxiety, depression, and suicide, are becoming increasingly prevalent in men, while concomitantly being underdiagnosed. More specifically, >6 million men suffer from depression symptoms such as fatigue, irritability, and loss of interest in work or hobbies. Subsequently, there has been a significant increase in incidences of suicide and substance abuse. Consequences of opioid misuse on public health have increased dramatically and this major source of morbidity and mortality spans gender, race, and income level. Men are significantly more likely to misuse and die from opioids. Moreover, opioid use can conduce hypogonadism.

OPIOID PRESCRIPTIONS

There appears to be a high degree of variability in the dispensing of pain medications. Most patients report using far less than is prescribed by their surgeons; however, **in patients undergoing cancer surgery with curative intent, the risk of new persistent opioid use was 10.4%.**

GONADAL DYSFUNCTION

Male gonadal function is affected by opioid use and abuse via suppression of the hypothalamic-pituitary-gonadal axis resulting in hypogonadism. **Clinicians who treat hypogonadism should consider chronic opioid use as a causative agent for symptomatic hypogonadism.** As part of integrative men's health, urologists will need to cultivate responsibility and should **initially prescribe the *lowest effective dose*** and offer repeat assessment rather than increasing dosage hastily.

16

Urinary Incontinence and Pelvic Prolapse: Pathophysiology, Evaluation, and Medical Management

ELIZABETH ROURKE AND W. STUART REYNOLDS

CONTRIBUTORS OF CAMPBELL-WALSH-WEIN, 12TH EDITION

Toby C. Chai, Lori A. Birder, Elizabeth T. Brown, Alan J. Wein, Roger R. Dmochowski, Alvaro Lucioni, Kathleen C. Kobashi, Riyad T. Al-Mousa, Hashim, Benjamin M. Brucker, Victor W. Nitti, Gary E. Lemack, Maude Carmel, Casey Cg Kowalik, Alan J. Wein, Roger R. Dmochowski, W. Stuart Reynolds, Joshua A. Cohn, Christopher R. Chapple, Nadir I. Osman, Stephen D. Marshall, Jeffrey P. Weiss, Karl-Erik Andersson, Diane K. Newman, Kathryn L. Burgio, John P.F.A. Heesakkers, and Bertil Blok

OVERVIEW AND PATHOPHYSIOLOGY OF URINARY INCONTINENCE AND PELVIC ORGAN PROLAPSE

Urinary Incontinence (UI)

Overview of Neurophysiology. UI is the symptomatic complaint of the involuntary loss of urine and can develop because of anatomic and functional abnormalities of the lower urinary tract **(LUT).** The LUT is composed of the bladder and urethra, supported by a complex system of neural innervation and musculofascial support in the lower pelvis. It functions with the integration of many components, including the central nervous system (CNS), the peripheral nervous system, bladder smooth muscle, bladder stroma, suburothelial and intradetrusor interstitial cells, bladder urothelium, urethral smooth muscle, pelvic floor striated muscles, and the external urethral sphincter (EUS).

Pelvic parasympathetic nerves arise at the sacral level of the spinal cord, stimulate the bladder, and relax the urethra. Lumbar sympathetic nerves inhibit the bladder body and stimulate the bladder base and urethra. Pudendal nerves stimulate the EUS. These nerves contain afferent (sensory) as well as efferent axons.

Urethral and Sphincter Pathophysiology and Anatomy. The urethra is part of the bladder outlet, along with the pelvic floor musculature. The urethra has components of smooth muscle and striated muscle (rhabdosphincter or EUS). The periurethral striated muscle is part of the pelvic floor muscle complex. The EUS is composed of two parts. The periurethral striated muscle of the pelvic floor contains fast-twitch and slow-twitch fibers. The striated muscle of the distal sphincter mechanism contains predominantly slow-twitch fibers and provides >50% of the static resistance. In addition to striated muscle, the EUS appears to contain smooth muscle, which receives noradrenergic innervation. Investigators have shown that stimulation of the hypogastric nerve elicits myogenic potentials in the EUS.

In the male, the membranous urethra extends from the prostatic apex through the pelvic floor musculature (including the EUS) until it becomes the bulbous and penile urethra at the base of the penis. The male EUS covers the ventral surface of the prostate in a crescent shape proximal to the verumontanum, then assumes a horseshoe shape distal to the verumontanum, and is crescent shaped at the bulbar urethra.

In women, the urethra extends throughout the distal third of the anterior vaginal wall from the bladder neck to the meatus. The bulk of the muscle responsible for sphincteric control in women is circular striated muscle located in the proximal urethra and/or mid-urethra. **A network of vascular subepithelial tissue/estrogen sensitive submucosa in women contributes to a urethral seal effect and promotes continence.** The female EUS covers the ventral surface of the urethra in a horseshoe configuration.

Urinary continence is maintained during elevations in intraabdominal pressure by means of passive transmission of abdominal pressure to the proximal urethra along with a guarding reflex involving an active contraction of striated muscle of the EUS. The most common causes of **intrinsic sphincteric deficiency (ISD)** are iatrogenic, although, less commonly, neurologic disease can directly affect sphincter function.

Types of Urinary Incontinence. Stress urinary incontinence (SUI) is the complaint of involuntary loss of urine with physical exertion (i.e., walking, straining, exercise, sneezing, coughing) or other activities that cause a rise in intraabdominal pressure. SUI in women is unlikely to be caused solely by anatomic laxity of the anterior vaginal wall and may be also due to poor intrinsic (physiologic) sphincteric function.

Urgency urinary incontinence (UUI) is the complaint of involuntary urine loss associated with urgency. It can, occasionally, be noted on physical exam as the observation of involuntary leakage from the urethra synchronous with the sensation of a sudden, compelling desire to void that is difficult to defer. This may be accompanied by detrusor overactivity incontinence, a urodynamic diagnosis, although this does not have to be present to establish a diagnosis of UUI. Any neurologic process interrupting the normal suprapontine inhibition of the pontine micturition center may result in neurogenic detrusor overactivity (NDO) and cause UUI.

Mixed urinary incontinence (MUI) is the complaint of involuntary urine loss associated with urgency as well as activities causing a rise in intraabdominal pressure. Postural UI is the complaint of involuntary urine loss associated with a change in position (typically from sitting or lying down to standing). Nocturnal enuresis is the complaint of involuntary urine loss occurring during sleep and should be distinguished from urgency incontinence. Continuous UI is the complaint of continuous urine loss, day and night, typically seen with fistula of the lower urinary tract involving the vagina (i.e., vesicovaginal and ureterovaginal fistulae). Insensible UI is the complaint of urine loss when the patient is unaware of how or precisely when the urine loss occurred. Coital incontinence is the complaint of involuntary loss of urine with sexual intercourse. It may occur with initial penetration, intromission, and/or during orgasm. Poor emptying from detrusor underactivity or detrusor areflexia (causing **overflow incontinence**) can also cause UI (Table 16.1).

Pelvic Organ Prolapse (POP)

Types of Prolapse. POP refers to the downward displacement of the pelvic organs, which results in protrusion of the uterus

Table 16.1 Standard International Urogynecological Association/ International Continence Society Terminology of Urinary Incontinence Symptoms

TERMINOLOGY	DESCRIPTION
Urinary incontinence	Complaint of any involuntary leakage of urine
Stress urinary incontinence	Complaint of involuntary leakage on effort or exertion or on sneezing or coughing
Urgency	Complaint of a sudden compelling desire to pass urine, which is difficult to defer
Urgency urinary incontinence	Complaint of involuntary leakage accompanied by or immediately preceded by urgency
Postural incontinence	Complaint of voluntary loss of urine associated with change of body position, for example, rising from a seated or lying position
Nocturnal enuresis	Complaint of involuntary loss of urine that occurs during sleep
Mixed incontinence	Complaint of involuntary leakage associated with urgency and with exertion, effort, sneezing, or coughing
Continuous urinary incontinence	Complaint of continuous leakage
Insensible incontinence	Complaint of urinary incontinence when the woman has been unaware of how it occurred
Coital incontinence	Complaint of involuntary loss of urine with coitus

From Abrams P, Cardozo L, Fall M, et al. The standardisation of terminology of lower urinary tract function: Report from the Standardisation Sub-Committee of the International Continence Society. *Neurourol Urodyn* 2002;21:167-178. (reprinted in *Urology* 2003;61:37-49); Haylen BT, de Ridder D, Freeman RM, et al. An International Urogynecological Association (IUGA)/International Continence Society (ICS) joint report on the terminology for female pelvic floor dysfunction. *Neurourol Urodyn* 2010;29:4-20.

and/or the different vaginal compartments and their surrounding organs, such as the bladder, the rectum, or the bowel. It results from the loss of support of one or more compartments of the vagina (Fig. 16.1). The levator ani muscles, and their interaction with endopelvic fascia, are an important component of the pelvic organ support.

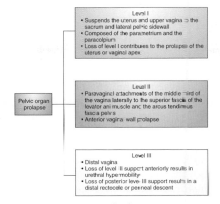

FIG. 16.1 Levels of support.

Anterior compartment prolapse corresponds to the descent of the anterior vaginal wall. Most commonly, this represents the descent of the bladder (**cystocele**), but it can also represent an anterior enterocele, especially after prior reconstructive surgery. **Apical prolapse** corresponds to the descent of the uterus (uterine or cervical prolapse) or, in a posthysterectomy patient, the vaginal cuff. It can include the small intestine (**enterocele**). **Posterior compartment prolapse** is a weakness of the posterior vaginal wall and can involve the rectum (**rectocele**) but can also include the small bowel or colon even in the presence of an intact uterus. **Procidentia** refers to total vaginal eversion with complete uterine or vaginal cuff prolapse. POP occurs most frequently in the anterior compartment, followed by the posterior compartment, and least commonly in the apex.

Risk Factors. Vaginal childbirth, advancing age, and obesity are the most established risk factors for POP. The risk of POP increases with every additional vaginal childbirth, and forceps delivery further increases the risk of developing POP. Cesarean section seems to be protective against prolapse, but the degree of protection is unclear. The incidence and the prevalence of POP increase with advancing age with women 60–69 and 70–79 years of age having a higher risk of prolapse than women ages 50–59 years. **Hysterectomy is associated with an increased risk of developing POP.** Additionally, POP is more common in white and Hispanic women than African American women.

EVALUATION OF URINARY INCONTINENCE AND PELVIC ORGAN PROLAPSE

The purpose of evaluation of patients with UI includes documentation and characterization of the UI, including consideration of the differential diagnosis, prognostication, and facilitation of treatment selection. Additionally, proper evaluation helps assess symptom bother and establish a patient's expectations of potential outcomes. It is helpful to determine the impact that the leakage has on the patient's daily life and activities and can be done so with patient reported outcome measures and quality of life questionnaires. The American Urological Association (AUA) guidelines emphasize the importance of establishing patient expectation of treatment and an understanding of the balance between the benefits and risks/burden of available treatment options. (https://www.auanet.org/guidelines/guidelines/stress-urinary-incontinence-(sui)-guideline)

Regarding POP specifically, important questions focus on whether the patient is aware of any prolapse and what, if any, symptomatology and bother the prolapse may be causing. Patients with POP should also be assessed for presence of SUI given the high cooccurrence of these conditions.

Past medical and surgical histories are vital to the assessment of incontinence and should include the following: neurologic conditions (Parkinson disease, multiple sclerosis, stroke, spinal cord injury), medical diagnoses (diabetes, dementia), history of radiation, pelvic trauma, gynecologic and obstetric history, and previous pelvic surgery. Medications, especially those that can affect the LUT, should be reviewed (Table 16.2 and Fig. 16.2).

The general appearance of a patient, including age, gait, stature, and fragility, can provide important information regarding performance status, neurologic status, and other factors that may direct proper treatment planning. Similarly, an abdominal examination evaluating incisions, hernias, organomegaly, bladder distension, and body habitus is important, particularly if abdominal surgery is considered. A comprehensive female pelvic exam should comment on the external genitalia, estrogen status, lesions, and labial size/adhesions.

The most common methodology to document SUI on examination is the supine cough stress test, although this can also be performed in the standing position if SUI is not demonstrated in the

Table 16.2 Pharmacologic Agents That Can Affect the Lower Urinary Tract

PHARMACOLOGIC EFFECTS	COMMON AGENTS	POTENTIAL EFFECTS ON URINARY TRACT
Sympathomimetics	Ephedrine, methylphenidate, cocaine, amphetamine	Can increase outlet resistance and exacerbate obstructive symptoms/ overactive bladder symptoms Can decrease detrusor contractility and precipitate retention
Sympatholytics	Terazosin, doxazosin tamsulosin, alfuzosin, silodosin	Can decrease outlet resistance and exacerbate stress incontinence
Anticholinergics	Oxybutynin, fesoteridine, solifenacin, trospium, darifenacin	Can contribute to urinary retention, particularly in patients with outlet obstruction
Diuretics	Furosemide, thiazides, spironolactone, triamterene, bumetanide	Do not affect bladder directly, but because of increased urine production, can aggravate incontinence problems

recumbent position (Table 16.3). For males, a digital rectal exam should be performed evaluating for an enlarged prostate gland.

Urethral position and mobility should be assessed at rest and during straining and coughing. Mobility may be estimated by direct visualization or, less commonly, using a small, lubricated Q-tip in the urethra. Hypermobility is defined as a Q-tip deflection angle of >30 degrees from horizontal or resting position.

Assessment of POP should include evaluation of each compartment (anterior, posterior, and apical) and the perineal body should be assessed for laxity. A complete systematic examination is performed using two posterior blades of a split Grave's speculum at rest and with straining. Several classification systems are used to quantify POP, with the **Baden-Walker classification and the Pelvic Organ Prolapse-Quantification system (POP-Q)** being the most common (Table 16.4 and Fig. 16.3).

Additional evaluation tools include urinalysis, micturition diaries, urine flow rate, post-void residual (PVR) volume, and measurement

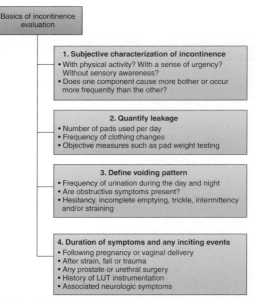

FIG. 16.2 History of present illness highlights for incontinence evaluation. *LUT,* Lower urinary tract.

of prostate specific antigen (PSA) in men. More advanced investigations may be performed to further elucidate the etiology of symptoms. These include computed tomography (CT)/magnetic resonance imaging (MRI)/ultrasound, cystoscopy (to evaluate for urethral stricture, outlet obstruction, or cause of hematuria), and urodynamics. Urodynamics may help to identify factors contributing to LUT dysfunction, predict consequences of LUT dysfunction on the upper tracts, predict consequences of interventions, and elucidate reasons for treatment failures. Urodynamics (UDS) may be performed before and after undergoing surgical intervention.

MEDICAL MANAGEMENT OF URINARY INCONTINENCE AND PELVIC ORGAN PROLAPSE

The approach to the treatment of incontinence is contingent on a clear understanding of the etiology and pathophysiology behind the patient's symptoms. The clinician must first determine whether the cause of the symptoms is a bladder or an outlet problem or a

Table 16.3 Components of a Focused Pelvic Examination[a]

Genitourinary Female

Pelvic examination (with or without specimen collection for smears and cultures), including:

- External genitalia (e.g., general appearance, hair distribution, lesions) and vagina (e.g., general appearance, estrogen effect, discharge, lesions, pelvic support, cystocele, rectocele)
- Urethra (e.g., masses, tenderness, scarring). Examination of bladder (e.g., fullness, masses, tenderness)
- Cervix (e.g., general appearance, lesions, discharge)
- Uterus (e.g., size, contour, position, mobility, tenderness, consistency, descent or support)
- Adnexa/parametria (e.g., masses, tenderness, organomegaly, nodularity)
- Anus and perineum

[a]At the time of this writing, all bullet points are required to be considered a complete female genitourinary examination. However, other organ systems/body areas not limited to the genitourinary system may be included in a report to accomplish the requirements of various levels of examination.

From CMS 97 guidelines for focused female pelvic examination. Documentation Guidelines for Evaluation and Management (E/M) Services, jointly approved by the American Medical Association and HCFA with revisions November, 1997.

Table 16.4 Baden-Walker Classification and the Pelvic Organ Prolapse-Quantification System (POP-Q) Staging Criteria

STAGE	CRITERIA
0	Aa, Ap, Ba, Bp at −3 cm, and C or D ≤ − (tvl − 2) cm
I	Stage 0 criteria not met and leading edge < −1 cm
II	Leading edge ≥ −1 cm but ≤ +1 cm
III	Leading edge > +1 cm but < + (tvl − 2) cm
IV	Leading edge ≥ + (tvl − 2) cm

combination of both. Therapeutic options should be considered with the goal of providing an individualized, patient-directed treatment plan based on patient's goals and risk-benefit and cost-benefit ratios.

Urgency Urinary Incontinence

Nonsurgical intervention for patients with UUI ranges from behavioral and dietary modification to biofeedback or pharmacotherapy. According to the overactive bladder (OAB) guidelines, behavioral

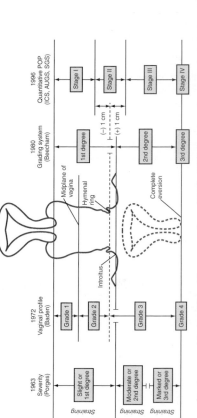

FIG. 16.3 Visual comparison of systems used to quantify pelvic organ prolapse (POP). *AUGS*, American Urogynecologic Society; *ICS*, International Continence Society; *SGS*, Society of Gynecologic Surgeons. (From Theofrastous JP, Swift SE. The clinical evaluation of pelvic floor dysfunction. *Obstet Gynecol Clin North Am* 1998;25:783-804.)

therapy (e.g., fluid management, dietary modification, and bladder training) is the first line of therapy (https://www.auanet.org/guidelines/guidelines/overactive-bladder-(oab)-guideline). Weight loss reduces SUI and may significantly reduce UUI episodes, as well. Medications (anticholinergics and/or β-3 adrenergic agonists) can be added subsequently but are technically considered second-line therapy. If recommending antimuscarinic medication, prescribers should educate the patient about potential side effects, including dry mouth, constipation, cognitive effects, and visual impairment. **Extended-release formulations are favored over short-acting formulations** because of lower rates of dry mouth.

Sacral neuromodulation (SNM), posterior tibial nerve stimulation (PTNS), intradetrusor injection of onabotulinumtoxinA, and augmentation cystoplasty (AC) may be considered in patients with refractory symptoms or who are not candidates for pharmacotherapy. For continuity, these surgical interventions for UUI are presented here, and surgical options for SUI and POP are in Chapter 17.

The posterior tibial nerve contains motor and sensory signals from the L4-S3 nerve roots. Stimulation of this nerve activates somatic afferent fibers, which send inhibitory signals to the sacral and central pontine micturition center allowing for bladder inhibition and improved storage. It is a relatively noninvasive treatment modality that consists of 12 (1–3 times weekly) treatments of 30 minutes each. Patients must be able/willing to come to the clinic to complete weekly induction treatments followed by a maintenance schedule to prevent symptom relapse after successful treatment. This often presents as a barrier to compliance with the treatment. Overall, **PTNS may produce a clinical response in approximately 60% to 80% of patients with medication-refractory OAB with limited risk of adverse events.**

OnabotulinumtoxinA is produced by *Clostridium botulinum*, an anaerobic, gram-negative bacterium. It is a potent neurotoxin that causes **inhibition of presynaptic acetylcholine release at the neuromuscular junction. This results in a flaccid paralysis.** The procedure can be performed in the office or operating room with either flexible or rigid cystoscopy. The recommended dose is 100 units for idiopathic OAB. Injections can result in a 59% decrease in daily incontinence episodes. The primary risks of onabotulinumtoxinA injection in clinical trials include symptomatic UTI in ~20% and the need to initiate intermittent catheterization in up to 12%.

SNM delivers electrical impulses to the S3 sacral nerve root that is responsible for innervation of the autonomic functions of the pelvic nerves and striated muscles. A test called a percutaneous nerve evaluation (PNE) can be performed in the office or an ambulatory setting and, if successful, can followed by a complete implant of a permanent lead and implantable generator (IPG). Alternatively, a permanent lead may be implanted for a longer test period (stage 1) followed by IPG implant, if successful (stage 2). SNM can also be utilized in the setting of nonobstructive urinary retention. SNM had 5-year success rates of 70%–80% and is often considered a more durable, long-term management option for OAB with/without incontinence. Drawbacks of SNM include a revision rate >30% at 5 years from undesirable changes in stimulation, pain, or inadequate efficacy.

In patients who have failed first- to third-line therapies, AC and/or urinary diversion (UD) (fourth-line OAB therapy) can be considered (https://www.auanet.org/guidelines/guidelines/overactive-bladder-(oab)-guideline). Ileum is the preferred bowel segment for AC and UD, and care must be taken to preserve the terminal ileum in order to prevent vitamin B_{12} and salt losses. Patients must also be able to demonstrate appropriate dexterity and willingness to catheterize the urethra or a concomitant catheterizable channel after AC. Contraindications to AC include impaired renal function, bowel disease (Crohn's, inflammatory bowel, short gut as seen in cloacal exstrophy, congenital abnormalities), and malignancy.

Female Stress Urinary Incontinence. Patients with SUI may benefit from conservative measures using pelvic floor muscle training (PFMT), biofeedback, electrical stimulation, and pharmacotherapy. Urethral bulking injection therapy can provide an intermediate option between nonsurgical and surgical therapies, but surgery remains the mainstay of treatment for SUI.

Continence pessaries are placed transvaginally and are designed to prevent urine loss by stabilizing and supporting the urethra and bladder neck, increasing urethral length, and providing gentle compression of the urethra against the pubic bone during increases in intraabdominal pressure. This structural arrangement can reduce, and often prevent, SUI. Uresta is a bell-shaped pessary (Fig. 16.4) with a handle at its base for easy insertion and removal. Its narrow tip allows for easy insertion into the vagina, like a tampon, and it positions itself so that the wide base

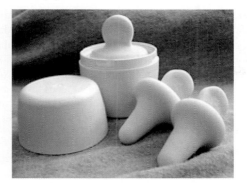

FIG. 16.4 Uresta kit.

provides support to the urethra. Impressa is a disposable single-use tampon-like device that has a core, cover, and applicator. Impressa is designed to prevent the device from moving within the vagina and to produce suburethral tension-free support whenever pressure is transferred from the abdominal cavity to the pelvic floor

Stress Urinary Incontinence in Males. Treatment must be tailored to the patient's needs, goals, and expectations and requires detailed counseling. Some men may be satisfied with protective garments and/or urine-collection devices, such as indwelling or condom catheters, or urethral plugs and external occlusion devices. Injection therapy has not proven a particularly viable option for the treatment of male SUI (which occurs most commonly after radical prostatectomy). The male sling and artificial urinary sphincter are discussed in Chapter 17.

Pelvic Organ Prolapse. The goal of POP repair is to restore the normal anatomy and function of the vagina and the lower urinary and gastrointestinal tracts. Vaginal pessaries have been used for centuries as a conservative treatment for POP. Pessaries are made of an inert plastic or silicone material to minimize odors and prevent absorption of vaginal secretions. There are very few contraindications to pessary use, but **a pessary should not be placed in those with an active pelvic or vaginal infection, severe ulceration, or allergy to silicone or latex, or in patients who are likely to be noncompliant with maintenance care and follow-up**

appointments. Common side effects include vaginal discharge and odor. Serious complications from pessaries are rare; however, vesicovaginal fistula, rectovaginal fistula, erosion, and subsequent impaction have been reported. Combined pessary and PFMT and PFMT alone can be equally effective in reducing symptoms and increasing muscle strength and should be considered for treatment. Patients that fail pessary use or who are not candidates for their use may be considered for surgical management. This is discussed in Chapter 17.

Suggested Readings

Abrams P, Cardozo L, Fall M, et al. The standardisation of terminology of lower urinary tract function: report from the Standardisation Sub-Committee of the International Continence Society. *Neurourol Urodyn* 2002;21:167-178.

Bump RC, Mattiasson A, Bo K, et al. The standardization of terminology of female pelvic organ prolapse and pelvic floor dysfunction. *Am J Obstet Gynecol* 1996;175:10-17.

Chapple C, Abrams P. Male lower urinary tract symptoms (LUTS): an international consultation on male LUTS. Montreal, Canada: Société Internationale d'Urologie, 2013.

Gormley EA, Lightner DJ, Burgio KL, et al. Diagnosis and treatment of overactive bladder (non-neurogenic) in adults: AUA/SUFU guideline. *J Urol* 2012;188(6 suppl): 2455-2463.

Haylen BT, de Ridder D, Freeman RM, et al. An International Urogynecological Association (IUGA)/International Continence Society (ICS) joint report on the terminology for female pelvic floor dysfunction. *Neurourol Urodyn* 2010;29:4-20.

Nambiar AK, Bosch R, Cruz F, et al. EAU guidelines on assessment and nonsurgical management of urinary incontinence. *Eur Urol* 2018;73:596-609.

17

Surgical Management of Urinary Incontinence and Pelvic Organ Prolapse

ELISABETH SEBESTA AND W. STUART REYNOLDS

CONTRIBUTORS OF CAMPBELL-WALSH-WEIN, 12TH EDITION

Siobhan M. Hartigan, Christopher R. Chapple, Roger R. Dmochowski, Jack C. Winters, Ryan M. Krlin, Barry Hallner, Alex Gomelsky, Roger R. Dmochowski, Anne P. Cameron, Dirk J.M.K. Deridder, Tamsin Greenwell, Lindsey Cox, Eric S. Rovner, Hunter Wessels, and Alex J. Vanni.

VAGINAL AND ABDOMINAL RECONSTRUCTIVE SURGERY FOR PELVIC ORGAN PROLAPSE (POP)

Preoperative Considerations

Because pelvic organ prolapse (POP) predominantly impacts quality of life, consideration must be given to prolapse stage, patient's symptoms, and the degree of bother. As patients' expectations and readiness to undergo surgery for POP impact their satisfaction and how they perceive their improvement, **success after POP surgery must consider patient satisfaction along with symptom improvement**.

Surgical Management of Pelvic Organ Prolapse (Table 17.1)

Anterior Compartment (Table 17.2). Since these are commonly combined central and lateral defects, an anterior colporrhaphy (Fig. 17.1) that corrects only central defects should be combined with a paravaginal repair (Fig. 17.2). Various grafts have been used to augment anterior compartment repair. It is essential for women

Table 17.1 Surgical Approach to Pelvic Organ Prolapse

POP-Q SITE	VAGINAL	ABDOMINAL
Aa Urethra	Anterior repair Bladder neck suspension Sling	Retropubic urethropexy
Ba Bladder	Anterior repair Paravaginal repair Colpocleisis	Wedge colpectomy Paravaginal repair ASC

C
Cervix/cuff
	Uterosacral ligament
	  suspension
	Iliococcygeus suspension
	Sacrospinous fixation
	Manchester operation
	Hysteropexy
	Vaginal hysterectomy
	Colpocleisis
		Abdominal hysterectomy
		Uterosacral ligament
		  suspension
		ASC
		Uterine suspension

D Cul-de-sac	McCall culdoplasty	Halban culdoplasty Moschcowitz culdoplasty
Ap	Rectovaginal plication (posterior repair) Site-specific repairs	Colpoperineopexy

ASC, Abdominal sacrocolpopexy; POP-Q, pelvic organ prolapse-quantification.

Table 17.2 Surgical Repairs for Anterior Compartment Pelvic Organ Prolapse

Anterior colporrhaphy	• Plication of pubocervical fascia to repair a central defect (Fig. 17.1) • Anatomic cure: 37%–100% • De novo/occult SUI: 41%–66%; de novo OAB: 5%–7% • Postoperative urinary retention or incomplete emptying—usually transient • Cystoscopy should be performed to rule out bladder or ureteral injuries • Dyspareunia: 3.1%–19%
Paravaginal repair	• Reattachment of the pubocervical fascia to the ATFP to repair a lateral compartment defect • Vaginal (Fig. 17.2) or abdominal (Fig. 17.3) approaches, including open, laparoscopic, or robotic • Anatomic cure: 67%–100%

Table 17.2 Surgical Repairs for Anterior Compartment Pelvic Organ Prolapse—cont'd

	More serious complications vs. colporrhaphy (bleeding requiring transfusion (12%), neuropathy from lithotomy, ureteral obstruction, vaginal abscesses)
Anterior colporrhaphy with grafts	• Augmented repair by attaching a graft to ATFP and/or obturator internus fascia laterally ± central plication sutures
	• Multiple graft materials have been used to augment anterior colporrhaphy
	• Lower objective failure rates than colporrhaphy alone but no difference in subjective cure
	Mesh complications: 11.4% extrusion, 6.8% requiring surgical intervention (see Complications Related to Mesh)

ATFP, Arcus tendineus fasciae pelvis; *OAB*, overactive bladder; *SUI*, stress urinary incontinence.

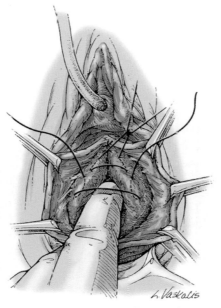

FIG. 17.1 Anterior colporrhaphy. The anterior fibromuscularis layer is imbricated with 2-0 delayed absorbable continuous or interrupted suture. (From Nichols DH. Cystocele. In: Nichols DH, ed. *Gynecologic and obstetric surgery*. St. Louis: Mosby, 1993:334-362.)

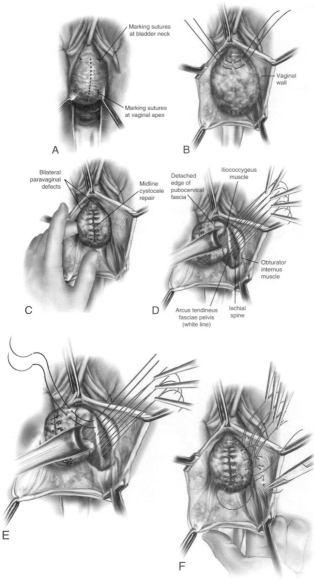

FIG. 17.2 Vaginal paravaginal repair. (A) Unopened anterior vaginal wall with marking sutures placed at anatomic level of bladder neck and vaginal apex. (B) Anterior vaginal wall opened via a midline incision. Sutures placed for midline cystocele repair. (C) Midline cystocele repair completed. Bilateral paravaginal defects identified. (D) Bladder retracted medially to expose lateral pelvic side wall. Permanent sutures have been passed through the white line. (E) Top two sutures have been passed through the detached edge of pubocervical fascia. (F) Three-point closure is completed with all sutures passed through the pubocervical fascia and inside wall of the vagina. (From Baggish M, Karram M. *Atlas of pelvic anatomy and gynecologic surgery*, 3rd ed. Philadelphia: Saunders, 2010.)

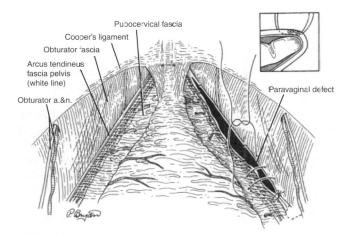

Puбocervical fascia
Cooper's ligament
Obturator fascia
Arcus tendineus fascia pelvis (white line)
Obturator a.&n.
Paravaginal defect

FIG. 17.3 Abdominal paravaginal repair. Paravaginal defect repair as viewed from the retropubic space: approximation of the pubocervical fascia medially to the arcus tendineus fascia pelvis laterally with 2-o braided nonabsorbable suture. Note the vertical orientation of the vaginal vessels in relation to the transverse orientation of the bladder vessels. *Inset* shows suture being passed beneath the vaginal vessels to ensure generous purchase of pubocervical fascia and control of hemostasis. *a*, Artery; *n*, nerve. (From Bruce RG, El-Galley R, Galloway NT. Paravaginal defect repair in the treatment of female stress urinary incontinence and cystocele. *Urology* 1999;54:647-651.)

with high-grade POP to undergo evaluation for stress urinary incontinence (SUI) with prolapse reduced, as the rate of occult SUI is 8.3%–66.1%. Antiincontinence surgery should be performed in select patients concomitantly with POP repair.

Apical Compartment (Table 17.3). The **vaginal apex is the cornerstone of vaginal support**, and failure to ensure apical support at the time of POP repair will increase the risk of recurrence exponentially. Surgical correction can be approached vaginally, abdominally, and robotically or laparoscopically, with or without uterine preservation (see Uterine Prolapse later). **In younger, sexually active, and more-physically active women, the data favor abdominal sacrocolpopexy (ASC) for its durability and preservation of functional vaginal length.** Women undergoing vaginal procedures are more likely to have SUI, dyspareunia, and recurrent prolapse necessitating repeat surgery.

Obliterative Procedures – In patients who no longer desire to be sexually active, a colpocleisis, with or without prior or concomitant hysterectomy, should be considered. Colpocleisis entails the removal of vaginal epithelium and use of purse-string sutures to sequentially reduce the prolapse proximally. The patient must still be screened for occult SUI, and urologists should offer concomitant antiincontinence procedures, as indicated.

Uterine Prolapse – **Vaginal hysterectomy alone is not an adequate treatment for a patient with uterine prolapse.** Vaginal apex suspension, or at minimum McCall culdoplasty (Fig. 17.4), should be performed at the time of hysterectomy for uterine prolapse to reduce the risk of recurrence. Barring contraindications, uterine-sparing approaches to POP repair are gaining popularity and may also be offered (Table 17.4).

Posterior Compartment (Table 17.5). Symptoms include vaginal bulging, defecatory dysfunction (stool trapping requiring vaginal splinting, urgency, constipation), and dyspareunia. Repair traditionally entails a midline posterior colporrhaphy, with or without graft augmentation. However, if a discrete defect in the fascia can be identified, a site-specific repair can be attempted. Although midline fascial plication remains the standard of care for posterior compartment prolapse, there is largely a lack of evidence comparing the two procedures. **Because of the increase in postoperative dyspareunia, plication of the levator ani muscles should not be**

Table 17.3 Surgical Repairs for Apical Compartment Pelvier

Uterosacral ligament suspension	• Suturing USL at the level of the ischial spine to pubocervical and rectovaginal fascia (Figs. 17.5–17.7) • Vaginal or abdominal approach • Minimizes injury to pudendal and gluteal vessels compared with SSL • Mean objective success rate: 85% (48%–96%) • Ureteral kinking/injury: 1%–11% Can be done as a hysteropexy if sparing uterus
Sacrospinous ligament fixation	• Unilateral (right side preferred) or bilateral suture fixation of the vaginal apex to the SSL medial to the ischial spine (Fig. 17.8) • Vaginal approach, either anteriorly or posteriorly • Alters vaginal axis if unilateral fixation • Success rates: 64%–96% • Gluteal pain—pudendal nerve entrapment: 15% • Particularly vulnerable to anterior compartment recurrence: 7.6%–92% (not all require surgery) Can be done as a hysteropexy if sparing uterus
Iliococcygeus suspension	• Bilateral anchoring of the vaginal vault through the pubocervical and rectocervical fascia to the fascia of the iliococcygeus muscle distal to the ischial spine near the insertion of the ATFP (Fig.17.9) • Vaginal approach, either anteriorly or posteriorly Cure rate: 53%–96%; buttock pain: 19%
Abdominal sacrocolpopexy	• Securing vaginal cuff to anterior longitudinal ligament at the sacral promontory with mesh or autologous fascial graft • Open, laparoscopic, or robotic approaches; success rates >90% • Minimally invasive approaches have lower complication rates • Vaginal mesh exposure: 0.8%–9.9% • Up to 20% recur with distal anterior/posterior defects requiring secondary vaginal repair

ASC, Abdominal sacrocolpopexy; *SSL*, sacrospinous ligament; *USL*, uterosacral ligament.

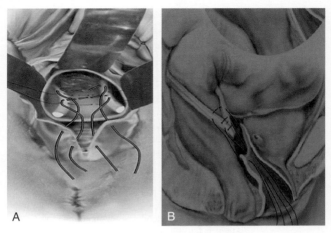

FIG. 17.4 (A and B) Internal and external McCall stitches are placed in a traditional fashion. Tying these sutures obliterates the cul-de-sac, supports the vaginal cuff, and increases posterior vaginal wall length. (From Walters M, Karram M. *Urogynecology and reconstructive pelvic surgery*, 4th ed. Philadelphia: Saunders, 2015:366.)

Table 17.4 Contraindications for Uterine Preservation

Postmenopausal bleeding
Current or recent cervical dysplasia
Familial cancer syndrome, *BRCA1* and *BRCA2*
Hereditary nonpolyposis colonic cancer syndrome
Tamoxifen therapy
Uterine abnormalities
Fibroids, adenomyosis, abnormal endometrial sampling
Abnormal uterine bleeding
Inability to comply with routine gynecologic surveillance
Cervical elongation (relative contraindication)

Modified from Ridgeway BM. Does prolapse equal hysterectomy? The role of uterine conservation in women with uterovaginal prolapse. *Am J Obstet Gynecol* 2015 Dec; 213(6): 802-809. doi: 10.1016/j.ajog.2015.07.035. Epub 2015 Jul 28. PMID: 26226554.

performed. If introital laxity is encountered, perineorrhaphy can be performed in conjunction with posterior repairs.

SURGERY FOR FEMALE SUI

SUI is the involuntary loss of urine on effort or physical exertion and with increased intra-abdominal pressure. **Two types of**

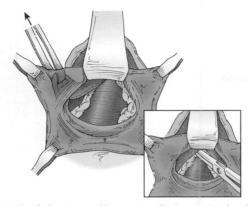

FIG. 17.5 To identify the uterosacral ligament, an Allis clamp is placed on the vaginal epithelium at the right apex and pulled straight upward. With the right uterosacral ligament on tension, the uterosacral ligament is visible in the pelvis. *Inset,* A long Allis clamp is used to grasp the right uterosacral ligament. (Modified from Walters MD, Muir TW. Surgical treatment of vaginal apex prolapse: transvaginal approaches. In: Vasavada S, Appell R, Sans P, Raz S, eds. *Female urology, urogynecology and voiding dysfunction.* New York: Marcel Dekker, 2005:663-676.)

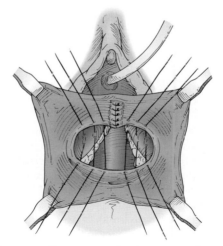

FIG. 17.6 High uterosacral ligament vaginal vault suspension. Three sutures are placed from lateral to medial in each uterosacral ligament. The sutures are brought through the vaginal muscularis anteriorly (pubocervical fascia) and posteriorly (rectovaginal fascia).

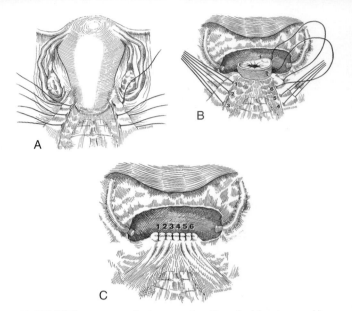

FIG. 17.7 (A) Three permanent sutures are placed in each of the uterosacral ligaments medial to the ischial spine. (B) One end of each of the six sutures is placed serially across vaginal apex through the anterior endopelvic fascia and the other end through the posterior endopelvic fascia. (C) All sutures are tied to reapproximate the anterior and posterior vaginal muscularis, to close any potential enterocele defect, and to elevate the vaginal apex toward the sacrum. (Copyright 2008 Loyola University Health System. Used with permission from Mary Pat Fitzgerald, MD.)

SUI have been suggested: urethral hypermobility (a hypermobile but otherwise healthy urethra, due to weakened support of the proximal urethra) and **intrinsic sphincter deficiency (ISD)** (a deficiency of the urethral sphincter mechanism). ISD is urodynamically defined as a leak point pressure (LPP) <60 cm H_2O or a maximum urethral closing pressure [MUCP] <20 cm H_2O. It is likely that ISD coexists with hypermobility in most cases. **However, there is no consistency in the existing data to support that ISD influences either the outcomes or type of surgical treatment.** Therapeutic options generally fall into one of seven categories (Box 17.1). Choice of surgery should take into account

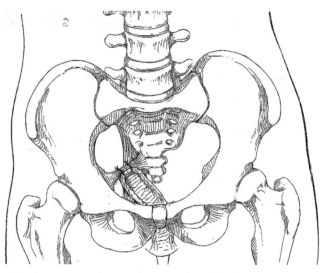

FIG. 17.8 Sacrospinous ligament fixation. With a unilateral suspension, the vagina is deflected to the right side and caudally. (From Richter K, Albright W. Long-term results following fixation of the vagina on the sacrospinous ligament by the vaginal route. *Am J Obstet Gynecol* 1981;141:811-816.

Table 17.5 Surgical Repairs for Posterior Compartment Pelvic Organ Prolapse

Posterior colporrhaphy	• Midline plication of the rectovaginal fascia (Fig. 17.10) • Anatomic cure: 82%–92% • Has been augmented with grafts; no studies show a benefit • Defecatory dysfunction (e.g., constipation, anismus) may persist
Site-specific repair	• Repair of discrete defect in rectovaginal fascia, most commonly transverse (Fig. 17.11) • A discrete defect may not always be identified • Anatomic cure: 56%–100% • Anatomic correction does not always correlate with symptom relief, but symptom relief should be the priority for surgical success

---

Box 17.1 Surgical Methods

Open retropubic colposuspension
Laparoscopic retropubic colposuspension
Suburethral sling procedure
Needle suspension
Periurethral injection
Artificial sphincter
Vaginal anterior repair (anterior colporrhaphy)

---

surgeon preference, coexisting problems, the patient's anatomic features, and her general health.

Retropubic Suspension Surgery

Retropubic colposuspension surgically lifts tissues near the bladder neck and proximal urethra behind the anterior pubic bone. Retropubic procedures have traditionally been used when hypermobility was thought to be the cause of a woman's SUI. If significant ISD is present, it is hypothesized, but unproven, that SUI will persist after retropubic suspension. In such circumstances, a colposuspension is less likely to be successful than a tight fascial sling or artificial sphincter.

Indications for Retropubic Suspension. Careful assessment of the patient is essential (Fig. 17.12). **A retropubic suspension is indicated when (1) a patient is undergoing laparotomy for concomitant abdominal surgery that cannot be performed vaginally and (2) there is limited vaginal access.**

Types of Surgical Repairs and Results (Table 17.6). There are four variations of retropubic colposuspension: Marshall-Marchetti-Krantz (MMK), Burch, vagino-obturator shelf (VOS) repair, and paravaginal procedures (Fig. 17.13A-E). **The Burch is regarded as the standard open retropubic colposuspension due to durable results and minimal complications. It is as effective as other primary or secondary surgery for resolving SUI.**

Complications. Postoperative voiding difficulty is common. Retention lasting more than 4 weeks occurs in 5% and is permanent in <5%, similar to pubovaginal slings (PVS). **Therefore, all patients should be counseled before surgery about the potential need for clean intermittent catheterization (CIC).** Preoperative storage

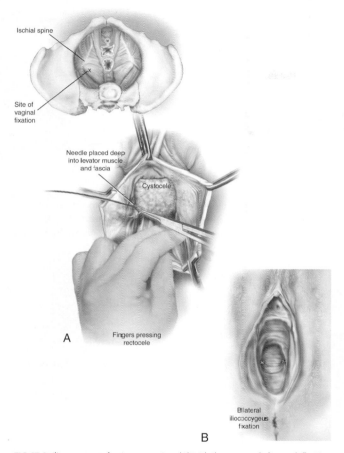

FIG. 17.9 Iliococcygeus fascia suspension. (A) With the surgeon's finger deflecting the rectum downward, the right iliococcygeus fascia sutures is placed. *Inset*, View of the dissected vagina. (B) Abdominal view of the endopelvic fascia. Approximate location of the sutures are delineated by the + sign. (From Walters M, Karram M. *Urogynecology and reconstructive pelvic surgery*, 3rd ed. Philadelphia: Mosby, 2006.)

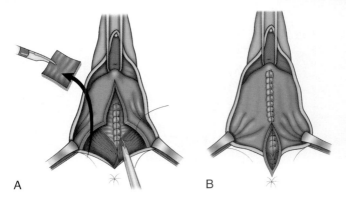

FIG. 17.10 (A and B) Technique of posterior colporrhaphy with rectovaginal tissue plication. (From Ginsberg D. Treatment of vaginal wall prolapse. In: Goldman H, Vasabada S, eds. *Female urology: a practical clinical guide.* Totowa, NJ: Humana Press, 2007:281-296.)

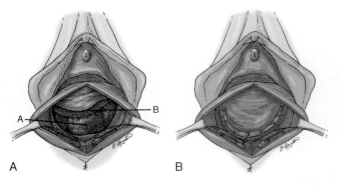

FIG. 17.11 Site-specific rectocele repair. (A) Identification of low transverse defect. (B) Primary repair. (From Richardson AC. The rectovaginal septum revisited: its relationship to rectocele and its importance in rectocele repair. *Clin Obstet Gynecol* 1993;36:976-983.)

symptoms should be appropriately evaluated but do not serve as a contraindication for a retropubic suspension for concomitant SUI. Risk of de novo urgency is ~11%, and 66% in those with preoperative urgency. Postoperative POP is possible and should be adequately evaluated preoperatively.

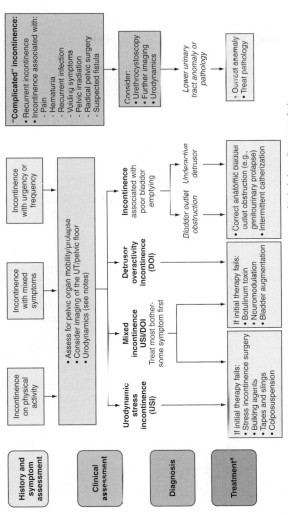

FIG. 17.12 Algorithm for the specialized management of stress urinary incontinence in women (after the Third International Consultation on Incontinence, Monaco, 2004). *UT, Urinary tract.*

[a]At any stage of the patient's care pathway, management may need to include continence products.

Content of figure:

History and symptom assessment

- Incontinence on physical activity
- Incontinence with mixed symptoms
- Incontinence with urgency or frequency

"Complicated" incontinence:
- Recurrent incontinence
- Incontinence associated with:
  - Pain
  - Hematuria
  - Recurrent infection
  - Voiding symptoms
  - Pelvic irradiation
  - Radical pelvic surgery
  - Suspected fistula

Clinical assessment

- Assess for pelvic organ mobility/prolapse
- Consider imaging of the UT/pelvic floor
- Urodynamics (see notes)

Consider:
- Urethrocystoscopy
- Further imaging
- Urodynamics

Lower urinary tract anomaly or pathology

Diagnosis

- Urodynamic stress incontinence (USI)
- Mixed incontinence USI/DOI — Treat most bothersome symptom first
- Detrusor overactivity incontinence (DOI)
- Incontinence associated with poor bladder emptying

Bladder outlet obstruction / *Underactive detrusor*

Treatment[a]

- If initial therapy fails:
  - Stress incontinence surgery
  - Bulking agents
  - Tapes and slings
  - Colposuspension

- If initial therapy fails:
  - Botulinum toxin
  - Neuromodulation
  - Bladder augmentation

- Correct anatomic bladder outlet obstruction (e.g., genitourinary prolapse)
- Intermittent catherization

- Correct anomaly
- Treat pathology

Table 17.6 Retropubic Colposuspensions for Treatment of Female Stress Urinary Incontinence

MMK	• Suspension of the vesicourethral junction toward the periosteum of the symphysis pubis (Fig. 17.13E) • Short-term subjective (88%) and objective (72%–100%) cure • Long-term data limited; decrease in continence with time (28%–71% at 10–17 years) • Overall complications 21%; osteitis pubis 0.9%–3.2% **No evidence to support the continued use of MMK over other procedures due to complications and decline in continence**
Burch	• Elevation of the anterior vaginal wall and paravesical tissues toward the iliopectineal line of the pelvic sidewall (Fig. 17.13A) • Care should be taken not to tie the sutures tightly • Overall continence: 85%–90% within the first year • More durable with longer follow-up: 70% continence at 5 years • Ureteral obstruction possible • Groin pain: 6.8%–12% • May aggravate posterior compartment prolapse, predisposing to enterocele: 3%–17% • Recurrent anterior prolapse: 11%
VOS repair	• Anchoring of the vagina to the internal obturator fascia (Fig. 17.13B) or the internal obturator and iliopectineal line (Fig. 17.13C) • Combination of the Burch and paravaginal defect repair Limited data, reported cure: 60%–86%
Paravaginal defect repair	• Closing a presumed fascial weakness laterally at the site of attachment of the pelvic fascia to the internal obturator fascia (Fig. 17.13D) Less effective than Burch (objective cure of 72% at 6 months vs. 100% with Burch); **not recommended for the treatment of SUI alone**

MMK, Marshall-Marchetti-Krantz; *VOS,* vagino-obturator shelf.

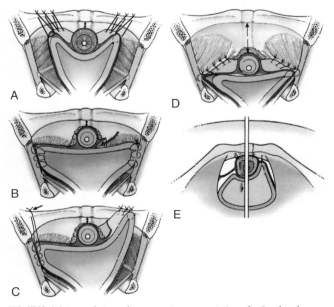

FIG. 17.13 (A) Coronal view, diagrammatic representation of a Burch colposuspension. (B) Coronal view, diagrammatic representation of a vagino-obturator shelf procedure. (C) Coronal view, diagrammatic representation of a vagino-obturator shelf procedure on the left, augmented by stitching to the iliopectineal line, and a Burch procedure on the right. (D) Coronal view, diagrammatic representation of a paravaginal repair. (E) Diagram demonstrating the sutures in a Marshall-Marchetti-Krantz procedure and their proximity to the urethra. (From Turner-Warwick R, Chapple CR. *Functional reconstruction of the urinary tract and gynaeco-urology: an exposition of functional principles and surgical procedures.* Oxford: Blackwell Science, 2002.)

Slings—Autologous, Biologic, Synthetic, and Mid-urethral

Suburethral slings are currently considered the procedure of choice for surgical correction of female SUI. Although slings have been performed for over a century, they only became the predominant surgery for SUI in the 1990s. In 1998 the Food and Drug Administration (FDA) approved the first mid-urethral sling (MUS) for the treatment of SUI, and, subsequently, sling surgery increased more than threefold.

Preoperative Assessment – The initial evaluation of a woman with SUI who is desiring surgical treatment includes:

- Focused history (**including degree of baseline urgency which correlates with poorer post-sling outcomes**)
- Physical examination (including focused neurologic and pelvic examination)
- Objective demonstration of SUI (via cough or Valsalva stress test, either supine or standing)
- Assessment of postvoid residual (PVR)
- Urinalysis (UA)

More extensive evaluation, including radiographic studies, cystourethroscopy, and urodynamic studies (UDS), may be occasionally performed. However, **UDS are not necessary in the work-up of clearly demonstrated SUI (https://www.auanet.org/guidelines/guidelines/stress-urinary-incontinence-(sui)-guideline).**

Preoperative Counseling – Most important, women should be counseled on the risk of transient and permanent postoperative voiding dysfunction, including difficulty emptying the bladder and de novo storage symptoms. Preoperative instruction in performing CIC in select patients may minimize the need for an indwelling urethral catheter postoperatively.

Pubovaginal Sling (PVS). **PVS using autologous fascia remains the gold standard for management of all forms of SUI.** PVS is a highly versatile surgical procedure for both uncomplicated and complicated SUI. This includes women who require CIC, those undergoing concomitant urethral reconstruction, and those who failed retropubic suspensions or MUS. The PVS is placed at the bladder neck to provide dynamic urethral compression without obstruction during times of increased intraabdominal pressure. Autologous slings are the gold standard and include **rectus abdominis fascia** (Fig. 17.14A) and **fascia lata** (Fig. 17.14B).

Surgical Considerations (Figs.17.15–17.20) – An inverted U-shaped incision is utilized to allow periurethral dissection to the level of the bladder neck. To pass the sling, Stamey/Cobb-Ragde needles or large clamps (i.e., tonsils) are passed from above. Cystourethroscopy should be performed to rule out bladder injury and examine for urine efflux. If bladder perforation occurs, the needles may be repassed. The vaginal incision should be closed and any additional vaginal procedures completed prior to sling

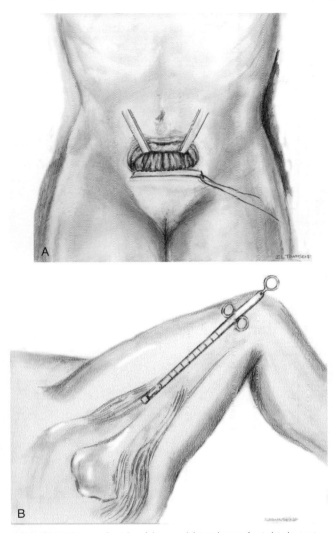

FIG. 17.14 (A) Rectus fascial graft harvest. (B) Autologous fascia lata harvest.

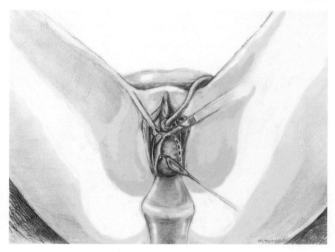

FIG. 17.15 Inverted-U incision.

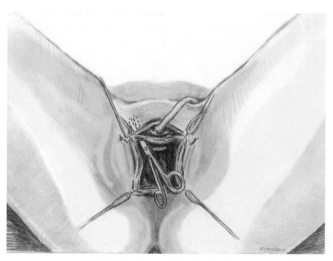

FIG. 17.16 Perforation of endopelvic fascia.

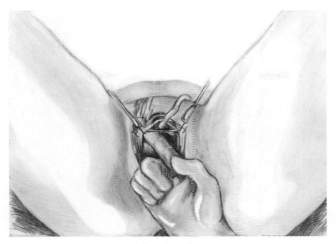

FIG. 17.17 Blunt dissection of retropubic space.

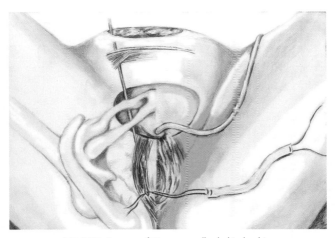

FIG. 17.18 Passage of Stamey needles behind pubis.

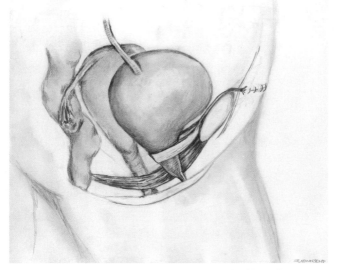

FIG. 17.19 Sagittal view of pubovaginal sling position at bladder neck in retropubic position.

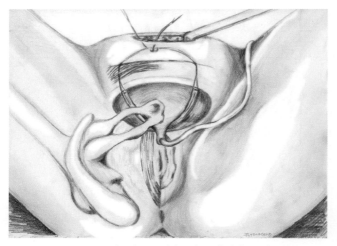

FIG. 17.20 Passage of and tying of sling through abdominal incision.

tensioning. The sling is loosely tied with a two-fingerbreadth distance above rectus fascia.

Outcomes – PVS is effective for primary and recurrent SUI. Success rates are generally high but vary due to variable outcome measures (24%–97%). Women with mixed urinary incontinence (MUI) have similarly high cure rates, but urge resolution may also involve medical anticholinergic therapy. Postoperative de novo urgency urinary incontinence rates (UUI) are 2%–22%.

Complications – Incidence of voiding dysfunction (including urinary tract infections [UTIs], difficulty voiding, and UUI) after PVS varies widely depending on definition (2.5%–35%). The presence of preoperative voiding dysfunction affects a woman's ability to empty after PVS; however, urodynamic findings like low detrusor pressures and Valsalva voiding should not exclude women from having a PVS. It is appropriate to initially treat voiding dysfunction conservatively. Surgical management of outlet obstruction usually involves a complete urethrolysis (65%–93% success) or sling incision (84%–100% success). Unlike with synthetic slings, urethral perforation and vaginal exposure rates after PVS are very low (<1%).

Mid-urethral Slings. MUSs work by impeding the movement of the posterior urethral wall above the sling, in addition to urethral compression. Unlike bladder neck slings, MUSs are placed loosely at the mid-urethra.

There are two basic types of multi-incision MUS: retropubic (RP) and **transobturator (TO)** (Table 17.7). Single-incision mid-urethral slings (SIMSs) are newer and can be placed via either RP or TO route. Currently, almost all MUS products are constructed from a soft, loosely woven, polypropylene monofilament mesh with a pore size >75 μm (type I mesh).

Surgical Considerations – Regardless of approach, cystourethroscopy must be performed to exclude trocar penetration of the lower urinary tract. If bladder perforation is noted, the trocar is withdrawn and repassed without long-term morbidity. If urethral injury is noted, the surgeon must abandon mesh placement. Tensioning is performed by inserting a clamp or sound between the sling and urethra.

Outcomes – Overall, outcomes are similar between RP and TO MUS in patients with predominantly SUI (Table 17.7). The AUA guidelines state that either RP or TO MUS may be

Table 17.7 Comparison of Mid-urethral Slings

Retropubic	• Trocars pass through space of Retzius and anchor into the endopelvic fascia (Fig. 17.21)
	• Top-down or bottom-top approach
	• TVT bottom-top MUS was the first sling available and has the most long-term data
	• Success rates for SUI: 48%–97%
	• Bladder perforation and major vascular injuries more common vs. TO
	• Higher rates of postoperative voiding dysfunction requiring surgical intervention vs. TO (2.7% vs. 0%)
Transobturator	• Trocars pass through obturator foramen and anchor to obturator internus and externus muscle and fascia (Fig. 17.22)
	• Outside-in or inside-out approach
	• Success rates for SUI: 43%–92%
	• Permanent and devastating groin pain (6.4%)
Single-incision	• Short trocars passed transvaginally; can be placed either in RP or TO fashion; no skin exit point (Fig. 17.23)
	• Should be tensioned slightly tighter than MUS
	• Newer; less long-term data
	• Higher risk of persistent or recurrent SUI
	• Higher rates of de novo urgency
	• Increased risk of vaginal exposure and urinary tract erosions

MUS, Mid-urethral sling; *RP,* retropubic; *SUI,* stress-urinary incontinence; *TO,* transobturator; *TVT,* tension-free vaginal tape.

offered in patients appropriate for MUS surgery and depends on surgeon preference (**https://www.auanet.org/guidelines/ guidelines/stress-urinary-incontinence-(sui)-guideline). Women with SUI have a higher cure rate than those with MUI; however, MUS procedures are still effective in those with MUI. There is less long-term data with SIMS, but there is some evidence of decreasing efficacy with longer follow-up.** It should be noted that the SIMS device primarily associated with higher incontinence rates has been removed from the market.

Complications – The incidence of complications with MUS is low. Bladder trocar injury (2.7%–3.8%) and voiding dysfunction (7.6%) are most common. Vaginal mesh exposure is rare (0.5%–8.1%),

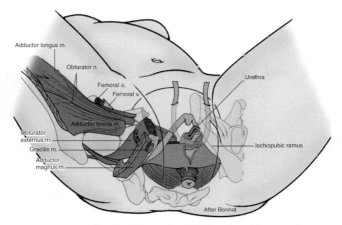

FIG. 17.21 Mid-urethral sling as placed via the retropubic approach.

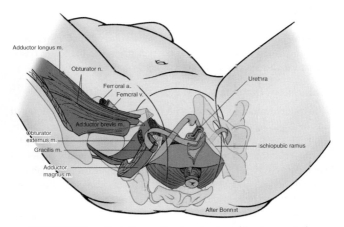

FIG. 17.22 Mid-urethral sling as placed via the transobturator approach.

especially with type I mesh slings. Observation should never be considered when there is urethral (0%–0.6%) or intravesical (0.5%–0.6%) mesh perforation. Voiding dysfunction is usually related to a sling placed too tightly, too proximally, or associated with unrecognized or de novo POP. Obstruction is often transient and may be

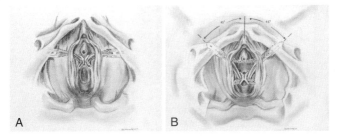

FIG. 17.23 Mid-urethral sling as placed via a single-incision approach. (A) Hammock style. (B) U position.

managed with CIC; however, surgical intervention is occasionally required. If sling division or excision is required for obstruction, the risk of recurrent SUI varies from 20%–74%, with one-third of women electing repeat surgery.

SURGICAL PROCEDURES FOR SPHINCTERIC INCONTINENCE IN MEN

Radical prostatectomy is the most common cause of sphincteric incontinence in men. **Surgical correction is the first-line treatment for the majority of cases.**

Evaluation, Diagnosis, and Indications for Surgery

The initial evaluation of men with incontinence requires a detailed history, physical examination, PVR, and UA ± urine culture (Fig. 17.24). It is important to differentiate between SUI and UUI as the treatment algorithm differs. **Although the finding of detrusor overactivity on UDS is not a contraindication to surgery**, it should be considered during patient counseling. Additionally, cystourethroscopy should be performed prior to surgical intervention to evaluate for unrecognized urethral and bladder neck pathology. **Artificial urinary sphincters (AUSs) and slings should be considered first-line therapy for sphincteric incontinence in men** (Fig. 17.25). **(https://www.auanet.org/guidelines/guidelines/incontinence-after-prostate-treatment)**

Male Slings

Male slings are either transobturator (Fig. 17.26A) or quadratic (Fig. 17.26B). Slings should not be performed in patients with

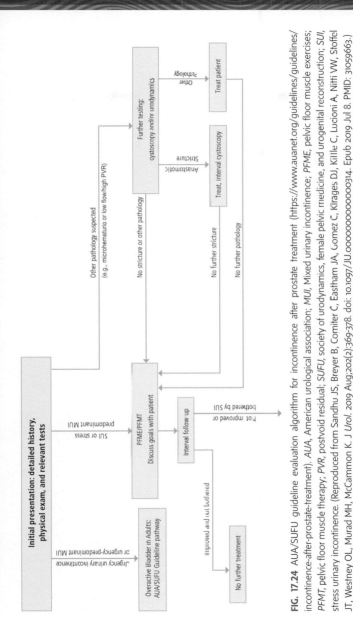

FIG. 17.24 AUA/SUFU guideline evaluation algorithm for incontinence after prostate treatment (https://www.auanet.org/guidelines/guidelines/incontinence-after-prostate-treatment). *AUA,* American urological association; *MUI,* Mixed urinary incontinence; *PFME,* pelvic floor muscle exercises; *PFMT,* pelvic floor muscle therapy; *PVR,* postvoid residual; *SUFU,* society of urodynamics, female pelvic medicine, and urogenital reconstruction; *SUI,* stress urinary incontinence. (Reproduced from Sandhu JS, Breyer B, Comiter C, Eastham JA, Gomez C, Kirages DJ, Kittle C, Lucioni A, Nitti VW, Stoffel JT, Westney OL, Murad MH, McCammon K. *J Urol.* 2019 Aug;202(2):369-378. doi: 10.1097/JU.0000000000000314. Epub 2019 Jul 8. PMID: 31059663.)

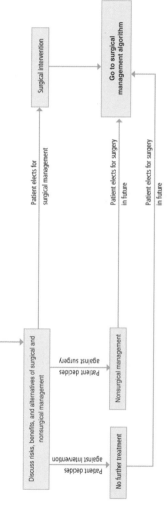

FIG. 17.24, cont'd

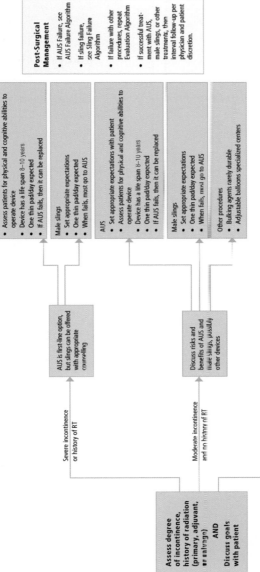

FIG. 17.25 AUA/SUFU algorithm for surgical management (https://www.auanet.org/guidelines/guidelines/incontinence-after-prostate-treatment). *AUS,* Artificial urinary sphincter; *PFME,* pelvic floor muscle exercises; *PFMT,* pelvic floor muscle therapy; *RT,* radiation therapy. (Reproduced from Sandhu JS, Breyer B, Comiter C, Eastham JA, Gomez C, Kirages DJ, Kittle C, Lucioni A, Nitti VW, Stoffel JT, Westney OL, Murad MH, McCammon K. *J Urol.* 2019 Aug;202(2):369-378. doi: 10.1097/JU.0000000000000314. Epub 2019 Jul 8. PMID: 31059665.)

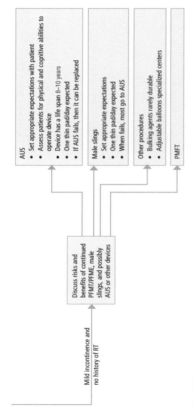

FIG. 17.25, cont'd

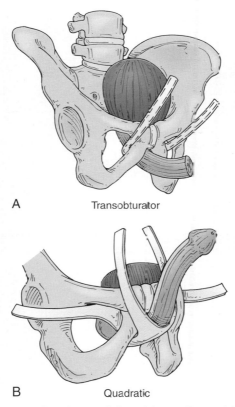

A   Transobturator

B   Quadratic

FIG. 17.26 Proposed mechanism of slings. (A) Transobturator. (B) Quadratic fixation.

severe SUI but instead should be considered alternatives in those who are not candidates for AUS. Complications include perineal pain, urinary retention, infection, and rare cases of erosion (1%–2%).

Artificial Urinary Sphincter

AUS remains the gold standard for the treatment of sphincteric incontinence in male patients because of its long-term durability and effectiveness in moderate and severe incontinence. The AUS consists of a fluid-filled cuff placed around the urethra and

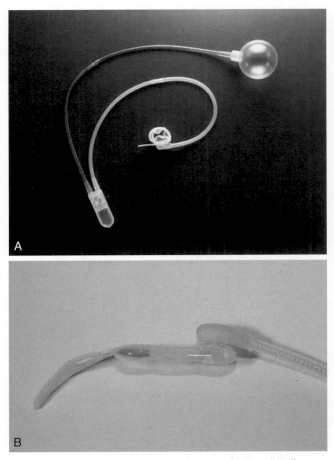

FIG. 17.27 AMS 800 narrow backed artificial urinary sphincter. (A) Cuff, pump, and pressure-regulating balloon. (B) Close-up view of a 3.5-cm cuff. Note the subtle folds of the three-cushion design unique to the 3.5-cm cuff.

provides circumferential compression (Fig. 17.27). The degree of compression is determined by the compliance of the pressure-regulating balloon. The standard is 61–70 cm H_2O for bulbar AUS filled with 23 mL. The most common cuff sizes are 4.0 or 4.5 cm for standard bulbar placement.

Table 17.8 Outcomes of Surgical Therapy for Male Sphincteric Urinary Incontinence

DEVICE	OUTCOMES (%)			
	CURED OR IMPROVED	CURED	IMPROVED	FAILED
Artificial urinary sphincter	82–89	73–76[a]	3–16	18–25
Transobturator sling	70–84	40–80[b]	3–30	16–30
Quadratic sling	32–100	32–70[c]	14–32	30–68

[a]Defined as 0–1 pad.
[b]Defined as no pads. Not included are results from series that included higher proportion of men with history of adjuvant radiotherapy.
[c]No consensus definition among studies

Based on Haab, 1997; Hajivassiliou, 1999; Montague, 2000; Venn, 2000; Montague, 2001; Dalkin, 2003; Raj, 2005; Eauer, 2009; Hudak 2011; Lai, 2012; Li, 2013; Rehder, 2012, 2013; Torrey, 2013; Brant, 2014; Comiter, 2014; Zuckerman, 2014; Kowalik, 2015; Simhan, 2015; McCall, 2016; Chen, 2017; Ferro, 2017; Wingate, 2017 Grabbert, 2019.

Long-term durability is well established (Table 17.8), with a revision rate of 16% and 28% at 2 and 5 years, respectively. Complications after AUS include urinary retention, infection (1%–3% for initial surgery), and erosion (5%–10% in average-risk patients). Both infection and erosion require explant. Urethral atrophy from chronic compression can be managed with revision. Finally, mechanical failure is common and device life is typically 7–10 years.

COMPLICATIONS RELATED TO THE USE OF MESH

The use of mesh in female pelvic surgery is a controversial topic. In spite of these challenges, well-trained urologists should not be dissuaded from using these effective products in the care of their patients.

The MUS is recognized as a standard procedure for the surgical treatment of SUI. The procedure is safe and effective and has improved the QoL for millions of women. MUS has been extensively studied, with 20-year follow-up with high success rates and low complications rates; however, patients must be appropriately counseled preoperatively. Several randomized controlled trials showed similar mesh exposure rates with the three configurations of slings (0.7%–4.4% at 1 year), **in contrast to the mesh used in vaginal POP repair, in which the rate is much higher at 10%–20%.**

Owing to severe mesh complications and extensive subsequent litigation, the FDA halted all sales of vaginal mesh products in April 2019. However, many patients already have these implants and may require treatment of their complications. Mesh exposures in the vagina can be treated conservatively, particularly if asymptomatic, there are no signs of infection, and the exposure is smaller than 0.5–1 cm. Excision is warranted if the exposure is symptomatic or large and fails to heal.

ASC with mesh is an extremely durable repair. The rate of mesh exposure after ASC was initially believed to be significantly lower than vaginal mesh placement. However, with longer follow-up in large, well-designed studies, the exposure rate approaches 10.5% of at 7 years in some series. Vaginal mesh excision after ASC is technically challenging, and an abdominal approach is warranted.

URINARY TRACT FISTULAE

In the industrialized world, most fistulae are iatrogenic. They may also occur from congenital anomalies, malignancy, inflammation and infection, radiation therapy, ischemia, parturition, and other processes. Fistulae can have devastating effects on the QoL and, therefore, active treatment of fistula is always warranted.

Vesicovaginal fistula (VVF) is the most common acquired fistula of the urinary tract. Causes of VVF (Box 17.2). **The most common complaint is constant urinary drainage from the vagina, often after the removal of a urethral catheter.**

The goal of VVF management is the rapid cessation of urinary leakage with return of normal urinary and genital function. Conservative management may be tried, but those with ongoing leakage require surgical repair. VVF may be repaired transvaginally or transabdominally (Table 17.9). **Overall, VVFs in the industrialized world are successfully repaired on the first attempt in >85% with prolonged postoperative urinary catheter drainage.** The presentation, workup, and management of VVF and other fistulae is summarized in Table 17.10.

BLADDER AND FEMALE URETHRAL DIVERTICULA

A bladder diverticulum is a herniation of the bladder urothelium through the muscularis propria of the bladder wall, resulting in a thin-walled outpouching. These may empty poorly during micturition, leaving a large PVR. They often occur in the

---

Box 17.2 Cause of Vesicovaginal Fistulae

Traumatic
    Postsurgical
    Abdominal hysterectomy
    Vaginal hysterectomy
    Antiincontinence surgery
    Anterior vaginal wall prolapse surgery (e.g., colporrhaphy)
    Vaginal biopsy
    Bladder biopsy, endoscopic resection, laser therapy
    Other pelvic surgery (e.g., vascular, rectal)
    External trauma (e.g., penetrating, pelvic fracture, sexual)
Radiation therapy
Advanced pelvic malignancy
Infectious or inflammatory cause
Foreign body
Obstetric
    Obstructed labor
    Forceps laceration
    Uterine rupture
    Cesarean section injury to bladder
Congenital

---

setting of bladder outlet obstruction (BOO) or neurogenic vesicourethral dysfunction. Urine cytology should be considered in most patients with bladder diverticula, as there is an increased risk of bladder cancer in diverticula attributed to urinary stasis and chronic inflammation (0.8%–10%).

Management (Fig. 17.29)

Observation with surveillance and CIC may be appropriate in some patients. **In cases of BOO, definitive treatment of the outlet is indicated before or simultaneously with formal diverticulectomy.** Endoscopic management with transurethral resection of diverticular neck may be considered in patients who are not suited for an open operative approach. Operative excision may be performed using open, laparoscopic, or robotic approaches.

    Urethral diverticula (UD) in female patients are urine-filled periurethral cystic structures connected to the urethra via an ostium. The prevalence of UD is 1%–6% in women. Repeated

Table 17.9 Abdominal versus Transvaginal Repair of Vesicovaginal Fistulae

	ABDOMINAL	TRANSVAGINAL
Incision	Abdominal incision	Vaginal incision(s) can be done immediately in the absence of infection or other complications.
Timing of repair (elapsed time from fistula creation)	Eventually within 2–3 weeks but often delayed 3–6 months	
Exposure	Fistula located low on the trigone or near the bladder neck may be difficult to expose transabdominally	Fistula located high at the vaginal cuff may be difficult to expose transvaginally.
Location of ureters relative to fistula tract	Fistula located near ureteric orifice may necessitate reimplantation	Reimplantation may not be necessary even if fistula tract is located near ureteric orifice.
Sexual function	No change in vaginal depth	Risk of vaginal shortening (e.g., Latzko technique)
Use of adjunctive flaps	Omentum, peritoneal flap, rectus abdominis flap	Labial fat pad (Martius fat pad), peritoneal flap, gluteal skin or gracilis myocutaneous flap
Relative indications	Large fistulae, location high in a deep narrow vagina, radiation fistulae, failed transvaginal approach, small-capacity bladder requiring augmentation, need for ureteral reimplantation, inability to place patient in the lithotomy position	Uncomplicated fistulae, low fistulae
Complications	Higher morbidity Increased length of stay Higher transfusion need Higher readmission rate Higher risk for sepsis	Vaginal shortening
Cost	High	Low

Table 17.10 Summary of Urologic Fistulae, Including Presentation, Evaluation, and Management

Vesicovaginal fistula	• Causes: obstetric complications (developing world) or bladder injury during pelvic surgery (60%–75%, industrialized world) • Presentation: constant vaginal urinary leakage • Workup: pelvic exam (± dye test), cystoscopy ± biopsy, cross-sectional imaging or VCUG + upper tract study; rule out concomitant ureteral injury and ureterovaginal fistula (Fig. 17.28) • Management: catheter drainage x 2–6 weeks (spontaneous healing 13%–23%), transvaginal or transabdominal repair, urinary diversion • Tissue flaps: transvaginal repair (labial fat/Martius flap or peritoneum); transabdominal repair (omental or peritoneal flap)
Ureterovaginal fistula	• Cause: distal ureteral injury during gynecologic surgery • Presentation: constant urinary leakage with normal voiding habits; bladder filling is maintained (unlike VVF) • Prompt stenting may be curative; percutaneous drainage to decompress upper tract may temporize • If surgery needed: end-to-end anastomosis, reimplant with Psoas hitch, Boari flap, or bowel interposition
Ureteroarterial fistula	• Potentially life threatening (7%–23% mortality rate) • Most commonly involves iliac artery • Presentation: intermittent gross hematuria, sudden onset of massive hematuria in patient with indwelling stent • Risk factors: previous iliac artery surgery, radiation • Angiography is diagnostic and therapeutic
Vesicouterine fistula	• Cause: bladder injury during cesarean section • Youssef syndrome: menouria, cyclic hematuria with associated apparent amenorrhea, infertility, urinary continence (due to sphincter-like activity of the cervix) • Treatment: prolonged bladder catheterization ± fulguration • Surgical management: often required and should respect the reproductive wishes of the patient • If patient no longer desires childbearing, then hysterectomy with bladder closure

Continued

Table 17.10 Summary of Urologic Fistulae, Including Presentation, Evaluation, and Management—cont'd

Urethrovaginal fistula	• Causes: obstructed labor, iatrogenic, trauma (pelvic fractures) • 20% associated with VVF • Presentation: complete incontinence or urinary spraying • Diagnosis: physical exam and cystourethroscopy • Surgical repair usually transvaginal • Flaps often used with urethral repair (vaginal advancement, Martius, muscle) • Repair of SUI may be performed concomitantly or staged
Uroenteric fistula	• Most common causes: diverticular disease (65%–75%, usually colovesical), Crohn's disease (5%–6%, usually ileovesical), malignancy (10%–15%) • Pneumaturia is most common presenting symptom (50%–70%) • Gouverneur syndrome: suprapubic pain, urinary frequency, dysuria, and tenesmus • CT findings: bladder wall thickening adjacent to loop of thickened colon, air in the bladder (in the absence of urinary tract instrumentation), colon diverticula • Nonoperative management: TPN, bowel rest, antibiotics • Single- or multi-stage operative management often required
Rectourethral fistula	• Most common causes: post-prostatectomy or other treatments for prostate cancer (cryotherapy, brachytherapy, external beam radiation) • Symptoms: fecaluria, hematuria, UTIs, nausea, vomiting, fever • Biopsy should be done in patients with history of pelvic malignancy • Diagnosis: VCUG or RUG • Usually require surgical repair, often staged with fecal diversion as the first stage • Transrectal, transanal, perineal, transabdominal approaches all possible
Renovascular or pyelovascular fistula	• Most common causes: percutaneous renal access (renal biopsy or PCNL) • Angiographic embolization is recommended • Rarely require flank exploration and partial/simple nephrectomy

PCNL, Percutaneous nephrolithotomy; *RUG*, retrograde urethrogram; *SUI*, stress urinary incontinence; *TPN*, total parenteral nutrition; *UTI*, urinary tract infection; *VCUG*, voiding cystourethrogram; *VVF*, vesicovaginal fistula.

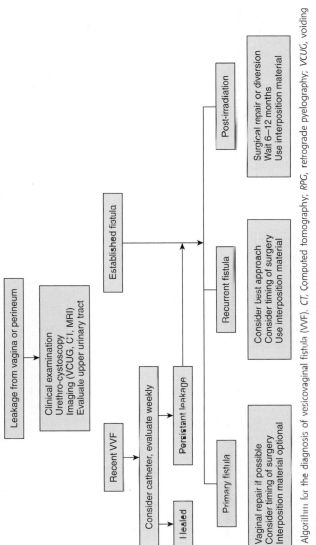

FIG. 17.28 Algorithm for the diagnosis of vesicovaginal fistula (VVF), *CT,* Computed tomography; *RPG,* retrograde pyelography; *VCUG,* voiding cystourethrogram.

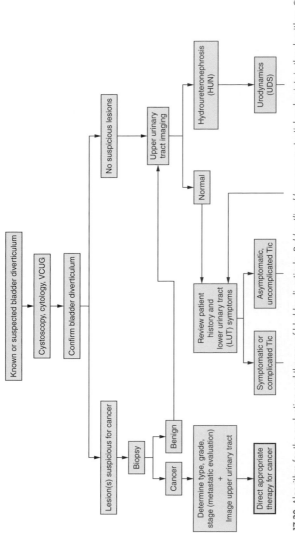

FIG. 17.29 Algorithm for the evaluation and therapy of bladder diverticula. *Bold-outlined boxes are potential end points in the algorithm. CIC,* Clean intermittent catheterization; *Tic,* bladder diverticulum; *VCUG,* voiding cystourethrogram. (Modified from Rovner ES, Wein AJ. Bladder diverticula in adults. In: Resnick M, Elder JA, Spirnak JP, eds. *Decision making in urology,* 3rd ed. Hamilton, Ontario: BC Decker, 2004:260–263.)

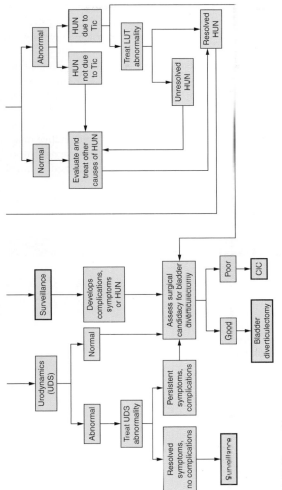

FIG. 17.29—cont'd

infection of these obstructed glands results in enlargement and an anterior vaginal wall mass on physical examination. Most UD are benign, but ~10% of diverticulectomy specimens have premalignant and malignant changes (most commonly adenocarcinoma). Calculi in UD are seen in 4%–10% of cases.

Presentation and Evaluation. The "three Ds"—dyspareunia, and dribbling—make up the classic presentation of UD. However, this presentation is only seen in 5%, and presentation may be variable (Box 17.3). Cystourethroscopy should be performed in an attempt to visualize the ostium, which is most often located posterolaterally; however, this can be difficult to identify. Preoperative imaging, including transvaginal ultrasound and pelvic magnetic resonance imaging (MRI), is important in diagnosis and planned surgery for UD.

Surgical Repair. Symptomatic patients should be offered surgical management. Seven to 16% of women with UD have SUI and

---

Box 17.3 Signs and Symptoms of Urethral Diverticula

Symptoms

Vaginal or pelvic mass
Pelvic pain
Urethral pain
Dysuria
Urinary frequency
Postvoid dribbling
Dyspareunia
Urinary urgency
Incontinence
Urinary hesitancy
Vaginal or urethral discharge
Double voiding
Sense of incomplete emptying

Signs

Recurrent urinary tract infection
Hematuria
Vaginal or perineal tenderness
Urinary retention
Vaginal mass
Urethral discharge with stripping of anterior vaginal wall

may undergo concomitant antiincontinence surgery at the time of diverticulectomy. **Synthetic materials should not be used.** Most commonly, complete excision and reconstruction is performed (Box 17.4). Complications include recurrent UTIs, urinary incontinence, persistent or recurrent UD (10%–22%), or urinary fistula (Table 17.11).

Box 17.4 Principles of Transvaginal Urethral Diverticulectomy

Mobilization of a well-vascularized anterior vaginal wall flap(s)
Preservation of the periurethral fascia as a separate layer
Identification and excision of the neck or ostium of the UD
Removal of entire UD wall or sac (epithelium)
Watertight urethral closure
Multilayered, nonoverlapping closure with absorbable suture
Closure of dead space
Preservation or creation of continence

UD, Urethral diverticulum.

Table 17.11 Complications of Transvaginal Urethral Diverticulectomy

COMPLICATION	RANGE OF REPORTED INCIDENCE
Urinary incontinence	1.7%–16.1%
Urethrovaginal fistula	0.9%–8.3%
Urethral stricture	0–5.2%
Recurrent urethral diverticula	10%–22%
Recurrent urinary tract infection	0–31.3%
Other:	
Hypospadias/distal urethral necrosis	Not available
Bladder or ureteral injury	Not available
Vaginal scarring or narrowing: dyspareunia, etc.	Not available

Modified from Dmochowski R. Surgery for vesicovaginal fistula, urethrovaginal fistula, and urethral diverticulum. In: Walsh PC, Retik AB, Vaughan ED Jr, et al., eds. *Campbell's urology,* 8th ed. Philadelphia: Saunders, 2002

Suggested Readings

Abrams P, Andersson KE, Birder L, et al. Fourth International Consultation on Incontinence Recommendations of the International Scientific Committee: evaluation and treatment of urinary incontinence, pelvic organ prolapse, and fecal incontinence. *Neurourol Urodyn* 2010;29:213.

American Urogynecologic Society (AUGS). Update on vaginal mesh for prolapse and incontinence. https://www.augs.org/update-on-vaginal-mesh-for-prolapse-and-incontinence.

FDA safety communication: UPDATE on serious complications associated with transvaginal placement of surgical mesh for pelvic organ prolapse. 2014. http://www.fda.gov/medicaldevices/safety/alertsandnotices/ucm262435.htm.

Food and Drug Administration. Urogynecologic surgical mesh: update on the safety and effectiveness of transvaginal placement for pelvic organ prolapse. 2011. https://www.fda.gov/media/81123/download

Ford AA, Rogerson L, Cody JD, Aluko P, Ogah JA. Mid-urethral sling operations for stress urinary incontinence in women. *Cochrane Database Syst Rev* 2017;7:CD006375.

Haylen BT, de Ridder D, Freeman RM, et al. An international urogynecological association (IUGA)/International continence society (ICS) joint report on the terminology for female pelvic floor dysfunction. *Neurourol Urodyn* 2010;29:4-20.

Herschorn S, Bruschini H, Comiter C, et al. Committee of the International Consultation on Incontinence. Surgical treatment of stress incontinence in men. *Neurourol Urodyn* 2010;29:179-190.

Kenton K, Stoddard AM, Zyczynski H, et al. 5-year longitudinal followup after retropubic and transobturator mid urethral slings. *J Urol* 2015;193:203-210.

Kobashi KC, Albo ME, Dmochowski RR, et al. Surgical treatment of female stress urinary incontinence: AUA/SUFU Guideline. *J Urol* 2017;198:875-883.

Lapitan MC, Cody JD, Grant A. Open retropubic colposuspension for urinary incontinence in women. *Cochrane Database Syst Rev* 2009;4:CD002912.

Maher C, Baessler K, Glazener CM, Adams EJ, Hagen S. Surgical management of pelvic organ prolapse in women. *Cochrane Database Syst Rev* 2007;4:CD004014.

Nambiar A, Cody JD, Jeffery ST, Aluko P. Single-incision sling operations for urinary incontinence in women. *Cochrane Database Syst Rev* 2017;7:CD008709.

Nygaard IE, McCreery R, Brubaker L, et al. Abdominal sacrocolpopexy: a comprehensive review. *Obstet Gynecol* 2004;104:805-823.

Richter HE, Albo ME, Zyczynski HM, et al. Retropubic versus transobturator midurethral slings for stress incontinence. *N Engl J Med* 2010;362:2066-2076.

Sandhu JS, Breyer B, Comiter C, et al. Incontinence after prostate treatment: AUA/SUFU guideline. *J Urol* 2019;202:369-378.

Terlecki RP, Flynn BJ. The use of surgical mesh for incontinence and prolapse surgery: Indications for use, technical considerations and management of complications. *AUA Update* 2010;29:14.

18

Surgery for Benign Disorders of the Penis, Urethra, and Scrotal Contents

EMILY F. KELLY AND ALEXANDER GOMELSKY

CONTRIBUTORS OF CAMPBELL-WALSH-WEIN, 12TH EDITION

Ramon Varasoro, Gerald H. Jordan, Kurt A. Mccammon, Dorota J. Hawksworth, Mohit Khera, and Amin S. Herati

SURGERY FOR BENIGN DISORDERS OF THE PENIS AND URETHRA

Tenets of Reconstructive Surgical Techniques

- The aims are to minimize tissue injury and promote healing.
- Delicate instruments, including fine tenotomy scissors, forceps, skin hooks, and needle holders, are necessary.
- The smallest possible absorbable sutures should be used to assure tension-free tissue alignment.
- Supine or prone position, rather than high lithotomy, is preferred.

PRINCIPLES OF RECONSTRUCTIVE SURGERY

- Extensibility, inherent tension, stress relaxation, and creep are important in predicting the behavior of transferred tissue.
- A **graft** is tissue transferred to a host bed, whereas a **new blood** supply develops by *take*.
- Urethral reconstruction may employ grafts from full-thickness skin (FTSG), oral mucosa (OMG), bladder epithelium, and rectal mucosa.

- Penile reconstruction employs split-thickness skin grafts (**STSGs**), with FTSGs rarely needed. Epidermis and superficial dermal plexus in an STSG convey favorable vascular characteristics. However, physical characteristics are not carried, and graft tends to less durable.
- In a **mesh graft**, systematic slits in different ratios are placed in an STSG and allow subgraft collections to vent. These conform better to irregular graft host beds, and increased levels of growth factors improve take.
- **FTSGs** have less predictable vascular characteristics but do not contract as much and are more durable (Fig. 18.1A).
- **OMGs** consist of nonkeratinized mucosa and have optimal vascular characteristics. They can be thinned without impacting the graft's vascular characteristics (Fig. 18.1B).
- Buccal mucosal graft (**BMG**) is harvested from the overlying buccinator muscle in the cheek. It is easy to harvest and handle, resilient to infections, and accustomed to wet environment. It is a standard for urethral reconstruction.
- A **flap** is transferred with the **blood supply preserved** or surgically reestablished at the recipient site (Figs. 18.2 and 18.3).

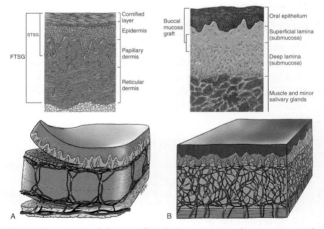

FIG. 18.1 Cross-sectional diagrams (histologic appearance above, microvasculature below) of the skin. (A) Cross-sectional diagrams of skin. (B) Cross-sectional diagrams of oral mucosa. *FTSG*, Full-thickness skin graft; *STSG*, split-thickness skin graft. (From Jordan GH, Schlossberg SM. Using tissue transfer for urethral reconstruction. *Contemp Urol* 1993;13:23.)

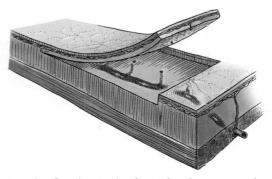

FIG. 18.2 Random flap. The arterial perforators have been interrupted, and flap survival depends on the intradermal and subdermal plexuses.

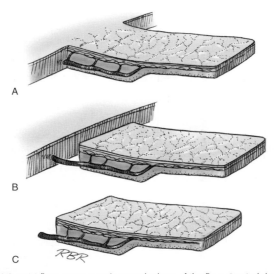

FIG. 18.3 Axial flaps. Large vessels enter the base of the flaps. Survival depends on these vessels and on the random distal vascularity. (A) Peninsula flap The vascular continuity and the cutaneous continuity in the flap base are intact. (B) Island flap. The vascular pedicle is intact; the cuticular continuity has been divided. These axial vessels are unsupported (dangling). (C) Microvascular free-transfer flap. The free-flap cuticular and vascular connections are interrupted at the base of the flap. Vascular continuity is reconstituted in the recipient area by a microsurgical anastomosis. (From Jordan GH, McCraw JB. Tissue transfer techniques for genitourinary reconstructive surgery. *AUA Update Series* 1988;7:lesson 10.)

- In complex cases, microvascular free-transfer technology is a mainstay. Skin islands based on dartos fascia or tunica dartos are used for urethral reconstruction. Dermal graft may be used to augment the tunica albuginea of the corpora cavernosa.
- Summary of surgical anatomy (Figs 18.4 through 18.12)

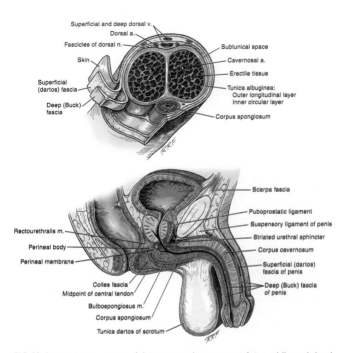

FIG. 18.4 *Top,* Cross section of the penis at the junction of its middle and distal thirds. The septum is correctly illustrated as strands that interweave with the tunica albuginea ventrally and dorsally. *Bottom,* Diagram of a sagittal section of the penis and perineum illustrating the fascial layers. *a.,* Artery; *m.,* muscle; *n.,* nerve; *v.,* vein.

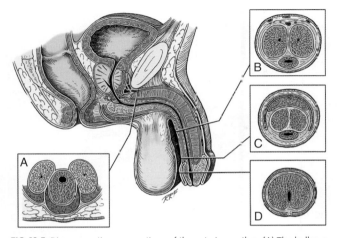

FIG. 18.5 Diagrammatic cross sections of the anterior urethra. (A) The bulbous urethra. The urethra is eccentrically placed in the corpus spongiosum. Proximally, the corpora cavernosa have split into individual crura, with the urethra lying against the triangular ligament. (B) In the shaft of the penis, the urethra is more centrally placed in relation to the corpus spongiosum, and the corpora cavernosa are intimately fused, separated only by septal fibers. (C) At the coronal margin, the urethra remains relatively centrally placed, and the corpora cavernosa are fused, again separated by septal fibers. The spongy tissue of the corpus spongiosum has become incorporated as the deep tissues of the glans. (D) The fossa navicularis widens in caliber and is totally surrounded by the spongy erectile tissue of the glans penis. The urethra here is relatively ventrally placed in relation to the body of the corpus spongiosum. (From Jordan GH. Complications of interventional techniques of urethral stricture disease: direct visual internal urethrotomy, stents and laser. In Carson C, ed. *Topics in clinical urology: complications of interventional techniques.* New York: Igaku-Shoin, 1996:86-94.)

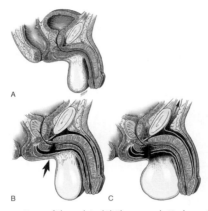

FIG. 18.6 Cross sections of the pelvis. (A) The normal attachment of the fasciae enveloping the penile structures. The dartos fascia is contiguous with the Scarpa fascia onto the abdomen, with the tunica dartos of the scrotum, with the Colles fascia on the perineum, and over the thigh, eventually to insert at the fascia lata. (B) With trauma to the pelvis or perineum, the corpus spongiosum is injured; however, the hematoma is confined by the attachment of the Buck fascia. (C) With trauma to the perineum or pelvis, the corpus spongiosum is injured, and the Buck fascia is violated; the hematoma can spread throughout the confines of the extended dartos fascia–tunica dartos system.

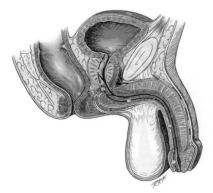

FIG. 18.7 Sagittal section of the pelvis. The urethra is subdivided into the following sections: *1*, fossa navicularis; *2*, pendulous or penile urethra; *3*, bulbous urethra; *4*, membranous urethra; *5*, prostatic urethra; and *6*, bladder neck. By common usage, the divisions of the fossa navicularis, pendulous urethra, and bulbous urethra compose the anterior urethra, and the divisions of the membranous urethra, prostatic urethra, and bladder neck compose the posterior urethra. (Modified from Devine CJ Jr, Angermeier KW. Anatomy of the penis and male perineum. *AUA Update Series* 1994;8:11)

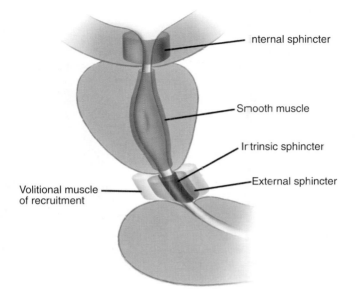

FIG. 18.8 Diagrammatic representation of the sphincters surrounding the male posterior urethra.

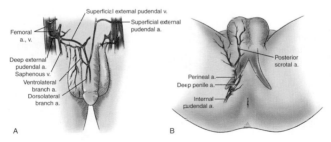

FIG. 18.9 The vasculature to the genital skin. (A) The superficial external pudendal vessels arborize to become the fascial blood supply contained in the dartos fascia of the penis. (B) The scrotal artery is a terminal branch of the deep internal pudendal artery. This artery is thought to arborize in the tunica dartos of the scrotum and Colles fascia of the perineum. The perineal artery continues lateral to the groin crease onto the thigh and extends toward the groin. a., Artery; v., vein.

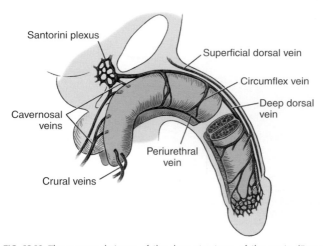

FIG. 18.10 The venous drainage of the deep structures of the penis. (From Horton CE, Stecker JF, Jordan GH. Management of erectile dysfunction, genital reconstruction following trauma and transsexualism. In: McCarthy JG, ed. *Plastic surgery*, vol 6. Philadelphia: Saunders, 1990:4213-4245.)

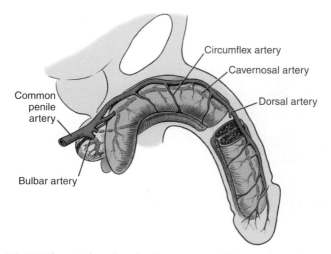

FIG. 18.11 The arterial supply to the deep structures of the penis. (From Horton CE, Stecker JF, Jordan GH. Management of erectile dysfunction, genital reconstruction following trauma and transsexualism. In: McCarthy JG, ed. *Plastic surgery*, vol 6. Philadelphia: Saunders, 1990:4213-4245.)

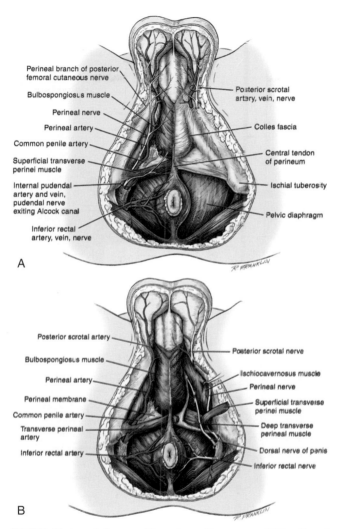

FIG. 18.12 "Peel-away" diagrams of the anatomy of the perineum. (A) The skin and subcuticular tissues have been removed. (B) In the anterior perineal triangle, Colles fascia has been removed. In the posterior anal triangle, the pelvic diaphragm has been removed. Note the division of the superficial transverse perineal muscle, exposing the deep transverse perineal muscle.

Continued

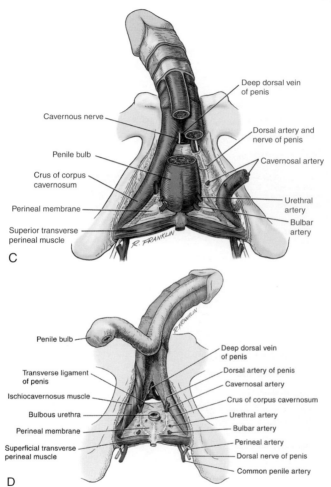

FIG. 18.12, cont'd (C) The anterior perineal triangle has been dissected to expose the erectile bodies. (D) The corpus spongiosum has been divided at the departure of the urethra from the penile bulb. The intracrural space is exposed. (From Devine CJ Jr, Angermeier KW. Anatomy of the pelvis and male perineum. *AUA Update Series* 1994;13:1015.)

SELECTED PROCESSES

- **Lichen Sclerosis (LS)** – Previously called balanitis xerotica obliterans; thought to be **premalignant for squamous cell carcinoma of the glans, so biopsy needed;** most common cause of meatal stenosis; management of LS-related strictures is complex and often suboptimal.
  - If only foreskin involved, circumcision may be curative.
  - Combination of topical steroids and tetracycline may stabilize inflammatory process.
  - Consider intermittent catheterization and 0.05% clobetasol when meatus is easily maintained at 14–16 Fr.
  - Surgical reconstruction is often with BMG and staged. **However, due to skin involvement with LS, genital flaps and grafts have a high failure rate in this population.**
- **Urethrocutaneous Fistula** – Epithelium-lined tract; may be a complication of urethral surgery or from periurethral infections, inflammatory strictures, or treatment of a urethral growth; treatment should focus on defect and underlying cause.
  - Small fistula may be closed with layered, watertight closure (6-0 or 7-0 absorbable sutures); avoid superimposed suture lines; maintain girth of urethral lumen.
  - For large fistula, utilize local flaps; tunica dartos provides tissue interposition and minimizes superimposed suture lines; suprapubic tube (SPT) urinary diversion.
- A **congenital urethral diverticulum** is a pouch lined with transitional cell epithelium; result of either segmental, urethral distention or attachment of a structure to urethra by narrow neck; in males, may result from incomplete development of anterior urethra or result of straddle trauma causing intracorporeal spongiosal hematoma; a **Müllerian duct remnant** may cause congenital diverticulum in the prostatic urethra; in proximal hypospadias, diverticulum represents an enlarged utricle.
- **Paraphimosis** is painful swelling of foreskin distal to phimotic ring; occurs when foreskin is retracted but not reduced.
- **Urethral meatal stenosis** in young boys is a consequence of circumcision; **ammoniacal meatitis** develops, which heals with a membrane across ventral meatus.
- All **failed hypospadias repairs** should be evaluated for urethral stricture disease.

URETHRAL STRICTURE DISEASE

- **Urethral Stricture** – Scarring that involves epithelium and corpus spongiosum in **anterior urethra** (Fig. 18.13); posterior urethral strictures are called **PFUIs** (pelvic fracture urethral injuries); strictures of prostatic urethra or bladder neck are contractures or stenoses.
- The **anterior urethra** is invested by corpus spongiosum; proximally, assumes eccentric position in relation to the corpus spongiosum; genital skin has dual and bilateral blood supply, forming fasciocutaneous vascular system; corpus spongiosum derives blood supply from **common penile artery**.
- **Symptoms** include obstructive voiding and urinary tract infections (UTIs), such as prostatitis and epididymitis, and are often long-standing.
- Treatment planning depends on length, location, depth, and density of the spongiofibrosis.
- Imaging options include contrast-enhanced studies (magnetic resonance imaging [MRI]), endoscopy, and selective penile

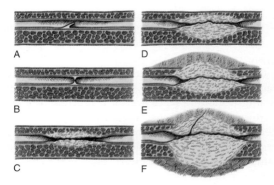

FIG. 18.13 The anatomy of anterior urethral strictures includes, in most cases, underlying spongiofibrosis. (A) Mucosal fold. (B) Iris constriction. (C) Full-thickness involvement with minimal fibrosis in the spongy tissue. (D) Full-thickness spongiofibrosis. (E) Inflammation and fibrosis involving tissues outside the corpus spongiosum. (F) Complex stricture complicated by a fistula. This can proceed to the formation of an abscess, or the fistula may open to the skin or the rectum. (From Jordan GH. Management of anterior urethral stricture disease. *Probl Urol* 1987;1:199-225.)

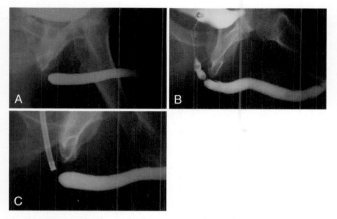

FIG. 18.14 Series of radiographs demonstrating the usefulness of the combination of contrast enhancement with endoscopy. (A) A retrograde urethrogram shows a totally obliterative process involving the proximal bulbous urethra. (B) The patient was successful in relaxing to void; however, there is suggestion of a wide-caliber annular area proximal to the obliterative process of the bulbous urethra. (C) Endoscopy through the suprapubic cystostomy tube clarifies the anatomy of the proximal urethra and demonstrates the length of the obliterative process.

ultrasonography; **endoscopy is imperative to evaluate urethra proximal and distal to stricture.**

- **Voiding cystourethrogram (VCUG)/retrograde urethrogram (RUG)** in steep lateral oblique position avoids underestimation of stricture length.
- Combined contrast studies (through SPT) with endoscopy help define stricture anatomy (Fig. 18.14).
- It may be beneficial to defunctionalize the urethra with SPT and reevaluate in 6–8 weeks.

TREATMENT OF URETHRAL STRICTURES

- Several options exist, so goals of treatment established before making treatment choice.
  - **Urethral Dilation** – Simplest treatment; stretches scar atraumatically; seldom curative; balloon dilation over wire is safest method.

- **Internal Urethrotomy** – Any transurethral incision (i.e., direct vision internal urethrotomy [DVIU]).
  - Success is higher with bulbous urethral location, stricture length <1.5 cm, and no dense, deep spongiofibrosis; results of laser urethrotomy are mixed; repeated dilation and urethrotomies diminish success rate of eventual open urethral reconstruction.
  - **Complications** – Stricture recurrence (most common); bleeding and extravasation of irrigation fluid; cavernosospongiosal fistula and cavernosal venoocclusive dysfunction.
  - Urethral catheter is placed for 3–5 days followed by frequent self-catheterization (may taper over 3–6 months).
- **Urethroplasty** – **gold standard** for anterior urethral strictures; may be offered as initial therapy for all strictures; goal is to excise scar and reconstruct the urethra.
  - **Excision with primary anastomosis (EPA)** – (Fig. 18.15); not recommended for penile urethral strictures >1 cm given increased risk of chordee and penile shortening; main surgical points include stricture resection, spatulation of urethral ends, and primary tension-free anastomosis; imperative to preserve the bulbar arterial supply.
  - Substitution of the scarred urethral tissue with either a flap or graft provides equivalent results.
- **BMG** is most common graft used; can be a one-stage (graft is not tubularized) or staged procedure (Johansson technique with second stage 3–6 months later) depending on the length, complexity, and quality of the urethral tissue.
- **Flaps** are more complex than grafts.
- **Augmented anastomosis** may be used with graft and flap onlay; results may exceed those of pure onlay.
- **Perineal urethrostomy** is a viable option in selected patients; addition of BMG may be useful in very proximal bulbar strictures.
- The treatment is based on size and location.
  - **Meatal or fossa navicularis** – initial treatment is dilation or meatotomy; urethroplasty if recurrent.
  - **Bulbar stricture** <2 cm – DVIU, dilation, or urethroplasty; 70% success with endoscopic techniques if stricture <1 cm; 80%–95% long-term success rates with urethroplasty.

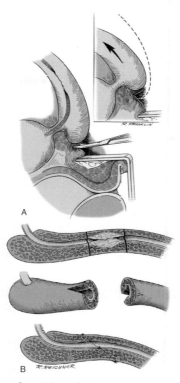

FIG. 18.15 Techniques for excision and primary reanastomosis of anterior urethral stricture. (A) The bulbospongiosus is released from its attachment to the perineal body. The arteries to the bulb are not divided. This technique allows the urethra to be mobilized distally. This technique combined with development of the intracrural space can shorten the path of the urethra by approximately 1 to 1.5 cm. (B) Technique of a primary spatulated anastomosis after excision of an anterior urethral stricture. (From Jorcan GH. Principles of plastic surgery. In: Droller MJ, ed. *Surgical management of urologic disease: an anatomic approach.* Philadelphia: Mosby, 1992:1218-1237.)

- **Bulbar stricture** >2 cm – primary urethroplasty ± graft.
- **Any stricture that failed DVIU/dilation** – urethroplasty.
- **Penile urethra (any length)** – urethroplasty (endoscopic treatment has high recurrence) with graft.

PELVIC FRACTURE URETHRAL INJURIES (PFUIS): URETHRAL DISTRACTION

- Result of blunt pelvic trauma; accompanies ~10% of pelvic fractures; often not a total distraction but a strip of epithelium may remain.
- Use of aligning catheters is controversial; may create an endoscopically manageable stenosis or facilitate subsequent reconstruction.
- Combination of contrast-enhanced studies with endoscopy and selective MRI is used to define anatomy; bladder neck appearance is not predictive of its ultimate function; simultaneous reconstruction of the bladder neck and the posterior urethra is usually not performed together.
- Resultant obliteration in PFUIs is typically short and amenable to mobilization of the corpus spongiosum and primary spatulated anastomosis of the proximal anterior urethra to apical prostatic urethra.

POSTPROSTATECTOMY VESICOURETHRAL DISTRACTION DEFECTS: VESICOURETHRAL STENOSIS

- **Options** – Indwelling SPT (short- or long-term); continent catheterizable bladder augmentation (long-term outcomes may exceed aggressive reconstruction); functional reconstruction using an above-and-below technique (laparotomy and posterior perineal triangle dissection).
- **Omental interposition** allows safe mobilization of rectum from the area of the distraction scar or from complex fistula.
- If patient was **irradiated**, any effects must settle, and tissue interposition should be used during repair. Functional reconstruction is often impossible and diversion is often safest and best option for ultimate urinary and bowel function.

CONGENITAL PENILE CURVATURE

- **Chordee Without Hypospadias** – meatus is orthotopic, but findings are suggestive of hypospadias (i.e., malformation of the ventral structures of the penis); not characterized by large, erect penis.
- **Congenital Curvature of the Penis** – related to nonsymmetrical expansion of the erectile bodies during tumescence;

patients have exceptionally large, erect penises; reconstruction involves artificial erection to demonstrate location of maximal curvature followed by excision with plicating closure or pure plication (e.g., Nesbit); use of grafts is not recommended due to possibility of graft-induced venoocclusive dysfunction.

Acquired penile curvature inevitably follows penile trauma. **Most are associated with Peyronie disease (PD)** which is covered in detail in Chapter 14.

SURGICAL ANATOMY AND VASCULATURE OF THE SCROTUM

- **Layers of Scrotal Wall** – hair bearing skin, dartos muscle, and internal and external spermatic fascia (separated by cremasteric muscle). **Dartos fascia prevents spread of necrotizing fasciitis to deeper structures in scrotum** (Figs. 18.16 and 18.17).
- Testes are encased by tunica albuginea and protected by layers of tunica vaginalis.

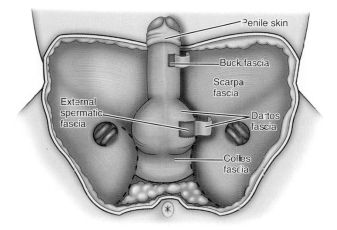

FIG. 18.16 Anatomic barriers to the spread of infection. (Modified from Kavoussi PK, Costabile RA. Disorders of scrotal contents: orchitis, epididymitis, testicular torsion, torsion of the appendages, and Fournier gangrene. In: Chapple CR, Steers WD, eds. *Practical urology: essential principles and practice*. London: Springer-Verlag, 2011.)

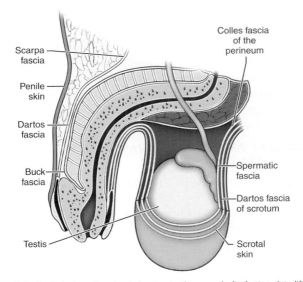

FIG. 18.17 Sagittal view of anatomic barriers to the spread of infection. (Modified from Kavoussi PK, Costabile RA. Disorders of scrotal contents: orchitis, epididymitis, testicular torsion, torsion of the appendages, and Fournier gangrene. In: Chapple CR, Steers WD, eds. *Practical urology: essential principles and practice.* London: Springer-Verlag, 2011.)

- The epididymis is posterolateral to testis and has a head (caput), body (corpus), and tail (cauda).
- The vas deferens is a continuation of the cauda epididymis and travels along the spermatic cord into the pelvis. The ampulla of the vas joins with the seminal vesicles (SVs) and forms the proximal ejaculatory duct.
- The appendix testis and the appendix epididymis are nonfunctional, vestigial structures.
- The scrotum derives blood supply anteriorly from the superficial and deep external pudendal arteries and posteriorly from the posterior scrotal artery. Venous drainage follows the arterial supply, which empty into the great saphenous vein and to the internal iliac veins, respectively.
- **The testicular blood supply is from the (1) testicular artery (off the aorta), (2) artery to the ductus deferens (from internal**

iliac artery), and (3) cremasteric artery (from external iliac artery). This redundancy allows testicular viability if one or two of the arteries are injured or ligated.

- The epididymis gets >80% of its blood supply from the superior epididymal artery (from the testicular artery) and the rest from the inferior epididymal artery (branches off the deferential artery and distal branches of the testicular artery). **The superior epididymal artery can be sacrificed to gain additional testicular mobilization during vasectomy reversal because of the vascular anastomoses between the superior and inferior epididymal artery.**

PREOPERATIVE CONSIDERATIONS AND SCROTAL ACCESS

- **Scrotal hair is removed using a disposable clipper on the day of surgery.** Skin is cleansed with an antiseptic.
- Patients with risk factors for infection should receive a single preprocedure dose of intravenous cephalosporin or clindamycin (https://www.auanet.org/guidelines/archived-documents/antimicrobial-prophylaxis-best-practice-statement).
- Preincisional local anesthetic injection and spermatic cord block may provide pain control.
- A transverse or a median raphe scrotal incision is used for benign indications.
- If scrotal malignancy is suspected, an inguinal approach is preferred. The spermatic cord is isolated and clamped with noncrushing clamps to prevent tumor seeding while awaiting frozen-section biopsies. If frozen section reveals no malignancy, the testis and spermatic cord can be spared and the remainder of the surgery is performed.
- Meticulous hemostasis is common to all techniques.

PARTIAL OR TOTAL SCROTECTOMY

- This is most commonly performed for severe infection such as Fournier's gangrene (FG). Due to its fulminant progression, urgent surgical debridement is required, and repeat debridement may be performed every 24–48 hours (Fig. 18.18).
- Partial scrotectomy is also required in patients with an inadvertent scrotal violation (via tumor aspiration, biopsy, exploration,

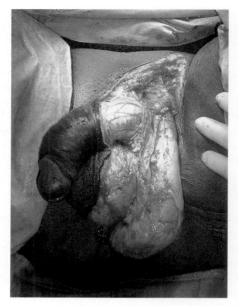

FIG. 18.18 Aggressive debridement of Fournier gangrene. (Modified from Kavoussi PK, Costabile RA. Disorders of scrotal contents: orchitis, epididymitis, testicular torsion, torsion of the appendages, and Fournier gangrene. In: Chapple CR, Steers WD, eds. *Practical urology: essential principles and practice.* London: Springer-Verlag, 2011.)

and/or orchiectomy) during an evaluation/treatment of testicular malignancy.
- Other scrotal nonmalignant conditions requiring partial scrotal excision include hidradenitis suppurativa, postradiation lymphedema, penoscrotal Paget disease, primary lymphangitis, and cosmesis to reduce scrotal descent.
- If immediate reconstruction is not performed, the testes are placed into medial thigh pockets with loose wound approximation until the scrotal reconstruction.

SCROTAL RECONSTRUCTION
- Small defects can be treated with wet-to-dry dressings.
- FG defects smaller than of the scrotum can heal by secondary intent, loose skin approximation with nonabsorbable

monofilament suture, and vacuum-assisted closure (VAC) device, which hastens recovery time, reduces wound surface area, and improves likelihood of skin graft take.

- Larger defects benefit from (1) local advancement flaps using either remaining scrotum or thigh tissues, (2) fasciocutaneous flaps from the superomedial or anterolateral thigh, or (3) meshed STSG. Thigh flaps cause less contracture-related effects than skin grafts.

HYDROCELECTOMY

- Hydroceles are excess fluid between the parietal and visceral layers of the tunica vaginalis.
- A **communicating hydrocele** is when peritoneal fluid drains through a patent processus vaginalis; ~80% resolve spontaneously by 18 months of age.
- **Acquired hydroceles** result from an imbalance between the production and reabsorption of fluid within the tunica vaginalis.
- Hydroceles are typically painless scrotal bulges and may extend into the inguinal canal.
- Ultrasonography may identify intratesticular malignancy in scrotal fluid collections and guide surgical approach.
- Observation is indicated unless there is significant discomfort, cosmetic concerns, or an underlying malignancy.
- Pyoceles require urgent drainage. Repair may utilize plication and **excisional techniques (lower rates of recurrence)**.
  Lord Plication – This is an **option for thin-walled and smaller hydroceles.** The hydrocele sac is opened along its anterior surface and plicated using interrupted, 2-0 chromic sutures in a circumferential fashion (Fig. 18.19). Since no excision is performed, plication has the **lowest risk for postoperative hematoma** and does not benefit from drain placement.
  Jaboulay (Winkelman) Technique – Some of the parietal tunica albuginea is resected, the parietal layer of the tunica behind the testis is everted, and the opposing parietal tunical edges are approximated to each other without compressing the spermatic cord. Alternatively, the cut edges can be oversewn with 3-0 chromic (Fig. 18.20)
  Bottleneck Technique – All but a 2-cm circumferential segment of tunica around the testis and cord structures is trimmed

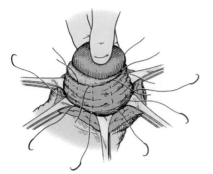

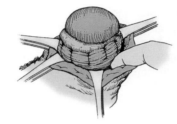

FIG. 18.19 Lord plication technique.

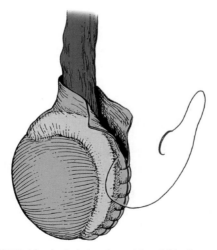

FIG. 18.20 Jaboulay technique for excision of thin, floppy sacs.

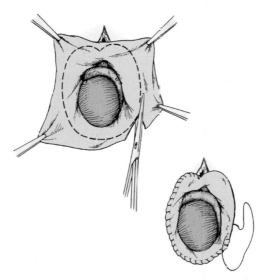

FIG. 18.21 Simple excision of the thick-walled hydrocele sac and oversewn edges.

and the tunical edges are tacked to each other, leaving the sac open (Fig. 18.21).

Window Technique – After a stab incision into the tunica to drain hydrocele fluid, a 2.5- × 2.5-cm cruciate incision ("window") is made into the parietal tunica vaginalis. The flaps of the cruciate incision are everted and stitched with 2-0 chromic.

Simple Orchiectomy

- Bilateral simple orchiectomy is an option to medical androgen deprivation therapy for hormonally responsive metastatic prostate cancer. Unilateral simple orchiectomy can be performed for severe testis trauma, prolonged ischemia from testicular torsion, and chronic orchalgia.
- Simple orchiectomy can be performed through a scrotal or inguinal incision; however, **the latter is associated with better pain-related outcomes in patients with orchalgia.**
- The spermatic cord is divided into two bundles that are double clamped proximally and distally. The cord is divided

between the clamps, and the proximal stump is suture ligated with 2-0 Vicryl.

- In an epididymis-sparing orchiectomy, the testis is sharply dissected off the epididymis and the superior, middle, and inferior epididymal arteries that perforate the testis must be located and suture ligated. The caput and cauda of the epididymis are adjoined with 4-0 chromic.

Excision of Epididymal Masses

- Epididymal cysts and spermatoceles arise from cystic accumulations of semen in the epididymal tubules, rete testes, or efferent ductules.
- Surgery is only indicated if there is discomfort, infection, disability from large size, or infertility.
- **Men of reproductive age run the risk of obstructive azoospermia after epididymal cyst surgery, particularly if it is located in the corpora or cauda.**
- The most common surgical approach is via a trans-scrotal incision and dissection to the level of the tunica vaginalis. **The tunica is sharply opened, and the epididymal cyst or spermatocele is exposed and dissected down to its stalk and ligated with 5-0 or 6-0 absorbable suture**
- **Epididymal masses with malignant potential should be approached via an inguinal incision like a radical orchiectomy to avoid lymphatic disruption.**
- A trans-scrotal approach is appropriate for biopsy-proven benign epididymal masses.
- A microsurgical approach is recommended to avoid injury to the testicular blood supply.

VASECTOMY

- While a safe, effective, and permanent method of male contraception, no one vasectomy technique is 100% effective.
- Repeat vasectomy may be indicated if (1) postvasectomy semen analysis (PVSA) demonstrates persistent live sperm, (2) recanalization of the two vasal ends results in pregnancy, and (3) there is 1%–2% risk for chronic postoperative scrotal pain.
- Local anesthesia with or without oral sedation is used, but intravenous sedation or general anesthesia is an option.
  - **Conventional vasectomy (CV)** may be appropriate with a history of prior scrotal surgery, trauma, or challenging

anatomy. A median raphe incision or bilateral paramedian scrotal incisions are made. The vas is trapped between the surgeon's thumb, index, and middle fingers, and the vasal sheath is pushed to the surface. The vas is grasped with a towel clamp and pulled out of the wound. A short vas segment is removed, and the free vasal ends are occluded with clips, sutures, and/or cautery. After ensuring hemostasis, the vas ends are dropped back into the scrotum, and the contralateral side is done. Skin closure is with absorbable suture.

- **Minimally invasive vasectomy (MIV)** is the **recommended method of vas isolation**, due to less discomfort and fewer complications; uses special vas dissecting instruments (Fig. 18.22) and/or ring-tipped vas clamps (Fig. 18.23). The incision is smaller than the CV. In the **open** approach, the perivasal tissues are minimally dissected through the skin incision, and the vas is grasped with a clamp. In the **closed** approach, the vas is grasped with a vas clamp before an incision is made. The incision is made afterward, and the remainder of the procedure is the same. MIV incisions may be left open.

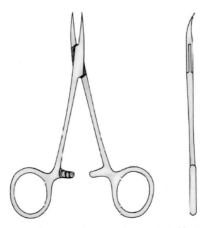

FIG. 18.22 Sharp, curved mosquito hemostat (From Li S, Goldstein M, Zhu J, et al. The no-scalpel vasectomy. *J Urol* 1991;145:341-344.)

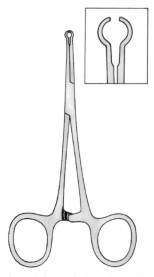

FIG. 18.23 Ring-tipped vas deferens fixation clamp. The cantilevered design prevents injury. (From Li S, Goldstein M, Zhu J, et al. The no-scalpel vasectomy. *J Urol* 1991;145:341-344.)

- **No-scalpel vasectomy (NSV) is a vas isolation technique and does not specify the vas occlusion method.** After the vas is grasped with the ring-tipped clamp, the overlying skin is punctured and spread with a sharp, curved mosquito hemostat (Figs. 18.24 and 18.25). Spreading continues until the vas is encountered, at which point the anterior vasal wall is pierced with the hemostat and lifted through the skin opening (Figs. 18.26 and 18.27). The partially transected vas is regrasped with the ring clamp, and the posterior wall is dissected and divided (see Figs. 18.15 and 18.16). After occlusion, the ends are dropped back into the scrotum. The skin perforation(s) may be left open or closed.
- Following vas division, the free ends may be separated by fascial interposition (FI) with the internal spermatic fascia, suture ligation, vas clipping or folding, and mucosal cauterization (MC). A partial ligation (open-ended) technique leaves the testicular vas open and the ends are separated by FI.

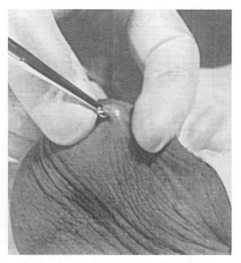

FIG. 18.24 Vas fixed in the ring clamp. The scrotal skin is tightly stretched over the most prominent portion of the vas. (From Li S, Goldstein M, Zhu J, et al. The no-scalpel vasectomy. *J Urol* 1991;145:341-344.)

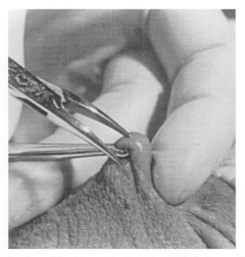

FIG. 18.25 Puncture of the skin, vas sheath, and wall into the lumen. (From Li S, Goldstein M, Zhu J, et al. The no-scalpel vasectomy. *J Urol* 1991;145:341-344.)

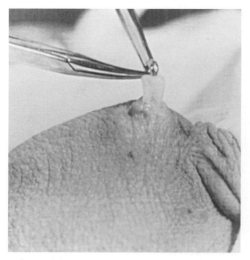

FIG. 18.26 Delivery of the clean vas. (From Li S, Goldstein M, Zhu J, et al. The no-scalpel vasectomy. *J Urol* 1991;145:341-344.)

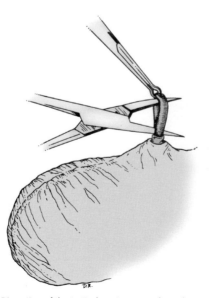

FIG. 18.27 Dissection of the testicular artery away from the vas deferens.

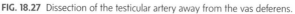

- The **AUA guidelines recommend four methods of vas occlusion with occlusive failure rates** ≤1%: nondivision with extended cautery; MC with FI and without clips or ligatures; MC without FI and without ligatures/clips; and unoccluded testicular end while the abdominal end is occluded with MC and FI (https://www.auanet.org/guidelines/guidelines/vasectomy-guideline)
- If vas excision is performed, a 1-cm segment of vas should be excised.

    Couples may stop using other contraception when the PVSA demonstrates azoospermia or ≤100,000 non-motile sperm/mL. **If the initial PVSA (after at least 10–20 ejaculations) has persistent motile sperm, repeat testing is recommended in 6 months. If this trend continues at the 6-month PVSA, the procedure is considered a failure.**

    Despite an initial negative PVSA, recanalization can occur and pregnancy rates following a successful vasectomy are 0.05%.

RETRACTILE TESTIS AND INTERMITTENT TESTICULAR TORSION (ITT)

- ITT is **characterized by acute, short-duration** (<2 hours) scrotal pain with rapid, spontaneous resolution.
- Orchiopexy in this population has low morbidity, excellent pain relief, and reduces future risk for testicular infarction. Several approaches to orchiopexy are available.
    - **Testicular fixation with suture** – The testis and cord are exposed by opening the parietal layer of the tunica vaginalis, and the tunica albuginea is sutured to the dartos muscle with an absorbable 3-0 suture.
    - **Dartos pouch procedure** – A transverse incision is made in the cranial aspect of the hemiscrotum, and the parietal layer of the tunica vaginalis is opened. A subdartos tunnel is made bluntly between the dartos and external spermatic fascia toward the dependent scrotum. The testis is then positioned in the pouch and secured with a purse-string suture around the spermatic cord.
    - **Risks of fixation** – Recurrent torsion (2.2% following prior fixation with suture), segmental or complete infarction

by entrapping the intratesticular arteries at the lower pole of the testis, intratesticular abscess formation, and potential negative impact on spermatogenesis. The latter risk may be diminished by placement of the testis in a dartos pouch or fixation with polytetrafluoroethylene suture

COMPLICATIONS OF SCROTAL SURGERY

- Hematoma is the main complication of scrotal surgery and should be drained if it is very large or infected. The spermatic artery can be controlled via a subinguinal incision if ongoing bleeding is encountered.
- **Retroperitoneal hemorrhage** is very rare but potentially lethal and should be promptly recognized and addressed. The subinguinal incision may need to be extended into the retroperitoneum for better access.
- **Chronic scrotal pain** following vasectomy may be seen in **2%** and rarely requires surgical treatment.
- **Early vasectomy failure** is usually from technical failure (i.e., occlusion of only one vas).
- **Late vasectomy failure** (recanalization) may occur in **0.05%.**
- **Short-term changes in semen parameters** may occur after hydrocelectomy and sclerotherapy but typically return to baseline levels at **12 months.**
- **Hydrocele recurrence** after successful repair is seen in **0%–2%.**
- **Infected hematoma** requires evacuation and healing via secondary intention.
- A **sperm granuloma** is an inflammatory nodule at the vasectomy site and forms in 5%. It is not considered a complication and is treated initially conservatively.
- If **postprocedural pain is localized to the terminal ends of the transected vasa**, repeat vasectomy or excision of the vasal edges may be offered.

19

Neoplasms of the Male Genitalia

BOGDANA SCHMIDT AND KIRSTEN L. GREENE

CONTRIBUTORS OF CAMPBELL-WALSH-WEIN, 12TH EDITION

Andrew J. Stephenson, Timothy D. Gilligan, Stephen Riggs, Kevin R. Rice, K. Clint Carey, Timothy A. Masterson, Richard S. Foster, Kris Gaston, Peter E. Clark, Christopher B. Anderson, James M. Mckiernan, Rene Sotelo, Luis G. Medina, Marcos Tobias Machado, Curtis A. Pettaway, Sr., Juanita M. Crook, and Lance C. Pagliaro

TESTIS CANCER

Neoplasms of the testis comprise a morphologically and clinically diverse group of tumors, more than 95% of which are germ cell tumors (GCTs). GCTs are broadly categorized as seminoma and nonseminoma (NSGCT) because of differences in natural history and treatment. **GCT is a relatively rare malignancy, accounting for 1%–2% of cancers among men in the United States.** Currently, the long-term survival for men with metastatic GCT is 80%–90%. With the successful cure of patients, an important treatment objective is minimizing treatment-related toxicity without compromising curability (Table 19.1, Box 19.1).

Epidemiology, Etiology, and Clinical Presentation

In the United States, testis cancer is the most common malignancy among men aged 2–40 years and the second most common cancer after leukemia among young men aged 15–19 years. The incidence rate rises rapidly after puberty, peaking at ages 25–35 years. The incidence of bilateral GCT is approximately 2%. The majority of bilateral GCTs are metachronous and occur over an average interval of 5 years. Incidence of GCT is

Table 19.1 Testis Cancer Subtypes

Seminoma	• Most common type of GCT • Occur at an older average age than NSGCT, with most cases diagnosed in the fourth or fifth decade of life
Spermatocytic tumor	• Rare and accounts for fewer than 1% of GCTs • Does not arise from GCNIS • Not associated with a history of cryptorchidism or bilaterality
Embryonal carcinoma	• The presence and proportion of EC has been associated with an increased risk of occult metastases • Can differentiate to other NSGCT cell types (including teratoma) within the primary tumor or at metastatic sites
Choriocarcinoma	• Rare and aggressive tumor that typically is seen with extremely elevated serum hCG levels • Choriocarcinoma commonly spreads by hematogenous routes, and common sites of metastases include lungs, liver, and brain
Yolk sac tumor	• More common in mediastinal and pediatric GCTs • Yolk sac tumors almost always produce AFP but not hCG
Teratoma	• Contain well or incompletely differentiated elements of at least two of the three germ cell layers: endoderm, mesoderm, and ectoderm • Associated with normal serum tumor markers but may cause mildly elevated serum AFP levels • Teratoma is resistant to chemotherapy • Teratomas may grow uncontrollably, invade surrounding structures, and become unresectable • On rare occasions, teratoma may transform into a somatic malignancy such as rhabdomyosarcoma, adenocarcinoma, or primitive neuroectodermal tumor

AFP, Alpha-fetoprotein; *EC,* embryonal carcinoma; *GCNIS,* germ cell neoplasia in situ; *GCT,* germ cell tumor; *hCG,* human chorionic gonadotropin; *NSGCT,* nonseminoma germ cell tumor.

highest in whites and lowest in African Americans. A stage migration of GCT has been observed in several countries partially because of an increased awareness and earlier diagnosis.

There are five well-established risk factors for testis cancer:
• White race

Box 19.1 Key Points

SEMINOMA versus NONSEMINOMA

- Compared with NSGCT, seminoma is associated with an indolent natural history with a lower incidence of metastatic disease and lower rates of occult retroperitoneal and distant metastases in patients with CS I and IIA-B, respectively.
- No poor-risk prognostic category exists for metastatic seminoma, and substantially more patients are classified as good risk by IGCCCG criteria compared with NSGCT.
- Seminoma is associated with increased sensitivity to radiation therapy and platin-based chemotherapy compared with NSGCT.
- Serum hCG is elevated in only 15% of patients with metastatic seminoma, and serum tumor marker levels are not used to guide treatment decisions.
- Teratoma at metastatic sites is less of a concern for seminoma compared with NSGCT but should be considered in patients who fail to respond to conventional therapy.

- Cryptorchidism (four to six times more likely to be diagnosed with testis cancer, but relative risk falls to two to three if orchidopexy is performed before puberty)
- Family history of testis cancer
- Personal history of testis cancer
- Germ cell neoplasia in situ (GCNIS)/intratubular germ cell neoplasia (ITGCN)

Physical Examination. The most common presentation of testis cancer is a painless testis mass. Regional or distant metastasis at diagnosis is present in approximately two-thirds of NSGCTs and 15% of pure seminomas, and symptoms related to metastatic disease are the presenting complaint in 10%–20% of patients. The physician should carefully examine the affected and the normal contralateral testis, noting their relative size and consistency and palpating for any testicular or extratesticular masses. The differential diagnosis of a testis mass includes epididymo-orchitis, torsion, hematoma, or paratesticular neoplasm (benign or malignant). In patients with a presumptive diagnosis of epididymo-orchitis, patients should be reevaluated within 2–4 weeks of completion of an appropriate course of oral antibiotics. A persistent mass or pain should be evaluated further.

Diagnostic Testing. In men with a testis mass, hydrocele, or unexplained scrotal symptoms or signs, bilateral scrotal ultrasonography should be considered an extension of the physical examination. Testis cancer is one of the few malignancies associated with serum tumor markers (lactate dehydrogenase [LDH], alpha-fetoprotein [AFP], and human chorionic gonadotropin [hCG]) that are essential in its diagnosis and management. Serum tumor marker levels should be obtained at diagnosis, after orchiectomy, to monitor for response to chemotherapy, and to monitor for relapse in patients on surveillance and after completion of therapy. Preorchiectomy serum tumor marker levels should not be used in management decisions (Table 19.2).

Initial Treatment: Radical Inguinal Orchiectomy. Patients suspected of having a testicular neoplasm should undergo a radical inguinal orchiectomy within 1–2 weeks of diagnosis with removal of the tumor-bearing testicle and spermatic cord to the level of the internal inguinal ring. A trans-scrotal orchiectomy or biopsy is contraindicated because it leaves the inguinal portion of the spermatic cord intact and may alter the lymphatic drainage of the testis, increasing the risk of local recurrence and pelvic or inguinal lymph node metastasis. In highly select patients, partial orchiectomy can be considered in cases in which the tumor is polar and measures 2 cm or smaller and in which the contralateral testicle is compromised or absent. For the rare patient with diffuse metastatic

Table 19.2 Tumor Markers

Alpha-fetoprotein (AFP)	• Half-life of AFP is 5–7 days
	• Embryonal and yolk sac tumors produce AFP
	• Mildly elevated AFP (<20) may not represent germ cell tumor
Beta-human chorionic gonadotropin (bHCG)	• Half-life of bHCG is 24–36 hours
	• bHCG is elevated in embryonal, choriocarcinoma and seminoma
Lactate dehydrogenase (LDH)	• Half-life of LDH is 24 hours
	• LDH nonspecific and is the most commonly elevated marker
	• Patients should not be treated due to elevated LDH alone

and/or symptomatic GCT requiring early initiation of systemic chemotherapy, diagnosis may be pursued via biopsy of a metastatic site or even made presumptively based on the clinical features and/or serologic studies. For such cases, a delayed radical orchiectomy is recommended for all patients regardless of response to therapy in the retroperitoneum.

Staging

The prognosis of GCT and initial management decisions are dictated by the clinical stage of the disease, which is based on the histopathological findings and pathological stage of the primary tumor, postorchiectomy serum tumor marker levels, and the presence and extent of metastatic disease as determined by physical examination and staging imaging studies, classified using the Tumor, Node, Metastases (TNM) system (Table 19.3).

Table 19.3 TNM Staging of Testicular Tumor: American Joint Committee on Cancer and Union Internationale Contre le Cancer

Primary Tumor (T)[a]	
The extent of primary tumor is usually classified after radical orchiectomy and, for this reason, a *pathological* stage is assigned.	
pTx	Primary tumor cannot be assessed
pTo	No evidence of primary tumor (e.g., histologic scar in testis)
pTis	Intratubular germ cell neoplasia (carcinoma in situ)
pT1	Tumor limited to testis and epididymis without vascular/lymphatic invasion; tumor may invade into tunica albuginea but not tunica vaginalis
pT2	Tumor limited to testis and epididymis with vascular/lymphatic invasion or tumor extending through tunica albuginea with involvement of tunica vaginalis
pT3	Tumor invades spermatic cord with or without vascular/lymphatic invasion
pT4	Tumor invades scrotum with or without vascular/lymphatic invasion

Regional Lymph Nodes (N)	
Clinical (as Determined by Noninvasive Staging)	
NX	Regional lymph nodes cannot be assessed
No	No regional lymph node metastasis

Continued

Table 19.3 TNM Staging of Testicular Tumor: American Joint Committee on Cancer and Union Internationale Contre le Cancer—cont'd

Regional Lymph Nodes (N)

N1	Metastasis with lymph node mass ≤2 cm in greatest dimension or multiple lymph nodes, none more than 2 cm in greatest dimension
N2	Metastasis with lymph node mass, >2 cm but not more than 5 cm in greatest dimension or multiple lymph nodes, any one mass >2 cm but not more than 5 cm in greatest dimension
N3	Metastasis with lymph node mass >5 cm in greatest dimension

Pathologic (pN) (as Determined by Pathologic Findings of RPLND Without Prior Chemotherapy or Radiotherapy)

pNX	Regional lymph nodes cannot be assessed
pN0	No regional lymph node metastasis
pN1	Metastasis with lymph node mass ≤2 cm in greatest dimension and ≤5 nodes positive, none more than 2 cm in greatest dimension
pN2	Metastasis with lymph node mass >2 cm but not more than 5 cm in greatest dimension; or >5 nodes positive, none more than 5 cm; or evidence of extranodal extension of tumor
pN3	Metastasis with lymph node mass >5 cm in greatest dimension

Distant Metastasis (M)

MX	Distant metastasis cannot be assessed
M0	No distant metastasis
M1	Distant metastasis
M1a	Nonregional nodal or pulmonary metastasis
M1b	Distant metastasis at site other than nonregional lymph nodes or lung

Serum Tumor Markers (S)

SX	Marker studies unavailable or not performed
S0	Marker study levels within normal limits
S1	LDH <1.5 × N[b] *and* hCG (MIU/mL) <5000 *and* AFP (ng/mL) <1000

Table 19.3 TNM Staging of Testicular Tumor: American Joint Committee on Cancer and Union Internationale Contre le Cancer—cont'd

S2	LDH 1.5-10 × N *or*
	hCG (MIU/mL) 5000–50,000 *or*
	AFP (ng/mL) 1000–10,000
S3	LDH >10 × N *or*
	hCG (MIU/mL) >50,000 *or*
	AFP (ng/mL) >10,000

Stage Grouping				
GROUP	**T**	**N**	**M**	**S (SERUM TUMOR MARKERS)**
Stage 0	pTis	N0	M0	S0
Stage I	pT1-4	N0	M0	SX
Stage IA	pT1	N0	M0	S0
Stage IB	pT2	N0	M0	S0
	pT3	N0	M0	S0
	pT4	N0	M0	S0
Stage IS	Any pT/Tx	N0	M0	S1-3
Stage II	Any pT/Tx	N1-3	M0	SX
Stage IIA	Any pT/Tx	N1	M0	S0
	Any pT/Tx	N1	M0	S1
Stage IIB	Any pT/Tx	N2	M0	S0
	Any pT/Tx	N2	M0	S1
Stage IIC	Any pT/Tx	N3	M0	S0
	Any pT/Tx	N3	M0	S1
Stage III	Any pT/Tx	Any N	M1	SX
Stage IIIA	Any pT/Tx	Any N	M1a	S0
	Any pT/Tx	Any N	M1a	S1
Stage IIIB	Any pT/Tx	N1-3	M0	S2
	Any pT/Tx	Any N	M1a	S2
Stage IIIC	Any pT/Tx	N1-3	M0	S3
	Any pT/Tx	Any N	M1a	S3
	Any pT/Tx	Any N	M1b	Any S

[a]Except for pTis and pT4, extent of primary tumor is classified by radical orchiectomy. Treatment may be used for other categories in the absence of radical orchiectomy.

[b]N indicates the upper limit of normal for the LCH assay.

AFP, α-Fetoprotein; *hCG,* human chorionic gonadotropin *LDH,* lactate dehydrogenase; *RPLND,* retroperitoneal lymph node dissection.

Data from AJCC. Testis. In: Edge SE, Byrd DR, Compton C, eds. *AJCC Cancer Staging Manual,* 7th ed, New York: Springer, 2010:469-473.

Management of Nonseminoma Germ Cell Tumor (NSGCT)

Clinical Stage (CS) I. The long-term survival associated with surveillance, retroperitoneal lymph node dissection (RPLND), and primary chemotherapy approaches 100%, thus any intervention after orchiectomy, represents overtreatment for the 70%–80% of patients with disease limited to the testis. The most common risk factors for occult metastasis are lymphovascular invasion (LVI) and a predominant component of embryonal carcinoma (EC). **In the absence of these two risk factors, the risk of occult metastasis is less than 20%.**

Surveillance – Surveillance offers the potential of reducing treatment-related toxicity by restricting treatment to those with a proven need for it. More than 90% of relapses occur within the first 2 years, but late relapses (>5 years) are seen in up to 1% of patients.

Retroperitoneal Lymph Node Dissection – The rationale for RPLND for CS I NSGCT is based on several factors:

- The retroperitoneum is the most common site of occult metastatic disease and the risk of associated systemic disease is low
- 15%–25% incidence of retroperitoneal teratoma (which is resistant to chemotherapy) is seen in those with occult metastasis
- Low risk of abdominal-pelvic recurrence after full, bilateral template RPLND, thereby obviating the need for routine surveillance computed tomography (CT) imaging
- High cure rates after RPLND alone for patients with low-volume (pN1) retroperitoneal malignancy and teratoma (pN1-3)
- Avoidance of chemotherapy in more than 75% of patients if adjuvant chemotherapy is restricted to those with extensive retroperitoneal malignancy (pN2-3)
- High salvage rate of relapses with good-risk, induction chemotherapy
- Low short- and long-term morbidity when a nerve-sparing RPLND is performed by experienced surgeons (Figs. 19.1 and 19.2)

Primary Chemotherapy – Bleomycin, etoposide, Platin (BEP) for 1 cycle, is associated with the lowest risk of relapse, but these relapses are less amenable to salvage therapy because they are chemo-resistant. In contrast, patients who relapse after RPLND or on surveillance are chemotherapy naïve and are cured with chemotherapy in virtually all cases.

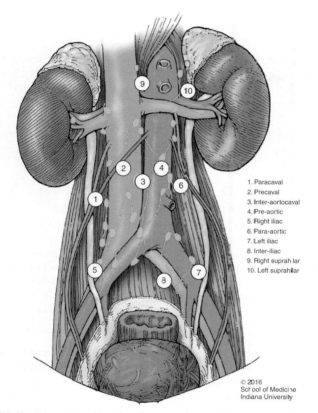

1. Paracaval
2. Precaval
3. Inter-aortocaval
4. Pre-aortic
5. Right iliac
6. Para-aortic
7. Left iliac
8. Inter-iliac
9. Right suprahilar
10. Left suprahilar

© 2016
School of Medicine
Indiana University

FIG. 19.1 Retroperitoneal lymph node regions. (Copyright 2016 Section of Medical Illustration in the Office of Visual Media at the Indiana University School of Medicine. Published by Elsevier Inc. All rights reserved.)

Clinical Stage IS. There is consensus that these patients should be treated similar to those with CS IIC-III and receive induction chemotherapy.

Clinical Stage IIA and IIB. The optimal management of CS IIA-B NSGCT is controversial. RPLND (with or without adjuvant chemotherapy) and induction chemotherapy (with or without postchemotherapy RPLND) are accepted treatment options with survival rates exceeding 95%. Thus there is consensus that CS IIA-B

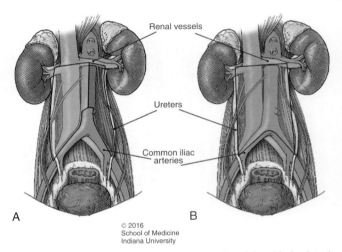

FIG. 19.2 Retroperitoneal lymph node dissection templates. (A) Modified unilateral templates—right-sided shaded in yellow, left-sided shaded in purple. (B) Modified bilateral template—shaded area. (Copyright 2016 Section of Medical Illustration in the Office of Visual Media at the Indiana University School of Medicine. Published by Elsevier Inc. All rights reserved.)

NSGCT patients with elevated tumor markers or bulky lymph nodes (>3 cm) should receive induction chemotherapy, while RPLND is preferred as initial therapy in those patients at risk for retroperitoneal teratoma **who are at otherwise low risk for systemic disease (normal serum tumor markers, lymphadenopathy <3 cm).**

Clinical Stage IIC and III. Induction chemotherapy with cisplatin-based regimens (BEP×3 or EP×4) is the initial approach used for the treatment of CS IIC and III NSGCT, based on risk stratification (Table 19.4).

Management of Postchemotherapy Residual Masses in NSGCT. Patients are classified into the following categories based on their response to chemotherapy.

- Complete response (CR), defined by normalization of serum tumor markers and resolution of radiographic disease (usually defined as residual masses ≤1 cm)
- Normalization of serum tumor markers with persistent radiographic tumor (partial remission–marker negative)

- Partial remission–marker positive
- Disease progression

Approximately 5%–15% of patients fall into categories 3 and 4 and are typically managed with second-line treatment (salvage chemotherapy). Between 38% and 68% of patients have residual masses larger than 1 cm after first-line chemotherapy, and there is clear consensus that they should undergo postchemotherapy

Table 19.4 International Germ Cell Cancer Collaborative Group Risk Classification for Advanced Germ Cell Tumor

NONSEMINOMA	SEMINOMA
Good Prognosis	
Testicular/retroperitoneal primary *and*	Any primary site *and*
No nonpulmonary visceral metastases	No nonpulmonary visceral metastases
and	*and*
Good markers—all of:	Normal AFP, any hCG, any LDH
AFP <1000 ng/mL *and* hCG <5000 IU/L (1000 ng/mL) *and* LDH <1.5 × *upper limit of normal (N)*	
56% of nonseminomas	90% of seminomas
5-year PFS, 89%	5-year PFS, 82%
5-year survival, 92%	5-year survival, 86%
Intermediate Prognosis	
Testicular/retroperitoneal primary *and*	Any primary site *and*
No nonpulmonary visceral metastases	Nonpulmonary visceral metastases
and	*and*
Intermediate markers—any of:	Normal AFP, any hCG, any LDH
AFP ≥1000–10,000 ng/mL and ≤10,000 ng/mL *or* hCG ≥5000–50,000 IU/L and ≤50,000 IU/L *or* LDH ≥1.5 × N and ≤10 × N	
28% of nonseminomas	10% of seminomas
5-year PFS, 75%	5-year PFS, 67%
5-year survival, 80%	5-year survival, 72%

Continued

Table 19.4 International Germ Cell Cancer Collaborative Group Risk Classification for Advanced Germ Cell Tumor—cont'd

NONSEMINOMA	SEMINOMA
Poor Prognosis	
Mediastinal primary	No patients classified as
or	poor prognosis
Nonpulmonary visceral metastases	
or	
Poor serum markers—any of:	
AFP >10,000 ng/mL or	
hCG >50,000 IU/L (10,000 ng/mL) or	
LDH >10 × upper limit of normal	
16% of nonseminomas	
5-year PFS, 41%	
5-year survival, 48%	

AFP, α-Fetoprotein; *hCG*, human chorionic gonadotropin; *LDH*, lactate dehydrogenase; *PFS*, progression-free survival.

Data from International Germ Cell Consensus Classification: a prognostic factor-based staging system for metastatic germ cell cancers. International Germ Cell Cancer Collaborative Group. *J Clin Oncol* 1997;15:594-603.

surgery (PCS). **On average, histology of resected specimens will demonstrate necrosis, teratoma, and viable malignancy (with or without teratoma) in 40%, 45%, and 15% of cases, respectively.** **Relapsed Nonseminoma Germ Cell Tumor.** Chemotherapy-naïve patients are treated with risk-based induction chemotherapy, and cure rates exceed 95%. Men who relapse after previously receiving first-line chemotherapy are treated with second-line (salvage) chemotherapy. Patients with serologic CR to second-line chemotherapy with residual masses should undergo postsalvage chemotherapy surgical resection (PSCS). Patients with viable malignancy in PCSC specimens have a particularly poor prognosis, and their survival is not improved with the use of postoperative chemotherapy. Late relapse after chemotherapy is defined as that occurring more than 2 years after treatment. Roughly 3% of NSGCT patients experience a late relapse. Late relapses can be divided into three histopathological categories: viable malignancy (54%–88%; yolk sac tumor is most common), teratoma (12%–28%), and malignant transformation (10%–20%; adenocarcinoma is most common).

Management of Seminoma

Clinical Stage I. Approximately 80% of patients with seminoma are CS I, and this is the most common presentation of testis cancer. The management of these patients has undergone substantial changes over the past 2 decades, and surveillance, primary radiotherapy, and primary chemotherapy with single-agent carboplatin are now accepted treatment options. The long-term cancer control with each of these modalities approaches 100% with guidelines recommending surveillance as the preferred approach.

Surveillance – Compared with NSGCT, surveillance for CS I seminoma is complicated by the limited utility of serum tumor markers to detect relapse and the need for long-term surveillance CT imaging because 10%–20% of relapses occur 4 years or more after diagnosis.

Primary Chemotherapy – The rationale for single-agent carboplatin is based on the 65%–90% reported CR rates observed among patients with advanced seminoma and its reduced toxicity compared with cisplatin.

Primary Radiotherapy – The optimal radiation dose has not been defined, and most centers use 20–25.5 Gray (Gy). The most common sites of recurrence are the thorax and left supraclavicular fossa. Virtually all recurrences are cured with first-line chemotherapy.

Clinical Stage IIA and IIB Seminoma. Approximately 15%–20% of seminoma patients have CS II disease, 70% of whom have CS IIA-B. Radiotherapy using 30 Gy or primary chemotherapy are recommended with relapses cured in almost all cases with first-line chemotherapy, and disease-specific survival approaches 100%.

Clinical Stage IIC and III Seminoma. As with NSGCT, patients with CS IIC and III seminoma are treated with induction chemotherapy, with the regimen and number of cycles determined by risk. Ninety percent of patients with advanced seminoma are classified as good-risk and should receive either BEPx3 or EPx4 chemotherapy.

Management of Postchemotherapy Residual Masses. After first-line chemotherapy, 58%–80% of patients have radiologically detectable residual masses. Spontaneous resolution of these masses is reported in 50%–66% of cases (30%–50% for masses >3 cm), and the median time to resolution is 12–18 months. The histology of residual masses is necrosis and viable malignancy in 90% and 10% of cases, respectively. Postchemotherapy radiotherapy has no role in the management of residual masses. The size of residual masses is an important predictor of viable malignancy; 13%–55% of discrete residual masses larger than 3 cm contain viable malignancy compared with 0%–4% for masses <3 cm. There is consensus that patients with discrete residual masses >3 cm should be evaluated further with fluorodeoxyglucose – positron emission tomography (FDG-PET) at least 6 weeks after completion of chemotherapy, and those who are PET-negative and those with masses <3 cm should be observed. For patients with FDG-PET positive residual masses larger than 3 cm, strong consideration should be given for post-chemotherapy (PC)-RPLND, particularly those with residual masses after second-line chemotherapy.

Relapsed Seminoma. Chemotherapy-naïve relapse occurs in men with CS I seminoma on surveillance and in those with CS I-IIB seminoma treated with primary radiotherapy. Patients who relapse after single-agent carboplatin are considered to have chemotherapy-naïve relapse and should receive first-line cisplatin-base chemotherapy. An estimated 15%–20% of advanced seminoma patients relapse after induction chemotherapy, including 10% who achieve an initial complete response. An important consideration for advanced seminoma patients who relapse after first-line chemotherapy is the potential for teratoma at the site of relapse. Patients with normal serum tumor markers should undergo biopsy before undergoing resection or second-line chemotherapy.

PENILE CANCER

Penile squamous cell carcinoma accounts for 0.4%–0.6% of all malignant neoplasms among men in the United States and Europe but represents up to 10% of malignant neoplasms in men in some Asian, African, and South American countries. Penile cancer is a disease of older men, with an increase in incidence in the sixth decade of life.

Epidemiology, Etiology, and Clinical Presentation

Penile cancer is rare in developed countries and varies worldwide with age, circumcision, human papillomavirus (HPV) status, and lifestyle and hygiene practices. Risk factors include lack of neonatal circumcision, phimosis, HPV-16 infection, exposure to tobacco products, lichen sclerosus, and penile trauma. Carcinoma of the penis is characterized by a relentless progressive course, causing death for the majority of untreated patients within 2 years. Rarely, long-term survival occurs, even with advanced local disease and regional node metastases.

Carcinoma of the penis usually begins with a small lesion that gradually extends to involve the entire glans, shaft, and corpora. The earliest route of dissemination from penile carcinoma is metastasis to the regional femoral and iliac nodes. Patients with cancer of the penis, more than patients with other types of cancer, seem to delay seeking medical attention (Fig. 19.3).

Most tumors of the penis are squamous cell carcinomas demonstrating keratinization, epithelial pearl formation, and various degrees of mitotic activity. Squamous carcinoma histologic subtypes are classified into two major groups by their relationship to

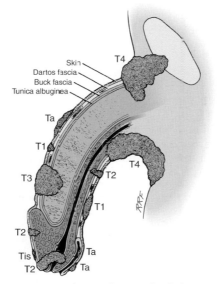

FIG. 19.3 Because treatment decisions for inguinal node dissections are based in part on the pathologic characteristics of the primary lesion (see section on treatment of inguinal nodes), determining the anatomic structure invaded is required. This diagram illustrates primary tumor (T) staging using the eighth edition TNM system.

HPV and show distinct morphologic features and clinical behavior (Box 19.2 and 19.3).

Physical Examination. Most lesions are confined to the penis, on the surface of the glans penis or in the preputial area, where it progressively enlarges. The penile lesion is assessed with regard to size, location, fixation, and involvement of the corporeal bodies.

Box 19.2 Key Points

PENILE LESIONS

A number of penile lesions must be considered in the differential diagnosis of penile carcinoma. These diseases can be identified by appropriate skin tests, tissue studies, serologic examinations, cultures, or specialized staining techniques.

- Condyloma acuminatum
- Buschke-Löwenstein tumor
- Balanitis xerotica obliterans
- Infectious lesions (e.g., chancre, chancroid, herpes, lymphopathia venereum, granuloma inguinale, tuberculosis)

Box 19.3 Key Points

NONSQUAMOUS MALIGNANT NEOPLASMS

- Basal cell carcinoma represents a highly curable variant with a relatively low metastatic potential.
- Sarcomas are prone to local recurrence; regional and distant metastases are rare. Superficial lesions can be treated with less radical procedures.
- Melanoma is an aggressive form of cancer but can be cured if diagnosed and treated with the appropriate surgical procedure at an early stage. Novel immunotherapy strategies may improve survival in recurrent or advanced disease.
- Extramammary Paget's disease (EMPD) disseminates by intraepidermal spread initially. Wide local excision to achieve negative margins is the therapy of choice. Invasive EMPD can be lethal.
- Penile metastases most often represent spread from a clinically obvious existing primary tumor. Prognosis is poor, and therapy should be directed toward the primary tumor site histology and local palliation.

Assessment of the inguinal area for adenopathy is important. A biopsy to confirm the diagnosis of carcinoma of the penis and assess the **depth of invasion, the presence of vascular invasion, and the histologic grade of the lesion** is important prior to initiation of any therapy.

Diagnostic Testing. The results of laboratory tests in patients with penile cancer are often normal. In patients with penile cancer the primary tumor and the inguinal lymph nodes are readily assessed by palpation. For small-volume glanular lesions, imaging studies offer little additional information to palpation in most patients. However, **for lesions thought to invade the corpus cavernosum, contrast-enhanced MRI may provide additional information**, especially when physical examination findings are equivocal and organ-sparing techniques are being considered. In patients with no palpable adenopathy, CT imaging offers no additional information over physical examination but may have a role in examination in obese patients or in those with prior inguinal surgery, in whom examination may be unreliable. Among patients with proven inguinal metastases, CT scan of the abdomen and pelvis may help to determine those patients with poor prognostic features for cure with surgery alone.

Staging

In the TNM staging system, the primary tumor stage is assigned by biopsy (or complete resection) and additional prognostic factors within the primary tumor included in the TNM system (i.e., tumor grade, the presence of vascular or perineural invasion, corpora cavernosum involvement). In most cases, the **presence of palpable adenopathy, along with the histologic features of the primary tumor, determines the need for additional imaging studies** (Table 19.5).

Management

Primary Tumor. Surgical amputation of the primary tumor remains the oncologic gold standard for rapid definitive treatment of the penile primary tumor; local recurrence rates range from 0% to 8%. Patients with penile primary tumors exhibiting favorable histologic features (stages Tis, Ta, T1; grade 1 and grade 2 tumors) are

Table 19.5 Definitions of AJCC TNM

Definition of Primary Tumor (T)

T CATEGORY	T CRITERIA
TX	Primary tumor cannot be assessed
T0	No evidence of primary tumor
Tis	Carcinoma *in situ* (Penile intraepithelial neoplasia [PeIN])
Ta	Noninvasive localized squamous cell carcinoma
T1	Glans: Tumor invades lamina propria
	Foreskin: Tumor invades dermis, lamina propria, or dartos fascia
	Shaft: Tumor invades connective tissue between epidermis and corpora regardless of location
	All sites with or without lymphovascular invasion or perineural invasion and is or is not high grade
T1a	Tumor is without lymphovascular invasion or perineural invasion and is not high grade (i.e., grade 3 or sarcomatoid)
T1b	Tumor exhibits lymphovascular invasion and/or perineural invasion or is high grade (i.e., grade 3 or sarcomatoid)
T2	Tumor invades into corpus spongiosum (either glans or ventral shaft) with or without urethral invasion
T3	Tumor invades into corpora cavernosum (including tunica albuginea) with or without urethral invasion
T4	Tumor invades into adjacent structures (i.e., scrotum, prostate, pubic bone)

Definition of Regional Lymph Node (N)

Clinical N (cN)

cN CATEGORY	cN CRITERIA
cNX	Regional lymph nodes cannot be assessed
cN0	No palpable or visibly enlarged inguinal lymph nodes
cN1	Palpable mobile or unilateral inguinal lymph node
cN2	Palpable mobile ≥ 2 unilateral inguinal nodes or bilateral inguinal lymph nodes
cN3	Palpable fixed inguinal nodal mass or pelvic lymphadenopathy unilateral or bilateral

Pathologic N (pN)

pN CATEGORY	pN CRITERIA
pNX	Lymph node metastasis cannot be established
pN0	No lymph node metastasis
pN1	≤ 2 unilateral inguinal metastases, no ENE

Table 19.5 Definitions of AJCC TNM—cont'd

pN CATEGORY	pN CRITERIA
Definition of Primary Tumor (T)	
pN2	≥3 unilateral inguinal metastases or bilateral metastases, no ENE
pN3	ENE of lymph node metastases or pelvic lymph node metastases
Definition of Distant Metastasis (M)	
M CATEGORY	**M CRITERIA**
M0	No distant metastasis
M1	Distant metastasis present

Used with the permission of the American College of Surgeons. Amin, M.B., Edge, S.B., Greene, F.L., et al. (Eds.) AJCC Cancer Staging Manual, 8th Ed. Springer New York, 2017.

at a lower risk for metastases and these patients are best suited for organ-sparing or glans-sparing procedures (Table 19.6).

Inguinal Nodes. Lymph node metastasis is a prognostic factor for cancer-specific survival for patients with penile cancer, and prompt treatment of the lymph nodes can provide both diagnostic and therapeutic advantages for these patients. **The lymph node metastatic spread follows that of the penile lymphatic drainage in a level-by-level fashion, starting with superficial inguinal, to deep inguinal, and then pelvic lymph nodes.** The presence and the extent of metastasis to the inguinal region are the most important prognostic factors for survival in patients with squamous penile cancer, affecting the prognosis of the disease more than tumor grade, gross appearance, and morphologic or microscopic patterns of the primary tumor. Historically, a course of antibiotics was recommended for patients with suspicious nodes to potentially discern metastasis from cancer; this practice is no longer advocated because it can delay treatment and in cases of clinical concern a biopsy can be performed.

The cure rate with inguinal lymph node dissection (ILND) when nodes are positive for malignancy may be as high as 80%, there is substantial morbidity the procedure can produce. Early complications of phlebitis, pulmonary embolism, wound infection, flap necrosis, and permanent and disabling lymphedema of the scrotum and lower limbs are frequent after inguinal and

Table 19.6 Treatment of the Primary Penile Tumor (Category 2A Recommendation)

STAGE	TREATMENT
Tis (glans)	Laser therapy, glans resurfacing; alternative: topical therapy
Ta, Tis (foreskin, shaft skin)	Surgical excision to achieve negative margin; alternatives: laser therapy, topical therapy (Tis only)
Ta, T1 grade 1–3 (glans)	Therapy based on size and position of lesion as well as potential side effects, excision, glans resurfacing procedures, glansectomy, radiotherapy (not indicated for Ta)
Ta, T1 grade 1–3 (foreskin, shaft)	Complete surgical excision to achieve negative margin
T2 or greater	Partial or total penectomy, radiotherapy, or chemoradiotherapy
T4 (adjacent structures)	Consider neoadjuvant chemotherapy with surgical consolidation for responding patients if baseline resectability is a concern
Local disease recurrence after conservative therapy	Complete surgical excision to achieve negative surgical margins; may require partial or total penectomy; select patients with superficial low-grade recurrences may be candidates for repeat penile-conserving procedure

ilioinguinal node dissections. One alternative to ILND for all patients has been to observe patients with normal findings on inguinal examination and intervene at time of early clinical suspicion. Patients with both Tis, Ta and stage T1, grade 1 tumors exhibit a relatively low incidence of positive lymph nodes overall (0%–16%) and are optimal candidates for surveillance strategies. Management options of T1 grade 2 tumors include observation or an inguinal staging procedure. The incidence of metastases among patients stage T1b or greater tumors ranges from 33% to more than 50%, so an inguinal staging procedure appears warranted. Patients exhibiting corporeal invasion (stage pT2) in the penile tumor exhibit a high risk for metastasis (Fig. 19.4A,B).

Fine-Needle Aspiration (FNA) Cytology – Fine-needle aspiration cytology of clinically negative groins **does not exhibit**

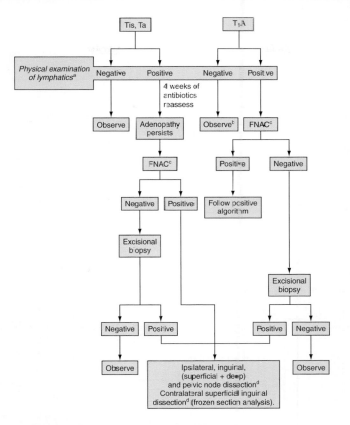

aIncludes physical examination and/or imaging studies.
bAlternative DSNB at experienced centers, superficial dissection if noncompliant patient.
cFine-needle aspiration cytology.
dIf two or more positive ipsilateral inguinal nodes or extranodal extension found.

FIG. 19.4 Management of regional disease. (A) Very low risk (left side) and low-intermediate risk (right side).

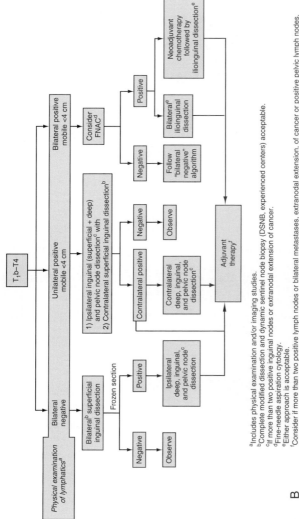

aIncludes physical examination and/or imaging studies.
bComplete modified dissection and dynamic sentinel node biopsy (DSNB, experienced centers) acceptable.
cIf more than two positive inguinal nodes or extranodal extension of cancer.
dFine-needle aspiration cytology.
eEither approach is acceptable.
fConsider if more than two positive lymph nodes or bilateral metastases, extranodal extension, of cancer or positive pelvic lymph nodes.

FIG. 19.4, cont'd (B) High-risk and lower-volume metastatic patients. (C) Bulky metastatic and distant disease.

high enough sensitivity to be relied on as a staging modality. However, direct aspiration of palpable inguinal nodes is easily performed, exhibited a sensitivity of 93%, and, if positive, provides immediate information with which to advise patients about further treatment.

Dynamic Sentinel Node Biopsy (DSNB) – DSNB helps define where in the inguinal lymph node field the sentinel lymph node resides using combination of visual (vital blue dyes) or gamma emission (hand-held gamma probe) techniques at the time of surgery. **When performed at high-volume centers using a standardized protocol, it has an acceptable sensitivity.**

Superficial and Modified Complete Inguinal Dissection – Superficial node dissection involves removal of those nodes superficial to the fascia lata. A complete ILND (removal of those nodes deep to the fascia lata contained within the femoral triangle as well as the pelvic nodes) is then performed if the superficial nodes are positive at surgery by frozen-section analysis. Either superficial or complete modified inguinal dissection should adequately identify microscopic metastases in patients with clinically normal inguinal examination findings, without the need for a pelvic dissection if the inguinal nodes are negative.

Inguinal and Ilioinguinal Lymphadenectomy – The goals are to eradicate all obvious cancer, to provide coverage for exposed vasculature, and to provide rapid wound healing. ILND should be bilateral for patients with unilateral adenopathy at initial presentation of the primary tumor due to **anatomic crossover of penile lymphatics with bilateral drainage and the finding of contralateral metastases in >50% of patients, even if the contralateral nodal region is normal on palpation.**

For patients undergoing ILND for curative intent (i.e., in whom preoperative studies reveal no pelvic adenopathy), PLND should routinely be considered in patients with two or more positive inguinal lymph nodes or when extracapsular nodal extension is present. PLND serves as a staging tool for identifying patients at increased risk for pelvic metastases in whom adjunctive therapy should be considered. PLND can be performed simultaneously with ILND in the setting of higher-volume inguinal metastases or as a secondary procedure after inguinal pathology is available. Alternatively, if pelvic nodal metastases are proven before lymphadenectomy (based on clinical findings), consideration should be given to neoadjuvant chemotherapeutic strategies followed by surgery or clinical trial enrollment (Fig. 19.5).

Radiation Therapy

External-Beam Radiotherapy (EBRT). Primary EBRT affords at least a 50% chance to control the primary tumor and avoid penile amputation with 5-year local control rates ranging from 55% to 70%, with penile preservation rates of 39% to 66%. EBRT is most frequently considered in patients who are not surgical candidates and those presenting with locoregionally advanced disease in which the primary region would be treated in contiguity with the nodal regions, including both groins and the pelvis.

Brachytherapy (BT). Brachytherapy involves a temporary implantation of interstitial needles in and around the primary tumor. Local control provided by BT appears superior to EBRT, with 5-year local control rates of 77% to 88%. Penile preservation rates are 74%–88% at 5 years and 67%–70% at 8–10 years (Boxes 19.4 and 19.5).

MALE URETHRAL CANCER

Male primary urethral cancer (PUC) is a rare disease that usually manifests after the sixth decade of life and is more common in African Americans than whites. The most common histologic subtypes are squamous cell carcinoma, urothelial carcinoma, and adenocarcinoma. The prognosis of male anterior PUC is variable and is strongly tied to tumor aggressiveness. Several tumor characteristics are associated with survival, including grade, stage, location, and histology.

Epidemiology, Etiology, and Clinical Presentation

Most patients with anterior PUC have a history of chronic urethral inflammation with urethral stricture disease being the most common risk factor, present in at least 50% of patients with PUC. Other risk factors for anterior **PUC include sexually transmitted diseases (HPV-16), lichen sclerosus, urethritis, pelvic radiation, trauma, and instrumentation**. Presenting symptoms include obstructive voiding symptoms, hematuria or bloody urethral discharge, and penile or perineal mass. Nearly all patients are symptomatic at the

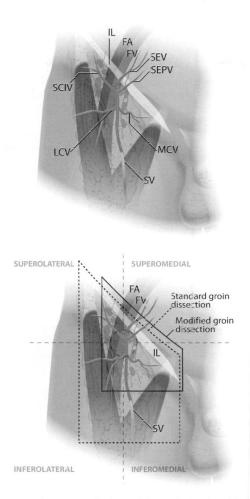

FIG. 19.5 Topographic anatomy plus limits of the standard and modified inguinal lymph node dissections. *FA,* Femoral artery; *FV,* femoral vein; *IL,* inguinal ligament; *LCV,* lateral cutaneous vein; *MCV,* medial cutaneous vein; *SCIV,* superficial circumflex iliac vein; *SEPV,* superficial external pudendal vein; *SEV,* superficial epigastric vein.

Box 19.4 Key Points

RADIATION THERAPY

- Radiation provides an effective penile-preserving approach for T1–T2 squamous cell carcinomas smaller than 4 cm using either external-beam radiotherapy or brachytherapy.
- Because 20% of recurrences occur after 5 years, continued follow-up is required becaue salvage penectomy for persistent or recurrent disease may be curative.
- The criteria for surgical staging of inguinal lymph nodes are the same whether patients undergo primary radiation or primary surgical management.
- Unresectable lymph nodes may be rendered operable by neoadjuvant chemotherapy or chemoradiation.
- Integration of radiation, surgery, and chemotherapy in advanced disease is being investigated in a prospective international randomized trial (InPACT: EA 8134).
- Palliative radiotherapy may be beneficial for metastatic disease.

Box 19.5 Key Points

CHEMOTHERAPY

- Neoadjuvant chemotherapy with a cisplatin-containing regimen should be considered for patients with lymph node metastases because responses in this setting may facilitate curative resection. In the absence of level 1 evidence, the optimal or standard multi-modal strategy remains undefined.
- The use of bleomycin in the treatment of men with metastatic penile cancer was associated with an unacceptable level of toxicity and is discouraged.
- Surgical consolidation to achieve disease-free status or palliation should be considered in fit patients with a proven objective response to systemic chemotherapy.
- Among patients who progress through chemotherapy, surgery is not recommended.

time of presentation, but a high index of clinical suspicion is required to diagnose these tumors.

The anterior urethra (bulbar urethra, pendulous urethra, and fossa navicularis) is lined by stratified and pseudostratified columnar epithelium, which transitions to stratified squamous epithelium in the very distal urethra. The posterior urethra (prostatic and membranous urethra) is lined by urothelium. **Because there is a change in cell type along the length of the urethra, male PUCs vary by site of origin** (Fig. 19.6). Among urethral cancers described in population-level studies, 50%–80% are urothelial carcinomas, 10%–30% are squamous cell carcinomas, and 5%–10% are adenocarcinomas (Table 19.7).

Male PUC can spread by direct extension to adjacent structures, including the corpus spongiosum and the periurethral tissues, or it can metastasize through lymphatic spread to regional lymph nodes. **The lymphatics from the anterior urethra drain into the inguinal lymph nodes, although the bulbar urethral can occasionally drain into the external iliac lymph nodes. The posterior urethra drains into the pelvic lymph nodes.** Palpable

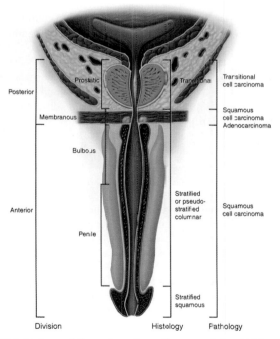

FIG. 19.6 Anatomy of the male urethra with corresponding histology and pathology.

Table 19.7 Grading System for Primary Urethral Carcinoma

G	DEFINITION
Urothelial Carcinoma	
LG	Low grade
HG	High grade
Squamous Cell Carcinoma, Adenocarcinoma	
Gx	Grade cannot be assessed
G1	Well differentiated
G2	Moderately differentiated
G3	Poorly differentiated

Data from Hansel D, Reuter VE, Bochner B, et al. Urethra. In: Amin MB, ed. *AJCC Cancer Staging Manual*, 8th ed. New York: Springer, 2017.

inguinal lymph nodes occur in approximately 20%–30% of cases and almost always represents metastatic disease in contrast to penile cancer, in which palpable inguinal nodes can be inflammatory.

Staging

The tumor, node, metastases (TNM) staging classification is based on depth of invasion of the primary tumor and presence or absence of regional lymph node involvement and distant metastasis. Transurethral or percutaneous needle biopsy of the primary lesion is necessary for a tissue diagnosis. MRI provides superior soft-tissue resolution and is the optimal imaging modality to characterize the local extent of disease (Table 19.8, Fig. 19.7).

Management

Aggressive local control is paramount in the management of localized PUC. The optimal method varies according to tumor location. Chemoradiation with or without surgical consolidation is an alternative to surgical resection of advanced urethral tumors (Table 19.9).

Carcinoma of the Pendulous Urethra. Tumors of the pendulous urethra and fossa navicularis are usually amenable to surgical resection. As opposed to patients with penile cancer, it is unclear if there is a survival benefit to prophylactic inguinal lymph node

Table 19.8 The American Joint Committee on Cancer Urethral Cancer Tumor, Node, Metastases (TNM) Staging System

Primary Tumor (T) (Male and Female)	
TX	Primary tumor cannot be assessed
T0	No evidence of primary tumor
Ta	Noninvasive papillary carcinoma
Tis	Carcinoma in situ
T1	Tumor invades subepithelial connective tissue
T2	Tumor invades any of the following: corpus spongiosum, periurethral muscle
T3	Tumor invades any of the following: corpus cavernosum, anterior vagina
T4	Tumor invades other adjacent organs (e.g., bladder)

Transitional Cell Carcinoma of The Prostate	
Tis	Carcinoma in situ, involvement of the prostatic urethra or periurethral prostatic ducts without stromal invasion
T1	Tumor invades urethral subepithelial connective tissue immediately underlying the urothelium
T2	Tumor invades the prostatic stroma surrounding ducts either by direct extension from the urothelial surface or by invasion from prostatic ducts
T3	Tumor invades the periprostatic fat
T4	Tumor invades other adjacent organs (e.g., bladder, rectum)

Regional Lymph Nodes (N)	
NX	Regional lymph nodes cannot be assessed
N0	No regional lymph node metastasis
N1	Single regional lymph node metastasis in the inguinal region or true pelvis (perivesical, obturator, internal [hypogastric] and external iliac), or presacral lymph node
N2	Multiple regional lymph node metastasis in the inguinal region or true pelvis (perivesical, obturator, internal [hypogastric] and external iliac), or presacral lymph node

Distant Metastasis (M)	
M0	No distant metastasis
M1	Distant metastasis

Data from Hansel D, Reuter VE, Bochner B, et al. Urethra. In: Amin MB, ed. *AJCC Cancer Staging Manual*, 8th ed. New York: Springer, 2017.

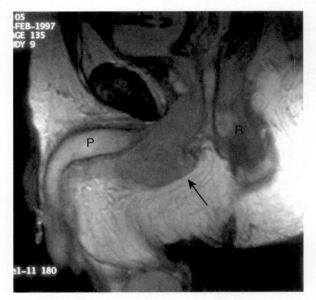

FIG. 19.7 Magnetic resonance image demonstrating a large proximal anterior urethral cancer *(arrow)*. *P,* Penis; *R,* rectum.

dissection in patients with anterior PUC without palpable inguinal lymph nodes.

Carcinoma of the Bulbar Urethra. Some low-stage lesions of the proximal anterior urethra may be treated by transurethral resection or segmental excision with an end-to-end anastomosis. Patients treated with transurethral resection should be considered for repeat transurethral resection to ensure accurate staging and a complete resection. The standard and most aggressive surgical management for advanced-stage bulbar urethral cancer is radical cystectomy, pelvic lymphadenectomy, and total penectomy. Because of the poor outcomes after surgery alone for advanced tumors of the urethra, surgical monotherapy has been deemed inadequate for advanced-stage PUC, particularly of the bulbar urethra, leading to increased interest in multimodal therapy, with chemoradiation a reasonable alternative for some patients.

Table 19.9 Summary of 2020 National Comprehensive Cancer Network Clinical Practice Guidelines on Primary Urethral Cancer of the Male Anterior Urethra (Category 2A recommendation)

STAGE		FIRST-LINE TREATMENT OPTIONS	ADJUVANT THERAPY
Tis, Ta, T1		Repeat TUR $\pm$ intraurethral BCG or chemotherapy	
Male T2	Pendulous urethra	Partial urethrectomy $\pm$ penectomy[a]	If positive margin: Chemoradiotherapy or Additional surgery or Radiotherapy
	Bulbar urethra	Urethrectomy $\pm$ radical cystoprostatectomy[a]	If $\geq$ pT3 or N+: Chemotherapy or Chemoradiotherapy
Female T2		Chemoradiotherapy or Urethrectomy + cystectomy or Distal urethrectomy (depending on location)	
$\geq$ T3	No	Chemoradiotherapy $\pm$ consolidative surgery or Neoadjuvant chemotherapy with consolidative surgery or radiation or Radiotherapy or Consolidative surgery alone for nonurothelial histology	

Continued

Table 19.9 Summary of 2020 National Comprehensive Cancer Network Clinical Practice Guidelines on Primary Urethral Cancer of the Male Anterior Urethra (Category 2A recommendation)—cont'd

STAGE	FIRST-LINE TREATMENT OPTIONS	ADJUVANT THERAPY
N+	Radiotherapy preferably with chemotherapy (preferred for SCC) OR Systemic therapy OR Chemoradiotherapy ± consolidative surgery	

aConsider neoadjuvant chemotherapy.

BCG, Bacille Calmette-Guérin; *TUR,* transurethral resection.

Data from Bladder Cancer, *NCCN Clinical Practice Guidelines in Oncology,* 2020: https://www.nccn.org/professionals/physician_gls/default.aspx.

Carcinoma of the Prostatic Urethra. Prostatic urethral carcinoma is commonly found in patients with a history of bladder cancer. **Approximately 20%–40% of patients with aggressive bladder cancer have synchronous involvement of the prostate at the time of cystectomy,** and up to 39% of patients with high-risk nonmuscle-invasive bladder cancer (NMIBC) can have recurring problems in the prostate after intravesical therapy. Given the rarity of primary prostatic urethral carcinoma, any patients found to have urothelial carcinoma in the prostate should be thoroughly evaluated for coexisting urothelial carcinoma of the bladder and upper tracts.

The management of male primary posterior urethral cancer is largely based on the treatment of patients with bladder cancer who have synchronous or metachronous prostatic involvement. Patients with prostatic urethral involvement were previously classified as stage T4 and historically managed with radical cystectomy; however, not all patients with prostatic involvement have a poor prognosis, and many could be managed with less aggressive measures. Those with high-grade superficial disease treated with Bacille Calmette-Guérin (BCG) can have prostatic response rates of at least 70% and an extensive transurethral

Table 19.10 Summary of 2020 National Comprehensive Cancer Network Clinical Practice Guidelines on Urothelial Carcinoma of the Prostate (Category 2A Recommendation)

TYPE	FIRST-LINE TREATMENT OPTIONS
Mucosal	TURP and BCG
Ductal or acinar	TURP and BCG OR Radical cystectomy ± urethrectomy
Stromal invasion	Radical cystectomy ± urethrectomy ± neoadjuvant chemotherapy

TURP, Transurethral resection of the prostate; *BCG,* bacille Calmette-Guerin.
Data from Bladder Cancer, *NCCN Clinical Practice Guidelines in Oncology,* 2020: https://www.nccn.org/professionals/physician_gls/default.aspx.

resection of the prostate (TURP) before treatment with BCG removes the majority of cancerous urothelium and likely improves exposure of prostatic tissue to BCG and increases response rates. Prostatic ductal involvement has been an indication for cystectomy for some; however, these patients can also be effectively managed with TURP and BCG, and their prognosis is similar to those with superficial prostatic involvement. Patients with prostatic urothelial carcinoma invasive into the stroma should be managed with radical cystectomy and pelvic lymphadenectomy with or without perioperative chemotherapy (Table 19.10).

Urethral Recurrence After Radical Cystectomy

The risk of urethral recurrence (UR) after radical cystectomy ranges from 1% to 15%, with larger series reporting rates near 5%, most occurring within 2 years of radical cystectomy. Risk factors for UR include
- Bladder tumor multifocality
- Presence of carcinoma in-situ (CIS)
- A history of NMIBC
- Involvement of the prostate with urothelial carcinoma
- A positive urethral margin
- Cutaneous diversion

Patients with orthotopic neobladders (ONBs) have a lower risk of UR than patients with cutaneous diversions. Although this may

> **Box 19.6** Key Points
>
> FEMALE URETHRAL CANCER
> - The three most common histologies for female urethral cancer are urothelial carcinoma, squamous cell carcinoma, and adenocarcinoma.
> - Compared with anterior urethral cancers, posterior cancers are found at a more advanced stage and are associated with worse survival.
> - Radiation and surgical excision are options for low-stage anterior tumors, each with high cure rates.
> - Surgery and radiation therapy for proximal female urethral tumors have poor outcomes when used alone; therefore, multimodal therapy is recommended.

reflect differences in selection criteria for urinary diversion, some theorize that ONBs are protective against UR because of changes in the local immune response, the antineoplastic effects of ileum, or the continued exposure of the urethra to urine.

The strongest indications for prophylactic urethrectomy are a positive urethral margin or gross urethral involvement. **A staged urethrectomy after radical cystectomy has similar outcomes compared with a planned urethrectomy at the time of radical cystectomy**. Patients who have a positive cytology or symptoms of urethral bleeding, discharge, or a palpable mass require evaluation with urethroscopy and biopsy. Patients with noninvasive URs can be managed successfully with endoscopic resection and topical therapy. Patients with invasive URs often have an aggressive disease course with a median survival of 17 months (Box 19.6).

Suggested Readings

Bladder cancer, NCCN Clinical Practice Guidelines in Oncology. 2020. https://www.nccn.org/professionals/physician_gls/default.aspx.

Diagnosis and treatment of early stage testicular cancer. AUA guideline. 2019. https://www.auanet.org/guidelines/testicular-cancer-guideline.

EAU guidelines: penile cancer. 2018. https://uroweb.org/guideline/penile-cancer/.

EAU guidelines: primary urethral carcinoma. 2020. https://uroweb.org/guideline/primary-urethral-carcinoma/.

EAU guidelines: testicular cancer. 2020. https://uroweb.org/guideline/testicular-cancer/.

Penile cancer, NCCN Clinical Practice Guidelines in Oncology. 2020. Https://www.nccn.org/professionals/physician_gls/default.aspx.

Testis cancer, NCCN Clinical Practice Guidelines in Oncology. 2020. Https://www.nccn.org/professionals/physician_gls/default.aspx.

20

Tumors of the Bladder

SUMIT ISHARWAL, KIRSTEN L. GREENE, AND ALAN W. PARTIN

CONTRIBUTORS OF CAMPBELL-WALSH-WEIN, 12TH EDITION

Sumit Isharwal, Max Kates, Trinity J. Bivalacqua, Joseph Zabell, Badrinath R. Konety, Thomas J. Guzzo, John P. Christodouleas, David J. Vaughn, Neema Navai, Colin P.N. Dinney, Anton Wintner, Douglas M. Dahl, Guarionex Joel Decastro, James M. Mckiernan, Mitchell C. Benson, Eila C. Skinner, Siamak Daneshmand, and Khurshid A. Guru

EPIDEMIOLOGY

- In the United States 81,400 patients will be diagnosed with bladder cancer (BlCa) in 2020, and 17,980 will die from their disease.
- The average age of diagnosis is 73 years in the United States with approximately 9 of 10 patients diagnosed after the age of 55 years.
- Although BlCa is more than three times as prevalent in men, women are more likely to be seen initially with more advanced tumors and less favorable prognosis.
- BlCa is most common among white Americans, with an incidence rate 1.5 times that of African Americans, twice that of Hispanic Americans, and six times that of Native Americans.

ECONOMIC IMPACT

- BlCa is the most expensive cancer to treat per patient over a patient's lifetime.

RISK FACTORS

- **Genetics** – The most-studied genes associated with BlCa are *N*-acetyltransferase 2 and a deletion of glutathione S-transferase μ.

Both of these genes are associated with the ability to metabolize aromatic amines and thus play an important role in the subset of individuals with environmental carcinogen exposure.

- **Hereditary** – Patients with Lynch syndrome are at increased risk of developing urothelial cancer. This increased risk is primarily found among the mismatch repair gene *MSH2* mutations carriers.
- **Tobacco** – This is the main known cause of BlCa and accounts for 30%–40% of all urothelial carcinomas. Aromatic amines are the primary carcinogens in tobacco smoke that lead to cancer.
- **Occupational Risk** – Particularly at-risk occupations that work with aromatic amines include tobacco, dye, and rubber workers; hairdressers; painters; and leather workers. Those who work with polycyclic aromatic hydrocarbons are also at risk, including chimney sweeps, nurses, waiters, petroleum workers, and seamen.
- **Medical Conditions** – Patients with neurogenic bladder and spinal cord injuries who have chronic indwelling catheters are at a modestly increased risk of developing squamous cell carcinoma of the bladder. Malignant potential of bladder exstrophy has been well documented, with adenocarcinoma accounting for >90% of cases and squamous cell and urothelial carcinoma account for the remaining 10%.
- **Schistosomiasis** – Schistosomiasis remains a major contributor to squamous cell carcinoma of the bladder in many tropical countries.
- **Radiation Exposure** – External beam radiation therapy for cervical cancer and prostate cancer is associated with higher incidence of BlCa with estimated latency period of 15–30 years.
- **Chemotherapy** – Cyclophosphamide that has been shown to cause BlCa and phosphoramide mustard is the primary mutagenic metabolite.
- **Environmental Pollution** – Exposure to arsenic in drinking water has been associated with the development of BlCa. The mechanism of arsenic-mediated carcinogenesis is thought to be multifactorial, including oxidative stress, epigenetic effects, and alterations in DNA repair.

PRESENTATION AND WORKUP

- Painless gross hematuria is present in 85% of patients with newly diagnosed BlCa, and microscopic hematuria is present in nearly all patients.

- Irritative voiding symptoms (e.g., frequency, urgency) also may be signs of BlCa, particularly carcinoma in situ (CIS).
- Workup includes a history and physical examination, cystoscopy, upper tract imaging, urine culture, and urine cytology in patients with gross hematuria.

Diagnosis

The gold-standard test for the diagnosis of BlCa is cystoscopy followed by biopsy/resection of tumor. Increasingly, blue light cystoscopy and narrow band imaging (NBI) are being used as adjuncts to cystoscopy in identifying occult malignancy.

PATHOLOGY

Staging and Grading

BlCa are staged using 8th edition of Tumor Node Metastasis/American Joint Committee on Cancer (TNM/AJCC) (Table 20.1).

Table 20.1 Definitions of AJCC TNM

Defination of Primary Tumor (T)	
T CATEGORY	**T CRITERIA**
TX	Primary tumor cannot be assessed
To	No evidence of primary tumor
Ta	Non-invasive papillary carcinoma
Tis	Urothelial carcinoma *in situ*: "flat tumor"
T1	Tumor invades lamina propria (subepithelial connective tissue)
T2	Tumor invades muscularis propria
pT2a	Tumor invades superficial muscularis propria (inner half)
pT2b	Tumor invades deep muscularis propria (outer half)
T3	Tumor invades perivesical soft tissue
pT3a	Microscopically
pT3b	Macroscopically (extravesical mass)
T4	Extravesical tumor directly invades any of the following: prostatic stroma, seminal vesicles, uterus, vagina, pelvic wall, abdominal wall
T4a	Extravesical tumor invades directly into prostatic stroma, seminal vesicles, uterus, vagina
T4b	Extravesical tumor invades pelvic wall, abdominal wall

Table 20.1 Definitions of AJCC TNM—cont'd

Definition of Regional Lymph Nodes (N)[a]

N CATEGORY	N CRITERIA
NX	Lymph nodes cannot be assessed
N0	No lymph node metastasis
N1	Single regional lymph node metastasis in the true pelvis (perivesical, obturator, internal and external iliac, or sacral lymph node)
N2	Multiple regional lymph node metastasis in the true pelvic (perivesical, obturator, internal and external iliac, or sacral lymph node metastasis)
N3	Lymph node metastasis to the common iliac lymph nodes

Definition of Distant Metastasis (M)

M CATEGORY	M CRITERIA
M0	No distant metastasis
M1	Distant metastasis
M1a	Distant metastasis limited to lymph nodes beyond the common iliacs
M1b	Non-lymph node distant metastases

Note: cTNM is the clinical classification, and pTNM is the pathologic classification.
[a]Regional lymph nodes include both primary and secondary drainage regions. All other nodes above the aortic bifurcation are considered distant lymph nodes.
Used with the permission of the American College of Surgeons. Amin, M.B., Edge, S.B., Greene, F.L., et al. (Eds.) AJCC Cancer Staging Manual, 8th Ed. Springer New York, 2017.

Clinical stage reflects findings in transurethral resection of bladder tumor (TURBT) as well as radiologic and physical exam findings with bimanual exam at time of TURBT. Pathological staging is based on surgical resection of the bladder via partial or radical cystectomy and pathological evaluation of pelvic lymph nodes. BlCa are graded using the 2004 World Health Organization/International Society of Urologic Pathologists (WHO/ISUP) grading system.

- High- and low-grade cancers are often considered essentially separate diseases based on disparate genetic development, biologic behavior, and management strategies.

- The most important risk factor for progression is grade.
- CIS is a precursor as well as a risk factor for progression, invasion, and metastasis.
- Deep penetration into the lamina propria, especially if involving muscularis mucosae, increases the risk of recurrence and progression.
- Hydronephrosis often indicates muscle invasion.

Histology

The majority of primary BlCa are urothelial carcinomas, representing more than 90% of all bladder tumors. Urothelial cancer has a propensity for divergent differentiation and include squamous, glandular, micropapillary, sarcomatoid, plasmacytoid, and nested variant histologies. Nonurothelial malignancy includes small cell carcinoma, pure squamous cell carcinoma, and adenocarcinoma. Small cell carcinoma should be treated as metastatic disease with chemotherapy (usually cisplatin and etoposide) followed by either radiation therapy or surgery for elimination of the local disease. Radical cystectomy is the mainstay treatment for squamous cell carcinoma and primary bladder adenocarcinoma. The standard treatment for urachal adenocarcinoma is en bloc resection of the bladder dome, urachal ligament, and umbilicus.

MANAGEMENT OF NONMUSCLE INVASIVE BLADDER CANCER

Approximately 70%–80% of BlCa cases are nonmuscle-invasive bladder cancer (NMIBC) at presentation with 60%–70% as stage Ta, 20%–30% as T1, and approximately 10% as CIS. Risk of recurrence is typically approximately 40%–60% but can be influenced by multiple clinical factors. Risk of progression, however, is of key concern in patients with NMIBC given the heterogeneity of tumors with rates of progression as low as 6% in patients with low-grade Ta lesions to as high as 17% in high-grade T1 tumors. There are several tools such as European Organization for Research and Treatment of Cancer risk calculator that can be used to predict risk of recurrence and progression. Table 20.2 shows American Urological Association (AUA) risk stratification for NIMBC.

Table 20.2 American Urological Association Risk Stratification for Nonmuscle-Invasive Bladder Cancer

LOW RISK	INTERMEDIATE RISK	HIGH RISK
LG solitary Ta ≤3 cm	Recurrence within 1 year, LG Ta	HG T1
PUNLMP	Solitary LG Ta >3 cm	Any recurrent, HG Ta
	LG Ta, multifocal	HG Ta, >3 cm (or multifocal)
	HG Ta, ≤3 cm	Any CIS
	LG T1	Any BCG failure in HG patient
		Any variant histology
		Any LVI
		Any HG prostatic urethral involvement

BCG, Bacille Calmette-Guérin; *CIS,* carcinoma in situ; *HG,* high grade; *LG,* low grade; *LVI,* lymphovascular invasion; *PUNLMP,* papillary urothelial neoplasm of low malignant potential. From Chang SS, Boorjian SA, Chou R, et al. Diagnosis and treatment of non-muscle invasive bladder cancer: AUA/SUO Guideline. *J Urol* 2016;196(4):1021-1029.

Endoscopic Surgical Management

Transurethral Resection of Bladder Tumor. TURBT is intended to be diagnostic and therapeutic by providing specimens to allow for pathological determination of stage and grade, while simultaneously removing and/or fulgurating all visible tumors. Traditionally, TURBT has been performed with monopolar loop using sterile water or glycine solution. The use of bipolar loop allows use of saline irrigation, which can decrease risk of transurethral resection (TUR) syndrome in cases of perforation and if the resection is prolonged.

The incidence of perforation can be reduced by avoiding overdistention of the bladder and using anesthetic paralysis during the resection of significant lateral wall lesions to lessen an obturator reflex response. Resection of diverticular tumors presents significant risk of bladder wall perforation, and accurate staging is difficult to achieve given the absence of underlying detrusor.

Complications of Transurethral Resection of Bladder Tumor and Bladder Biopsy. Minor bleeding and irritative symptoms are common side effects in the immediate postoperative period. The major complications of uncontrolled hematuria and clinical bladder perforation occur in 1%–6.7% of cases. The majority of perforations are extraperitoneal; however, intraperitoneal rupture is possible when tumors are resected at the dome. Extraperitoneal bladder perforation during TURBT can typically be managed with prolonged urethral catheter drainage. Intraperitoneal perforation is less likely to close spontaneously and usually requires open or laparoscopic surgical repair. TUR syndrome from fluid absorption is uncommon, particularly with the use of bipolar energy, and managed in the same manner as during transurethral resection of the prostate.

Repeat Transurethral Resection of Bladder Tumor. AUA guidelines recommend repeat TURBT of primary tumor site, to include muscularis propria, within 6 weeks of the initial TURBT in patients with incomplete initial resection, and patients with stage T1 disease. These guidelines also recommend consideration of repeat TURBT in patients with high-risk, high-grade Ta tumors.

Enhanced Cystoscopic Techniques: Fluorescence Cystoscopy, Narrow Band Imaging. Blue light cystoscopy with cysview uses the photosensitizing agent hexaminolevulanic acid with preferential accumulation of photoactive porphyrins in malignant cells. Under blue light, cancer cells emit red fluorescence resulting in better tumor visualization (Fig. 20.1). When blue light cystoscopy with cysview is used, small papillary tumors and almost one-third more cases of CIS overlooked on white light cystoscopy are identified.

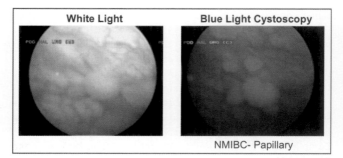

FIG. 20.1 White light cystoscopy reveals apparent normal-appearing mucosa juxtaposed with blue light cystoscopy demonstrating visual evidence of bladder cancer. Blue light cystoscopy reveals accumulation of hexaminolevulinate in the same area, ultimately found to contain nonmuscle-invasive bladder cancer (NMIBC). (Image courtesy Dr. Siamak Daneshmand.)

NBI is an optical image enhancement technology intended to improve the visibility of blood vessels inherent to neoplastic processes. NBI light is composed of two specific wavelengths that are absorbed by hemoglobin; 415-nm light penetrates only the superficial mucosal layers, whereas 540-nm light penetrates more deeply. The combination allows improved visualization of tumors and enables distinguishing blood vessels on and below the surface from tumors.

Intravesical Therapy

Perioperative Intravesical Therapy. AUA guidelines recommend that in a patient with suspected or known low- or intermediate-risk BlCa, a clinician should consider administration of a single postoperative instillation of intravesical chemotherapy (e.g., gemcitabine, mitomycin C) within 24 hours of TURBT. A meta-analysis of 18 randomized controlled trials showed that a single dose of intravesical chemotherapy within 24 hours after TUR of NMIBC resulted in a 13% absolute reduction in tumor recurrence from 50%–37%, yielding a number needed to treat of 7.2. Although local irritative symptoms are the most common complications of postoperative instillation, serious sequelae and rare deaths have also occurred, especially in patients with perforation during resection. Chemotherapy should be withheld in patients with extensive resection or when there is concern about perforation.

Intravesical Immunotherapy. Bacille Calmette-Guérin (BCG): Intravesical BCG treatment leads to cytokine induction with preferential upregulation of IFN-γ, IL-2, and IL-12 reflects induction of a T-helper type-1 (Th1) response. This immunologic response activates cell-mediated cytotoxic mechanisms believed to underlie the efficacy of BCG. Intravesical BCG decreases both tumor recurrence and progression.

Treatments are typically started 2–4 weeks after tumor resection, allowing time for reepithelialization of the bladder after TURBT, thereby minimizing the potential for intravasation of live bacteria. Patients receive a 6-week induction course followed by three weekly instillations at 3 and 6 months and every 6 months thereafter for 3 years. Recent data suggest that 1-year course of maintenance BCG can be considered for intermediate risk disease instead of 3 years. Contraindications to BCG therapy and management of infectious complications of BCG is shown in Boxes 20.1 and 20.2.

> **Box 20.1** Contraindications to Bacille Calmette-Guérin (BCG) Therapy
>
> **ABSOLUTE CONTRAINDICATIONS**
>
> Immunosuppressed and immunocompromised patients[a]
> Immediately after transurethral resection on the basis of the risk of intravasation and septic death
> Personal history of BCG sepsis
> Gross hematuria (intravasation risk)
> Traumatic catheterization (intravasation risk)
> Total incontinence (patient will not retain agent)
>
> **RELATIVE CONTRAINDICATIONS**
>
> Urinary tract infection (intravasation risk)
> Liver disease (precludes treatment with isoniazid if sepsis occurs)
> Personal history of tuberculosis (risk theorized but unknown)
> Poor overall performance status
> Advanced age
>
> **NO OR INSUFFICIENT DATA ON POTENTIAL CONTRAINDICATIONS**
>
> Patients with prosthetic materials have not been shown to have increased risk of infectious or other complications in limited literature (Rosevear et al., 2010)
> Ureteral reflux
> Antitumor necrosis factor medications (theoretically predispose to BCG sepsis)
>
> ---
> [a]Recent small series suggest this may not be an absolute contraindication (Herr, 2012).
> From Ehlers S. Why does tumor necrosis factor targeted therapy reactivate tuberculosis? *J Rheumatol (Suppl)* 2005;74:35-39.

Intravesical Chemotherapy. The agents are summarized in Table 20.3. Optimization of mitomycin delivery can be achieved by eliminating residual urine volume, fasting overnight, using sodium bicarbonate to reduce drug degradation, and increasing concentration to 40 mg in 20 mL.

AUA guidelines states that in a low-risk patient, a clinician should not administer induction intravesical therapy. In an intermediate-risk patient a clinician should consider administration of a 6-week course of induction intravesical chemotherapy or immunotherapy. In

Box 20.2 Management of Bacille Calmette-Guerin (BCG) Toxicity

GRADE 1: MODERATE SYMPTOMS <48 HOURS

Mild or moderate irritative voiding symptoms, mild hematuria, fever <38.5°C

Assessment

Possible urine culture to rule out bacterial urinary tract infection

Symptom Management

Anticholinergics, topical antispasmodics (phenazopyridine), analgesics, nonsteroidal antiinflammatory drugs

(Asymptomatic prostatic granulomas that occur after BCG therapy can occasionally mimic prostate cancer clinically and/or radiographically. There is no evidence to support treatment in this setting [Suzuk et al., 2013].)

GRADE 2: SEVERE SYMPTOMS AND/OR >48 HOURS

Severe irritative voiding symptoms, hematuria, or symptoms lasting >48 hours

All maneuvers for grade 1, plus the following:

Assessment

Urine culture, chest radiograph, liver function tests

Management

Consider dose reduction to one-half to one-third of dose when instillations resume.

Treat culture results as appropriate.

Can also consider pretreating with a single dose of isoniazid before each subsequent instillation

Antimicrobial Agents

Administer isoniazid and rifampin orally until symptom resolution.

Also use vitamin B6 or pyridoxine.

Do not use monotherapy.

Observe for rifampin drug-drug interactions (e.g., warfarin).

Monitor liver function tests.

GRADE 3: SERIOUS COMPLICATIONS (HEMODYNAMIC CHANGES, PERSISTENT HIGH-GRADE FEVER)

Allergic Reactions (Joint Pain, Rash)

Perform all maneuvers described for grades 1 and 2, plus the following:

Isoniazid and rifampin, depending on response.

Also use vitamin B6 or pyridoxine.

Continued

> **Box 20.2** Management of Bacille Calmette-Guérin (BCG)
> Toxicity—cont'd
>
> ***Solid Organ Involvement (Liver, Lung, Kidney)***
>
> Stop BCG instillations. Initiate antimycobacterial therapy with
> isoniazid, rifampin. If symptoms persist, consult with infectious
> disease specialist with expertise in antituberculous therapy. Can
> add ethambutol.
>
> Cycloserine often causes severe psychiatric symptoms and is to be
> strongly discouraged.
>
> BCG is almost uniformly resistant to pyrazinamide, so this drug has
> no role.
>
> Consider prednisone when response is inadequate or for septic shock
> (never given without effective antibacterial therapy).

a high-risk patient with newly diagnosed CIS, high-grade T1, or high-risk Ta urothelial carcinoma, a clinician should administer a 6-week induction course of BCG.

Management of Refractory High-Grade Disease

- If the initial treatment was intravesical chemotherapy, a course of BCG should be considered. BCG has demonstrated superiority to repeat courses of chemotherapy in this setting because the latter will lead to only an approximately 20% disease-free survival.
- For patients who have failed BCG, a second course still gives a 30%–50% response. A second course of BCG is recommended for patients with intermediate- or high-risk disease if persistent or recurrent Ta disease or CIS is noted after a single course of intravesical BCG.
- Patients who cannot tolerate BCG for any reason may be considered for salvage chemotherapy, but the risk of failure and progression is high.
- The Food and Drug Administration has approved pembrolizumab for the treatment of patients with BCG unresponsive high-risk NMIBC with CIS with or without papillary tumors who are ineligible for or have elected not to undergo cystectomy. The complete response rate in patients with high-risk

Table 20.3 Comparisons Among Intravesical Agents

AGENT	PERIOPERATIVE USE	RISK GROUP	CYSTITIS (%)	OTHER TOXICITY	DROPOUT (%)	CONCENTRATION AND DOSE
Doxorubicin (Adriamycin)	Yes	Low to intermediate	20–40	Fever, allergy, contracted bladder, 5%	2–16	50 mg/50 mL
Epirubicin	Yes	Low to intermediate	10–30	Contracted bladder rare	3–6	50 mg/50 mL
Thiotepa	Yes	Low to intermediate	10–30	Myelosuppression, 8%–19%	2–11	30 mg/30 mL
Mitomycin	Yes	Low to intermediate	30–40	Rash, 8%–19%; contracted bladder; 5%	2–14	40 mg/20–40 mL
BCG	No	Intermediate to high	60–80	Serious infection, 5%	5–10	1 vial/50 mL
Interferon	No	Salvage	<5	Flulike symptoms; 20%	Rare	50–100 MU/50 mL
Gemcitabine	Yes	Salvage	Mild	Occasional nausea	<10	1–2 g/50–100 mL
Valrubicin	No	Salvage	Mild	UTI, abdominal pain, asthenia	<10	800 mg/55 mL

BCG, Bacille Calmette-Guérin; UTI, urinary tract infection.
Modified from O'Donnell MA. Practical applications of intravesical chemotherapy and immunotherapy in high-risk patients with superficial bladder cancer. Urol Clin North Am 2005;32:121-131.

BCG-unresponsive NMIBC with CIS was 41% and median response duration was 16.2 months.

Role of "Early" Cystectomy

Current AUA guidelines suggest radical cystectomy in patients who are fit for surgery and have persistent high-grade T1 disease on repeat resection or T1 tumors with associated CIS, LVI, or variant histologies. These guidelines also suggest cystectomy in high-risk patients with persistent or recurrent disease within 1 year after treatment with two induction cycles of BCG or BCG maintenance.

Surveillance and Prevention

The AUA guidelines recommend cystoscopic surveillance based on risk stratification of the tumor into low-, intermediate- and high-risk categories. The recommended surveillance schedule is shown in Table 20.4.

MANAGEMENT OF MUSCLE-INVASIVE BLADDER CANCER

Twenty percent to 30% of patients present with muscle-invasive bladder cancer (MIBC) at the time of initial presentation. MIBC is a highly lethal entity and if left untreated will result in mortality within 2 years of diagnosis in 85% of cases.

TUR is the gold standard method for establishing the diagnosis of MIBC. Bimanual examination under anesthesia remains an important aspect of primary tumor assessment. Cross-sectional imaging plays an important adjuvant role to TUR and physical examination in the assessment and staging of patients with MIBC. A high suspicion for extravesical disease is warranted when hydronephrosis is noted on cross-sectional imaging.

Radical Cystectomy and Pelvic Lymph Node Dissection for Muscle-Invasive Bladder Cancer

For patients with cT2–T4a, N0, M0 disease, radical cystectomy and bilateral pelvic lymph node dissection remains the gold standard therapy. In men, radical cystectomy includes excision of the surrounding perivesical soft tissue, prostate, and seminal vesicles. In women, anterior pelvic exenteration is often used and includes the ovaries, uterus with cervix, and anterior vagina.

Table 20.4 2016 AUA/SUO Guideline Suggested Surveillance Strategies

RISK	TUMOR STATUS	CYSTOSCOPY SCHEDULE	UPPER TRACT IMAGING
Low	Solitary Ta low grade	3 months after initial resection Annually beginning 9 months after initial surveillance if no recurrence Consider cessation at 5 or more years Consider cytology or tumor markers	Not necessary unless hematuria present
Intermediate	Multiple Ta low grade Large tumor Recurrence at 3 months	Every 3–6 months for 1–2 years Every 6–12 months for subsequent 2 years Annual cystoscopy thereafter Consider cytology or tumor markers Restart clock with each recurrence	Consider imaging at 1- to 2-years intervals, especially for recurrence Imaging for hematuria
High	Any high grade (including CIS)	Every 3–4 months for 2 years Semiannually for 2 years Annually for lifetime Cytology at same schedule Consider tumor markers Restart clock with each recurrence	Imaging annually for 2 years, then consider lengthening interval

CIS, Carcinoma in situ.
Modified from Chang SS, Boorjian SA, Chou R, et al. Diagnosis and treatment of non-muscle invasive bladder cancer: AUA/SUO Guideline. *J Urol* 2016;196(4):1021-1029.

Vaginal sparing is appropriate in the absence of locally advanced tumors.

The RAZOR study, a randomized phase 3 trial, showed that robotic cystectomy is noninferior to open cystectomy for 2-year progression-free survival. Potential benefits of robotic cystectomy include decreased blood loss, decreased transfusion rates, and shorter hospital stay.

Early recovery after surgery (ERAS) protocols have reduced perioperative gastrointestinal complications and hospital stays. These protocols vary but include avoiding bowel preparation and nasogastric tubes, decreasing narcotic pain management (including epidural narcotics), instituting early feeding, and using a μ-opioid antagonist that blocks the effects of narcotics on the bowel.

Bilateral Pelvic Lymph Node Dissection. Bilateral pelvic lymphadenectomy should be performed in all patients, including those with unilateral bladder wall involvement, due to documented crossover risk to the contralateral lymphatic chain. It is well established that approximately 25% of patients will have pathologic lymph node metastases at the time of cystectomy, and increasing nodal yield at the time of pelvic lymph node dissection improves the sensitivity of detecting nodal metastasis.

Anatomic Extent of Pelvic Lymph Node Dissection and Landing Zones. A standard pelvic lymph node dissection template is bounded distally by the circumflex iliac vein and Cloquet's node, laterally by the genitofemoral nerve, medially by the bladder and internal iliac vessels, posteriorly by the obturator fossa, and proximally by the bifurcation of the common iliac artery. An extended template dissection includes the tissue extending above the common iliac bifurcation to the aortic bifurcation and presacral region. A superextended template lymph node dissection includes tissue up to the level of the inferior mesenteric artery. It is not yet known whether extended pelvic lymphadenectomy is more effective than standard pelvic lymphadenectomy. We await the results of the SWOG S1011 prospective, randomized trial comparing survival in cystectomy patients undergoing extended or standard pelvic lymph node dissection.

Intraoperative Decision Making

Grossly Positive Nodes and T4b Disease. For patients with clinically positive lymph nodes, the standard of care is cisplatin-based systemic chemotherapy. Patients who have a radiographic complete or partial response to systemic therapy are candidates for and should be evaluated for cystectomy. Those undergoing cystectomy have been noted to have a complete pathologic response typically in the 14%–25% range. Patients who do achieve a complete response appear to have a significant survival advantage with 5-year cancer-specific survival rates of 63%.

If adenopathy is encountered at the time of cystectomy, a frozen section should be taken to confirm metastasis, and an extended lymph node dissection and radical cystectomy should be completed when feasible. Cystectomy is not performed when lymph node metastases are unresectable because of bulk, when there is evidence of extensive periureteral disease, when the bladder is fixed to the pelvic sidewall, or when the tumor is invading the rectosigmoid colon.

Intraoperative Frozen Sections of the Ureter. The role of intraoperative frozen-section analysis of the ureters at the time of cystectomy remains somewhat controversial. When frank tumor is encountered, it should be resected to a negative margin. When CIS only is encountered, maximal resection without compromising ureteral length for urinary diversion is advocated because it is debatable whether a negative CIS margin reduces upper tract recurrence or is definitively associated with poorer outcome.

Oncologic Outcomes Following Radical Cystectomy. Table 20.5 illustrates the reported oncologic outcomes of large surgical series. Pathologic tumor stage and presence of nodal metastasis are the strongest predictors of recurrence and survival following cystectomy.

Neoadjuvant Therapy for Muscle-Invasive Bladder Cancer. Based on the randomized trial results and subsequent meta-analyses, cisplatin-based neoadjuvant chemotherapy is associated with an overall survival advantage of 5%–6% and a pathologic complete response rate of 30%–40%. AUA guideline recommends cisplatin-based neoadjuvant chemotherapy to eligible radical cystectomy patients prior to cystectomy. Clinicians should not prescribe carboplatin-based neoadjuvant chemotherapy for clinically resectable stage cT2-T4aN0.

Adjuvant Therapy for Muscle-Invasive Bladder Cancer. Adjuvant chemotherapy trials have been hampered by small overall numbers and difficult patient accrual, which has limited the ability to draw definitive conclusions regarding the overall effectiveness of this approach. Current AUA guidelines favor neoadjuvant chemotherapy instead of adjuvant chemotherapy based on higher-level evidence data. However, guidelines suggest considering adjuvant chemotherapy in the setting of pT3/T4 or node-positive disease based on the available data.

Table 20.5 Percentage of 5-Year Disease-Specific Survival (DSS) by Pathologic Stage After Radical Cystectomy With and Without Pelvic Lymph Node Metastasis: Selected Series Reporting DSS (2000–2012)

SELECTED SERIES	PATIENTS (n)	≤P1	P2A	P2	P2B	P3A	P3	P3B	P4A, B	N NEG	N+
Stein et al., 2001	1054	88		81		68		47	44	78	35
Madersbacher et al., 2003	507	76		74			52		36	—	33
Hautmann et al., 2006	788	90		72			43		28	75	21
Shariat et al., 2006b	888	81		72			44		28	80	35
Ghoneim et al., 2008	2720	82	75		53		40		29	62	27
Manoharan et al., 2009	432	81		70			44		16	72	29

Urinary Diversion

In patients undergoing radical cystectomy, conduit, continent cutaneous, and orthotopic neobladder urinary diversions should all be discussed. The current body of published literature is insufficient to conclude that any form of urinary diversion is superior to another on the basis of health-related quality-of-life outcomes.

Conduit. The ileal conduit is the most commonly utilized urinary diversion using a short segment of distal ileum. The preservation of the most distal 15 cm can reduce issues related to absorption of vitamin B_{12}, fat-soluble vitamins, and bile salts. It is not advisable to use ileum for a conduit in patients with a short bowel syndrome, in patients with inflammatory small bowel disease, and in those whose ileum has received extensive irradiation often as a consequence of prior radiation therapy for a pelvic malignant neoplasm. Transverse colon is used for the conduit when one wants to be sure that the segment of conduit used has not been irradiated in individuals who have received extensive pelvic irradiation. The sigmoid conduit is a good choice in patients undergoing a pelvic exenteration who will have a colostomy as no bowel anastomosis is required.

Long-term complications of ileal and colon conduits include stomal stenosis, peristomal hernia, pyelonephritis, calculus formation, ureteral obstruction, and renal deterioration. Metabolic complications of intestine interposed in the urinary tract include electrolyte abnormalities, altered sensorium, abnormal drug metabolism, osteomalacia, growth retardation, persistent and recurrent urinary tract infection, formation of calculi, short gut, and development of urothelial or intestinal cancers. Specific abnormalities for each segment of intestine are summarized in Table 20.6.

Continent Cutaneous Urinary Diversion. Because the ability to self-catheterize is essential to the patient undergoing continent diversion, the patient must be assessed for the ability to care for themself. While there are many techniques for creating continent catheterizable reservoirs, the Indiana pouch remains one of the most reliable of all catheterizable reservoirs. The major long-term problems with continent cutaneous diversion relate to function of the efferent continence mechanism, and surgical revision is often required. This type of reservoir is used in patients who want to avoid a stoma appliance and preserve continence but either are not candidates for or do not want a neobladder.

Table 20.6 Electrolyte Disturbances Associated with Bowel Segments used for Urinary Diversion

| SEGMENT | SYNDROME | BLOOD | | | ASSOCIATED ABNORMALITIES | SYMPTOMS | TREATMENT |
| | | Na⁺ | K⁺ | Cl⁻ | pH | | |

SEGMENT	SYNDROME	Na⁺	K⁺	Cl⁻	pH	ASSOCIATED ABNORMALITIES	SYMPTOMS	TREATMENT
Stomach	Severe metabolic alkalosis	—	↓	↓	↑	Elevated aldosterone	Lethargy, muscle weakness, respiratory insufficiency, seizures, ventricular arrhythmia	H_2 blocker, proton pump inhibitor; if life threatening, arginine hydrochloride infusion and/or removal of segment
Jejunum	Hyperkalemic, hypochloremic metabolic acidosis	↓	↑	↓	↓	Elevated renin and angiotensin	Lethargy, nausea, vomiting, dehydration, muscle weakness	Intravenous hydration, sodium bicarbonate, thiazide; if life threatening, removal of segment
Ileum/colon	Hyperchloremic metabolic acidosis	—	↓	↑	↓	Total-body potassium depletion, hypocalcemia	Fatigue, anorexia, lethargy, weakness	Potassium citrate, sodium citrate, citric acid, sodium bicarbonate, chlorpromazine, nicotinic acid

Orthotopic Urinary Diversion. If orthotopic neobladder is planned, adequate urethral length must be maintained and a frozen section analysis of the urethral margin performed. In the presence of a positive urethral margin, orthotopic neobladder should not be performed, and the patient should be made aware of this possibility during preoperative counseling. An algorithm for patient selection is presented in Fig. 20.2. The bowel segment used for the reservoir should be completely detubularized and reconstructed into a

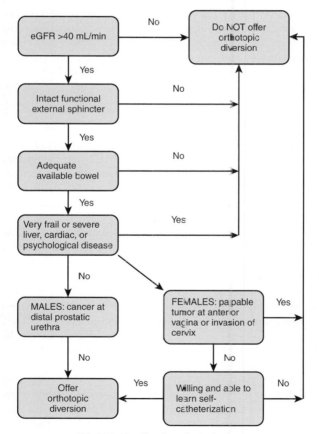

FIG. 20.2 Algorithm for patient selection.

spherical shape. The ultimate storage volume of the mature pouch should be at least 300–500 mL at low pressure. The two most popular configurations are the Hautmann W-neobladder and the Studer pouch neobladder. With orthotopic diversion, most patients void by Valsalva maneuver with relaxation of the external sphincter. Daytime continence develops gradually over 3–6 months in most patients and is ultimately achieved in 80%–90% of both male and female patients. Persistent nocturnal incontinence is common, observed in 20%–50% of patients. Nocturnal continence may continue to improve beyond 12 months from surgery and may improve with timed voiding. Factors influencing continence rates include age, intestinal segment used, and application of a prostate-sparing technique. The primary late complications of orthotopic diversion that are directly related to the diversion itself include incontinence, urinary retention, urinary tract infection, ureteroileal or afferent limb obstruction, urethral stricture, upper tract and pouch stones, vaginal fistula, and pouch rupture.

Bladder Preservation

Bladder preserving therapy should be offered to patients with newly diagnosed MIBC who desire to retain their bladder and for those with significant comorbidities for whom radical cystectomy is not a treatment option. Choices include multimodal therapy, maximal TURBT, partial cystectomy with lymphadenectomy, and primary radiation therapy.

Trimodality therapy – It involves a maximal safe complete TUR, chemotherapy (cisplatin, or 5-fluorouracil, and mitomycin), and radiation. Appropriate candidates are those with a limited disease burden and adequate normal bladder function. In general, a patient is considered to have a limited disease burden if the bladder tumor is unifocal and small (<4 cm in maximal dimension) without frank extravesicular extension on imaging (i.e., not cT3b), is not causing hydronephrosis, and can be gross totally resected by TUR. The major chemoradiation bladder preservation trials for surgically fit patients are summarized in Table 20.7.

Partial Cystectomy – Ideal candidates for partial cystectomy include those with small, solitary tumors amenable to wide resection with 2 cm margins. It is imperative that the tumor is in a location that allows for complete resection while maintaining adequate functional bladder capacity. The presence of CIS is considered by

Table 20.7 Major Prospective Trimodal Bladder Preservation Studies

STUDY	PATIENTS (n)	STAGE	CHEMOTHERAPY	RT (Gy)	CR RATE (%)	SALVAGE CYSTECTOMY RATE (%)	SURVIVAL
Housset et al., 1993	54	T2–4No–1Mx	Cisplatin + 5-FU + 4	44	74	NA	3-year CSS, 62%; OS, 59%
Shipley et al., 1998	62	T2–4NoMx	Cisplatin + 3	64.8	60	25.8	5-year OS, 49%
Tunio et al., 2012	200	T2–4NoMx	Weekly cisplatin	65	93		5-year OS, 52%
James et al., 2012	182	T2–4aNoMx	5-FU, MMC + 2	55 or 64		11.4	5-year OS, 48%
Gogna et al., 2006	113	T2–4NoMx	Weekly cisplatin	64	70	13	5-year OS, 50%
Kaufman et al., 2009a, 2009b	50	T2–4aNoMx	Weekly cisplatin + paclitaxel	64.3	87		5-year OS, 56%; 5-year CSS, 71%

CR, Complete response; CSS, cause-specific survival; 5-FU, 5-fluorouracil; MMC, mitomycin C; OS, overall survival.

most to be a contraindication to partial cystectomy, and random bladder biopsies can be performed preoperatively.

MANAGEMENT OF METASTATIC BLADDER CANCER

Systemic cisplatin-based combination chemotherapy is the standard of care for patients with metastatic urothelial cancer (Table 20.8). Although the majority of patients with metastatic disease (40%–70%) will experience an initial response to chemotherapy, most will ultimately progress with a median survival of 14 months and overall 5 year survival rates of 5%–20%. Patients who meets any of the following criteria are not cisplatin candidates: a World Health Organization or Eastern Cooperative Oncology Group performance status >2, creatinine clearance <60 mL/min, ≥ grade 2 audiometric hearing loss, ≥ grade 2 peripheral neuropathy, or a New York Heart Association class III or higher heart failure. When cisplatin therapy is contraindicated, carboplatin has been substituted with the benefit of improved tolerability but with the cost of decreased efficacy.

Second-Line Chemotherapy

Salvage chemotherapy in this setting with conventional agents typically has a suboptimal response rate Table 20.9. Multiple novel single agents have been evaluated in patients with advanced BlCa, typically with modest response rates of <20% Table 20.10.

Immune Checkpoint Inhibitor Therapy

Programmed cell death-1 (PD-1) is a molecule expressed on activated T cells that binds to PD-L1 to modulate the immune response. Tumor cells may express PD-L1 as a mechanism to neutralize T-cell activation. These immune checkpoint inhibitors result in an increase in T-cell activation and proliferation, which may result in an antitumor response. The anti–PD-L1 and anti–PD-1 agents have been approved for platinum-resistant and cisplatin-ineligible metastatic urothelial cancer (Table 20.11). Recently, avelumab has been approved as a maintenance therapy in patients with unresectable locally advanced or metastatic urothelial cancer who did not have disease progression with first-line chemotherapy.

Table 20.8 Randomized Trials of Front-Line Chemotherapy for Metastatic Urothelial Cancer

GROUP	PATIENTS (n)	TREATMENT/ CONTROL ARM	RELATIVE RISK (%)	MEDIAN SURVIVAL (MONTHS)	P VALUE
Intergroup (Loehrer et al., 1992)	269	MVAC/Cis	39 vs. 12	12.5 vs. 8.2	.0001
MDAH (Logothetis et al., 1990)	110	MVAC/CISCA	65 vs. 46	11.1 vs. 8.3	.0003
EORTC (Sternberg et al., 2006b)	263	HD-MVAC/MVAC	72 vs. 58	14.9 vs. 15.1	.0417
Lilly (von der Maase et al., 2005)	405	GC/MVAC	49 vs. 46	14.0 vs. 15.2	.66
Greece (Bamias et al., 2004)	220	DC/MVAC	37 vs. 54	9.3 vs. 14.2	.026
EORTC (Bellmunt et al., 2012)	626	GC/PCG	46 vs. 57	12.7 vs. 15.8	.03
Dreicer et al., 2004	85	CaP/MVAC	28 vs. 36	13.8 vs. 15.4	.65

CaP, Carboplatin and paclitaxel; *Cis,* cisplatin; *CISCA,* cisplatin, cyclophosphamide, and doxorubicin (Adriamycin); *DC,* docetaxel and cisplatin; *EORTC,* European Organization for Research and Treatment of Cancer; *GC,* gemcitabine and cisplatin; *HD-MVAC,* high-dose MVAC; *MDAH,* MD Anderson Hospital; *MVAC,* methotrexate, vinblastine, doxorubicin (Adriamycin), and cisplatin; *N,* number of patients; *NR,* not reported; *PCG,* paclitaxel, cisplatin, and gemcitabine.

Table 20.9 Salvage Chemotherapy for Metastatic Urothelial Cancer

DRUG	AUTHOR (REFERENCE)	N	ELIGIBILITY	RR (%)	MEDIAN PFS (MONTHS)	MEDIAN OS (MONTHS)
Paclitaxel (24-hour)	Dreicer et al., 1996	9	One prior regimen	56	—	—
Paclitaxel (weekly)	Vaughn et al., 2002	31	One prior regimen for advanced disease, prior adjuvant chemotherapy and taxanes allowed	10	2.2	7.2
Docetaxel (every 3 weeks)	McCaffrey et al., 1997	30	One prior cisplatin regimen, prior taxanes not allowed	13	—	9.0
Gemcitabine	Lorusso et al., 1998	35	One prior platinum regimen	22.5	—	5.0
Gemcitabine	Albers et al., 2002	30	One prior cisplatin regimen	11	4.9	8.7
Gemcitabine-paclitaxel	Sternberg et al., 2001a	41	One prior cisplatin regimen including perioperative therapy	60	—	14.4

N, Number of patients; *OS*, overall survival; *PFS*, progression-free survival; *RR*, response rate.

Table 20.10 Salvage Trials With Single-Agent Chemotherapeutic and Novel Agents for Metastatic Urothelial Cancer

AGENT	AUTHOR	N	PRIOR	RR (%)	MEDIAN PFS (MONTHS)	MEDIAN OS (MONTHS)
Gemcitabine	Lorusso et al., 1998	35	One prior platinum regimen	23	3.8	5
Gemcitabine	Albers et al., 2002	30	One prior cisplatin regimen	11	4.9	8.7
Paclitaxel	Vaughn et al., 2002	31	One prior regimen for advanced disease, prior adjuvant chemotherapy and taxanes allowed	10	2.2	7.2
Ifosphamide	Witte et al., 1997	56	One prior cytotoxic regimen	20	2.5	5.5
Docetaxel	McCaffrey et al., 1997	30	One prior cisplatin regimen, prior taxanes not allowed	13		9
Nab-Paclitaxel	Ko et al., 2013	48	One prior platinum regimen	32	6	10.8
Abraxane	Sridhar et al., 2011	47	One prior platinum regimen	32	6	10.8
Eribulin	Quinn et al., 2010	40	One prior platinum regimen	38	3.9	9.4
Vinflunine	Culine et al., 2006	51	One prior platinum regimen	18	3.0	6.6
Vinflunine	Bellmunt et al., 2013	370	One prior platinum regimen	28		6.9
Pemetrexed	Sweeney et al., 2006	47	One prior regimen including perioperative therapy within 12 months	27.7	2.9	9.6
Pemetrexed	Galsky et al., 2007	12	One prior regimen	8		—
Ixabepilone	Dreicer et al., 2007	42	One prior platinum regimen, prior taxane allowed	11.9	2.7	8.0
Oxaliplatin	Winquist et al., 2005	18	One prior regimen for advanced disease, prior adjuvant chemotherapy >6 months earlier not counted	6	—	—

N, Number of patients; *OS,* overall survival; *PFS,* progression-free survival; *RR,* response rate.

Table 20.11 Food and Drug Administration–Approved Checkpoint Inhibitors for Platinum-Resistant Metastatic Urothelial Cancer as a Second-Line Treatment and Cisplatin-Ineligible Metastatic Urothelial Cancer as a First-Line Treatment

INDICATION	TARGET	TREATMENT	TRIAL	PHASE	N	MEDIAN FOLLOW-UP (MONTHS)	OBJECTIVE RESPONSE RATE (95% CI)	
							ALL	PD-L1 HIGH
Platinum resistant	PD-L1	Avelumab	Javelin	Ib	242	9.9	17% (11–24)	24% (14–36)
		Durvalumab	Study 1108	I/II	191	5.8	18% (13–24)	28% (19–38)
		Atezolizumab	IMVigor 210	II	310	11.7	15% (11–20)	27% (19–37)
			IMVigor 211	III	459	17	13% (10–17)	23% (16–32)
	PD-1	Nivolumab	Check Mate 032	I/II	78	15.2	24% (15–35)	24% (9–45)
			Check Mate 275	II	265	7	20% (15–25)	28% (19–40)
		Pembrolizumab	Keynote-045	III	270	14.1	21% (16–27)	22% (13–33)
Cisplatin ineligible	PD-L1	Atezolizumab	IMVigor 210	II	119	17.2	23% (16–31)	28% (14–47)
	PD-1	Pembrolizumab	Keynote-052	II	370	5	24% (20–29)	38% (29–48)

Fibroblast Growth Factor Receptor Therapy

Erdafitinib is a kinase inhibitor approved for patients with locally advanced or metastatic BlCa that has susceptible genetic alteration in FGFR3 or FGFR2 and that has progressed during or following prior platinum-containing chemotherapy. A recent phase 2 clinical trial showed that patients who received erdafitinib had response rate of 40% and median duration of response was 5.6 months.

Suggested Readings

Advanced Bladder Cancer (ABC) Meta-analysis Collaboration: Neoadjuvant chemotherapy in invasive bladder cancer: update of a systematic review and meta-analysis of individual patient data. *Eur Urol* 2005;48:202-205.

Advanced Bladder Cancer (ABC) Meta-analysis Collaboration: Adjuvant chemotherapy in invasive bladder cancer: a systematic review and meta-analysis of individual patient data. *Eur Urol* 2005;48:189-199.

Chang SS, Boorjian SA, Chou R, et al. Diagnosis and treatment of non-muscle invasive bladder cancer: AUA/SUO guideline. *J Urol* 2016;196:1021-1029. https://www.auanet.org/guidelines/bladder-cancer-non-muscle-invasive-guideline.

Chang SS, Bochner BH, Chou R, et al. Treatment of non-metastatic muscle-invasive bladder cancer: AUA/ASCO/ASTRO/SUO guideline. *J Urol* 2017;198:552-559. https://www.auanet.org/guidelines/bladder-cancer-non-metastatic-muscle-invasive-guideline.

James ND, Hussain SA, Hall E, et al. Radiotherapy with or without chemotherapy in muscle invasive bladder cancer. *N Engl J Med* 2012;366:1477-1488.

Messing EM, Tangen CM, Lerner SP, et al. Effect of intravesical instillation of Gemcitabine vs saline immediately following resection of suspected low-grade non-muscle-invasive bladder cancer on tumor recurrence: SWOG S0337 randomized clinical trial. *JAMA* 2018;319:1880-1888.

Parekh DJ, Reis IM, Castle EP, et al. Robot-assisted radical cystectomy versus open radical cystectomy in patients with bladder cancer (RAZOR): an open-label, randominzed, phase 3 non-inferiority trial. *Lancet* 2018;391:2525-2536.

Patel VG, Oh WK, Galsky MD. Treatment of muscle-invasive and advanced bladder cancer in 2020. *CA Cancer J Clin.* 2020. doi:10.3322/caac.21631.

Robertson AG, Kim J, Al-Ahmadie H, et al. Comprehensive molecular characterization of muscle-invasive bladder cancer. *Cell* 2017;171:540-556.

Von der Maase H, Sengelov L, Roberts JT, et al. Long-term survival results of a randomized trial comparing gemcitabine plus cisplatin, with methotrexate, vinblastine, doxorubicin, plus cisplatin in patients with bladder cancer. *J Clin Oncol* 2005;23: 4602-4608.

21

Benign Prostatic Hyperplasia

JONATHAN T. WINGATE, ALAN W. PARTIN AND
KIRSTEN L. GREENE

CONTRIBUTORS OF CAMPBELL-WALSH-WEIN, 12TH EDITION

Paolo Capogrosso, Andrea Salonia, Francesco Montorsi, Sevann Helo, R. Charles Welliver Jr., Kevin T. Mcvary, Misop Han, Claus G. Roehrborn, and Douglas William Strand

EPIDEMIOLOGY AND PATHOBIOLOGY

Benign prostatic hyperplasia (BPH), a noncancerous enlargement of the prostate gland, is the most common benign tumor found in men. BPH is a pathologic process but certainly not the only cause of lower urinary tract symptoms (LUTS) in aging men. Despite intense research efforts to elucidate the underlying etiology of BPH, cause-and-effect relationships have not been established. Previously held notions that the clinical symptoms of male LUTS are caused by a mass-related increase in urethral resistance are too simplistic. It is now clear that symptoms are caused by age-related detrusor dysfunction and other conditions such as polyuria, sleep disorders, and a variety of systemic medical conditions unrelated to the prostate-bladder unit.

It is well recognized that voiding symptoms poorly correlate with underlying pathophysiology. This has led to the recognition that LUTS may commonly be related to bladder outlet obstruction (BOO) as a result of benign prostatic obstruction (BPO), which is often associated with benign prostatic enlargement resulting from the histologic condition of BPH (Fig. 21.1). Failure to empty can be related either to an outlet obstruction, detrusor under activity of the bladder, or a combination of both. Postmicturition symptoms, such as post void dribbling, are very troublesome and may cause significant interference with quality of life.

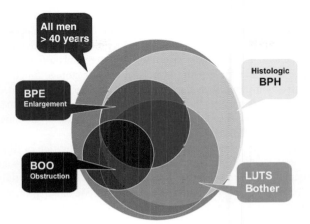

FIG. 21.1 Diagram showing the relationship between histologic hyperplasia of the prostate (BPH), lower urinary tract symptoms (LUTS), benign prostate enlargement (BPE), and bladder outlet obstruction (BOO). The size of the circles does not represent actual proportions but rather illustrates the partial overlap between the different disease definitions. (From Roehrborn CG. Pathology of benign prostatic hyperplasia. *Int J Impot Res* 2008;20[suppl 3]:S11-S18.)

LUTS symptoms are encompassed by the term *overactive bladder (OAB) syndrome*, which is defined as **urgency, frequency, nocturia, and urgency incontinence (irritative symptoms)**, and are believed to be correlated with an underlying detrusor over activity. These symptoms tend to be more bothersome, especially if they are associated with incontinence. **Storage (obstructive) symptoms include hesitancy, intermittent stream, straining to void, prolonged micturition, feeling of incomplete emptying, and dribbling**. LUTS (both irritative and obstructive) can also be associated with urinary infections or, more rarely, with other conditions, such as bladder stones, carcinoma, or carcinoma in situ in the bladder and must be differentiated.

Histopathologically, BPH is characterized by an increased number of epithelial and stromal cells in the periurethral area of the prostate. The precise molecular etiology of this hyperplastic process is uncertain. Androgens, estrogens, stromal-epithelial interactions, growth factors, and neurotransmitters may play a role, either singly or in combination, in the etiology of the hyperplastic process.

The pathophysiology of BPH is complex. Prostatic hyperplasia increases urethral resistance, resulting in compensatory changes in bladder function. However, the elevated detrusor pressure required to maintain urinary flow in the presence of increased outflow resistance occurs at the expense of normal bladder storage function. Obstruction-induced changes in detrusor function, compounded by age-related changes in both bladder and nervous system function, lead to urinary frequency, urgency, and nocturia, the most bothersome BPH-related complaints.

There is no globally accepted epidemiologic definition of BPH since the pathological manifestation and the clinical symptom complex poorly coincide in many men. The prevalence of BPH thus can either be calculated based on histologic criteria (autopsy prevalence) or clinical criteria (clinical prevalence). Numerous other demographic and environmental factors have been suggested as risk factors or contributors to the disease process, including religion, socioeconomics, sexual activity, vasectomy, alcohol use, liver disease, hypertension, smoking, and obesity.

As is true for prostate cancer, BPH occurs more often in the West compared with Eastern countries, such as Japan and China, and may be more common among blacks. Not long ago, a study found a possible genetic link for BPH in men younger than age 65 years who have a very enlarged prostate: Their male relatives were four times more likely than other men to need BPH surgery at some point in their lives, and their brothers had a six fold increase in risk.

CLINICAL MANIFESTATIONS

The presentation of LUTS is often that of BOO secondary to BPH. Symptoms may significantly and impair health-related quality of life and are classified as voiding (hesitancy, weak stream, straining, and prolonged voiding), storage (frequency, urgency, nocturia, urge incontinence, and voiding of small volumes), or postmicturition (post void dribble, incomplete emptying). Most men who have LUTS present with a combination of these symptoms. Although rare in the present day, some men present with urinary retention as the initial sign of BPH/LUTS, and this often heralds the need for surgical intervention.

The American Urological Association (AUA)/IPSS (International Prostate Symptom Score) (0–35) and associated bothersome index score (0–6) (Fig. 21.2) are routinely utilized and documented

International Prostate Symptom Score (I-PSS)

Patient name: _____ Date of birth: _____Date completed _____

In the past month:	Not at all	Less than 1 in 5 times	Less than half the time	About half the time	More than half the time	Almost always	Your score
1. Incomplete emptying How often have you had the sensation of not emptying your bladder?	0	1	2	3	4	5	
2.Frequency How often have you had to urinate less than every two hours?	0	1	2	3	4	5	
3. Intermittency How often have you found you stopped and started again several times when you urinated?	0	1	2	3	4	5	
4. Urgency How often have you found it difficult to postpone urination?	0	1	2	3	4	5	
5. Weak stream How often have you had a weak urinary stream?	0	1	2	3	4	5	
6. Straining How often have you had to strain to start urination?	0	1	2	3	4	5	
	None	**1 time**	**2 times**	**3 times**	**4 times**	**5 times**	
7. Nocturia How many times did you typically get up at night to urinate?	0	1	2	3	4	5	
Total I-PSS Score							

Score: 1–7: *Mild*   8–19: *Moderate*   20–35: *Severe*

Quality of Life Due to Urinary Symptoms	Delighted	Pleased	Mostly satisfied	Mixed	Mostly dissatisfied	Unhappy	Terrible
If you were to spend the rest of your life with your urinary condition just the way it is now, how would you feel about that?	0	1	2	3	4	5	6

FIG. 21.2 American Urological Association/International Prostate Symptom Score (IPSS).

into the medical record to gauge the degree of risk (low [0–7], moderate [8–19], or high [20–35]) and degree of bother related to the symptoms. This risk level can guide management (conservative, medical or surgical) and be used to gauge success of therapy or progression of disease.

> ## Key Points
>
> - The autopsy prevalence of benign prostatic hyperplasia (BPH) increases linearly starting at 40 years of age and is remarkably similar across cultures and ethnicities.
> - Cross-sectional studies suggest increases KEY in lower urinary tract symptoms (LUTS) severity, frequency, bother, and quality-of-life impairment with age that are fundamentally similar in all societies studied.
> - Analytical studies have failed to reveal significant risk factors for the development of BPH and LUTS.
> - The natural history of BPH in individual patients is highly variable and measured primarily by prostate volume growth
> - Inter individual variability is also noted in secondary physiologic measures such as urinary flow and residual urine, the development of complications, the risk for urinary retention and the need for surgery.
> - There are certain baseline factors allowing an assessment of risk for volume growth, progression, and risk for complications.

DIAGNOSIS AND TESTING

Physical examination and a complete history are an important first step in the basic workup of every patient complaining of LUTS and should not be neglected. Assessment should begin with a medical history and review of medications. The history should include questions related to any causes that may lead to bladder dysfunction, such as cerebrovascular disease, previous surgical procedures, and history of prostatic disease (inflammatory, benign, and cancer). Document onset and duration of symptoms, sexual history, and previously attempted treatment(s).

Medications, such as diuretics, and over-the-counter preparations, such as nasal decongestants and antihistamines, exacerbate urinary symptoms. Additionally, dietary factors such as water intake, caffeine, and alcohol use can contribute to the clinical manifestations of LUTS symptoms.

The exam should accurately assess the male pelvis, mostly to identify disorders potentially associated with LUTS. To this aim, examine the suprapubic area and palpate for a bladder; inspect the penis for evidence of a urethral stricture or phimosis and the scrotum and testicles. An elevated body mass index and signs suggestive for metabolic syndrome should be noted. In addition, the motor/sensory functions of the perineum and the lower limbs should be assessed to rule out neurologic alterations. As the last step of the physical assessment, a digital rectal examination should be performed to estimate volume and texture of the prostate.

Additionally, voiding charts and diaries can provide useful information. Urinalysis (dipstick and microscopic exam) is performed looking for blood, pyuria, and crystals. Urine cytology may be ordered if history of smoking indicates. Serum prostate-specific antigen (PSA) can be ordered to estimate prostate volume (PSA <1.6, >2, and >2.3 predicts prostate volume >40 cc for men in their 50s, 60s, and 70s, respectively) and need for further prostate cancer evaluation (if history of 5-α-reductase use PSA will be lower). Uroflowmetry (normal >15 cc/sec), postvoid residual measurement, (normal <30 cc - severe >300 cc), and pressure-flow studies may be ordered in select patients. Urodynamic studies are considered optional and best suited for patients who demonstrate LUTS in which the diagnosis of BOO is unclear.

Before surgical intervention, clinicians should consider assessment of prostate size and shape via abdominal or transrectal ultrasonography (TRUS) or cross-sectional imaging (i.e., magnetic resonance imaging [MRI] or computed tomography [CT]). Cystourethroscopy should be reserved for those with gross hematuria, history or suspicion of bladder cancer, recurrent severe urinary tract infection (UTI), crystals suggestive of bladder stone, or trauma.

Key Points

- Assessing symptom severity is the first step in the workup of patients with lower urinary tract symptoms.
- The prostate-specific antigen test should be considered for patients with a life expectancy longer than 10 years.
- Ultrasound imaging and uro-flow measurement should be considered for patients with moderate to severe symptoms.
- Invasive urodynamic tests should be considered if bladder motility alterations are suspected.

TREATMENT

LUTS should be carefully assessed according to diagnostic algorithms (Figs. 21.3 and 21.4) aimed to evaluate symptom severity and better understand the underlying pathologic condition. The clinical management is based on patients' symptoms and expectations; besides conservative strategies, medical therapy and surgical interventions all play a major role throughout treatment management for men with BPH/LUTS. Physicians should maintain a careful balance between the potential benefits (symptom relief) and harm (adverse events) associated with each treatment modality and discuss with the patients appropriately.

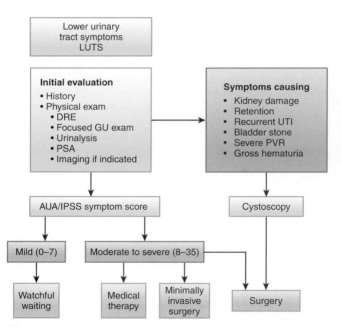

FIG. 21.3 Overview treatment management for lower urinary tract symptoms (LUTS). *AUA/IPSS,* American Urological Association/International Prostate Symptom Score; *DRE,* digital rectal exam; *GU,* genitourinary; *PSA,* prostate-specific antigen; *PVR,* postvoid residual; *UTI,* urinary tract infection.

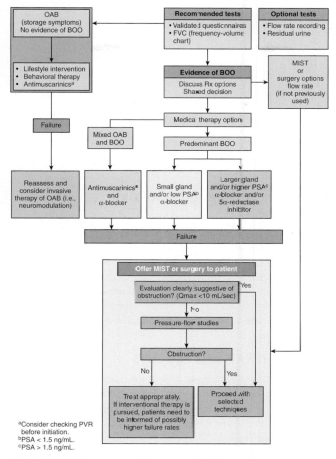

FIG. 21.4 Detailed management for persistent, bothersome lower urinary tract symptoms (LUTS) after basic management. *BOO,* Bladder outlet obstruction; *MIST,* minimally invasive surgical treatment; *OAB,* overactive bladder; *PSA,* prostate-specific antigen; *PVR,* postvoid residual; *Rx,* treatment. (Modified from Campbell-Walsh-Wein Chapter 146 Figure 2.)

RELATIONSHIP OF BENEFIT TO HARM

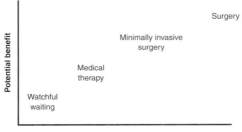

WATCHFUL WAITING OR CONSERVATIVE MANAGEMENT

Conservative management is the preferred approach for patients with mild symptoms (IPSS 0–7) and without complicating factors. Watchful waiting is based on patient education, lifestyle interventions, and disease monitoring. Lifestyle modifications include proper daily fluid intake; tea, caffeine, and alcohol avoidance or restriction; and concurrent medication adjustment. Patients should be followed up yearly to detect worsening of symptoms or the occurrence of complications.

MEDICAL TREATMENT FOR LUTS

Medical therapy plays a major role in the management of patients with LUTS. **The current drug armamentarium** (Table 21.1) **includes** α-adrenergic blockers (α1-blockers), 5-α reductase

Key Points

- Conservative management is the preferred approach for patients with mild symptoms and without complicating factors.
- Watchful waiting is based on patient education, lifestyle interventions, and disease monitoring.
- Lifestyle modifications include proper daily fluid intake; tea, caffeine, and alcohol avoidance or restriction; and concurrent medication adjustment.
- Patients should be followed up early to detect worsening of symptoms or the occurrence of complications.

Table 21.1 Minimally Invasive and Surgical Options for Treatment of Lower Urinary Tract Symptoms

ANTIMUSCARINIC DRUGS	AVAILABLE FORMULATION	RECOMMENDED DAILY DOSE
Darifenacin ER	7.5-, 15-mg capsule	1 × day
Fesoterodine ER	4-, 8-mg capsule	1 × day
Oxybutynin ER	5-, 10-, 15-mg[b] capsule	1 × day (up to 20 mg/day)
Oxybutynin IR	2.5-, 5-mg[a] capsule	3–4 × day (max, 20 mg/day)
Propiverine ER (no US)	30-mg capsule	1 × day
Propiverine (no US)	15-mg capsule	2–3 × day
Solifenacin	5-, 10-mg capsule	1 × day
Tolterodine IR	1-, 2-mg capsule	2 × day
Tolterodine ER	2-mg[b], 4-mg capsule	1 × day
		1 × day
Trospium IR	20-mg capsule	2 × day
Trospium ER	60-mg capsule	1 × day
β3 Agonist		
Mirabegron	25-mg capsule	1 × day

CLASS OF α-BLOCKERS	AVAILABLE FORMULATION	RECOMMENDED DAILY DOSE	RECOMMENDED ADMINISTRATION
Nonselective			
Terazosin	1[d], 2, 5, 10[d] mg capsule	5 or 10 mg qi	Initial dose is 1 mg at bedtime. The dose should be titrated up to 5 or 10 mg.
Doxazosin IR	1-, 2-, 4-mg capsule	2–8 mg qd	Initial dose is 2 mg at bedtime. The dose should be titrated up to 4 or 8 mg.
Doxazosin SR	4-, 8-mg capsule	4 or 8 mg qd	Initial dose is 4 mg after breakfast, eventually increased to 8 mg.
Uroselective			
Alfuzosin ER[b]	10-mg capsule	10 mg qd	Initial dose is 10 mg with the same meal each day.
Tamsulosin	0.4, 0.8[d] mg capsule	0.4–0.8 mg qd	Initial dose is 0.4 mg with the same meal each day.
Silodosin	4-, 8-mg capsule	8 mg qd	Initial dose is 8 mg with the same meal each day.

Continued

Table 21.1 Minimally Invasive and Surgical Options for Treatment of Lower Urinary Tract Symptoms—cont'd

FIVE α-REDUCTASE INHIBITORS	RECOMMENDED DAILY DOSAGE	COMMENTS
Finasteride	5 mg qd. Treatment is recommended for at least 6 months	• PSA levels decrease by approximately 50% • Finasteride is not indicated for PCa prevention -increased risk for high-risk disease • Patients should be warned regarding risk for sexual dysfunction and depression
Dutasteride	0.5 mg qd. Treatment is recommended for at least 6 months	• PSA levels decrease by approximately 50% • Dutasteride is not indicated for PCa prevention because of an observed increased risk for high-risk disease • Patients should be warned regarding risk for sexual dysfunction and depression

inhibitors (5-ARIs), antimuscarinic drugs, phosphodiesterase type 5 inhibitors (PDE5Is), β3-agonists, and numerous plant extracts (not listed). Of note, different combinations of medical compounds (α-blocker + 5-α-reductase inhibitor) also play a relevant role in the management of LUTS (Fig. 21.5).

5-ARIs block conversion of testosterone to dihydrotestosterone by inhibiting type I and/or type II 5-α reductase. Finasteride inhibits type II 5-α reductase, whereas dutasteride inhibits types I and II 5-α reductase. Use of 5-ARIs may result in prostate volume reduction of 25%. It important to note that a decrease in serum PSA of ~50% will be noted after 1 year and has been shown to continue with time thus interfering with use of PSA for prostate cancer screening. For men with enlarged prostates (e.g., >50 g), 5-ARI use has been demonstrated to lower risk of acute urinary retention (AUR), improve symptoms, increase flow rate, and decrease the risk of surgery. Side effects include decreased libido, ejaculatory dysfunction (volume), impotence, and gynecomastia (rare).

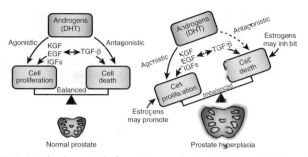

FIG. 21.5 Molecular control of prostate growth. Prostate hyperplasia is most likely due to an imbalance between cell proliferation and cell death. Androgens play a necessary but probably permissive role. Growth factors are more likely to be sites of primary defects.

Alpha-blockers relieve LUTS by reducing smooth muscle tone and have been demonstrated to markedly improve AUA/IPSS symptom scores and both irritative and obstructive symptoms, as well as quality of life. Urinary flow rates often increase. Alpha-blockers provide little or no reduction in the risk of AUR or risk of requiring minimally invasive surgical treatments (MISTs) or surgery. Side effects include dizziness, tired felling, orthostasis, congestion, and retrograde ejaculation.

Combination Therapy – Treatment of LUTS with a combination of the α-blockers and 5-ARI medications is common in clinical practice. Clinical trials have shown α-blocker and 5-ARI treatment to be synergistic for men.

PDE5-Is are known to be effective in the treatment of erectile dysfunction and have been found to improve BPH symptom in clinical studies. Although daily use of these medications is expensive, men with concomitant erectile dysfunction may derive benefit from PDE5-I treatment for their LUTS as well.

Supplements – Numerous alternatives to traditional pharmaceutical medical therapies have been proposed for the treatment of LUTS, including saw palmetto, stinging nettle, pumpkin seed, and African star grass. None of these supplements has demonstrated a significant benefit for patients with BPH.

If watchful waiting and medical management prove ineffective in a man who is unable to withstand the rigors of a surgery, urethral obstruction and incontinence may be managed by intermittent catheterization or an indwelling Foley. The catheter can stay in place indefinitely (in which case, it is usually changed regularly).

The gold standard surgical treatment for LUTS/BPH has been for decades, trans-urethral resection of the prostate (TURP; Figs. 21.6 and 21.7). A less extensive transurethral approach for smaller glands; transurethral incision of the prostate (TUIP) addresses a high riding bladder

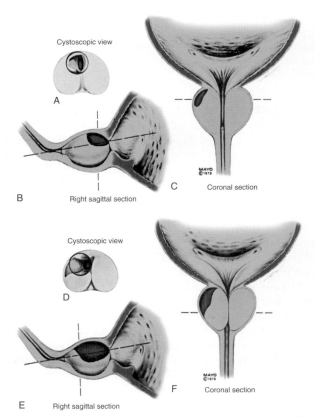

FIG. 21.6 Approach to transurethral resection of the prostate by starting the resection anteriorly. (A to C) First stage of resection of the prostate. The resection is begun at the 12 o'clock position, and the tissue at the bladder neck and the adjacent adenoma are resected in quadrants. (D) The midportion of the gland is resected starting at the 12 o'clock position and carried down to the 9 o'clock position. (E and F) Sagittal and coronal sections.

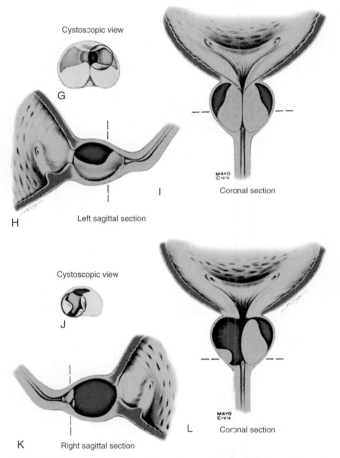

Cystoscopic view

G

Left sagittal section

H

I

MAYO
©1978

Coronal section

Cystoscopic view

J

Right sagittal section

K

L

MAYO
©1978

Coronal section

FIG. 21.6, cont'd (G) The resection is now begun at the 12 o'clock position, and the left side of the patient's gland in the midfossa is resected down to the 3 o'clock position. (H and I) Sagittal and coronal sections. (J) The midportion of the gland is resected farther down from the 9 o'clock position to the 6 o'clock position. (K and L) Sagittal views.

Continued

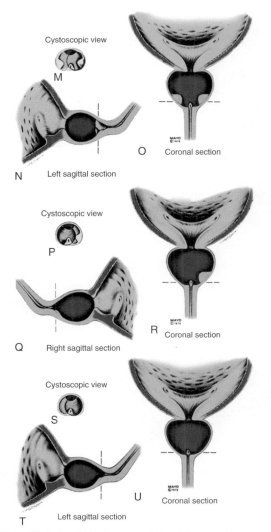

FIG. 21.6, cont'd (M to O) The tissue remaining at the apex is now resected. Resection is initiated next to the verumontanum and carried toward the 12 o'clock position. (P to R) Residual tissue is carefully cleared on the patient's right side. (S to U) The remaining residual tissue is cleared from the patient's left side, leaving an unobstructed view from the verumontanum through the bladder neck into the bladder. (©1978, the Mayo Foundation.)

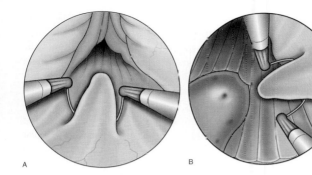

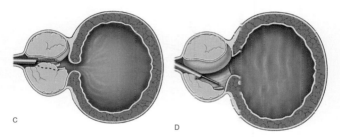

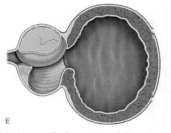

FIG. 21.7 Approach to transurethral resection of the prostate starting with the prostate floor. (A) View from resectoscope with an electrosurgical loop resecting prostate floor. (B) Resecting a lateral lobe. (C) Sagittal view of resection of the prostate floor. (D) Continuing resection down to the capsule. (E) Completed resection of this section of prostate, leaving some residual apical tissue to avoid injury to the external sphincter. (Modified from May F, Hartung R. Surgical atlas: transurethral resection of the prostate. *BJU Int* 2006;98(4):921-934.)

neck and primarily irritative symptoms (Fig. 21.8). The MIST and more invasive surgical treatment options (simple open and robotic) have greatly expanded over the past three decades. Newer minimally invasive procedures include (to name a few) Urolift (Figs. 21.9 and 21.10), visual laser ablation of the prostate, transurethral electro-vaporization (TVP) (Figs. 21.11 to 21.14) of the prostate, transurethral needle ablation (TUNA) (Figs. 21.15 to 21.17), transurethral microwave thermotherapy (TUMT) (Figs. 21.18), interstitial laser coagulation, bipolar transurethral resection of the prostate (bipolar

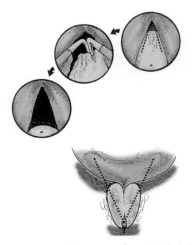

FIG. 21.8 Transurethral incision of the prostate. The incision is started at the ureteral orifice and carried through the bladder neck up to the verumontanum. This procedure is done bilaterally. (From Mebust WK. A review of TURP complications and the National Cooperative Study. Lesson 24, volume 8. *AUA Update Series* 1989;189190.)

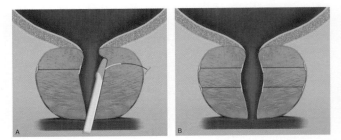

FIG. 21.9 (A and B) Placement of Urolift devices. (Courtesy of NeoTract, Inc.)

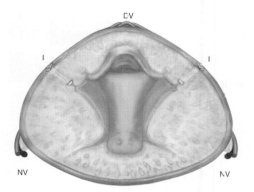

FIG. 21.10 Placement of implants (I) in the anterolateral position in the prostate between the dorsal veins (DV) and neurovascular bundles (NV). (Courtesy of NeoTract, Inc.)

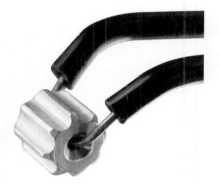

FIG. 21.11 VaporTrode electrode. (Courtesy of Olympus, Inc.)

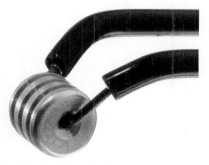

FIG. 21.12 Fluted electrode. (Courtesy of Olympus, Inc.)

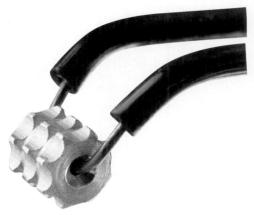

FIG. 21.13 Spiked electrode. (Courtesy of Olympus, Inc.)

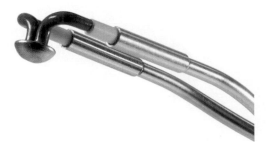

FIG. 21.14 PlasmaButton electrode. (Courtesy of Olympus, Inc.)

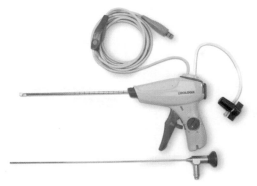

FIG. 21.15 Transurethral needle ablation handpiece. (Courtesy of Urologix, Inc.)

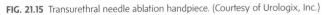

TURP), and transurethral incision of the prostate. These approaches are usually reserved for men with moderate symptoms and a small- to medium-sized (up to 75 g) prostate gland. For larger prostate glands, open (Figs. 21.19 to 21.30) and robotic-assisted simple prostatectomy has been frequently performed. Lately, holmium laser enucleation of the prostate (HoLEP) with the holmium:yttrium-aluminum-garnet

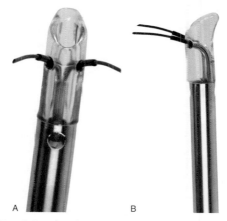

A   B

FIG. 21.16 (A and B) Deployed transurethral needle ablation needles. (Courtesy of Urologix, Inc.)

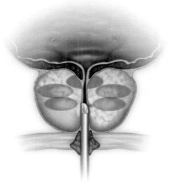

FIG. 21.17 The treated prostate in transurethral needle ablation. (Courtesy of Kevin T. McVary.)

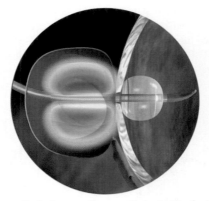

FIG. 21.18 Transurethral microwave therapy catheter treating the transition zone of the prostate. (Courtesy of Kevin T. McVary.)

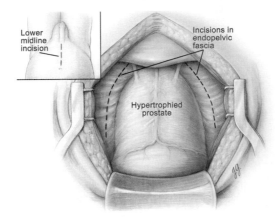

FIG. 21.19 Retropubic simple prostatectomy. The space of Retzius has been opened, and the periprostatic adipose tissue has been dissected free from the superficial branch of the dorsal vein complex. The endopelvic fascia is incised bilaterally *(dotted lines)*, and the puboprostatic ligaments are transected bilaterally. (© Brady Urological Institute.)

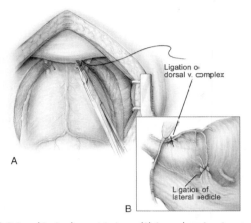

FIG. 21.20 Retropubic simple prostatectomy. (A) A 2-0 chromic suture on a -inch circle-tapered needle is passed in the avascular plane between the urethra and the dorsal vein complex at the apex of the prostate. A tie is grasped and tied around the dorsal vein complex. (B) With 2-0 chromic suture material on a CTX needle, a figure-of-8 suture is placed through the prostatovesicular junction just above the level of the seminal vesicles to control the main arterial blood supply to the prostate gland. When placing this suture, care must be taken to avoid entrapment of the neurovascular bundles located posteriorly and slightly laterally. (© Bracy Urological Institute.)

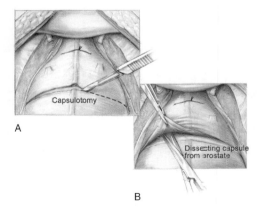

FIG. 21.21 Retropubic simple prostatectomy. (A) With the superficial branch of the dorsal vein complex secured proximally and distally, a no. 15 blade on a long handle is used to make the transverse capsulotomy. (B) Metzenbaum scissors are used to develop the plane anteriorly between the prostatic adenoma and the prostatic pseudocapsule. (© Brady Urological Institute.)

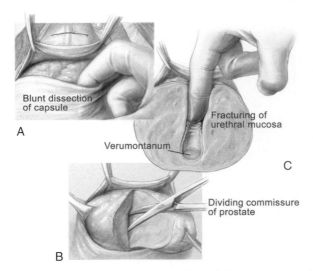

FIG. 21.22 Retropubic simple prostatectomy. (A) With blunt dissection with the index finger, the prostatic adenoma is dissected free laterally and posteriorly. (B) Metzenbaum scissors are used to divide the anterior commissure to visualize the posterior urethra and verumontanum. (C) The index finger is then used to fracture the urethral mucosa at the level of the verumontanum. With this last maneuver, extreme care is taken not to injure the external sphincteric mechanism. (© Brady Urological Institute.)

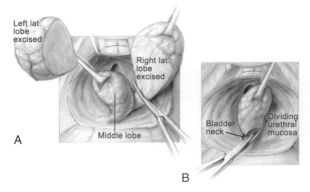

FIG. 21.23 Retropubic simple prostatectomy. (A) After removal of the left lateral lobe of the prostate, the right lateral lobe is excised with the aid of a tenaculum and Metzenbaum scissors. (B) Finally, the median lobe is removed under direct vision. (© Brady Urological Institute.)

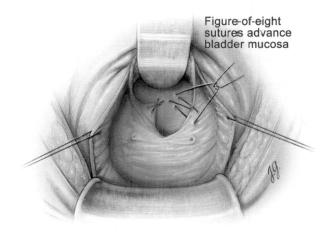

FIG. 21.24 Hemostatic maneuver during open simple prostatectomy. After enucle-ation of the entire prostatic adenoma, a o-chromic suture is used to place two figure-of-8 sutures to advance bladder mucosa into the prostatic fossa at the 5-o'clock and 7-o'clock positions at the prostatovesicular junction to ensure control of the main arterial blood supply to the prostate. (© Brady Urological Institute.)

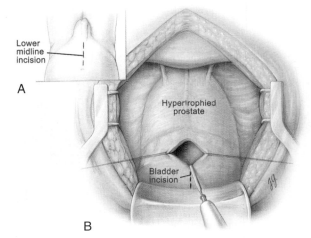

FIG. 21.25 Suprapubic simple prostatectomy. (A) A lower midline incision is made from the umbilicus to the pubic symphysis (B) After developing the prevesical space, a small, longitudinal cystotomy is made with electrocautery. (© Brady Urological Institute.)

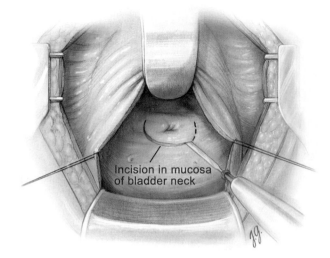

FIG. 21.26 Suprapubic simple prostatectomy. With adequate exposure of the bladder neck, a circular incision in the bladder mucosa is made distal to the trigone using electrocautery. (© Brady Urological Institute.)

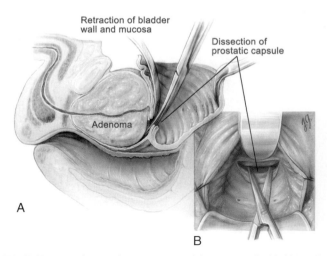

FIG. 21.27 Suprapubic simple prostatectomy. (A) Starting at the bladder neck posteriorly, Metzenbaum scissors are used to develop the plane between the prostatic adenoma and the prostatic pseudocapsule (lateral view). (B) Anterior view of the same maneuver. (© Brady Urological Institute.)

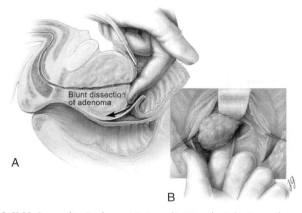

FIG. 21.28 Suprapubic simple prostatectomy. (A) Using the index finger, the prostatic adenoma is enucleated from the prostatic fossa (lateral view). (B) Anterior view of the same maneuver. With extremely large prostate glands, the left, right, and median lobes should be removed separately. (© Brady Urological Institute.)

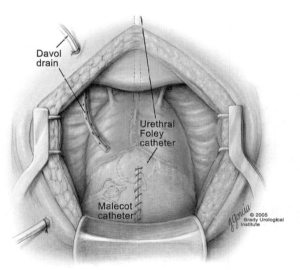

FIG. 21.29 Closure during suprapubic simple prostatectomy. After placement of a urethral catheter and a Malecot suprapubic tube, the cystotomy is closed in two layers using a running 2-0 Vicryl suture, enforced by tying multiple interrupted 3-0 Vicryl stay sutures. A closed Davol suction drain is placed on one side of the bladder and exits via a separate stab incision. (© Brady Urological Institute.)

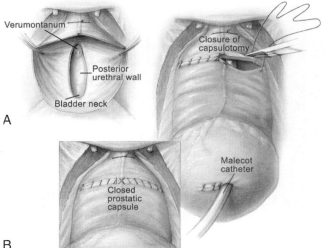

FIG. 21.30 Closure during retropubic simple prostatectomy. (A) View of the prostatic fossa and posterior urethra after enucleation of all the prostatic adenoma. Note that the verumontanum and a strip of posterior urethra remain intact. (B) After placement of a urethral catheter and, if needed, a Malecot suprapubic tube, the transverse capsulotomy is closed with two running 2-0 chromic sutures. The two sutures are tied first to themselves and then to each other across the midline to create a watertight closure of the prostatic pseudocapsule. (© Brady Urological Institute.)

(Ho:YAG) laser has been performed as a minimally invasive alternative to open surgery. However, the learning curve with HoLEP is steep. Table 21.2 lists the commonly used MIST and simple prostatectomy procedures with some associated comments.

PROGNOSIS

Over a variable period, sometimes months to years, the symptoms of BPH/LUTS often increase, requiring adding/changing medications, a MIST or more invasive surgical procedure. Patients should be counseled about the likelihood of progression, the natural history of LUTS related to BPH, and the treatment options that can be offered. Regular office visits (6–12 months) can help monitor progression and need for changing therapies.

Table 21.2 Minimally Invasive and Surgical Options for Treatment of Moderate to Severe Lower Urinary Tract Symptoms

TECHNIQUE	COMMENT	EVIDENCE LEVEL
• TURP (monopolar)	• Requires nonionic irrigant (glycine or sorbitol)	B
	• TUR syndrome serious risk (Box 21.1): hyperosmolar dilutional hypernatremia	
	• BNC, 2%	
	• Urethral stricture, 4%	
	• General anesthesia	
	• LOS, 0–2 days	
	• Catheterization, 1–3 days	
	• Retrograde ejaculation ~70%	
	• ED not common	
	• Incontinence, 0%–5%	
	• AUR, 5%–7%	
TURP (bipolar)	• Can use saline for irrigant	B
	• In general somewhat lower complication rates; presently preferred method	
Prostatic urethral lift (PUL) - Urolift	• Trans prostatic implant sutures delivered by a handheld device through a cystoscope to mechanically open the prostatic urethra by compressing prostate	C
	• Minimizes impact of ED and ejaculatory dysfunction	
	• Minimal learning curve	

Continued

Table 21.2 Minimally Invasive and Surgical Options for Treatment of Moderate to Severe Lower Urinary Tract Symptoms—cont'd

TECHNIQUE	COMMENT	EVIDENCE LEVEL
Convection radiofrequency (RF) REZUM	• Transurethral water vaporization injection (>100°C) • Minimal complications	C
Transurethral electro-vaporization of prostate: Vaportrode	• Current vaporization of prostate tissue • Both mono- and bipolar • Not routinely performed since early 2000s • Similar complications to TURP	B
Transurethral microwave therapy (TUMT)	• Transurethral thermo ablation (>65°C) (microwave) of prostate tissue • Tolerated under local anesthesia • Retreatment rates greater than TURP • BNC, 2% • Incontinence, 2% • Retention, 12% • UTI, 13% • ED <5%	C
Transurethral needle ablation (TUNA)	• Ejaculatory dysfunction >40% • Tolerated under local anesthesia • 3- to 7-day catheterization • Retreatment rate >TRUP • Irritative voiding symptoms, 7%–25% • UTI, 14% • ED, 6% • Ejaculatory dysfunction, 54%	NOT RECOMMENDED EXPERT OPINION

Transurethral incision of prostate (TUIP)	• Better for small (<50-g) prostates • "High-riding" bladder neck • IPSS scores high with smaller prostates • Complication rates <TURP	B
Laser: holmium: YAG (HOLEP)	• Laser light vaporization of the prostate • Laser safety important • Large gland enucleation • Requires morcillation • Long learning curve • Transfusion rate <2% • Incontinence <1% • BNC, 0%–3% • Ejaculatory dysfunction 70%–80%	B
Laser: KTP, LBO (GREENLIGHT), Nd: YAG, VLAP, PVP	• Better hemostasis than HOLEP and TURP • Can use for patients on anticoagulants • Minimal or no TUR syndrome • Irritative voiding symptoms (0%–30%) • UTI, 1%–2%; epididymitis, 5% • Long-term ED minimal	B

Continued

Table 21.2 Minimally Invasive and Surgical Options for Treatment of Moderate to Severe Lower Urinary Tract Symptoms—cont'd

TECHNIQUE	COMMENT	EVIDENCE LEVEL
Laser: thallium aquablation (Aquabeam™): hydrodissection	• Continuous as opposed to pulsed laser • Robotically controlled handpiece • High-velocity saline water jet • Requires general anesthesia	B C
Prostate embolization	• Selective embolization of prostatic arteries • Alcohol or microspheres • Complications: pain or fever, 0%–20% • Technically challenging • Performed by interventional radiology	EXPERT OPINION
Simple prostatectomy: open, laparoscopic, robotic	• Option for larger (75-g) prostates • General anesthesia • Catheter, 3–7 days • LOS, 1–3 days • ED, 3%–5% • Ejaculatory dysfunction, 90% • BNC, 2%–5%	C

[a]Level of evidence strength ratings: A, high; B, moderate; C, low. See https://www.auanet.org/guidelines/benign-prostatic-hyperplasia-(bph)-guideline. *AUR,* Acute urinary retention; *BNC,* bladder neck contracture; *ED,* erectile dysfunction; *HOLEP,* holmium laser enucleation of the prostate; *LOS,* length of stay; *TUR,* transurethral; *UTI,* urinary tract infection.

Box 21.1 TUR Syndrome

- Hyperosmolar fluid absorption
- Use of Ionic irrigate (glycine or sorbitol)
- Hyponatremia (<120 mmol/L)
- **Symptoms**
  - EKG changes
  - Fatigue
  - Vomiting
  - Confusion
  - Visual changes
  - Coma
- **Diagnosis**
  - Glasgow Coma Scale score
  - Measure sodium and potassium (STAT)
- **Treatment**
  - Supportive
  - Monitored bed
  - Oxygen: high flow
  - Intravenous hypertonic (3%) saline <100 cc/hr
  - Diuretics
  - Raise Na by 1 mmol/L per hour

Suggested Readings

Abrams P, Cardozo L, Fall M, et al. The standardization of terminology in lower urinary tract function: report from the standardization sub-committee of the International Continence Society. *Urology* 2003;61(1):37-49.

American Urological Association. Guideline: management of benign prostatic hypertrophy (BPH). 2010. http://www.auanet.org/guidelines/benign-prostatichyperplasia

Cornu JN, Ahyai S, Bachmann A, et al. A systematic review and meta-analysis of functional outcomes and complications following transurethral procedures for lower urinary tract symptoms resulting from benign prostatic obstruction: an update. *Eur Urol* 2015;67(6):1066-1096.

Foster HE, Barry MJ, Dahm P, et al. Surgical management of lower urinary tract symptoms attributed to benign prostatic hyperplasia: AUA guideline.

Issa MM. Technological advances in transurethral resection of the prostate: bipolar versus monopolar TURP. *J Endourol* 2008;22(8):1587-1595.

Kim EH, Larson JA, Andriole GL, et al. Management of benign prostatic hypertrophy. *Annu Rev Med* 2016;67:137-151.

Sotelo R, Clavijo R, Carmona O, et al. Robotic simple prostatectomy. *J Urol* 2008;179(2):513-515.

22

Prostate Cancer

SAMUEL WASHINGTON III, ALAN W. PARTIN
AND KIRSTEN L. GREENE

CONTRIBUTORS OF CAMPBELL-WALSH-WEIN, 12TH EDITION

Samuel L. Washington Iii, Andrew J. Stephenson, Robert Abouassaly, Eric A. Klein, Simpa S. Salami, Ganesh S. Palapattu, Alan W. Partin, Todd M. Morgan, Edouard J. Trabulsi, Ethan J. Halpern, Leonard G. Gomella, Onathan I. Epstein, Stacy Loeb, James A. Eastham, Samir S. Taneja, Marc A. Bjurlin, Laurence Klotz, Edward M. Schaeffer, Herbert Lepor, Li-Ming Su, Brandon J. Otto, Anthony J. Costello, Ryan Phillips, Sarah Hazell, Daniel Y. Song, Kae Jack Tay, Thomas J. Polascik, Maxwell V. Meng, Peter R. Carroll, Eugene K. Lee, J. Brantley Thrasher, Scott Eggener, Emmanuel S. Antonarakis, and Michael A. Carducci

PROSTATE CANCER INCIDENCE AND MORTALITY

- Most common noncutaneous malignancy in US men: 191,930 cases per year.
- Second most common cause of cancer death in the United States: 33,330 per year.
- Globally second most common cancer, fifth leading cause of cancer deaths.
- Age-adjusted incidence rate 104.1 per 100,000 men per year.

RACIAL DISPARITIES IN PROSTATE CANCER

- African American men have a 76% higher incidence and 60% higher cancer-specific mortality rate than white men.
- The incidence of prostate cancer in other ethnic groups is lower than that of whites and African Americans (Table 22.1)
- Differences in treatment patterns explain nearly half (48%) of the cancer-specific survival disparity after adjustments for

Table 22.1 Prostate Cancer Incidence and Mortality by Race/Ethnicity, United States, 2009–2013

	INCIDENCE[a]	MORTALITY RATE[a]
White	114.8	18.7
African American	198.4	42.8
Hispanic/Latino	104.9	16.5
Asian American and Pacific Islander	63.5	8.8
American Indian and Alaska Native	85.1	19.4

[a]Per 100,000, age adjusted to the 2000 US standard population.

demographics, tumor characteristics, and socioeconomic factors.

SCREENING CONTROVERSY, INCIDENCE, AND MORTALITY

- Screening is recommended by the American Urological Association (AUA) guidelines for men between 55 and 69 years of age who have at least a 10-year life expectancy and who wish to be screened.
- Shared decision making about whether to screen for prostate cancer is recommended uniformly.
- Prostate-specific antigen (PSA) and digital rectal exam (DRE) and used to screen for prostate cancer.
- PSA levels may be affected by age, gland size, infection/inflammation, medications such as 5-α reductase inhibitors, recent diagnostic procedures, and prostate-directed treatments.

Trials

The US Prostate, Lung, Colorectal, and Ovarian (PLCO) cancer screening trial found no difference in prostate cancer mortality between the screening and control groups through 15 years of follow-up. Concerns surrounding high rates of contamination, with an estimated 90% of patients in the control arm having received at least one PSA before or during the trial, question whether the trial actually compared annual screening versus none or whether it has been more accurately described as a comparison of organized screening versus opportunistic screening.

The European Randomized Study of Screening for Prostate Cancer (ERSPC) compared randomized between PSA screening every 4 years or no screening and men in the screening arm had a 57% (95% confidence interval [CI], 51–62) increased incidence of prostate cancer compared with controls and a 21% (95% CI, 9–31) relative reduction in death from prostate cancer (4.3 vs. 5.4 cancer deaths per 10,000 person-years) after a median follow-up of 13 years.

Soon after publication of the PLCO and ERSPC, the US Preventive Services Task Force (USPSTF) in 2012 recommended against routine PSA but later in April 2017 partially reversed its course and submitted new draft recommendations, giving a grade of C to prostate cancer screening in men 55–69 years of age (offered for selected patients) but keeping the grade of D for men 70 years of age and older (discouraging its use) at least partially in response to modeling studies suggesting an estimated 46%–57% increase in metastatic cases at presentation, leading to as much as a 20% increase in prostate cancer deaths.

RISK FACTORS AND CHEMOPREVENTION

- **Familial** – Relative risk increases according to the number of affected family members, their degree of relatedness, and the age at which they were affected (Table 22.2)
- **BRCA-Associated Cancers** – Especially BRCA2, more likely to present with higher-grade, locally advanced, and metastatic disease and have poorer cancer-specific and metastasis-free survival after prostatectomy.
- **Diet** – No clear association between dietary fat intake and prostate cancer risk.
- **Obesity** – Associated with higher rates of biochemical failure after treatment and 15%–20% increase per 5 kg/m^2

Table 22.2 Family History and Risk for Prostate Cancer

FAMILY HISTORY	RELATIVE RISK	95% CONFIDENCE INTERVAL
Father affected at any age	2.35	2.02–2.72
Brother(s) affected at any age	3.14	2.37–4.15
One affected first-degree relative diagnosed at any age	2.48	2.25–2.74
Affected first-degree relatives diagnosed <65 years	2.87	2.21–3.74
Affected first-degree relatives diagnosed ≥65 years	1.92	1.49–2.47
Second-degree relatives diagnosed at any age	2.52	0.99–6.46
Two or more affected first-degree relatives diagnosed at any age	4.39	2.61–7.39

increase in body mass index (BMI) in prostate-specific cancer mortality.

- **The Selenium and Vitamin E Cancer Prevention (SELECT) Trial** – A randomized, placebo-controlled, population-based primary chemoprevention trial designed to test the efficacy of selenium and vitamin E alone and in combination in the prevention of prostate cancer, demonstrated no effect on the risk for prostate cancer by either agent alone or in combination.
- **Finasteride** – The Prostate Cancer Prevention Trial (PCPT) showed a 25% reduction in the period prevalence of prostate cancer in men taking finasteride (18.4%) compared with placebo (24.4%) across all groups as defined by age, ethnicity, family history of prostate cancer, and PSA at study entry. However, a significant increase in the prevalence biopsy Gleason score 7 to 10 cancers was observed in men receiving finasteride (280 [37%]) compared with placebo (237 [22%]), particularly for biopsy Gleason score 8 to 10 cancers. In a secondary analysis of PCPT that adjusted for the effects of finasteride on the detection of prostate cancer, the adjusted prostate cancer rates were estimated to be 21.1% for the placebo group and 14.7% in the finasteride group, a 30% risk reduction for all cancers (hazard ratio [HR], 0.70; 95% CI, 0.64–0.76) and a nonstatistically significant 14% increase in high-grade cancer. Accounting for the increased probability of upgrading to pathologic Gleason 7 to 10 cancer at radical prostatectomy among men with biopsy Gleason 2 to 6 cancers in the placebo arm, the investigators estimated the rate of true high-grade cancer to be 6% in the finasteride arm and 8.2% in the placebo arm, representing a 27% relative risk reduction in the rate of true high-grade cancers in men treated with finasteride (HR, 0.73; 95% CI, 0.56–0.96).
- **Reduction by Dutasteride of Prostate Cancer Events (REDUCE) Trial** – Randomized, placebo-controlled primary chemoprevention trial using dutasteride, which reduced the risk for prostate cancer over 4 years by 23%.

PROSTATE CANCER BIOMARKERS

- **PSA Isoforms** – Free PSA, pro PSA, human kallikrein, mRNA, and *TMPRSS2:ERG* fusion products have been measured and integrated into commercially available serum and urine tests for additional prognostication and decision making prior to biopsy (Figs. 22.1 to 22.4)

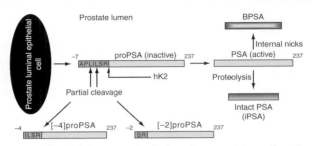

FIG. 22.1 Differential cleavage and activation of pro–prostate-specific antigen (PSA). ProPSA is released from the prostate epithelial cell with a 7–amino acid leader sequence. hK2 cleaves the amino acid leader to activate PSA. Active PSA undergoes proteolysis to yield inactive PSA (iPSA) and may also undergo internal degradation to form benign PSA (BPSA). Partial cleavage of the 7–amino acid leader sequence yields inactive forms of proPSA (i.e., [–2]pPSA or [–4]pPSA).

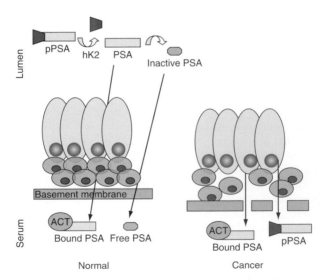

FIG. 22.2 Prostate-specific antigen (PSA) synthesis in normal versus cancer tissue. ProPSA is secreted into the lumen, where the 7–amino acid leader sequence is cleaved by hK2 to yield active PSA. Some of the active PSA diffuses into the serum, where it is bound to proteases such as α_1-antichymotrypsin (ACT). The luminal active PSA undergoes proteolysis, and the resulting inactive PSA (iPSA) may also enter the circulation to circulate in the unbound or free state. In prostate cancer, loss of the tissue architecture may permit a relative increase in bound PSA and proPSA in serum.

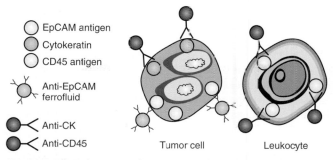

FIG. 22.3 CellSearch CTC: Circulating Tumor Cell (Veridex) cell enumeration system. *CD45*, CD stands for *cluster of differentiation*, which was originally called *leukocyte common antigen*. The anti-EpCAM ferrofluid captures the cells, and they are then validated with cytokeratin-positive and CD45-negative staining. *CK*, Cytokeratin; *EpCAM*, epithelial cell adhesion molecule.

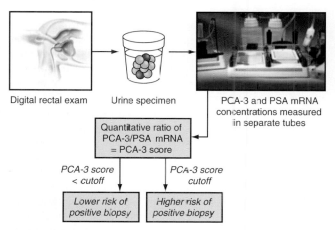

FIG. 22.4 PCA3 assay protocol. After "attentive" digital rectal exam, urine is collected. RT-PCR determines the mRNA levels for PCA3 and PSA. The ratio between PCA3/PSA determines the PCA3 score. Prostate cancer risk level suggests need for biopsy. (From Groskopf J, Aubin SM, Deras IL, et al. APTIMA PCA3 molecular urine test: development of a method to aid in the diagnosis of prostate cancer. *Clin Chem* 2006;52:1089-1095.)

- PSA density (defined as the PSA value divided by the prostate gland size) predicts reclassification on surveillance biopsy.

GENOMICS

- **Most Frequent Genomic Alterations** – Fusions of androgen-regulated promoters with ERG and other ETS-family transcription factors, accounting for 53% of the cases.
- *PTEN* deletions in *ERG* fusion–positive cases and that tumors with *SPOP* mutations (accounting for ≈10% of cases).
- **Most Common Fusion** – *TMPRSS2* or other promoters (*SLC45A3* and *NDRG*) fused to *ERG* (ETS-related gene) in 50%–60% of patients.
- Data are mixed on whether the presence of *TMPRSS2:ERG* fusions affect prognosis.

PROSTATE BIOPSY

Organizations such as the AUA recommend shared decision making for men 55–69 years of age considering PSA-based screening, a target age group for whom benefits may outweigh harms. Most organizations are relying increasingly on risk stratification approaches and changes in PSA level over time. The National Comprehensive Cancer Network (NCCN) advocates the selective use of biomarkers, including PSA derivatives, tissue assays of stromal hypermethylation (Confirm MDx), as well as urinary assays for ERG (MiPS, ExoDx) and PCA3 in the decision to perform TRUS biopsy.

- Significant coagulopathy, severe immunosuppression, and acute prostatitis are all contraindications to prostate biopsy.
- Antibiotic choice for prophylaxis is best guided by knowledge of local antibiotic resistance patterns. Refer to recent AUA guidelines on antimicrobial prophylaxis for more detail.
- Extended 12-core systematic biopsy incorporating apical and far-lateral cores in the template distribution allows maximal cancer detection and avoidance of a repeat biopsy while minimizing the detection of insignificant prostate cancers.
- Fewer than 12 cores constitutes undersampling and an inadequate biopsy.

Risks and Complications of Biopsy

- Bleeding is the most common complication seen after prostate biopsy. Hematuria, hematochezia, and hematospermia should be expected.

Infection				5–7%
	Hospitalization			1–3%
Bleeding				
	Hematuria			50%
		Needs intervention		<1%
	Rectal bleeding			30%
		Needs intervention		2.5%
	Hematospermia			50%
		Prolonged (>4 weeks)		30%
Other				
	LUTS	Transient	(~1 month)	6–25%
	Urinary retention			0.2 –2.6%
	ED	Transient	(~1 month)	<1%

FIG. 22.5 AUA White Paper: The prevention and treatment of the more common complications related to prostate biopsy update. https://www.auanet.org/guidelines/prostate-needle-biopsy-complications.

- Urinary retention is a rare occurrence.
- Infection ranging from cystitis and orchitis to sepsis is the most serious side effect of biopsy and antibiotic prophylaxis and early identification and treatment of postbiopsy infection is critical.
- The AUA white paper on the prevention and treatment of common biopsy complications provides details on the frequency of complications (Fig. 22.5).

PATHOLOGY

Staging Classification

The clinical staging of prostate cancer uses pretreatment parameters to predict the extent of disease, both for assessment of prognosis and to inform decisions regarding appropriate treatment (Fig. 22.6). Clinical staging is the assessment of disease extent

Discrete well-formed glands (Gleason pattern 3)

Cribriform, poorly formed, fused glands (Gleason pattern 4)

Sheets, cords, single cells, solid nests, necrosis (Gleason pattern 5)

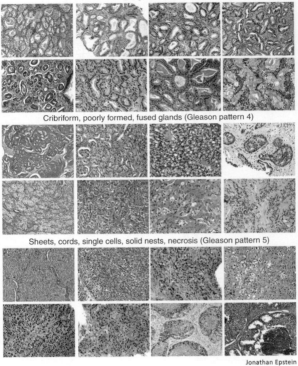

Jonathan Epstein

FIG. 22.6 The Gleason grading system and correlates with grade group morphologies. *From left to right: First row:* Closely packed, uniformly sized and shaped large glands; large variably sized and shaped glands, some with infolding; uniform medium-sized glands; and variably sized glands. *Second row:* Occasional tangentially sectioned glands among well-formed small glands; occasional tangentially sectioned glands among well-formed glands with open lumina; back-to-back discrete glands; and branching glands. *Third row:* Large irregular cribriform glands with well-formed lumina; irregular cribriform glands with slitlike lumina, glomeruloid structures, and fused glands; irregular cribriform glands with small round lumina; and small round cribriform glands. *Fourth row:* Poorly formed glands with peripherally arranged nuclei; small poorly formed glands; small poorly formed glands; and fused poorly formed glands. *Fifth row:* Sheets of cancer; sheets of cancer with rosette formation; small nests and cords of tumor with scattered clear vacuoles; and individual cells. *Sixth row:* Nests and cords of cells with only a vague attempt at lumina formation; solid nests of cancer; solid nests with comedonecrosis; and cribriform glands with central necrosis.

using pretreatment parameters (DRE, PSA values, needle biopsy findings, and radiologic imaging), whereas pathologic stage is determined after prostate removal and involves histologic analysis of the prostate, seminal vesicles, and pelvic lymph nodes if lymphadenectomy is performed.

GRADING ON PROSTATE BIOPSY

- Architectural patterns are identified and assigned a grade from 1 to 5, with the *most common* and *highest-grade* patterns on a given core added to result in the Gleason score.
- See Box 22.1 for grade group definitions.
- A tertiary (third) grade pattern is recorded typically when there is a nodule with Gleason score 3 + 4 = 7 or 4 + 3 = 7 and a minor (<5%) component of Gleason pattern 5.

HIGH-GRADE PROSTATIC INTRAEPITHELIAL NEOPLASIA

- For patients diagnosed with unifocal high-grade prostatic intraepithelial neoplasia on extended initial core sampling, a repeat biopsy within the first year is unnecessary in the absence of other clinical indicators of cancer.

Box 22.1 Grade Group Definitions

- Grade group 1 (Gleason score 3 + 3 = 6): only individual discrete well-formed glands
- Grade group 2 (Gleason score 3 + 4 = 7): predominantly well-formed glands with lesser component of poorly formed, fused, cribriform glands
- Grade group 3 (Gleason score 4 + 3 = 7): predominantly poorly formed, fused, cribriform glands with lesser component of well-formed glands
- Grade group 4 (Gleason score 8)
    - Poorly formed, fused, cribriform glands or
    - Predominantly well-formed glands and any lesser component lacking glands
    - Predominantly lacking glands and second most common component of well-formed glands
- Grade group 5 (Gleason scores 9 and 10): lack gland formation (or with necrosis) with or without poorly formed, fused, cribriform glands

IMAGING OF THE PROSTATE

Multiparametric Magnetic Resonance Imaging of the Prostate

The Prostate Image Reporting and Data System (PIRADS) categorization represents a consensus opinion to allow the systematic evaluation of lesions detected on multiparametric magnetic resonance imaging (mpMRI) to estimate their potential risk for prostate cancer. PIRADS is a standardized lexicon for reporting the results of these examinations while maintaining the Likert scale from 1 to 5 (Box 22.2).

- The PRECISION trial, a multicenter trial in Europe and North America, found that MRI-targeted biopsy had a higher detection rate of clinically significant disease and lower detection rate of clinically insignificant disease compared with standard transrectal ultrasound (TRUS) biopsy.

Prostate-Specific Membrane Antigen (PSMA)

A folate hydrolase, PSMA is found embedded within the cell membrane of all prostatic epithelial cells. ^{68}Gallium prostate-specific membrane antigen positron emission tomography (^{68}Ga-PSMA PET) has become an increasingly used diagnostic tool in the setting of biochemical recurrence after primary therapy.

Metastatic Workup

- Bone scan is indicated for patients with clinical stage T1 and a PSA level >20 ng/mL, clinical stage T2 and a PSA level >10 ng/mL, a Gleason score of 8 to 10 (Grade group 4–5), clinical stage

---

Box 22.2 PI-RADS v2 Categories

- PI-RADS 1: very low (clinically significant cancer is highly unlikely to be present)
- PI-RADS 2: low (clinically significant cancer is unlikely to be present)
- PI-RADS 3: intermediate (the presence of clinically significant cancer is equivocal)
- PI-RADS 4: high (clinically significant cancer is likely to be present)
- PI-RADS 5: very high (clinically significant cancer is highly likely to be present)

T3 or T4, or clinical symptoms. Routine bone scans are not necessary for men with low-risk prostate cancer.
- Computed tomography (CT) is recommended for high-risk patients, such as those with clinical stage T3 or greater disease or >10% nomogram probability of lymph node metastases.
- Fluciclovine F 18 and PSMA positron emission tomography (PET) have seen increasing investigation and incorporation into the metastatic workup clinical setting.
Table 22.3 shows risk stratification and indicated staging by risk category.

Key Points

DIAGNOSIS AND STAGING OF PROSTATE CANCER

- The combination PSA level, DRE, and other clinical factors (e.g., age, race, family history) can be used in combination to predict the risk that prostate cancer is present. The presence of prostate disease (prostate cancer, BPH, and prostatitis) is the most important factor affecting serum levels of PSA.
- PSA testing increases detection rates of prostate cancer and leads to the detection of prostate cancers that are more likely to be organ-confined when compared with detection without the use of PSA.
- The future risk for prostate cancer detection and the chance of finding cancer on a prostate biopsy increase incrementally with serum PSA level.
- Biochemical recurrence-free survival and cancer-specific survival are both inversely related to the pathologic stage of disease.
- Pathologic criteria that predict prognosis after radical prostatectomy are tumor grade, surgical margin status, presence of extracapsular disease, seminal vesicle invasion, and pelvic lymph node involvement.
- The Gleason grading system is the most commonly used classification scheme for the histologic grading of prostate cancer.

MANAGEMENT OF LOCALIZED PROSTATE CANCER

- The burden of overdiagnosis and overtreatment must be considered and discussed with the patient.
- In consideration of the necessity for treatment and the appropriate type of treatment, the patient's baseline urinary, bowel,

Table 22.3 Risk Stratification and Staging Workup

NCCN RISK GROUP	CLINICAL/PATHOLOGIC FEATURES	IMAGING
• Very low	• T1c AND • Gleason score ≤6/grade group 1 AND • PSA <10 ng/mL AND • Fewer than three prostate biopsy fragments/cores positive, ≤50% cancer in each fragment/core AND • PSA density <0.15 ng/mL/g	• Not indicated
• Low	• T1–T2a AND • Gleason score ≤6/grade group 1 AND • PSA <10 ng/mL	• Not indicated
• Favorable intermediate	• T2b–T2c OR • Gleason score 3+4=7/grade group 2 OR • PSA 10–20 ng/mL AND • Percentage of positive biopsy cores <50%	• Bone imaging: not recommended for staging • Pelvic ± abdominal imaging: recommended if nomogram predicts >10% probability of pelvic lymph node involvement
• Unfavorable intermediate	• T2b–T2c OR • Gleason score 3+4=7/grade group 2 or Gleason score 4+3=7/grade group 3 OR • PSA 10–20 ng/mL	• Bone imaging: recommended if T2 and PSA >10 ng/mL • Pelvic ± abdominal imaging: recommended if nomogram predicts >10% probability of pelvic lymph
• High	• T3a OR • Gleason score 8/grade group 4 or Gleason score 4+5=9/grade group 5 OR • PSA >20 ng/mL	• Bone imaging: recommended • Pelvic ± abdominal imaging: recommended if nomogram predicts >10% probability of pelvic lymph
• Very high	• T3b–T4 OR • Primary Gleason pattern 5 OR • >4 cores with Gleason score 8–10/grade group 4 or 5	• Bone imaging: recommended • Pelvic ± abdominal imaging: recommended if nomogram predicts >10% probability of pelvic lymph

PSA, Prostate-specific antigen.

and sexual function are critical considerations because of their influence on quality of life. Shared decision making is critical.

- Risk stratification nomograms take into account clinical variables such as age, PSA, Gleason grade, clinical stage, and volume of disease to help classify patients into risk categories. Table 22.4 shows commonly used risk assessment tools and nomograms.
- Table 22.5 summarizes national guidelines recommendation for prostate cancer by risk category.
- **Oncologic Outcomes** – Cancer-specific and overall mortality are considered to be the most valid end points for comparisons of efficacy but require a protracted follow-up given the known long lead-time from diagnosis to death.

Table 22.4 Online Risk Stratification Nomograms for Prostate Cancer

CLINICAL STATE	TITLE	WEBSITE
Risk for prostate cancer	Prostate Cancer Prevention Trial Prostate Cancer Risk Calculator	Https://prostatecancerinfolink net/risk-prevention/pcpt-prostate-cancer-risk-calculator/
Pretreatment	Memorial Sloan Kettering Pretreatment Nomogram	Https://www.mskcc.org/nomograms/prostate/pre_op
	Partin tables	https://www.hopkinsmedicine.org/brady-urology-institute/specialties/conditions-and-treatments/prostate-cancer/fighting-prostate-cancer/partin-table.html
	UCSF CAPRA score	https://urology.ucsf.edu/research/cancer/prostate-cancer-risk-assessment-and-the-ucsf-capra-score
Posttreatment	Memorial Sloan Kettering Posttreatment Nomogram	https://www.mskcc.org/nomograms/prostate/post_op

PSA, Prostate-specific antigen (test); *UCSF CAPRA*, University of California, San Francisco Cancer of the Prostate Risk Assessment.

Table 22.5 National Guidelines Treatment Recommendations

ORGANIZATION	RECOMMENDATIONS FOR LOW-RISK PROSTATE CANCER	RECOMMENDATIONS FOR INTERMEDIATE-RISK PROSTATE CANCER	TESTS RECOMMENDED FOR ACTIVE SURVEILLANCE MONITORING	RECOMMENDATIONS REGARDING OTHER TESTS
ASCO (Schroder et al., 2014)	AS is preferred management	Active treatment; active surveillance for select patients	PSA every 3–6 months DRE annually Systematic biopsy within 6–12 months of diagnostic biopsy, then every 3–5 years	Other tests remain investigational
NCCN (Tsodikov et al., 2018)	Very low-risk prostate cancer: AS is preferred management Low-risk prostate cancer: all therapies are options	Active treatment; active surveillance for select patients	PSA every 6 months Biopsy ≤ annually	Consider MRI for aggressive cancer suspected or PSA increases with negative systematic biopsy
AUA (Andriole et al., 2009; Wilt et al., 2012)	Very low-risk prostate cancer: AS is preferred management Low-risk prostate cancer: AS is preferred management. May offer definitive treatment to select patients with high probability of progression	Active treatment; active surveillance for select patients	Routine PSA and DRE Biopsy within initial 2 years	Should have accurate disease staging including systematic biopsy with ultrasound or MRI-guided imaging Consider prostate MRI as component of AS

NICE (Andriole et al., 2012)	AS is preferred management	Radical treatment for disease progression	PSA every 3–4 months, monitor kinetics DRE annually Systematic biopsy within 6–12 months of diagnostic biopsy, then every 3–5 years	MRI on enrollment

AS, Active surveillance; ASCO, American Society of Clinical Oncology; AUA, American Urological Association; DRE, digital rectal exam; MRI, magnetic resonance imaging; NCCN, National Comprehensive Cancer Network; NICE, National Institute for Health and Care Excellence; PSA, prostate-specific antigen

- Several studies have evaluated the comparative effectiveness of radiation therapy and radical prostatectomy in localized disease such as The Scandinavian Prostate Cancer Group Study Number 4 (SPCG-4), PIVOT, and ProtecT trials (Fig. 22.7).

Active Surveillance for Prostate Cancer

Active surveillance has been widely adopted as a safe and effective strategy for men with low-risk prostate cancer. It is considered the

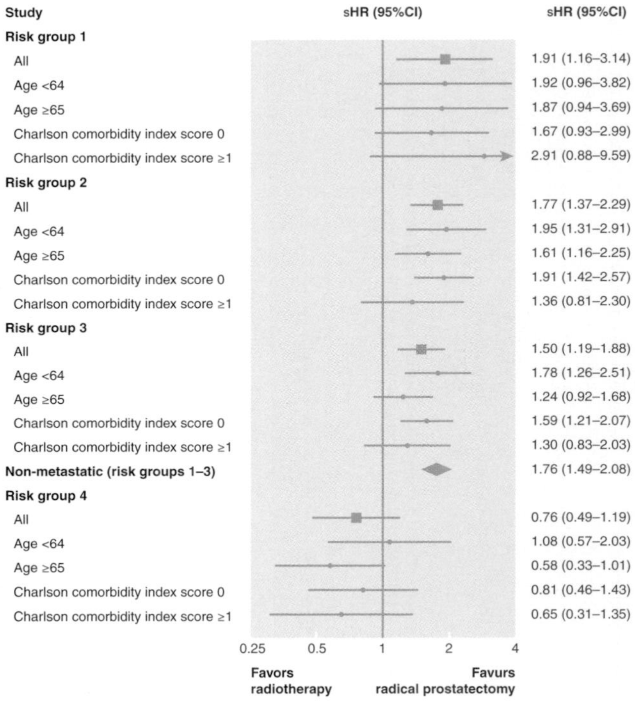

Study	sHR (95%CI)
Risk group 1	
All	1.91 (1.16–3.14)
Age <64	1.92 (0.96–3.82)
Age ≥65	1.87 (0.94–3.69)
Charlson comorbidity index score 0	1.67 (0.93–2.99)
Charlson comorbidity index score ≥1	2.91 (0.88–9.59)
Risk group 2	
All	1.77 (1.37–2.29)
Age <64	1.95 (1.31–2.91)
Age ≥65	1.61 (1.16–2.25)
Charlson comorbidity index score 0	1.91 (1.42–2.57)
Charlson comorbidity index score ≥1	1.36 (0.81–2.30)
Risk group 3	
All	1.50 (1.19–1.88)
Age <64	1.78 (1.26–2.51)
Age ≥65	1.24 (0.92–1.68)
Charlson comorbidity index score 0	1.59 (1.21–2.07)
Charlson comorbidity index score ≥1	1.30 (0.83–2.03)
Non-metastatic (risk groups 1–3)	1.76 (1.49–2.08)
Risk group 4	
All	0.76 (0.49–1.19)
Age <64	1.08 (0.57–2.03)
Age ≥65	0.58 (0.33–1.01)
Charlson comorbidity index score 0	0.81 (0.46–1.43)
Charlson comorbidity index score ≥1	0.65 (0.31–1.35)

0.25 0.5 1 2 4
Favors radiotherapy — Favurs radical prostatectomy

FIG. 22.7 Forest plot depicting propensity score adjusted subdistribution hazard ratios (sHRs) for radiotherapy versus radical prostatectomy for cancer-specific mortality stratified by risk group, and substratified by age and Charlson comorbidity index score. (Data from Sooriakumaran P, Nyberg T, Akre O, et al. Comparative effectiveness of radical prostatectomy and radiotherapy in prostate cancer: observational study of mortality outcomes. *BMJ* 2014;348:g1502.)

primary treatment for most of these men by numerous national organizations, including the American Urological Association (AUA) and the American Society of Clinical Oncology (ASCO). It is an important antidote to the dilemma of overtreatment that accompanies screening and early detection.

- Long-term active surveillance cohorts report a 15-year prostate cancer mortality rate of between 0.5% and 5%.
- About 25% of patients are offered definitive therapy at 5 years and 40% by 10 years.
- Table 22.6 summarizes active surveillance protocols across the largest trials in North America.
- The safety and efficacy of active surveillance hinges upon the assumption that initial diagnosis and risk assessment is accurate and that occult higher risk disease is not present.
- Periodic PSA testing (at least every 6 months), imaging with magnetic resonance imaging (MRI) or TRUS, and repeat biopsy

Table 22.6 Selection Criteria for Active Surveillance

	CLINICAL STAGE	PSA LEVEL	GLEASON SCORE ON BIOPSY	PSA DENSITY	NUMBER OF POSITIVE BIOPSY CORES
University of Toronto (Schroder et al., 2014)	T1c/T2a	≤10–15 ng/mL	≤3+3=6	Not included	Not included
Multicenter European study (PIRAS) (Tsodikov et al., 2018)	T1c/T2a	≤10 ng/mL	≤ 3+3=6	≤ 0.2 ng/mL/cm (Wit et al., 2012)	2
Johns Hopkins (Wilt et al., 2012)	T1c	Not included	≤3+3=6	≤0.15 ng/mL/cm (Wilt et al., 2012)	2
Canary Collaboration (Andriole et al., 2009)	T1/T2	Any	≤7	Any	Any

is warranted. Patients must be carefully counseled regarding the inherent risks and benefits of surveillance, and this must be carefully differentiated from the strategy of watchful waiting, which does not seek to preserve the option of treatment for cure, if and when it is ultimately indicated.

Key Points

ACTIVE SURVEILLANCE

- Newly diagnosed men on active surveillance should have a confirmatory biopsy within 1 year, targeting the undersampled areas of the prostate.
- After this, they should have PSA every 6 months and periodic repeat biopsy (every 3–5 years).
- MRI and targeted biopsy may replace serial systematic biopsies in very-low-risk men. Because the NPV of MRI is a function of underlying risk, those at higher risk still warrant systematic biopsies.
- Cancer deaths reported in men with low-risk cancer managed conservatively are thought to be caused by the coexistence of higher-grade cancer missed on the diagnostic biopsy.
- Three randomized trials comparing radical intervention to conservative management have shown little or no benefit to intervention in the low-risk group.
- Ten prospective active surveillance series have confirmed a very low rate of metastasis and prostate cancer mortality with an initial conservative approach. The disease-specific mortality varies between 0.5% and 5% at 15 years, depending on eligibility criteria.
- Approximately 25% of patients are reclassified to higher risk and managed with definitive therapy at 5 years. This figure is similar among all cohorts.
- Misattribution of grade (25%–30% of cases) is much more common than true biologic progression from Gleason 3 to 4 or 5 (1%–2.3% per year).
- Factors that increase the risk for coexistent higher-grade cancer include PSA density (>0.15), race (African-American), and volume of cancer on biopsy (number of positive cores, extent of core involvement).

SURGICAL MANAGEMENT OF PROSTATE CANCER

- Robotic-assisted laparoscopic radical prostatectomy has become the most frequent surgical approach in the United States.
- Intraoperative considerations include development of the space of Retzius, ligation of the dorsal vein complex (DVC), identification and transection of the bladder neck, dissection of the seminal vesicles, control of the prostatic pedicles, preservation of the neurovascular bundle, and apical dissection of the prostate with care to maintain as much urethral length as possible.
- The extent of pelvic lymphadenectomy and its diagnostic versus therapeutic value remains controversial but can be tailored based on cancer risk categorization.
- Postoperative complications include positional neural injuries, hemorrhage, bowel injury, ureteral injury, open conversion, urine leak, and bladder neck contracture formation. If pelvic lymphadenectomy is performed, then potential complications include lymphocele formation, deep venous thrombosis, lower extremity edema, obturator nerve injury, and ureteral injury.

Treatment Morbidity and Quality of Life Outcomes

- Urinary incontinence recovers in most men over the first year, although residual stress incontinence is common.
- Erective dysfunction has a 2- to 3-year course of recovery. Treatments range from PDE5 inhibitors to intracavernous injection, vacuum erection device, and penile prosthesis placement
- Penile shortening, dry ejaculate, infertility, and climacturia should be discussed.

RADIATION THERAPY FOR PROSTATE CANCER

Intensity-Modulated Radiation Therapy (IMRT)

IMRT employs more complex, dynamic beam shapes wherein the intensity of radiation is varied across the beam to allow for finer control of spatial variations in dose and can produce steeper dose gradients with improved sparing of normal tissues, particularly when tumors or tissues have complex, convex, or concave shapes

External Beam Radiation Treatment

Fractionated treatment is based on the idea that tumor control could be achieved with less normal tissue injury when the radiation dose is split into many small fractions. Additionally, late-responding normal tissues are generally more sensitive than early responding tissues (i.e., tumor) to increases in fraction size. EBRT has been routinely delivered in a fractionated manner using daily doses of 1.8 to 2.0 Gray.

Stereotactic Body Radiation Therapy

Moderate hypofractionation is generally considered to be that which uses doses of 2.4–4 Gy per day, whereas ultra (or extreme) hypofractionation uses doses of 6–10 Gy per fraction.

Heavy Particle Beams and Proton Therapy

No randomized clinical trial has directly compared patient outcomes of proton therapy versus IMRT for prostate cancer.

Brachytherapy

Prostate brachytherapy can be performed using either low dose rate (LDR) (permanent seed implant) or high dose rate (HDR) (temporary catheter) approaches. Postimplant dosimetry after LDR brachytherapy is important to assess implant quality. Combined brachytherapy and EBRT is not indicated for patients with low-risk disease but is supported by data for a role in the management of high-risk disease.

Patients who have preexisting obstructive uropathy (IPSS >20 or Qmax <10 cc/s) are relatively contraindicated for brachytherapy.

Role of Androgen Deprivation with Radiation Therapy

Randomized controlled trials have shown a survival benefit to the combination of radiation and hormonal therapy relative to either radiation or hormonal therapy alone for men with intermediate- to high-risk disease. For men with locally advanced, high-risk disease, 28–36 months of hormonal therapy appears superior to 4–6 months for reducing death from prostate cancer.

TREATMENT MORBIDITY AND QUALITY-OF-LIFE OUTCOMES

- Most rectal bleeding that occurs after radiation therapy (RT) is mild and self-limited or manageable with suppositories or enemas.
- Recently developed rectal-sparing strategies such as injectable hydrogel can reduce the risk for radiation proctitis.
- Urinary incontinence is uncommon after either EBRT or brachytherapy.
- PDE5Is are frequently effective in patients who experience post-RT ED.

Postradiation Follow-Up and Response

Nadir PSA value is a significant predictor of outcome, but no absolute nadir threshold can or should be used to define cure. Three sources of PSA potentially contribute to the nadir: residual benign prostatic epithelium, residual local prostate cancer cells, and subclinical disseminated micrometastases. The longer the time to nadir and the lower the absolute nadir, the more likely it is that only benign prostatic epithelium remains.

The **postnadir doubling time** of the PSA level also correlates with the type of failure, with distant failures having shorter PSA doubling times of 3 to 6 months, whereas doubling times for those with local failures are 1 year or more.

Focal Therapy for Prostate Cancer

The goal of focal therapy is to treat only those foci of cancer within the prostate gland that will affect the patient's survival or quality of life while preserving surrounding tissue and structures and in turn the patient's sexual and urinary function. Ablation modalities include cryotherapy, high-intensity focal ultrasonography (HIFU), and brachytherapy, among others.

- After prostate focal therapy, PSA, which is a traditional marker of therapeutic success, is less relevant because its levels are affected by the amount of residual prostate epithelium that may continue to grow.
- MRI and prostate biopsies are recommended to assess the treated (infield) area and the untreated (outfield) area.

Biochemical Recurrence of Prostate Cancer

- The AUA Guidelines Panel ultimately defined PSA recurrence as a value of ≥ 0.2 ng/mL with a second confirmatory laboratory value.

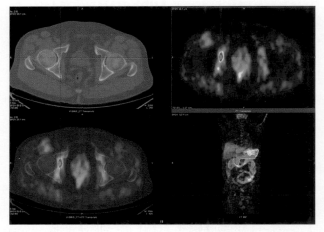

FIG. 22.8 ¹¹C-acetate positron emission tomography scan in biochemical recurrence.

- Not all men with a detectable PSA after surgery are destined to clinical progression (i.e., metastatic disease), need for second-line treatment, or death from prostate cancer.
- Some men have detectable PSA postoperatively that plateaus and does not subsequently rise.
- 50% of patients will not have clinical failure after a median follow-up of 9.4 years. Several nomograms are available that can aid in estimating one's risk of biochemical recurrence postprostatectomy and can be used in patient counseling (Fig. 22.8).

IMAGING IN BIOCHEMICAL RECURRENCE

Identifying patients with local failure only is critical to initiate salvage therapies while sparing those with distant metastatic disease the burden of local salvage therapy.

- CT and bone scan remain standard of care.
- Novel PET imaging (fluciclovine and PSMA) has demonstrated promise in the detection of prostate cancer recurrence; however, its cost and **variable clinical utility at extremely low PSA levels** currently limit its widespread usage.
- Compared with PET/CT, mpMRI performs better in identification of local recurrence, especially at low levels of biochemical failure.

Salvage Radiation Therapy after Radical Prostatectomy

Salvage radiation therapy remains the best chance for long-term freedom from progression in men with PSA recurrence after radical prostatectomy

PSA Recurrence after Definitive Radiotherapy

- The Phoenix definition, PSA nadir +2 ng/mL was found to be a significant predictor of metastatic disease, disease-specific mortality, and overall mortality on multivariable analysis.
- **Biopsy After Radiotherapy** – The goal is to identify the presence or absence of locally residual or recurrent disease and to identify grade of remaining disease.

Salvage Radical Prostatectomy

- Patients selected for salvage radical prostatectomy should have biopsy-proven recurrent prostate cancer, at least 10 years of life expectancy, lack of identifiable metastasis on imaging, and a PSA <10 ng/mL.
- Salvage prostatectomy is associated with a higher rate of urinary incontinence, ED, and rectal injury following salvage prostatectomy compared with robotic assisted laparoscopic radical prostatectomy (RALRP) performed in the primary setting.

Salvage Cryotherapy

Patients best suited for cryotherapy are those with localized treatment failure after radiation therapy with biopsy-proven disease. This is a reasonable approach with adequate disease-specific outcomes and limited morbidity.

Salvage Brachytherapy

Modern techniques such as high-dose rate brachytherapy demonstrate improved cancer control outcomes but also have comparable morbidity outcomes to cryotherapy and surgery.

Salvage HIFU

Although short- to intermediate-term follow-up has been demonstrated with HIFU, further studies are necessary to establish its place as a viable alternative in the radio-recurrent setting.

Androgen Deprivation Therapy after Biochemical Recurrence Following Radiation Therapy to the Prostate

- Defining the patient population who is at highest risk is important to treat the patients with early androgen deprivation therapy (ADT) who are likely to benefit while sparing the significant side effects to those who are at low risk to fail.
- Patients with PSA doubling times <12 months benefit from ADT with freedom from distant metastatic disease of 57% versus 78%.

TREATMENT OF CASTRATION-RESISTANT PROSTATE CANCER

Nonmetastatic Castration-Resistant Prostate Cancer

- Patients start ADT at the first sign of a rising PSA after local therapy, before clinical and radiographic evidence of metastasis is present.
- Apalutamide and enzalutamide have recently been approved for use in this clinical space.

Metastatic Castration-Resistant Prostate Cancer

Patients with metastatic castrate resistant prostate cancer (mCRPC) represent a heterogeneous population with respect to their clinical and disease characteristics at the time of disease progression on ADT.

Cytotoxic Chemotherapy

- Docetaxel is the standard first-line chemotherapy for mCRPC. It prolongs progression-free and overall survival, ameliorates pain, and improves quality of life. Toxicity of docetaxel includes myelosuppression, fatigue, peripheral edema, neurotoxicity, hyperlacrimation, and nail dystrophy.
- Cabazitaxel is as a second-line chemotherapy option for patients with mCRPC who have had progressive disease during or after docetaxel treatment. Side effects with cabazitaxel include neutropenia (including febrile neutropenia) and diarrhea but generally not neuropathy.
- Mitoxantrone has been approved to palliate symptoms associated with metastatic disease. It is sometimes used in patients

who have previously received docetaxel and/or cabazitaxel or in those who would not tolerate these agents.

- Platinum agents are indicated in patients with small cell prostate cancer and perhaps in other subsets of mCRPC patients (e.g., those with combined TP53 and PTEN inactivation or DNA repair deficiency mutations)

Next-Generation Hormonal Therapies

There is mounting evidence that CRPC is not androgen-independent and continues to rely on androgen/androgen receptor signaling.

- Abiraterone is a CYP17 inhibitor that depletes adrenal and intratumoral androgens. It is approved for the treatment of mCRPC before and after chemotherapy (but not for nonmetastatic CRPC).
- Enzalutamide is an androgen receptor (AR) signaling inhibitor that antagonizes the AR and prevents nuclear translocation and DNA binding. It was shown to improve survival in men with mCRPC in the prechemotherapy and postchemotherapy settings and to improve metastasis-free survival for men with M0 CRPC. Enzalutamide is approved for any patient with CRPC, regardless of metastatic status.
- Apalutamide is a second AR signaling inhibitor that has shown superiority to placebo in men with nonmetastatic (M0) CRPC and has received approval for this indication. Apalutamide is not approved for use in metastatic CRPC.
- Additional CYP17-inhibiting agents (e.g., orteronel) and AR-targeting agents (e.g., darolutamide) are in clinical development.
- AR-V7 is a blood-based biomarker that may be used to aid in the choice of therapy for mCRPC patients. AR-V7(+) patients may benefit more from taxane chemotherapy, whereas AR-V7(−) men may benefit similarly from either AR-directed therapy or chemotherapy.

Immunotherapy

Sipuleucel-T was the first therapeutic vaccine to be approved by the Federal Drug Administration (FDA) for the treatment of any cancer, and it is indicated for men with asymptomatic or minimally symptomatic mCRPC without visceral metastases or cancer-related pain requiring narcotics.

Pembrolizumab is a PD-1 inhibitor that is indicated for mCRPC patients with an MSI-high and/or MMR-deficient phenotype, although this may only reflect 2%–5% of prostate cancers.

Palliative Management

Pain and Spinal Cord Compression. Patients with back pain and a history of bone metastases should be evaluated for spinal cord compression. This clinical syndrome often includes one of the following signs and symptoms: back pain, focal neurologic deficit (motor, sensory), or changes in bladder or bowel control.

The first therapeutic intervention in patients with suspected or documented cord compression should include the administration of high doses of intravenous glucocorticoids followed by evaluation for neurosurgical decompression (emergent cases with spinal cord compression), radiation therapy (nonemergent cases), or both.

Zoledronic acid and denosumab are both reasonable treatment options for the prevention of skeletal-related events in patients with castration-resistant bone metastases.

Radium-223 is a novel alpha-emitting radiopharmaceutical that has received FDA approval for the treatment of symptomatic bone metastases in CRPC patients without visceral metastases or bulky lymph node disease.

Suggested Readings

Advanced Prostate Cancer: AUA/ASTRO/SUO Guidelines. https://www.auanet.org/guidelines/advanced-prostate-cancer.

Ahmed HU, El-Shater Bosaily A, Brown LC, et al. Diagnostic accuracy of multi-parametric MRI and TRUS biopsy in prostate cancer (PROMIS): a paired validating confirmatory study. *Lancet* 2017;389(10071):815-822.

Andriole G, Bostwick DG, Brawley OW, et al. Effect of dutasteride on the risk of prostate cancer. *N Engl J Med* 2010;362(13):1192-1202.

Andriole GL, Crawford ED, Grubb RL 3rd, et al. Prostate cancer screening in the randomized Prostate, Lung, Colorectal, and Ovarian Cancer Screening Trial: mortality results after 13 years of follow-up. *J Natl Cancer Inst* 2012;104(2):125-132.

AUA Castration-Resistant Prostate Cancer (2018). https://www.auanet.org/guidelines/prostate-cancer-castration-resistant-guideline.

AUA Early Detection of Prostate Cancer (2018). https://www.auanet.org/guidelines/prostate-cancer-early-detection-guideline.

Clinically Localized Prostate Cancer: AUA/ASTRO/SUO Guideline (2017). https://www.auanet.org/guidelines/prostate-cancer-clinically-localized-guideline.

Coleman MP, Quaresma M, Berrino F, et al. Cancer survival in five continents: a worldwide population-based study (CONCORD). *Lancet Oncol* 2008;9(8):730-756.

DeSantis CE, Miller KD, Sauer AG, et al. Cancer statistics for African Americans, 2019. *CA Cancer J Clin* 2019;69(3):211-233.

Ellis L, Canchola AJ, Spiegel D, et al. Racial and ethnic disparities in cancer survival: the contribution of tumor, sociodemographic, institutional, and neighborhood characteristics. *J Clin Oncol* 2018;36(1):25-33.

Epstein JI, Amin MB, Reuter VE, et al. Contemporary Gleason grading of prostatic carcinoma: an update with discussion on practical issues to implement the 2014 International Society of Urological Pathology (ISUP) Consensus Conference on Gleason Grading of Prostatic Carcinoma. *Am J Surg Pathol* 2017;41(4):e1-e7.

Kasivisvanathan V, Rannikko AS, Borghi M, et al. MRI-targeted or standard biopsy for prostate-cancer diagnosis. *N Engl J Med* 2018;378(19) 1767-777.

Klein EA, Thompson IM Jr, Tangen CM, et al. Vitamin E and the risk of prostate cancer: the Selenium and Vitamin E Cancer Prevention Trial (SELECT). *JAMA* 2011;306(14): 1549-1556.

Kumar-Sinha C, Tomlins SA, Chinnaiyan AM. Recurrent gene fusions in prostate cancer. *Nat Rev Cancer* 2008;8(7):497-511.

National Comprehensive Cancer Network: Guidelines. Version 2, 2013. Prostate cancer early detection. https://www.nccn.org/professionals/physician_gls/pdf/prostate_detection.pdf.

Pierorazio PM, Walsh PC, Partin AW, et al. Prognostic Gleason grade grouping: data based on the modified Gleason scoring system. *BJU Int* 2013b;111(5):753-760.

Pinsky PF, Prorok PC, Yu K, et al. Extended mortality results for prostate cancer screening in the PLCO trial with median follow-up of 15 years. *Cancer* 2017;123(4):592-599.

Schröder FH, Hugosson J, Roobol MJ, et al. Screening and prostate cancer mortality: results of the European Randomised Study of Screening for Prostate Cancer (ERSPC) at 13 years of follow-up. *Lancet* 2014;384(9959):2027-2035.

Siegel RL, Miller KD, Jemal A. Cancer statistics, 2020. *CA Cancer J Clin* 2020;70(1):7-30.

Thompson IM, Goodman PJ, Tangen CM, et al. The influence of finasteride on the development of prostate cancer. *N Engl J Med* 2003;349(3):215-224.

23

Urologic Complications of Renal Transplantation

RAMASAMY BAKTHAVATSALAM AND ROBERT M. SWEET

CONTRIBUTORS OF CAMPBELL-WALSH-WEIN, 12TH EDITION

Mohammed Shahalt, Stephen V. Jackman, and Timothy D. Averch

HEMATURIA

Postoperative hematuria is usually related to the urothelial trauma from ureterovesical anastomosis, stents, and catheters. This risk is increased in patients taking anticoagulation and antiplatelet agents. **Mostly it is self-limiting. Significant hematuria is uncommon and requires careful bladder irrigation due to the fresh ureterovesical anastomosis and rarely requires cystoscopy for clot evacuation and fulguration.** Hematuria is more frequent after the Politano-Leadbetter type of implantation.

After renal biopsy, hematuria requires immediate evaluation with ultrasound to rule out arteriovenous (AV) fistula. About 70% of AV fistula resolve spontaneously. If an AV fistula persists, it will require angiogram and selective embolization. Acute onset hematuria with pain and tenderness over the graft associated with low urine output requires urgent evaluation with ultrasound (US) to rule out vascular thrombosis.

Evaluation of asymptomatic microscopic hematuria (AMH) follows the American Urology Association (AUA) guidelines for general population; with the additional differential diagnoses of a retained stent, ureteritis and hemorrhagic cystitis from viruses (BK, adeno virus, and cytomegalovirus [CMV]). Viral cytopathic changes could be seen on cytology and confirmed by urine BK virus titer.

URETERAL STENT MANAGEMENT

Ureteral stenting in transplantation is known to protect against ureteric obstruction and urine leak. But there is risk of microbial colonization of the stent and urinary tract infection (UTI), including pyelonephritis and graft dysfunction irrespective of the dwell time.

Early stent removal before the third postoperative week has been shown to reduce the incidence of UTI without discernible effect on the incidence of urine leak and obstruction. Most patients are on cotrimoxazole for prophylaxis against pneumocystis, but patient-specific antimicrobial prophylaxis for high-risk patients is recommended.

Stenting and timing of removal should be individualized based on various factors, including the quality of ureter, bladder, bladder outflow issues; integrity of the anastomosis; difficulty of the surgery from body habitus; scarring from prior radiation or surgery; and comorbidities.

RETAINED STENT

Difficulty in removing a stent could be secondary to error of including the stent in the suture line and requires delayed removal after dissolution of the suture. If earlier removal is required, there is a need endoscopic suture transection. Routine removal of stents with accelerated encrustation could be difficult.

Stents left in for prolonged periods (either intentionally or forgotten) are uncommon and lead to encrustation. **Patients rarely manifest the classical symptoms of ureteral obstruction due to the denervation of kidney graft.** Common presentations are recurrent UTIs, decrease in urine output, progressive decline in renal function, and pain or discomfort from graft swelling and peritoneal irritation.

Prevention

Documentation and effective communication and timely removal of the stent are essential to avoid this iatrogenic complication.

Diagnosis and Treatment

Computed tomography (CT) scan should be performed to assess the burden of encrustation and management planning. **Percutaneous** nephrostomy will be required initially to relieve the obstruction and improve the renal function, which could be used for antegrade access for further procedures if required. A combination of various modalities is used in managing the encrusted stents (percutaneous nephrolithotomy, antegrade/retrograde intrarenal surgery, and extracorporeal wave shock lithotripsy) (Fig. 23.1, UNN Box 23.1).

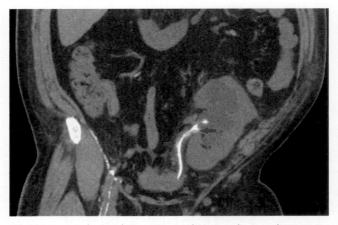

FIG. 23.1 Encrusted ureteral stent. Computed tomography scan demonstrates deposition of stone-like material *(arrows)* in the upper ureter. It is no longer functional (i.e., side holes and lumen are occluded).

Key Points

HEMATURIA AND URETERAL STENT MANAGEMENT

Majority of postop hematuria is self-limiting.

Consider duplex ultrasound for severe or persistent hematuria after renal biopsy to rule out arteriovenous (AV) fistula.

Sudden onset of anuria and hematuria requires evaluation with ultrasound to rule out vascular thrombosis

Ureteral stent decreases ureteral stricture and urinary leak.

Individualized plan for stent removal 2–3 weeks posttransplantation.

URINARY LEAK

Urine leak and ureteric obstruction comprise the most early urologic complication. **The risk factors are ureteric ischemia from various causes (long ureter, multiple arteries), procurement and implantation techniques, and bladder dysfunction** (Box 23.1).

Diagnosis

Urine leak should be suspected when the drain output is high with diminished urine output and raising serum creatinine. Other manifestations are leaking edematous wound, swelling of the scrotum and thigh, wound dehiscence, and disproportionate pain. US/CT scan will show edematous wound and fluid collection. Creatinine of the fluid from the wound/drain will be significantly higher than serum creatinine. CT cystogram and radionuclide studies may be required.

Treatment

The initial management is urinary diversion and drainage of the collection from the surgical site to protect the vascular anastomoses and to improve graft function and the condition of the patient. This is achieved by a Foley catheter and a percutaneous nephrostomy with antegrade stenting of the ureter if the ureter is not stented. Retrograde stent placement can be challenging with potential for further disruption of the anastomosis. Monitoring the drain output and graft function will guide further management. Periodic imaging may be required. The Foley catheter and nephrostomy tube can be removed on resolution of leak. Persistent urine leak despite adequate diversion and drainage requires exploratory surgery for ischemic ureter or a major leak.

Box 23.1 Causes of Urinary Leak

- Excessively long ureter and lower pole artery: ischemia
- Premature removal of bladder and/or ureteric drainage
- Technical problem such as suture dehiscence, ureteric twisting, or kinking
- Acute urine retention or bladder catheter obstruction
- Necrosis of renal parenchyma, ischemia, multiple arteries

Early exploration and reconstruction should be considered in patients with persistent leak despite maximal drainage because of the lower success rate of conservative management, the ease of early surgery secondary to lack of significant adhesions and fibrosis, and the decreased risk of subsequent ureteric stricture. The surgical option depends on the quality of the transplanted ureter, native ureter, and bladder. They are revision of ureterovesical anastomosis if the ureteric remnant is vascular and healthy, ureteroureterostomy to the native ureter, Boari flap, and pyelovesicostomy.

URETERAL OBSTRUCTION

Ureteral obstruction can be early (<3 months) or late (>3 months). The causes of early obstruction are mostly technical from defective anastomosis, edema, lack of stent, redundant ureter, and extrinsic compression (seroma, lymphocele, hematoma, and abscess). Diagnosis is made with US showing hydronephrosis with renal dysfunction (Box 23.2).

Treatment of the early obstruction involves percutaneous nephrostomy and antegrade stenting if not stented with possible balloon dilatation. Extrinsic compression from seroma or hematoma, requires drainage and surgical evacuation. Complete resolution is expected with this management. Surgical revision may be required in cases of redundant ureter.

Box 23.2 Common Causes of Ureteral Obstruction

EARLY URETERAL OBSTRUCTION (<3 MONTHS)
- Technical error during ureteroneocystostomy anastomosis
- Forgoing ureteral stent
- Anastomotic edema
- Redundant ureter
- Extrinsic compression (lymphocele, hematoma, abscess)

LATE URETERAL OBSTRUCTION (>3 MONTHS)
- Stones
- Ureteral strictures
- Lymphocele
- Fibrosis: postoperative scarring, ischemia, and infection related

Late ureteral obstruction is mostly caused by stones and stricture. The stones are either derived with the kidney at donation or formed after transplantation. The primary etiology for the stricture is ischemia, with others being chronic infection and periureteral scarring from urine leak and ureteritis from rejection and BK and CMV viral infection. Ureteric structure rates are similar across different types of ureterovesical anastomosis

Initial management of late strictures include percutaneous nephrostomy to decompress the collecting system and improve the renal function followed by evaluation of the stricture by nephrostogram. Voiding cystogram is helpful to rule out nonobstructive hydronephrosis secondary to reflux.

Decision for endoscopic or open surgical management depends on several factors: length and location of the stricture, function of the kidney, status of the bladder, patient's performance status and comorbidities, and available technology and expertise.

Endourologic options include double-J stent insertion, ureteral dilation, and endo ureterotomy (cold knife, holmium laser).

Open surgeries include uretero-ureterostomy to the native ureter, Boari flap, appendix or ileal interposition, or pyelovesicostomy. These procedures could also be performed successfully with minimally invasive techniques. Open surgery is very effective in terms of long-term outcome (Fig. 23.2).

Proximal ureteral stricture: Antegrade nephrostogram reveals hydronephrosis in the allograft without visualization of the ureter.

Key Points

URETERAL STRICTURE

Strictures are the predominant cause of ureteral obstruction in patients >3 months posttransplantation.

The primary cause of ureteral stricture development is ischemia of ureter.

Stricture should be suspected in patients with hydronephrosis and decreased graft function.

A variety of endourologic treatment options have been described to treat ureteral strictures however, open reconstructive surgery offers superior long-term results.

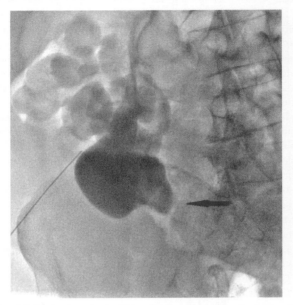

FIG. 23.2 Proximal ureteral stricture. Antegrade nephrostogram reveals hydronephrosis in the allograft without visualization of the ureter.

VESICOURETERAL REFLUX

The reported incidence of vesicoureteral reflux (VUR) varies widely (10.5%–86%), but the incidence of symptomatic or clinically significant VUR is <1% independent of the technique of ureterovesical anastomosis. The clinical consequences of VUR are unclear but may include a higher incidence of hypertension and urosepsis in the long term.

Diagnosis

Patients with recurrent UTIs should be evaluated for VUR by voiding cystourethrography. This will confirm the diagnosis and assess the severity of reflux in the transplant and native ureters. After the diagnosis of VUR is established, **a comprehensive workup to rule out bladder outlet obstruction and high-pressure bladder is recommended.**

Treatment

Initial management of VUR consists of treating the primary causes such as bladder outlet obstruction and a high-pressure, noncompliant bladder. In **patients with persistent symptomatic reflux, the antireflux measures could be considered.** Cystoscopic submucosal injections of various composites (Teflon or Macroplastique) are successful in low-grade reflux (90% in grade 1 and II and 30% in grade 3). Open surgical reconstruction is considered for high-grade reflux and failed endoscopic therapy.

LYMPHOCELE

Lymphocele is a lymph-containing perinephric pseudocyst with a variable incidence (0.6%–33.9%). Usually present in few weeks to 6 months. The source of the lymph is from perivascular and hilar lymphatics of the iliac vessels and kidney. Other risk factors include retransplantation, obesity, recipient age, duration of dialysis treatment, warm ischemia time, use of prophylactic low-molecular-weight heparin, delayed graft function, acute rejection, and use of mTOR inhibitors for immunosuppression.

Most of the lymphoceles are small and asymptomatic. Their proximity to the vessels, ureter, and bladder can cause pressure effects leading to unilateral limb edema, ureteric obstruction, or deep venous thrombosis. US will show the collection, and CT with contrast is useful in defining the relative position of ureter and vascular structures when operative intervention is planned. Diagnostic fine-needle aspiration under image guidance is useful to differentiate lymphocele from urinoma, seroma, or abscess.

Treatment

Using a prevention strategy of meticulous attention in securing the perivascular and hilar lymphatics during transplantation is essential. Treatment modalities for symptomatic lymphoceles are aspiration with or without sclerotherapy, percutaneous drainage, and laparoscopic or open fenestration with peritoneal window. **Adequate percutaneous or open drainage is essential for infected lymphocele.** The success rates for aspiration alone, sclerotherapy, drain placement, laparoscopic, and open surgery are 41%, 69%, 50%, 92%, and 84%, respectively.

NEPHROLITHIASIS

Stones in transplanted kidneys are uncommon with an incidence of 1%. Clinical implications are significant in is a solitary functioning kidney. Stones are either donor gifted or de novo. Most of the stones are calcium based like in general population (67%), and the rest are struvite (20%) and uric acid (13%). The risk factors are secondary hyperparathyroidism, recurrent UTIs, and metabolic abnormalities such as hypercalciuria, hyperuricosuria (cyclosporine), hypocitraturia, and hyperoxaluria (cyclosporine and tacrolimus).

The clinical presentation is usually a vague abdominal discomfort, hematuria, decrease in urine output, increasing creatinine, and UTI. US and CT imaging are diagnostic, defining the location, size of the stone, and presence of obstruction.

Asymptomatic patients with stones <4 mm could be followed for progression with serial US and graft function. Initial management of patients with infection or obstruction include immediate percutaneous nephrostomy and treatment of infection. Definitive treatment is undertaken after the control of infection and improvement in graft function. This includes variable combinations of extracorporeal shock wave lithotripsy, ureteroscopic surgery, and percutaneous nephrolithotomy. Donor-gifted stones can be removed successfully by ex vivo endoscopy prior to implantation. Posttreatment surveillance for development of silent hydronephrosis from ureteric scarring is essential. Comprehensive metabolic screening and treatment of underlying metabolic abnormalities if present is required.

LOWER URINARY TRACT COMPLICATIONS

Successful transplantation requires a functional lower urinary tract (continent, compliant, sterile, low-pressure reservoir with easy complete emptying; free from infection, stones, and malignancy). Obstructive nephropathies comprise the fourth major cause of renal failure in the United States (4.9%). Comprehensive pretransplant evaluation of symptomatic patients include outflow studies (uroflowmetry, urodynamics), imaging, and **counseling regarding the possible posttransplant requirement (clean intermittent catheterization [CIC] and or surgery)**.

Posttransplant voiding dysfunction is common due to factors such as a small-volume bladder from oliguria, abnormal anatomy, and various medications. Bladder volume tends to increase gradually after transplantation. Patients incapacitated from frequency may be treated with standard anticholinergics. Standard AUA guidelines should be followed in evaluation and management. Bladder augmentation or ileal conduit could be considered for persistent low-volume, high-pressure bladder.

BENIGN PROSTATIC HYPERPLASIA

Benign prostatic hypertrophy (BPH) is common in men after renal transplantation (10% at 3 years) and is an independent risk factor for UTI and graft loss. Prophylactic measures of starting on an alpha-blocker, adequate pain relief, and an aggressive bowel regimen should be considered prior to Foley removal. Pre-transplant surgery for BPH increases the risk of bladder neck contracture secondary to low urine output. Transurethral resection of the prostate (TURP) during the first 2 weeks should be avoided due the risk of rupturing the fresh ureterovesical anastomosis and ureteric reflux and sepsis with the indwelling stent. TURP using various energy devises could be safely performed 3 weeks posttransplant.

URINE INCONTINENCE

The estimated prevalence among female recipients is about 28%. The diagnosis and treatment of stress incontinence is same as in nontransplant patients with the caveat that the retropubic plane had been traversed during transplantation, and the ureter is in the anterior position. Several reports have described the feasibility and safety of tension-free vaginal tape (TVT), transobturator tape (TOT), sacral neuromodulation, laparoscopic sacrocolpopexy in female recipients, and insertion of an artificial urinary sphincter in men. **A management plan for patients with total incontinence ideally should be made prior to transplantation.**

GENITOURINARY MALIGNANCIES

Renal Cell Carcinoma

The risk of renal cell carcinoma (RCC) among kidney transplant recipients is higher compared with the general population (4.6% of

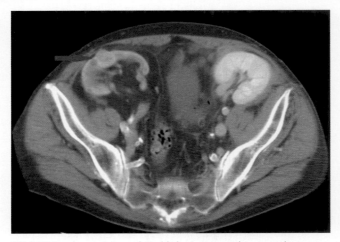

FIG. 23.3 Renal mass in transplanted kidney. Computed tomography scan reveals exophytic renal mass *(arrow)* in nonfunctioning allograft in an 80-year-old patient. Biopsy was performed, and low-grade papillary renal cell carcinoma, type 1, was found. Cryotherapy was used to ablate this mass.

cancers vs. 3%) especially for papillary histology (32% vs. 10%). The incidence is bimodal affecting only 10% of the grafts (58% papillary RCC). They are of low grade (I and II in 80%) and low stage (pT1a in 90%) (Fig. 23.3).

Management of RCC in kidney transplant patients is similar to that of general population (Fig. 23.4).

Renal Cell Carcinoma Management in Kidney Transplant Patients. No specific guidelines available for modifications of immunosuppression. With metastatic disease from RCC of the graft, consensus is allograft nephrectomy and discontinuing immunosuppression for the recipient immunity to recover and reject the donor-associated cancer cells provided the patient could tolerate the surgery.

Currently, no recommendations exist for posttransplant screening of native kidneys, but it is advisable to screen the high-risk groups: prior RCC, analgesic nephropathy, tuberous sclerosis, and known acquired cystic disease.

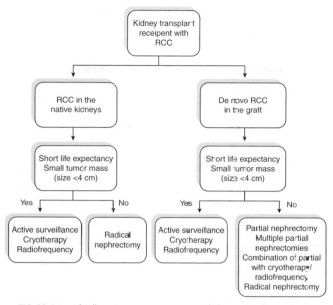

FIG. 23.4 Renal cell carcinoma management in kidney transplant patients.

Bladder Cancer

The risk of bladder cancer is increased compared with the general population (SIR = 3.18; 95% confidence interval, 1.34–7.53; $P = .008$). Urothelial carcinoma is the commonest type, and the risk factors include smoking and BK virus infection. Disease tend to be aggressive in nature with higher risks of recurrence, progression, and metastasis. The mean time of presentation ranges between 2.8 and 4 years post-transplantation. The common presentation is with microscopic or gross hematuria. Standard AUA guidelines for evaluation and management in the general population should be followed. Immunosuppression and associated comorbidities add to the challenge. **Intravesical bacillus Calmette-Guerin/chemotherapy can be used in selected patients with high-risk nonmuscle-invasive bladder cancer.** Chemo-radiotherapy and radical cystoprostatectomy and urinary diversion could be performed for muscle invasive disease. The graft with its blood vessels and ureter should be protected during surgery.

Prostate Cancer

The incidence of prostate cancer is comparable to the general population, and no specific screening recommendations is available for transplant recipients. Age appropriate prostate cancer screening (prostate-specific antigen) following the current guidelines for the general population is performed during pretransplant workup.

The challenges of management include the proximity of the transplant ureter, renal vessels, and kidney; postoperative scarring; and the increased risk of infection and poor healing secondary to the immunosuppression. Surgical modalities have been used safely. **The most common modality of treatment is radical prostatectomy, followed by radiation therapy and active surveillance.** Oncologic outcomes observed are comparable to those of the nontransplant patients.

Renal transplant patients pose additional risk due to the comorbidity of renal failure and immunosuppression requiring diligent and timely intervention of urologic complications. Management algorithm of malignancies in these patients are comparable to the general population with special considerations as described earlier. Urologic expertise is crucial and should play an active role in managing this unique patient population.

Suggested Readings

Alberts VP, Idu MM, Legemate DA, et al. Ureterovesical anastomotic techniques for kidney transplantation: a systematic review and meta-analysis. *Transpl Int* 2014;27(6):593-605.

Arpali E, Al-Qaoud T, Martinez E, et al. Impact of ureteral stricture and treatment choice on long-term graft survival in kidney transplantation. *Am J Transplant* 2018;18(8):1977-1985.

Berli JU, Montgomery JR, Segev DL, et al. Surgical management of early and late ureteral complications after renal transplantation: techniques and outcomes. *Clin Transplant* 2015;29(1):26-33.

Boissier R, Hevia V, Bruins HM, et al. The risk of tumour recurrence in patients undergoing renal transplantation for end-stage renal disease after previous treatment for a urological cancer: a systematic review. *Eur Urol* 2018 Jan;73(1):94-108.

Branchereau J, Karam G. Management of urologic complications of renal transplantation. *Eur Urol Suppl* 2016;15:408-414.

Branchereau J, Timsit MO, Neuzillet Y, et al. Management of renal transplant urolithiasis: a multicentre study by the French Urology Association Transplantation Committee. *World J Urol* 2018;36(1):105-109.

Hickman LA, Sawinski D, Guzzo T, Locke JE. Urologic malignancies in kidney transplantation. *Am J Transplant* 2018;18(1):13-22

Kälble T, Lucan M, Nicita G, et al. European Association of Urology. EAU guidelines on renal transplantation. *Eur Urol* 2005;47(2):156-156.

Kasiske BL, Zeier MG, Chapman JR, et al. Kidney Disease: Improving Global Outcomes. KDIGO clinical practice guideline for the care of kidney transplant recipients: a summary. *Kidney Int* 2010;77(4):299-311.

Lange D, Bidnur S, Hoag N, Chew BH. Ureteral stent-associated complications—where we are and where we are going. *Nat Rev Urol* 2015;12(1):17-25.

24

Principles and Acute Management of Upper Urinary Tract Obstruction

MICHAEL S. BOROFSKY AND ROBERT M. SWEET

CONTRIBUTORS OF CAMPBELL-WALSH-WEIN, 12TH EDITION

Casey A. Dauw, Stuart J. Wolf, Craig A. Peters, and Kirstan K. Meldrum

CLINICAL PRESENTATION

Upper urinary tract obstruction refers to the blockage of urinary flow from the renal calyces to the level of the ureterovesical junction. It is distinct from lower urinary tract obstruction (i.e., bladder through urethra); however, it can occur secondarily to lower urinary tract obstruction or dysfunction (i.e., urinary retention). Proper functioning of the lower urinary tract should always be considered in the differential.

Upper urinary tract obstruction can have a variable presentation. It can be symptomatic or asymptomatic, acute or chronic, and unilateral or bilateral, and it has a broad differential diagnosis. Obstructive uropathy accounts for approximately 10% of all cases of renal failure. On a population level, hydronephrosis tends to be more prevalent in women ages 20–60 years owing to pregnancy and gynecologic malignancies. After the age of 60 years, men are more likely to have hydronephrosis owing to the presence of prostatic diseases.

The most common presenting symptom associated with acute upper urinary tract obstruction is flank pain owing to stretching of the renal capsule. This can radiate to the lower abdomen, testicles, or labia and can cause severe degrees of discomfort along with nausea and vomiting. Chronic upper urinary tract obstruction, on the other hand, tends to have a milder course and in some cases can be painless.

Upper urinary tract obstruction can be associated with renal functional damage, particularly if left untreated. This is particularly concerning when present in childhood because congenital obstruction can prevent the kidneys from normal development. Acquired obstruction can similarly be determinantal to existing renal function in the mature adult as well.

HEMODYNAMIC CHANGES

Ureteral obstruction can lead to numerous functional changes that affect renal hemodynamics. Such changes depend on whether the obstruction is unilateral or bilateral. There is a triphasic response of renal blood flow in unilateral ureteral obstruction. In phase 1 (initial 2 hours), there is an increase in renal tubular pressure as a result of obstruction, leading to a decrease in glomerular filtration rate (GFR). The renal vasculature attempts to compensate for this decrease in GFR by increasing renal blood flow mediated by the release of vasodilators such as prostaglandin E2 and nitric oxide. During phase 2 (6–24 hours), the ureteral pressure remains elevated, and renal blood flow diminishes. In phase 3 (>24 hours), renal pelvic pressures trend down but remain elevated, and renal blood flow continues to diminish (Fig. 24.1), leading to renal ischemia.

In the case of bilateral ureteral obstruction (or solitary kidney obstruction), there is only a modest initial increase in renal blood flow followed by a more rapid decline, which can exacerbate the potential for renal function damage (Fig. 24.2). This is of clinical importance because timely decompression is of the essence.

FUNCTIONAL CHANGES

Upper urinary tract obstruction can damage the kidneys in several ways. Some of the functional change can be transient and relieved when the pressure is relieved; however, there is also the potential for permanent damage in cases with longstanding obstruction if associated with high pressures. It is likely that the risk of permanent damage to the affected kidney is related to the duration, degree, and severity of obstruction, though this these parameters are poorly defined.

One unique functional sequelae that occurs upon relief of bilateral ureteral obstruction or obstruction in a solitary kidney is **postobstructive diuresis.** This condition refers to polyuria that occurs as a result or in relation to osmotic diuresis of accumulated

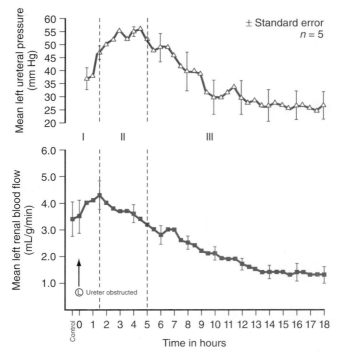

FIG. 24.1 Triphasic relationship between ipsilateral renal blood flow and left ureteral pressure during 18 hours of left ureteral obstruction. The three phases are designated by Roman numerals and separated by *vertical dashed lines*. In phase I, renal blood flow and ureteral pressure rise together. In phase II, the renal blood flow begins to decline, and ureteral pressure remains elevated. In phase III, the blood flow and ureteral pressure decline together. (From Moody TE, Vaughan ED JR, Gillenwater JY. Relationship between renal blood flow and ureteral pressure during 18 hours of total ureteral occlusion. Implications for changing sites of increased renal resistance. *Invest Urol* 1975;13:246-251.)

solutes, impaired tubular concentrating ability and reabsorption, as well as an increase in production of atrial natriuretic factor (ANP), which stimulates sodium wasting. Although this condition is typically self-limited, it is important to monitor electrolytes and ensure that the patient can self-hydrate to account for the potential of excess fluid losses. This condition is unlikely to occur in the

Unilateral obstruction

Bilateral obstruction or solitary kidney

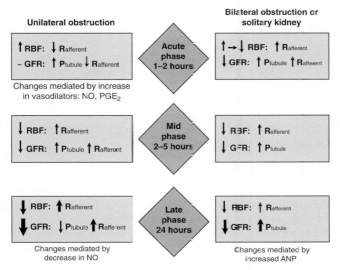

↑ RBF: ↓ R_afferent

~ GFR: ↑ P_tubule ↓ R_afferent

Changes mediated by increase in vasodilators: NO, PGE_2

↑ → ↓ RBF: ↑ R_afferent

↓ GFR: ↑ P_tubule ↑ R_afferent

Acute phase 1–2 hours

↓ RBF: ↑ R_afferent

↓ GFR: ↑ P_tubule ↑ R_afferent

↓ RBF: ↑ R_efferent

↓ GFR: ↑ P_tubule

Mid phase 2–5 hours

↓ RBF: ↑ R_afferent

↓ GFR: ↓ P_tubule ↑ R_afferent

↓ RBF: ↑ R_efferent

↓ GFR: ↑ P_tubule

Late phase 24 hours

Changes mediated by decrease in NO

Changes mediated by increased ANP

FIG. 24.2 Summary of the functional changes during ureteral obstruction. *~*, Little change; *ANP*, atrial natriuretic peptide; *GFR*, glomerular filtration rate; *NO*, nitric oxide; *PGE_2*, prostaglandin E_2; *Ptubule*, tubular hydrolic pressure; *Rafferent*, afferent arteriolar resistance; *RBF*, renal blood flow. *Refferent*, efferent arteriolar resistance.

setting of a normal contralateral kidney, which would otherwise be expected to maintain fluid and electrolyte balance.

DIAGNOSIS AND TESTING

Laboratory Studies

Urinalysis. Can provide an estimation of osmolality, evidence of urinary tract infection, insight into stone formation based on crystals that may be present in the urine, and the possible presence of medical renal disease with the presence of protein and/or cellular casts.

Fractional Excretion of Sodium (FENa). Can help differentiate between the three types of acute renal injury: prerenal, intrinsic, and postrenal. FENa = $(P_{Cr} \times U_{Na}) / (P_{Na} \times U_{Cr})$. FENa <1% suggests prerenal causes, >1% suggests intrinsic causes, >4% suggests postrenal causes (i.e., bilateral ureteral obstruction).

Assessment of Renal Function. Measurement of GFR is considered the gold standard, though is commonly estimated using serum creatinine levels. Creatinine is a waste product of muscle metabolism and can be influenced by age, muscle mass, and gender. In general, a GFR >90 mL/min/1.73 m^2 is considered normal, between 60 and 90 mL/min/1.73 m^2 is considered a mild decline in renal function, between 30 and 60 mL/min/1.73 m^2 is a moderate decline in renal function, between 15 and 30 mL/min/1.73 m^2 is a severe decline in renal function, and <15 mL/min/1.73 m^2 is considered renal failure.

IMAGING STUDIES (Tables 24.1 and 24.2)

Renal ultrasonography is considered a first-line modality in the evaluation of suspected upper urinary tract obstruction. Advantages include low cost, widespread availability, and lack of ionizing radiation. The information obtained by ultrasound is primarily anatomic and can provide renal size, cortical thickness, corticomedullary differentiation, and the grade of collecting system dilation (hydronephrosis). **Although the presence of hydronephrosis is suggestive of underlying obstruction, it is important to recognize that hydronephrosis is an anatomic finding, not a functional diagnosis, and that hydronephrosis alone does not indicate urinary tract obstruction.** The main downside of renal ultrasonography is that it is often unable to visualize the etiology of a potential obstruction, which often is located in the ureter, an area more challenging to confidently image via ultrasonography alone. Duplex Doppler sonography, which allows for identification of arterial waveforms, has been postulated as a tool to help detect

Table 24.1 Median Reported Sensitivity and Specificity for Diagnosis of Ureteral Calculi Relative to Noncontrast

MODALITY	MEDIAN SENSITIVITY (%)	MEDIAN SPECIFICITY (%)
Conventional radiography	57	76
Ultrasound	61	97
Intravenous pyelography	70	95
MRI	82	98.3
CT (not as gold standard)	98	97

CT, Computed tomography; *MRI*, magnetic resonance imaging.
(Adapted from Fulgham PF, Assimos DG, Pearle MS, Preminger GM. Clinical effectiveness protocols for imaging in the management of ureteral calculous disease: AUA technology assessment, 2012).

urinary obstruction via calculation of a **resistive index** (peak systolic velocity-end diastolic velocity/peak systolic velocity). In general, a resistive index of 0.70 is considered to be the upper limits of normal in adults; however, a wide variety of factors have been found to influence this measurement, limiting its widespread applicability. **Color Doppler ultrasonography** has also demonstrated utility in distinguishing obstructive from nonobstructive causes of obstruction by helping identify the presence of a ureteral jet in the bladder.

Computed Tomography (CT)

Cross-sectional imaging with a CT scan is considered the standard in the evaluation of urinary stone disease. CT has the advantage of speed, safety, and accuracy with reported

Table 24.2 Estimated Effective Radiation Dose by Type of Imaging Examination[a]

TYPE OF EXAM		EFFECTIVE DOSE (MSV)
Ultrasound (US)	Abdomen and pelvis US	0
Magnetic resonance imaging (MRI)	Abdomen and pelvis MRI	0
Conventional radiography		
	KUB	0.7
	KUB with tomograms	3.9
	IVU	3.0
Computed tomography (CT)		
	Noncontrast CT, abdomen and pelvis	10.0
	Without and with contrast CT, abdomen and pelvis (two-phase)	15.0
	Without and with contrast CT, abdomen and pelvis (three-phase)	20.0
	Noncontrast CT, abdomen and pelvis (low-dose protocol)	3.0
	Ultra-low dose protocol CT	<1.9

[a]Rob S, Bryant T, Wilson I, Somani BK. Ultra-low-dose, low-dose, and standard-dose CT of the kidney, ureters, and bladder: Is there a difference? Results from a systematic review of the literature. *Clin Radiol* 2017;72:11-15. Crossref, Medline, Google Scholar.
Adapted from Fulgham PF, Assimos DG, Pearle MS, Preminger GM. Clinical effectiveness protocols for imaging in the management of ureteral calculous disease: AUA technology assessment, 2012.

sensitivity rates of 96% for stone detection and specificity and positive predictive values of 100%. CT can detect most urinary stones with rare exceptions (i.e., protease inhibitor stones). It has also demonstrated the ability to identify a wide spectrum of alternative diagnoses, around 10% in patients being evaluated for renal colic. When a stone is not identified as being a source of upper urinary tract obstruction, CT urography (CTU) may be considered. Conventional CTU involves three phases: an unenhanced noncontrast phase, a nephrogenic phase at 100–120 seconds after contrast administration, and an excretory phase obtained several minutes afterward after the kidneys have had an opportunity to drain. The primary drawback of CT scanning is radiation exposure. Low-dose and ultra-low dose radiation protocols may be used with similar performance capabilities, especially in the case of stones and when the body mass index (BMI) is low (Fig. 24.3).

Magnetic Resonance Urography (MRU)

MRU is the best cross-sectional alternative to a CT scan because it is also able to provide excellent anatomic information without ionizing radiation. The main drawbacks of this diagnostic modality are that it is more costly and more restricted and does not directly identify most urinary stones. MRU can provide some unique functional information related to obstruction because the administration and uptake of contrast have been shown to correlate well with differential renal function, but contrast excretion has been shown to correlate well with renal scintigraphy (measured as renal transit time). **One concern when considering MRU is the potential for nephrogenic systemic fibrosis (NSF),** which has been linked to gadolinium-based agents and can occur in patients with severe renal impairment. Group II agents are not contraindicated.

Nuclear Renography

Nuclear medicine renography is the only imaging modality that can provide noninvasive information about dynamic renal function. The most commonly performed nuclear medicine scan for this purpose is technetium-99m-mercaptoacetyltriglycine (^{99m}Tc-MAG3) because it has high excretion by the kidneys, rapid clearance, low radiation dose, and tubular secretion. It is

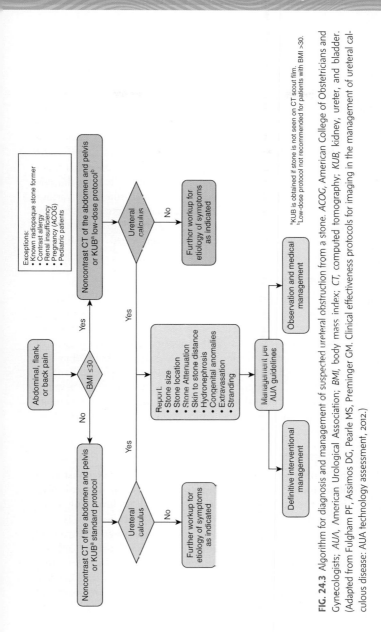

FIG. 24.3 Algorithm for diagnosis and management of suspected ureteral obstruction from a stone. *ACOG*, American College of Obstetricians and Gynecologists; *AUA*, American Urological Association; *BMI*, body mass index; *CT*, computed tomography; *KUB*, kidney, ureter, and bladder. (Adapted from Fulgham PF, Assimos DG, Pearle MS, Preminger GM. Clinical effectiveness protocols for imaging in the management of ureteral calculous disease: AUA technology assessment, 2012.)

preferred over technetium-99m-diethylenetriaminepentaacetic acid (^{99m}Tc-DTPA) because it has a higher renal uptake. Renal obstruction is most commonly determined based on the T1/2 (time for one half of the tracer to leave the collecting system). By convention, if the T1/2 is <10 minutes, the kidney is considered unobstructed. If the T1/2 is >20 minutes, the kidney is considered obstructed, and if the T1/2 is between 10 and 20 minutes, the results are considered equivocal. One possible false positive to watch for is the potential for prolonged washout times in the setting of massive collecting system dilation or poor renal function. This can be minimized with the administration of a diuretic during the study (furosemide) to accelerate urine flow. Various protocols exist, and it is important to take this into consideration when interpreting results and particularly comparing them to prior studies, which may have been performed with different protocols.

Excretory Urography

Before the advent and widespread availability of CT scans, excretory urography (intravenous pyelography) was the imaging modality of choice to diagnose upper urinary tract obstruction. Some of the downsides of this approach include the lack of detailed anatomic imaging of structures around the kidney and ureters as well as the fact that the test itself is dependent on GFR. Further, it requires instillation of contrast, which may not be feasible in patients with renal insufficiency or contrast allergies or in those whom radiation exposure is a concern (i.e., pregnancy).

Whitaker Test

The primary rationale for performing a Whitaker test is to differentiate obstructive from nonobstructive hydronephrosis. This test requires a percutaneous needle or nephrostomy in the collecting system through which contrast is infused at 10 mL/min. Intrapelvic pressures are monitored, as are intravesical pressures, which are obtained from a urodynamic catheter placed in the bladder. Measurements are taken by subtracting the intravesical pressures from the intrapelvic pressures as urine passes the ureteropelvic junction (UPJ) and then ureterovesical junction (UVJ). Pressures <15 cm H_2O are considered normal,

>22 cm H_2O is indicative of obstruction, and between 15 and 22 cm H_2O is considered indeterminate.

ACUTE MANAGEMENT

Two of the critical decisions upon the identification of upper urinary tract obstruction are symptom control and the need for drainage. In the event of symptomatic obstruction, characterized by renal colic, there is a need for analgesia. Non-narcotic treatment should be first-line therapy. Nonsteroidal antiinflammatory drugs (NSAIDs) can be very effective. They work by decreasing renal blood flow and subsequently renal pelvic pressure, which can lead to pain relief. **They have been clinically shown to be superior to opioids with a greater decrease in pain scores, lesser instance of gastrointestinal side effects, and decreased need for second-line analgesia.** It is important to be aware of the patient's renal function prior to NSAID administration because the reduction of renal blood flow can be detrimental, particularly in the setting of acute or chronic renal insufficiency. Other treatments for renal colic include acetaminophen, alpha blockers, cortico-steroids, and opioids. Additionally, antiemetics can be used in the event of concomitant nausea or vomiting, which occurs quite frequently in the setting of ureteral obstruction.

The second consideration that should be made in each case of obstruction is an assessment as to whether or not acute drainage is indicated. Typically, drainage can be achieved either by retrograde ureteral stenting, antegrade nephrostomy tube placement or by relieving the primary source of obstruction (such as in the case of a ureteral stone). The decision of whether acute drainage is warranted should be based on several factors. Acute drainage or decompression of an obstructed upper urinary tract should occur promptly in the setting of infection and has shown the potential to be lifesaving therapy in the event of severe infection or sepsis. In such instances, it is advisable to achieve drainage alone and temporize the obstruction because excess manipulation of the infected, obstructed urinary tract could exacerbate the underlying illness. Another scenario in which prompt drainage should be performed is in the event of bilateral renal obstruction or obstruction of a solitary kidney because there is a greater potential risk of renal injury without a contralateral functioning kidney to compensate. Similarly, prompt drainage should be considered whenever any degree of obstruction (with high intrarenal pressures) is suspected in the setting of infected urine, immunocompromised patients or risk for renal failure.

Methods of Upper Urinary Tract Drainage

Retrograde Ureteral Stent Placement. Retrograde ureteral stent placement is typically preferred for most cases of ureteral obstruction. Advantages of retrograde ureteral stent placement include the utilization of existing anatomy and orifices, a completely internal drainage without the need of any external drains or appliances, and in most cases a high degree of success that can be achieved with minimal sedation. Additionally, retrograde stenting can be performed on patients at high risk of bleeding. Disadvantages of retrograde stenting include the need to use cystoscopy and identify the ureteral orifice in order to place the stent and achieve renal decompression. Certain scenarios may make this challenging such as reconstructed lower urinary tract anatomy (ileal conduits, neobladders, transplant) or the presence of lower extremity contractures or anatomy precluding the ability to be placed in lithotomy. Other scenarios in which a retrograde ureteral stent may not be effective is in the event of severe obstruction such as with a densely impacted stone or stenosis whereby the passage to the kidney is completely obscured. Similarly, high-grade extrinsic compression as may be seen in the case of advanced malignancy or iatrogenic injury with a suture or clip may make retrograde passage impossible.

Technique. Prior to placement of a ureteral stent, AUA guidelines may recommend antibiotic prophylaxis (see Chapter 3). The procedure can be performed under local anesthesia, but sedation or general anesthesia is generally preferable. The procedure begins with placement of a cystoscope into the bladder. When in the bladder, a guidewire is used to cannulate the ureteral orifice of the affected kidney and attempt passage to the renal collecting system. Various guidewires exist and differ in their degree of stiffness and coatings. Typically, less stiff hydrophilic wires are safer with a decreased risk of inadvertent ureteral perforation and may be better suited to bypass obstruction. Conversely, stiffer wires allow for more secure retrograde access and can make it easier to pass a stent. Wires can be exchanged through open-ended catheters. Hybrid wires (PTFE coated

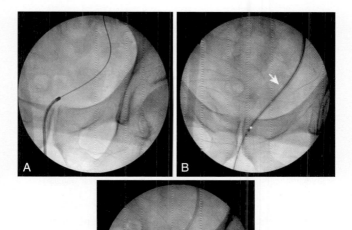

FIG. 24.4 (A) Cystoscope in bladder plus guidewire in ureter. (B) Stent placed in ureter through 10-Fr sheath (*asterisk* indicates radiopaque marker of pusher; *arrow* indicates 10-Fr sheath). (C) Guidewire and 10-Fr sheath removed; distal stent section coiled in bladder.

nitinol shaft with hydrophilic tip) offer the benefits of both of these features. When the wire is in the kidney, the open-ended catheter can be passed over it to perform retrograde pyelography with gentle instillation of contrast medium. This can be useful in detailing the renal collecting system anatomy and characterizing the degree of obstruction. It is also advisable to obtain a urine culture from the kidney at this time, especially in cases of suspected infection. The working wire should then be replaced and the stent placed coaxially until there is a curl in the kidney as well as in the bladder to ensure it stays in position (Fig. 24.4).

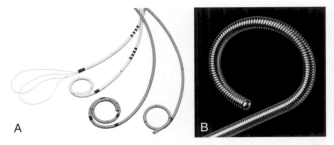

FIG. 24.5 Different stent designs. (A) Polaris Loop stent, Polaris Ultra stent, Percuflex Plus stent, and Contour VL stent. (B) Resonance metal stent. (A, Courtesy of Boston Scientific, Marlborough, MA; B, Courtesy of Cook Medical, Bloomington, IN.)

Ureteral Stents. Most stents are made of flexible polymers such as polyurethane or silicone. Metallic stents are available for use in instances of severe external compression and have been shown to be more resistant to obstruction. Although most stents have a double-J configuration, other designs exist as well, including single-J stents with only a proximal curl and other novel distal ends in an effort to decrease stent related lower urinary tract symptoms (Fig. 24.5). Ureteral stent symptoms are common and typically include flank discomfort, especially with voiding, bladder pain, hematuria, and dysuria, as well as urinary frequency and urgency. There is a validated ureteral stent symptom questionnaire designed to help characterize stent symptoms and identify meaningful ways to minimize them. To date, there are varying opinions on whether stent length and position are associated with worsened symptoms; however, alpha blockers and antimuscarinics have been shown to improve stent tolerability.

Antegrade Nephrostomy Tube Placement. Percutaneous nephrostomy tube insertion into the kidney is the other primary method of achieving upper tract drainage (Fig. 24.6). Advantages of this approach are the fact that it is potentially more definitive by addressing the kidney directly and can be achieved most rapidly and most definitively. One of the disadvantages to percutaneous nephrostomy tube insertion is the fact that it is more invasive and requires placement of a needle and tube directly through the renal

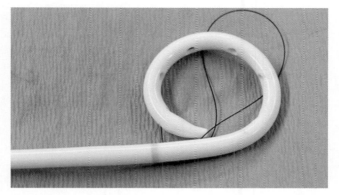

FIG. 24.6 Cope catheter with the retention string loosened for demonstration.

parenchyma. As a result there is higher potential for bleeding, and as such, this approach is contraindicated in patients with untreated coagulopathy.

The decision on whether or not to place a retrograde stent or antegrade nephrostomy tube depends on the indication, the patient's medical condition and anatomy, and preferences of both the patient and physician. Both approaches have been found to be effective in their potential to resolve fevers in patients with obstruction and infection. Another important consideration is patient quality of life in which temporary nephrostomy tubes have been found to have an improvement in health-related quality of life.

Technique. A majority of percutaneous nephrostomy tubes are placed by interventional radiologists, although communication between the urologist and interventional radiologist is important, especially in cases in which percutaneous tube placement may ultimately be used at a later date for an antegrade procedure such as percutaneous nephrolithotomy. Antimicrobial prophylaxis should be administered prior to the procedure, and all anticoagulation should be held. Local or general anesthesia may be used.

Patients may be positioned in either the prone or supine position. The prone position (Fig. 24.7) offers the advantage of optimizing

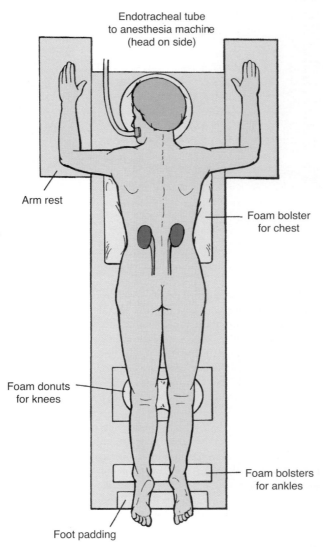

FIG. 24.7 Padding for prone positioning.

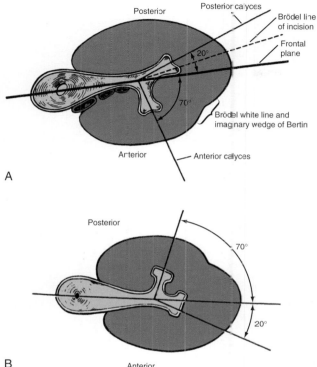

FIG. 24.8 Relation of anterior and posterior calyces to renal parenchyma in Brödel-type kidney (A) and Hodson-type kidney (B). The optimal site of percutaneous entry from the posterior aspect of the kidney is into a posterior calyx because the path into the renal pelvis is fairly straight. If entry is into an anterior calyx (from the posterior aspect of the kidney), then an acute angulation must be made to enter the renal pelvis, which may not be possible with rigid instrumentation. (From Smith AD. *Controversies in endourology.* Philadelphia: Saunders, 1995.)

potential sites of puncture into the kidney, particularly along the posterior calyces (Fig. 24.8). The upper pole in particular is favorable in the prone position owing to the posterior orientation of the upper pole in general (Fig. 24.9). Another advantage of the prone position is that it affords the operator access to both kidneys as may be warranted in the event of bilateral obstruction. One of the disadvantages

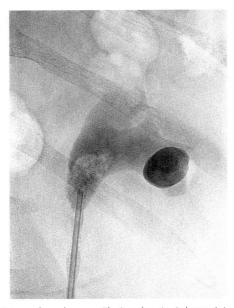

FIG. 24.9 Retrograde pyelogram with air and contrast shows air in upper pole compound calyx and posterior lower pole calyx.

of the prone position is the potential for decreased cardiac index and higher peak inspiratory pressures, though there is conflicting evidence to support this (Fig. 24.3). When placing patients in the supine position, typically the patient is positioned with the ipsilateral side toward the most lateral aspect of the table and the flank elevated with a bolster or 3-L bag of saline underneath the lumbar fossa. One advantage is the potential to more easily work from a retrograde position simultaneously in the absence of the availability of split leg table adaptors which allows for simultaneous antegrade/retrograde access in the prone position. Disadvantages include a lesser surface are for renal puncture and potential difficulty reaching the upper pole.

Access may be guided either via fluoroscopy or ultrasound. One advantage to fluoroscopy is that the full renal anatomy can be visualized at once. Further, access needles and tubes that are radiopaque can be confidently visualized, and there is potential to see stones, which are a common source of obstruction (Fig. 24.10). Disadvantages include exposure to the patient, surgeon, and

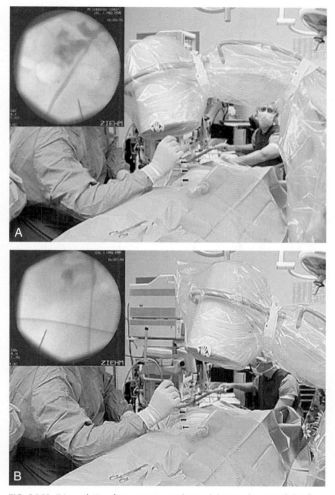

FIG. 24.10 Triangulation fluoroscopic guidance. (A) With the top of the fluoroscopy unit rotated laterally and cephalad, adjust the access needle *(arrows)* to a mediolateral orientation of the needle. (B) After rotating the top of the fluoroscopy unit medially and while keeping mediolateral orientation of the needle constant, move the needle in the cephalo-caudad plane until the needle is again aimed toward the desired calyx. (From Miller NL, Matlaga BR, Lingeman JE. Techniques for fluoroscopic percutaneous renal access. *J Urol* 2007;178:15-23.)

operating room personnel to radiation as well as a lack of three-dimensional imagery, which can make it challenging to interpret the position of the needle relative to the kidney and desired point of access. One of the main limitations is also the need for opacification of the collecting system. In some cases, this can be achieved via retrograde instillation of contrast through an open-ended catheter. Alternatively, a combined approach is commonly utilized whereby ultrasound is used to advance a needle into the kidney to achieve access and then contrast is instilled for the purpose of using fluoroscopy to guide the ultimate nephrostomy tube into a selected calyx. Ultrasound-guided access offers decreased radiation and lesser cost. It is additionally advantageous in providing a better three-dimensional perspective and can also identify surrounding viscera such as lung, pleura, spleen, liver, and bowel. Further, no opacification of the renal collecting system is necessary. One of the disadvantages of ultrasound is that it can be challenging to gain a confident image of the kidney, especially in obese patients with high BMIs.

Suggested Readings

Assimos D, Krambeck A, Miller NL, et al. Surgical Management of kidney stones, AUA/Endourology Society Guideline. 2016.

Fulgham PF, Assimos DG, Pearle MS, Preminger GM. Clinical effectiveness protocols for imaging in the management of ureteral calculous disease: AUA technology assessment. 2012.

Nord RG, Cubler-Goodman A, Bagley DH. Prone split-leg position for simultaneous retrograde ureteroscopic and percutaneous nephroscopic procedures. *J Endourol* 1991;5(1):13-16. http://doi.org/10.1089/end.1991.5.13.

25

Definitive Treatment Options for Ureteral Obstruction

MICHAEL S. BOROFSKY AND ROBERT M. SWEET

CONTRIBUTORS OF CAMPBELL-WALSH-WEIN, 12TH EDITION

Stephen Y. Nakada, and Sara L. Best

CLINICAL PRESENTATION

Upper urinary tract obstruction has a variable presentation depending on the etiology and acuity of the obstruction. Workup most commonly involves cross-sectional imaging and, in many cases, a temporizing procedure with either ureteral stent or nephrostomy tube drainage with concurrent retrograde or antegrade studies to further delineate the degree and nature of the obstruction prior to planning definitive management (see Chapter 24). One of the most common causes of obstruction is urinary stone disease (see Chapter 27). However, numerous non stone related causes of obstruction exist as well and can occur anywhere from the kidney to the bladder.

INDICATIONS FOR REPAIR

While temporizing measures such as stents and nephrostomy tubes with scheduled changes can offer a definitive solution in select situations such as end-of-life care and poor surgical candidates, in general, the goal in managing upper urinary tract obstruction should be a definitive repair that reestablishes normal drainage from the kidney to the bladder and avoids the needs for stents or nephrostomy tubes. Indications for repair include the presence of symptoms, impairment in renal function, development of stones and/or urinary tract infection (UTI) and in rare cases hypertension. The goal of repair should be symptom relief and preservation of renal function. In asymptomatic patients without apparent functional impairment to the kidney, observation with serial imaging and renal scans can be considered. Occasionally, nephrectomy is a more suitable treatment option rather than definitive repair. This can be considered in the event of diminished or absent renal function and a normal contralateral kidney, especially in the setting of chronic infection and/or pain. In general, differential renal function below 15%–20% is the threshold at which the kidney is considered nonsalvageable.

URETEROPELVIC JUNCTION OBSTRUCTION (UPJO)

Most cases of UPJO are congenital in nature but may not be identified until later in life. Other etiologies include stone-related or postoperative strictures, neoplastic obstruction, fibroepithelial polyps, or extrinsic compression. Cases of congenital UPJO typically result from intrinsic disease characterized by an aperistaltic segment of the ureter. Histologically, this segment of ureter often has abnormal longitudinal muscle or fibrous tissue distinct from the expected spiral musculature that is usually present. The resulting defect often leads to a ureter that looks grossly normal but does not function appropriately. Other less common etiologies include true ureteral strictures characterized by abnormal collagen deposition or kinks/valves in the ureter that preclude normal antegrade propulsion of urine. Aberrant crossing vessels are also associated with UPJO, having been identified in 63% of patients with UPJO but only 20% among individuals with normal kidneys.

Diagnosis

The routine use of maternal prenatal ultrasonography has led to a dramatic increase in the identification of prenatal hydronephrosis and ultimately UPJO. The diagnosis and management of UPJO in pediatric patients can be found in Chapter 7. The presentation of UPJO in adolescents, teenagers, and adults is more likely to include intermittent abdominal or flank pain with nausea and vomiting, hematuria, UTI or in rare cases hypertension. Typically, provocative testing with diuretic renography accompanied by Lasix administration confirms the diagnosis. Cross-sectional imaging with computed tomography (CT) and/or magnetic resonance imaging (MRI) can also be utilized to gain anatomic information and identify the presence of a crossing vessel. Ultimately, retrograde pyelography

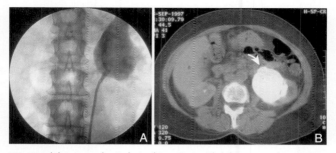

FIG. 25.1 (A) Retrograde study in this patient with left ureteropelvic junction obstruction reveals a "high insertion" of the left ureter. (B) Computed tomography scan in the same patient reveals the ureter inserting on the anatomically anterior aspect of the renal pelvis. A marsupializing incision must be made in a true posterior direction from the ureter into the renal pelvis.

can be used to confirm the diagnosis, though this is commonly accomplished at the time of definitive repair (Fig. 25.1).

Pyeloplasty

When treatment is indicated, the procedure of choice is a pyeloplasty (open, laparoscopic, robotic), though endourologic incisional procedures can be considered as well, particularly in the case of secondary UPJO. Pyeloplasty is most commonly performed in a dismembered fashion whereby the abnormal portion of ureter is fully incised, and the healthy end of the ureter is reanastomosed to the renal pelvis. This is the only approach that allows for complete excision of the diseased area of ureter. It also allows for transposition of the UPJ anterior to or posterior to potential crossing vessels. This can be achieved either by open or minimally invasive laparoscopic or robotic approaches with relatively equivocal outcomes.

Technique. In the classic Anderson-Hynes technique, the proximal ureter is dissected to the level of the renal pelvis. The abnormal UPJ tissue is excised, and the proximal ureter is spatulated and anastomosed to the renal pelvis in a watertight fashion, typically over a ureteral stent (Fig. 25.2). Reduction pyeloplasty can be performed in cases of extremely capacious renal collecting systems but is typically unnecessary. Contraindications for dismembered pyeloplasty include small intrarenal pelvis and

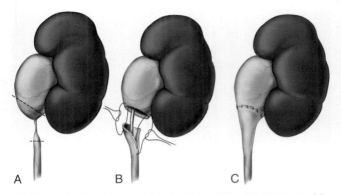

A   B   C

FIG. 25.2 (A) Traction sutures are placed on the medial and lateral aspects of the dependent portion of the renal pelvis in preparation for dismembered pyeloplasty. A traction suture is also placed on the lateral aspect of the proximal ureter, below the level of obstruction. This will help maintain proper orientation for the subsequent repair. (B) Ureteropelvic junction is excised. The proximal ureter is spatulated on its lateral aspect. The apex of this lateral, spatulated aspect of the ureter is then brought to the inferior border of the pelvis while the medial side of the ureter is brought to the superior edge of the pelvis. (C) Anastomosis is then performed with fine interrupted or running absorbable sutures placed full thickness through the ureteral and renal pelvis walls in a watertight fashion. In general, we prefer to leave an indwelling internal stent for adult patients. The stent is removed 4 to 6 weeks later.

long segment of diseased ureter typically 2 cm or greater. Open pyeloplasty is typically performed via an extraperitoneal flank approach. Laparoscopic pyeloplasty can be performed via a transperitoneal or retroperitoneal approach. One advantage of a transperitoneal approach for laparoscopic repair is larger working space and familiar anatomy. Most commonly, patients stay in hospital overnight with Foley catheter, and surgical drain left in place from 24–36 hours. If drain output increased after the Foley catheter is removed, this is suggestive of ureteral leak from reflux, and the catheter should be replaced for 7 days. The ureteral stent is typically removed 4–6 weeks after surgery. Success rates have been estimated at 95% for open or lap/robotic approaches with the majority of failures occurring in the first

2 years. If failure is identified, repeat pyeloplasty (86% success rate) or endopyelotomy (70% success rate) can be considered.

Special Situations

In the case of a small intrarenal pelvis, a ureterocalicostomy can be performed by transecting the lower pole of the kidney and anastomosing the ureter to the lower pole calyx (Fig. 25.3). If stones are present in the kidney, they can be removed at the time of repair via pyelolithotomy. If performed laparoscopically or

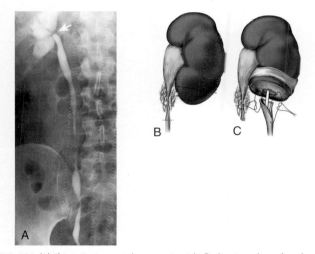

FIG. 25.3 (A) This patient reported progressive right flank pain and was found on this retrograde study to have a ureteropelvic junction obstruction *(arrow)* associated with a small intrarenal pelvis. This situation may be best managed with a ureterocalicostomy. (B) The ureter is identified in the retroperitoneum and dissected proximally as far as possible. The kidney is mobilized as much as necessary to gain access to the lower pole and to subsequently perform the anastomosis without tension. A lower pole nephrectomy is performed, removing as much parenchyma as necessary to widely expose a dilated lower pole calyx. (C) The proximal ureter is spatulated laterally. The anastomosis should subsequently be performed over an internal stent, and consideration should also be given to leaving a nephrostomy tube. The initial sutures are placed at the apex of the ureteral spatulation, and the lateral wall of the calyx with a second suture is placed 180 degrees from that.

Continued

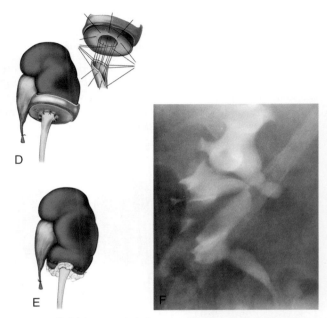

FIG. 25.3, cont'd (D) Anastomosis is then completed in an open fashion, placing each suture circumferentially *(inset)* but not securing them until the anastomosis has been completed. (E) Renal capsule is closed over the cut surface of the parenchyma whenever possible. However, the capsule should not be closed near the anastomosis because that may compromise the lumen by extrinsic compression. Instead, the anastomosis should be protected with a graft of perinephric fat or a peritoneal or omental flap. (F) Intravenous urogram 2 months after right ureterocalicostomy reveals a widely patent ureterocalyceal anastomosis at the lower pole *(arrow)*.

robotically, endoscopic stone retrieval can be achieved either with laparoscopic instruments or occasionally with passage of a flexible endoscope through one of the working ports. Alternatives to dismembered pyeloplasty typically include creation of flaps out of redundant renal pelvis. Such approaches can be utilized to address a high insertion of the ureter (Foley Y-V plasty) (Fig. 25.4) or long segments of diseased ureter (Culp-DeWeed spiral flap) (Fig. 25.5).

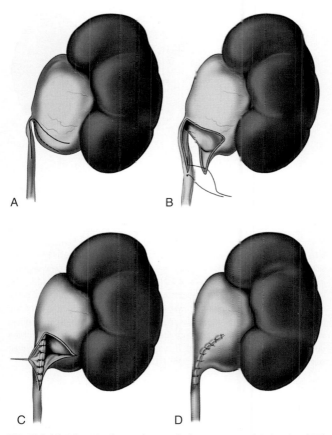

FIG. 25.4 (A) Foley Y-V plasty is best applied to a ureteropelvic junction (UPJ) obstruction associated with a high insertion of the ureter. The flap is outlined with tissue marker or stay sutures. The base of the V is positioned on the dependent, medial aspect of the renal pelvis and the apex at the UPJ. The incision from the apex of the flap, which represents the stem of the Y, is then carried along the lateral aspect of the proximal ureter well into an area of normal caliber. (B) The flap is developed with fine scissors. The apex of the pelvic flap is then brought to the most inferior aspect of the ureterotomy incision. (C) The posterior walls are then approximated using interrupted or running fine absorbable suture. (D) The anastomosis is completed with approximation of the anterior walls of the pelvic flap and ureterotomy.

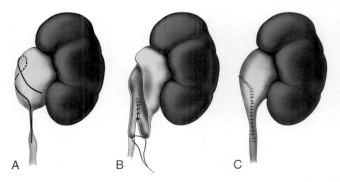

FIG. 25.5 (A) A spiral flap may be indicated for relatively long areas of proximal ureteral obstruction when the ureteropelvic junction (UPJ) is already in a dependent position. The spiral flap is outlined with the base situated obliquely on the dependent aspect of the renal pelvis. The base of the flap is positioned anatomically lateral to the UPJ, between the ureteral insertion and the renal parenchyma. The flap is spiraled posteriorly to anteriorly or vice versa. The anatomically medial line of incision is carried down completely through the obstructed proximal ureteral segment into normal-caliber ureter. The site of the apex for the flap is determined by the length of flap required to bridge the obstruction. The longer the segment of proximal ureteral obstruction, the farther away is the apex because this will make the flap longer. However, to preserve vascular integrity of the flap, the ratio of flap length to width should not exceed 3:1. (B) Once the flap is developed, the apex is rotated down to the most inferior aspect of the ureterotomy. (C) The anastomosis is then completed, usually over an internal stent, again using fine absorbable sutures.

Endopyelotomy

This is typically achieved by using an endoscope to make a full-thickness lateral incision at the level of the UPJ and allowing postprocedural healing over a ureteral stent. This can be performed in an antegrade or retrograde fashion. Antegrade may be preferred in the case of coexisting stones whereby the stones can be addressed simultaneously via percutaneous nephrolithotomy. Typically, stones should be removed prior to the endopyelotomy so that fragments do not migrate into the incision site.

Technique. Incision can be achieved using a laser, cautery wire balloon, or percutaneously guided cold knife. The incision should be made laterally to avoid vascular structures. A safety wire should

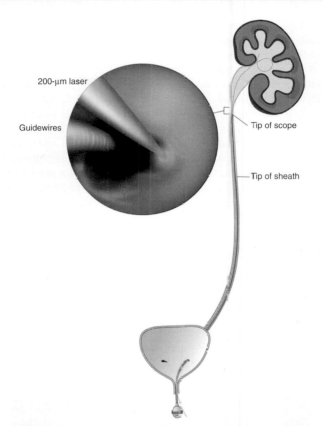

FIG. 25.6 Flexible ureteroscopic endopyelotomy using holmium laser, demonstrating endoscopic view of the ureteropelvic junction *(inset)*. A safety wire is in place, and the ureteroscope is passed through a ureteral access sheath as a lateral incision is being made under endoscopic view, using holmium laser fiber. A properly sited, complete incision is straightforward with this direct visualization technique.

always be used to ensure the ability to pass a stent once the incision is made (Fig. 25.6). After incision is made, balloon dilation can be considered up to 24 Fr to ensure a full-thickness incision. Similarly, contrast instillation can be performed to look for extravasation which confirms an adequately deep incision has been made.

Endopyelotomy stents may be considered for drainage that have different sized proximal and distal diameters such as to facilitate wider healing of the lumen. There is controversy as to whether the size of the stent leads to improvements in success rates. There is little known difference in outcomes among the various techniques. Outcomes for primary endopyelotomy can be variable (40%–70%) and are lower in the presence of a crossing vessel or in cases of high-grade obstruction. Outcomes are typically better for secondary UPJO. Contraindications for endopyelotomy include a long segment of obstruction (>2 cm), active infection, and untreated coagulopathy. Due to the low success rate and increase in bleeding risk, UPJO with a crossing vessel shouldn't be primarily managed in this way. Typically, if a primary endopyelotomy has failed, operative intervention with a laparoscopic or open approach should be considered.

RETROCAVAL URETER

Retrocaval ureter is a rare congenital abnormality whereby the course of the ureter wraps around the inferior vena cava and can result in obstruction. It is caused by abnormal persistence of the posterior cardinal veins during embryologic development. It can be diagnosed either via cross-sectional imaging or via retrograde pyelography based on the classic S shaped deformity that is seen upon opacification of the ureter (Fig. 25.7).

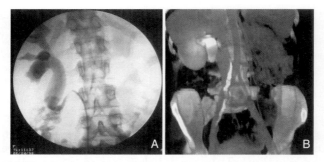

FIG. 25.7 (A) Retrograde pyelography in a patient with right-sided hydronephrosis. This study reveals a typical S-shaped deformity secondary to the ureter coursing laterally to medially posterior to the inferior vena cava. (B) Three-dimensional spiral computed tomography demonstrates the presence of a retrocaval ureter.

Pyelopyelostomy

The classic repair for a retrocaval ureter is achieved by dismembering the ureter via standard open or laparoscopic techniques and transposing it to its normal anatomic position anterior to the vena cava. The free ends are then anastomosed using absorbable sutures in a tension free watertight fashion.

URETERAL STRICTURE DISEASE

Ureteral strictures can occur as a result of many factors, including prior surgery, radiation, ischemia, fibrosis, malignancy, and congenital causes (Figs. 25.8 and Box 25.1). The location and length of the stricture are critical considerations when planning surgical repair.

Diagnosis

The location of a ureteral stricture can be identified on antegrade or retrograde pyelogram, CT urography, or diagnostic ureteroscopy. Often a combination of these will be utilized to fully characterize the length of the stricture as well. In cases in which the etiology of the stricture is unclear, a biopsy should be considered to rule out malignancy. Further, it is important to ensure adequate function of the ipsilateral renal unit prior to planning repair.

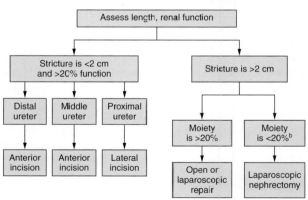

OPTIMAL THERAPY FOR BENIGN URETERAL STRICTURES[a]

[Assess length, renal function]

Stricture is <2 cm and >20% function → Distal ureter → Anterior incision; Middle ureter → Anterior incision; Proximal ureter → Lateral incision

Stricture is >2 cm → Moiety is >20% → Open or laparoscopic repair; Moiety is <20%[b] → Laparoscopic nephrectomy

[a]Consider balloon if transplant on immunosuppression.
[b]Pediatric patients and select patients with renal insufficiency may warrant repair.

FIG. 25.8 Algorithm for management of benign ureteral stricture disease.

> **Box 25.1** Differential Diagnosis for Etiology of Ureteral Stricture
>
> - Malignancy (e.g., transitional cell carcinoma, cervical cancer)
> - Ureteral calculus
> - Radiation
> - Ischemia or trauma caused by surgical dissection
> - Periureteral fibrosis caused by abdominal aortic aneurysm or endometriosis
> - Endoscopic instrumentation
> - Renal ablation injury
> - Infection (tuberculosis)
> - Idiopathic condition

Balloon dilation of ureteral strictures is another endoscopic management option whereby a balloon catheter is passed over the length of the stricture and expanded under high pressure to 15 to 24 Fr. This can be achieved either in antegrade or retrograde fashion. Typically, a stent is left for several weeks following the dilation (Fig. 25.9). Reported success rates range from 50%–76% and success has been found to be more likely when treating shorter, nonanastomotic strictures. As such, long strictures ≥2 cm in length are considered a contraindication for endoscopic approaches. Another endourologic technique is endoureterotomy. In this procedure, a ureteroscope is passed to the level of the stricture, and a full-thickness incision is made in the ureter most commonly using a holmium laser. This can be combined with balloon dilation to enlarge the incision. Success rates for endoureterotomy range from 66% to 83%. The position of the incision should be chosen depending on the segment of ureter involved. One rare situation in a completely obliterative stricture is a combined antegrade and retrograde approach whereby the light shining from one side of the stricture is identified and used as a target to make a blind incision in the ureter in hopes of identifying and reestablishing the true lumen. This "cut to the light" approach should be reserved for poor surgical candidates desiring internalization of urinary drainage.

Surgical Management

Definitive surgical repair of ureteral strictures is generally preferable to chronic stent changes when patients are otherwise acceptable surgical candidates. In such cases, the surgical approach will

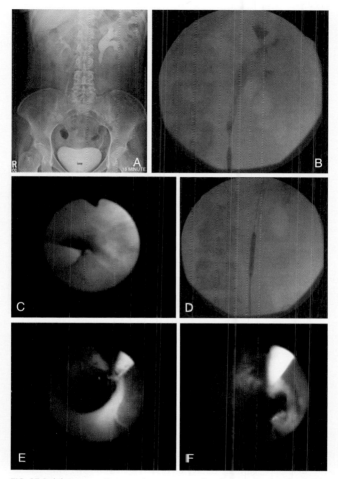

FIG. 25.9 (A) Preoperative excretory urogram showing proximal ureteral stricture after ureteral injury. (B) Fluoroscopic image of flexible ureteroscope at stricture. (C) Corresponding endoscopic image of stricture. (D) Fluoroscopic image of balloon dilation to enable incision of ureteral stricture. (E) Endoscopic image of strictured area after balloon dilation (note resultant full-thickness, lateral incision). (F) Endoscopic view completing laser incision of stricture.

Continued

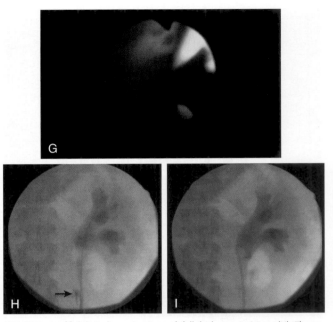

FIG. 25.9, cont'd (G) Endoscopic view of full-thickness incision. (H) Fluoroscopic image demonstrating extravasation *(arrow)*. (I) Fluoroscopic image after stent placement.

be determined based on the location and length of the stricture. In all cases, the surgeon should seek to reestablish ureteral continuity through creation of a tension-free, watertight repair. In the case of short segmental strictures, this may be accomplished by excising the diseased segment of ureter and reanastomosing the healthy proximal and distal segments (ureteroureterostomy, ureteroneocystotomy). Additional ureteral mobility can be achieved proximally by performing renal descensus and distally by mobilization of the bladder (psoas hitch, Boari flap). When the defect is exceedingly long, the ureter can be rerouted to the contralateral side (transureteroureterostomy), grafted with a tissue flap (buccal mucosal grafting), or substituted with a segment of bowel (ileal ureteral substitution). Autotransplantation of the kidney to the pelvis

Table 25.1 Available Surgical Techniques to Provide Additional Ureteral Mobility During Ureteral Stricture Repair

TECHNIQUE	URETERAL DEFECT LENGTH (cm)
Ureteroureterostomy	2–3
Ureteroneocystostomy	4–5
Psoas hitch	6–10
Boari flap	12–15
Renal descensus	5–8

is another treatment option in cases of severe ureteral stricture disease (Table 25.1).

Ureteroureterostomy. Ideally suited for short segment strictures (2–3 cm) in the proximal or mid ureter. Open or laparoscopic or robotic approaches are suitable. The ureter should be handled delicately, and a layer of adventitia should be preserved to avoid devascularization in the process of ureteral dissection. A Penrose drain or vessel loop may be used to assist in atraumatic handling. Upon identification of the diseased segment, it is excised, and the healthy ends of ureter are spatulated 180 degrees apart. Fine, absorbable suture should then be used to anastamose the ureter over a ureteral stent (Fig. 25.10). Retroperitoneal fat or omentum may be used to cover the anastomosis. Success rates are high (90%+).

Ureteroneocystotomy. This is the most appropriate surgical management option for ureteral stricture involving the distal 3–4 cm of the ureter. It can be performed either with open or laparoscopic or robotic approaches. This procedure can also be performed either as refluxing or nonrefluxing anastomosis with no significant difference in renal functional preservation or recurrence of stricture.

Psoas Hitch. Can help decrease tension on ureteroneocystotomy anastomosis by hitching the bladder superiorly and laterally toward the affected side. May provide an additional 5 cm of length compared with ureteroneocystotomy alone. Achieved by ligating and dividing the vascular pedicle of the bladder on the contralateral side. The remaining bladder is then hitched to the psoas tendon on the ipsilateral side while carefully avoiding injury to the genitofemoral nerve. This maneuver is contraindicated in the context of a small contracted bladder.

Boari Flap. Can further aide in achieving ureteral mobility by refashioning a portion of the bladder to act as a bridge toward the

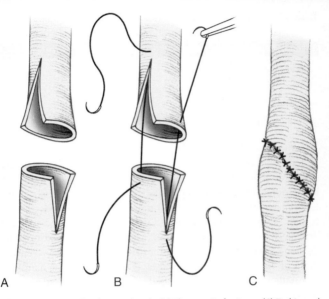

FIG. 25.10 (A) Spatulated ureteral ends. (B) Placement of sutures. (C) End-to-end ureteroureterostomy.

ureter. This maneuver can provide an additional 10–15 cm of length. It is performed by creating a flap of bladder tissue and rotating it cephalad then tubularizing it to connect to the ureter. It can be combined with a psoas hitch as well. As with a psoas hitch, a small bladder capacity is considered a contraindication for this approach.

Renal Descensus. Complete mobilization of the kidney can provide additional ureteral mobility. To achieve descensus, the lower pole is secured to the retroperitoneal muscle and can provide up to 8 cm of additional ureteral length. Length is typically dependent on the renal vessels, and there have been reports of renal vein ligation with reanastamosis more inferiorly to the vena cava.

Transureteroureterostomy. Can be considered for injured or diseased ureter with insufficient length to reach bladder. In this case, the ipsilateral diseased ureter is anastomosed to the contralateral side. Relative contraindications are any process that may affect both ureters including stones, retroperitoneal fibrosis, urothelial malignancy, or recurrent infection. Similarly, vesicoureteral reflux of the recipient ureter should be ruled out because this could lead to functional decline and infection of both kidneys.

Ileal Ureteral Substitution. Reserved for extensive ureteral stricture that cannot be addressed through listed repairs that use urothelial tissue. Distal ileum is used in an isoperistaltic fashion to replace the diseased segment of ureter. This can potentially be utilized anywhere from the renal pelvis to the bladder (Fig. 25.11). Contraindicated in patients with baseline renal insufficiency, bladder dysfunction, inflammatory bowel disease, or radiation enteritis.

Buccal Mucosa Grafting. Increasingly considered for long proximal ureteral strictures. In this case, the buccal mucosal graft is performed as an onlay to the affected portion of ureter after being spatulated at the diseased segment. An omental flap is sewn to the graft to provide blood supply.

Autotransplantation. Can be considered for extensive ureteral stricture in the context of a poorly functioning or absent contralateral kidney. The kidney is harvested in the fashion of a donor

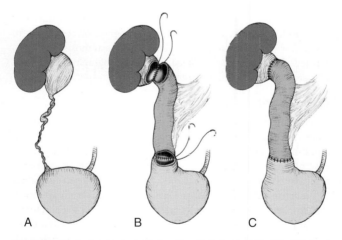

FIG. 25.11 (A) In ileal ureteral substitution, the affected ureter is first identified and dissected; this is followed by removal of the diseased portion. (B) A piece of ileum is brought through the colonic mesentery to bridge the renal pelvis and the bladder. (C) Proximal and distal anastomoses are completed in a full-thickness, watertight, tension-free manner.

nephrectomy and then transplanted into the pelvis with the renal vessels anastomosed to the iliac vessels and the ureter anastomosed to the bladder. In extensive ureteral stricture disease, the renal pelvis may be directed anastomosed to the bladder.

URETEROENTERIC ANASTOMOTIC STRICTURE

Ureteroenteric strictures may occur any time intestine is used for the purpose of urinary diversion. Long-term follow-up data suggest a 4%–9% rate of stricture among urinary conduits, and 2%–25% among patients with continent diversions. Strictures are more common on the left side owing to the fact that the left ureter typically requires a greater degree of dissection to provide more length such that it can be brought underneath the sigmoid mesentery at the time of diversion.

Diagnosis

Although typically benign, neoplasm should always be considered, especially in the case of prior malignancy. In such scenarios, a biopsy is warranted prior to any definitive type of repair. Another consideration is that many patients with urinary diversions have an element of chronic hydronephrosis. One unique test that may be considered in such scenarios is a loopogram or cystogram to assess for reflux (assuming a refluxing anastomosis was performed). If no reflux is visualized, diuretic renography can be used to assess for functional obstruction.

Management

Ureteroenteric strictures can be treated in a similar fashion as routine ureteral strictures with balloon dilation, endoureterotomy, and cautery balloons. One unique consideration that differs in the case of ureteroenteric strictures is that an antegrade approach is typically favored owing to a more challenging route to the ureter in the setting of prior diversion. Unique consideration is also merited for left-sided strictures, which tend to have a lower success rate and pose the risk of hemorrhage owing to the sigmoid mesentery that can be in close proximity. Success rates are widely variable based on reports but endourologic approaches are considered to have slightly less efficacy in the setting of ureteroenteric strictures than convention ureteral strictures. Success rates are inferior to definitive repairs, and definitive repair should be considered in

OPTIMAL THERAPY FOR URETEROENTERIC ANASTOMOTIC STRICTURES[a]

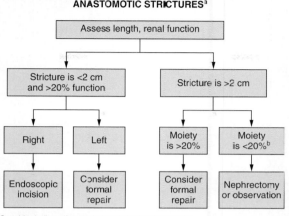

aConsider balloon if transplant on immunosuppression.
bPediatric patients and select patients with renal insufficiency may warrant repair.

FIG. 25.12 Algorithm for management of ureteroenteric anastomotic stricture disease.

any patient with a stricture length >1 cm or with prior failure of an endourologic intervention. Formal repair most commonly requires creation of a new ureteroenteric anastomosis (Fig. 25.12).

RETROPERITONEAL FIBROSIS (RPF)

RPF is characterized by inflammation and fibrosis in the retroperitoneum that leads to compression and local obstruction. RPF is most common between ages 40 and 60 years and tends to have a male predominance. It can involve the entirety of the retroperitoneum and is typically centered around the aorta at L4 to L5 and encompassing the ureters (Fig. 25.13). This process can cause the typical symptoms of obstruction but may also coexist with systemic symptoms such as weight loss, anorexia, fevers, malaise, hypertension, and anuria. Deep vein thrombosis (DVTs) and lower extremity edema can occur with inferior vena cava (IVC) compression. The etiology of RPF is typically idiopathic. Known causes include use of certain medications such as methysergide and other ergot alkyloids, beta blockers, and phenacetin. Lymphoma is another consideration that can coexist or cause RPF. Laboratory evaluation may include elevated erthyrocyte

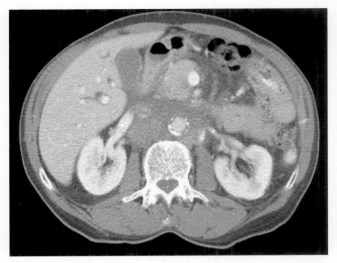

FIG. 25.13 Typical computed tomographic findings of retroperitoneal fibrosis. The study demonstrates the presence of a homogeneous mass obliterating the outline of the great vessels at the lumbar area.

sedimentaion rate, C-reactive protein, leukocytosis and possible anemia, and renal insufficiency. CT imaging typically demonstrated hydronephrosis with a retroperitoneal soft tissue mass enveloping the great vessels and ureters. MRI may be used to further risk stratify the diagnosis. In RPF, the fibrotic mass often has low signal intensity on T1-weighted imaging with variable T2 signal that tends to high in active disease. This can be a useful way to evaluate treatment efficacy because T2 signal intensity often diminishes with efficacious treatment (Fig. 25.14). When the diagnosis is in question, a biopsy may be obtained percutaneously or at the time of surgery to confirm.

Medical Management

The most common medical treatment for RPF is steroid therapy, which has been estimated to lead to some clinical response in 80% of patients. Immunosuppressive agents may be used in the case of steroid failure.

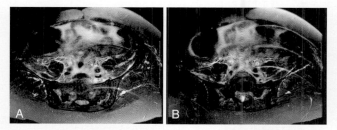

FIG. 25.14 (A) T2-weighted magnetic resonance image of a symptomatic patient demonstrating retroperitoneal fibrosis with enhancement and thus active disease. (B) Same patient after 1 month of medical therapy; note the decrease in enhancement on this corroborative T2-weighted image.

Surgical Management

Ureteral obstruction from RPF is most commonly managed with open or laparoscopic ureterolysis. Although hydronephrosis may only be present or more noticeable on one side, bilateral ureterolysis should be considered because RPF is typically a bilateral process. Dissection of the ureters should be performed by incising the rind encompassing the ureter over a right angle via a "split and roll" technique. Once the ureters are mobilized, they should be excluded from the fibrosis so that they do not become reencapsulated. This can be achieved through intraperitonealization of the ureters or omental wrapping that creates physical separation.

Suggested Readings

Link RE, Bhayani SB, Kavoussi LR. A prospective comparison of robotic and laparoscopic pyeloplasty. *Ann Surg* 2006;243:486.

Pipitone N, Vaglio A, Salvarani C. Retroperitoneal fibrosis. *Best Pract Res Clin Rheumatol* 2012;26(4):439-448. doi:10 1016/j.berh.2012.07.004.

Schöndorf D, Meierhans-Ruf S, Kiss B, et al. Ureteroileal strictures after urinary diversion with an ileal segment—is there a place for endourological treatment at all? *J Urol* 2013;190:585.

Turner-Warwick RT, Worth PH. The psoas bladder-hitch procedure for the replacement of the lower third of the ureter. *Br J Urol* 1969;41:701.

26

Urological Trauma in Adults and Children

GREGORY M. AMEND AND BENJAMIN N. BREYER

CONTRIBUTORS OF CAMPBELL-WALSH-WEIN, 12TH EDITION

Bruce J. Schlomer, Micah A. Jacobs, Steven B. Brandes, Jairam R. Eswara, Allen F. Morey, and Jay Simhan

RENAL TRAUMA

The kidney is the **most commonly injured urologic organ** in both children and adults. In the United States, blunt trauma accounts for 80%–90% of renal injuries, whereas 10%–20% are penetrating. Direct transmission of kinetic energy with rapid deceleration forces from a fall or an automobile accident place the kidneys at risk. **Significant deceleration can cause the kidney to tear at retroperitoneal points of fixation**, such as the renal hilum or ureteropelvic junction, resulting in renal artery thrombosis, renal vein disruption, renal pedicle avulsion, or ureteropelvic junction (UPJ) disruption. Penetrating renal injuries come from **gunshots (86%)** and stab wounds (14%). More than 77% of patients with penetrating renal injuries have associated abdominal injuries. As a result, it is important to consider concurrent intraabdominal injuries to the liver, intestine, and spleen in such trauma.

Children have up to 50% higher risk for renal trauma than adults after blunt abdominal injury and 33% higher risk for high-grade injury. The pediatric kidney is protected by less perirenal fat and less-developed abdominal wall muscles. The pediatric kidney also sits lower and is less protected by the rib cage. Last, the pediatric vertebral column is more pliable, leading to more stretch injuries on the ureters.

The best indicators of significant urinary system injury are **gross and microscopic hematuria** (>5 red blood cells/high-power field [RBCs/HPF] or positive dipstick finding), especially when associated with **acceleration/deceleration injury, penetrating trauma, or hypotension in the field** or emergency room (systolic blood pressure <90 mm Hg). The degree of hematuria and the severity of the renal injury do not consistently correlate.

In children, the **presence of hematuria may be a less sensitive indicator of renal injury**. Some studies have found that up to two-thirds of children sustaining ≥grade II renal injury have a normal urinalysis. Children have a **high catecholamine output after trauma, which maintains blood pressure until approximately 50% of blood volume has been lost**. This allows children to maintain their blood pressure with blood loss longer than adults, which would make hypotension a less reliable indicator of significant blood loss from a renal injury.

RENAL IMAGING

The indications for obtaining **imaging** in cases of suspected renal trauma are **penetrating trauma, blunt trauma with significant acceleration/deceleration mechanism and/or gross hematuria and/or microhematuria with hypotension, and in pediatric patients with >5 RBCs/HPF**. Contrast-enhanced computed tomography **(CT) with immediate and delayed images is the best** method for genitourinary imaging in renal trauma. Quick, highly sensitive, and specific, CT provides the most definitive staging information regarding parenchymal lacerations and extravasation of contrast-enhanced urine.

CT findings suspicious for significant renal injury include (1) medial hematoma (vascular pedicle injury), (2) medial urinary extravasation (renal pelvis or UPJ injury), (3) lack of contrast enhancement of the parenchyma (main renal arterial injury), and (4) active intravascular contrast extravasation (arterial injury with brisk bleeding). Perinephric hematoma size provides a rough estimate of the magnitude of renal bleeding. A hematoma >4 cm has been associated with higher intervention rates and should raise the suspicion that immediate intervention is needed (Fig. 26.1).

There is a limited role for intraoperative "one-shot" intravenous pyelogram (IVP). Its main purpose is to assess the presence of a functioning contralateral kidney when the surgeon encounters an unexpected retroperitoneal hematoma during abdominal exploration in an unstable trauma patient without a previous CT scan and is contemplating renal exploration or nephrectomy.

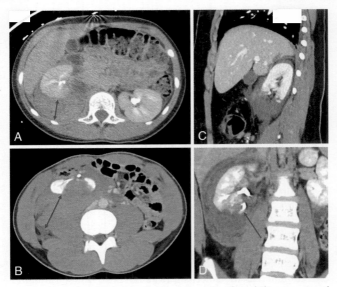

FIG. 26.1 Examples of high-risk criteria for intervention. (A and B) Large perirenal hematomas. *Arrows* indicate the size of the perirenal hematoma. (C) Significant amount of devascularized parenchyma. (D) Medial extravasation of contrast on delayed phase. The *arrow* indicates medial extravasation of contrast.

Sonography has poor specificity in adult patients with renal injuries. Sonography can confirm the presence of two kidneys and detect a retroperitoneal collection. It cannot differentiate between a hematoma and a urine leak. American Urological Association urotrauma guidelines state that ultrasonography can be used for the initial evaluation of renal trauma in children, but CT is preferred (https://www.auanet.org/guidelines/guidelines/urotrauma-guideline). The European Association of Urology (EAU) pediatric urology guidelines state that ultrasonography can be used as a screening tool for renal injury but that CT scan is the best imaging modality for diagnosis and staging.

RENAL TRAUMA CLASSIFICATION

Based on accurate grading by contrast-enhanced CT and updated in 2018, the kidney American Association for the Surgery of

Table 26.1 American Association for the Surgery of Trauma Organ Injury Severity Scale for the Kidney

GRADE[a]	TYPE	DESCRIPTION
I	Contusion	Microscopic or gross hematuria, urologic studies normal
	Hematoma	Subcapsular, nonexpanding without parenchymal laceration
II	Hematoma	Nonexpanding perirenal hematoma confined to renal retroperitoneum
	Laceration	<1 cm parenchymal depth of renal cortex without urinary extravasation
III	Laceration	>1 cm parenchymal depth of renal cortex without collecting system rupture or urinary extravasation
IV	Laceration	Parenchymal laceration extending through renal cortex, medulla, and collecting system
	Vascular	Main renal artery or vein injury with contained hemorrhage
V	Laceration	Completely shattered kidney
	Vascular	Avulsion of renal hilum, devascularizing the kidney

[a]Advance one grade for bilateral injuries up to grade III.
Data from Moore EE, Shackford SR, Pachter HL, et al. Organ injury scaling: spleen, liver, and kidney. *J Trauma* 1989;29:1664-1666.

Trauma (AAST) injury severity scale has been validated in multiple series as a predictive tool for clinical outcomes, such as the need for surgical or angiographic intervention or the rate of nephrectomy (Table 26.1).

CONTEMPORARY MANAGEMENT OF RENAL TRAUMA (Fig. 26.2)

Observation

Nonoperative management is the standard of care in hemodynamically stable, well-staged patients with AAST grades I–IV renal injuries, regardless of mechanism. Most experts agree that patients with grade IV/V injuries more often require surgical exploration. However, **even these high-grade injuries can be managed without renal operation if carefully staged and selected**. Overall,

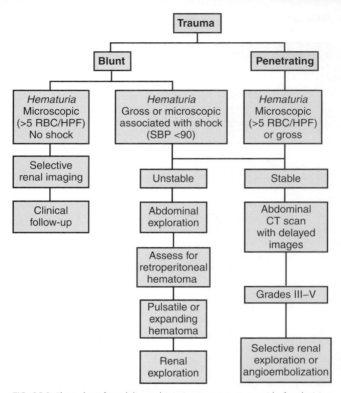

FIG. 26.2 Flow chart for adult renal injuries to serve as a guide for decision making. *CT,* Computed tomography; *IVP,* intravenous pyelography; *RBC/HPF,* red blood cells per high-power field; *SBP,* systolic blood pressure.

>90% can be successfully managed without surgery. Bluntly injured kidneys often heal well when managed conservatively, even in the setting of urinary extravasation and nonviable tissue (Fig. 26.3). The nephrectomy rate is higher with surgical exploration compared with nonoperative management.

All patients with high-grade injuries selected for nonoperative management should be closely observed with serial hematocrit readings and vital signs. Routine follow-up CT imaging for grade IV/V renal injuries is prudent at 48–72 hours post injury to evaluate for a troublesome urinoma or hematoma. A follow-up ultrasound

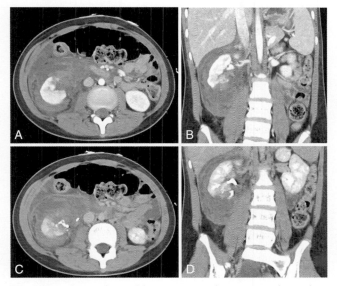

FIG. 26.3 Grade IV right renal laceration. Immediate contrast phases show laceration (A and B) with delayed phases showing extravasation of contrast from collecting system (C and D).

(US) can be obtained in children in lieu of CT. Conservative management rarely fails (2.7%) within the first 24 hours. **Risk factors for failure include renal injury grade, nonrenal abdominal injuries, and penetrating injuries**.

Persistent urinary extravasation can result in urinoma, perinephric infection, and, rarely, renal loss. In a high percentage, the extravasation resolves spontaneously. The classic triad of ipsilateral flank pain, ileus, and low-grade fever heralds a symptomatic, persistent urinoma after renal trauma. If persistent, placement of an internal ureteral stent often corrects the problem. Placement of a percutaneous drain can be used if a ureteral stent does not resolve symptoms from a urinoma.

After successful conservative management, the patient should undergo blood pressure monitoring for up to 1 year post injury because hypertension can occur. The **basic mechanisms for arterial hypertension as a complication of trauma are** (1) renal vascular injury, leading to stenosis or occlusion of the main renal artery or one of its branches (Goldblatt kidney), (2) compression of the renal parenchyma with extravasated blood or urine (Page kidney), and (3) posttrauma arteriovenous fistula (AVF). In these instances, the renin-angiotensin axis is stimulated by partial renal ischemia, resulting in hypertension.

In pediatric patients, the risk for renal scarring is likely negligible after a grade I/II injury, and repeat imaging is not recommended (AUA urotrauma guidelines). The risk for renal scarring is approximately 60% for grade III injures and closer to 100% for grade IV/V injuries, with some decline in differential function. Typically, renal scans are obtained if there is concern about significant loss of function and/or if hypertension is present during follow-up.

Angioembolization

Renal arteriography and embolization are commonly used in renal trauma to stop significant renal bleeding without the need for laparotomy. Its indications are increasing. Persistent bleeding after injury is typically caused by the injured blood vessels failing to tamponade. Delayed bleeding can be caused by the development of an AVF or a pseudoaneurysm in an injured artery that ruptures. Delayed bleeds typically develop 1–2 weeks and up to 1 month postinjury.

Superselective angioembolization has a high success rate for resolution of persistent and delayed bleeding, with most series reporting >80% success in adults and children. Even if initial angioembolization is not successful, a repeat angioembolization can be successfully performed.

Complications of renal angioembolization include postembolization syndrome, persistent bleeding, and postembolization abscess. Postembolization syndrome is a self-limited condition, which includes flank pain, fever, and possible ileus, and occurs in <10% of patients. The symptoms typically resolve within 3–4 days. If the fever persists, evaluation for postembolization abscess is indicated.

Surgery

Patients who are hemodynamically unstable from the kidney require exploration and subsequent nephrectomy/renorrhaphy. **The only absolute intraoperative indication for kidney exploration** is a pulsatile and expanding retroperitoneal hematoma that suggests a life-threatening renal artery laceration.

For early control of vessels, an incision is made in the posterior mesentery medial to the inferior mesenteric vein over the aorta, and vessel loops are applied around the renal vessels and tightened if needed (Fig. 26.4). If the renal injury is too severe to

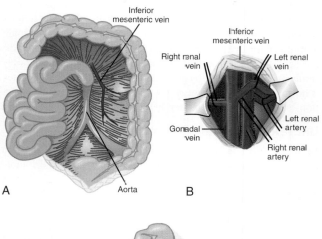

A — Inferior mesenteric vein / Aorta

B — Inferior mesenteric vein / Right renal vein / Left renal vein / Left renal artery / Right renal artery / Gonadal vein

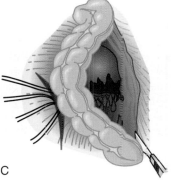

C

FIG. 26.4 The surgical approach to the renal vessels and kidney. (A) Retroperitoneal incision over the aorta medial to the inferior mesenteric vein. (B) Anatomic relationships of the renal vessels. (C) Retroperitoneal incision lateral to the colon, exposing the kidney.

repair or would leave a very small portion of remaining kidney, nephrectomy should be performed. In addition, if the patient is unstable and it is safest to expedite surgery with nephrectomy to save the life of the patient because of hypothermia, coagulopathy, or ongoing blood loss, nephrectomy should be performed. In a penetrating injury, especially high-velocity gunshot wounds, it is important to inspect the ipsilateral ureter for any injury and repair if found.

Although initial observation is warranted for patients with renal injury and urinary extravasation, a renal pelvis avulsion or proximal ureteral avulsion injury requires prompt surgical repair. Main renal artery thrombosis from blunt trauma occurs most often secondary to deceleration injuries. Revascularization rarely results in a successful salvage. As long as the contralateral kidney is normal, observation is often the best management because portions of the kidney will frequently reperfuse.

URETERAL TRAUMA

Ureteral injuries are often subtle, and clinicians must maintain a high index of suspicion to prevent a delay in diagnosis and comorbidity. More than 90% of trauma patients with ureteral injuries have a concurrent abdominal or retroperitoneal organ injury. Absence of hematuria does not reliably rule out ureteral injury. CT urography with delayed images is the best study for detecting ureteral injuries, manifesting with absence of contrast in the ureter on delayed images (Fig. 26.5).

When possible in a stable patient, repair of the injured ureter should be performed at the same time as the initial laparotomy. Immediate repair of the ureter is often not appropriate in an unstable, complex polytrauma patient. Ureteral blood supply is tenuous, and urine leakage that can result in patient debility, nephrectomy, and, in rare cases, even death, can be a sequela of imperfect repair. Principles of management of the injured ureter are in Box 26.1.

URETERAL INJURY MANAGEMENT

Ureteral avulsion from the renal pelvis can be managed by reimplantation of the ureter directly into the renal pelvis. These can be performed open or in a delayed fashion, laparoscopically or robotically. Ureteroureterostomy is used in acute injuries to the upper two-thirds of the ureter. Autotransplantation of the kidney has

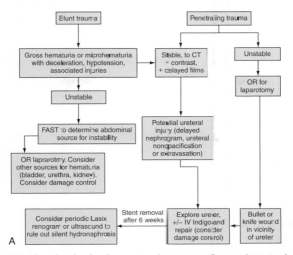

FIG. 26.5 Algorithm for the diagnosis and treatment of ureteral injuries from external violence. *CT*, Computed tomography *IVP*, intravenous pyelography; *OR*, operating room.

Box 26.1 Principles of Management in Ureteral Trauma

1. After penetrating injury, determine the course of the knife or bullet tract to ensure that the ureter is not at risk.

2. Mobilize the injured ureter carefully, sparing the adventitia widely.

3. Debride the ureter minimally but judiciously until edges bleed, especially in high-velocity gunshot wounds.

4. Repair ureters with spatulated, tension-free, stented, watertight anastomosis using fine absorbable sutures and retroperitoneal drainage.

5. Retroperitonealize the ureteral repair by closing peritoneum over it.

6. Do not tunnel ureteroneocystostomies.

7. With severely injured ureters, blast effect, concomitant vascular surgery, and other complex cases, consider omental interposition to isolate the repair.

8. If immediate repair is not possible, or the patient is hemodynamically unstable: (a) ligate the ureter with long permanent suture, and delayed repair or (b) place a nephrostomy tube after intensive care unit resuscitation (damage control).

9. Another option is a temporary cutaneous ureterostomy over a single-J stent or pediatric feeding tube with a suture tied around the ureter proximal to the injury site to secure the stent and prevent urinary leakage.

been used after profound ureteral loss or after multiple attempts at ureteral repair have failed.

Ureteroneocystostomy is used to repair distal ureteral injuries that occur so close to the bladder that the bladder does not need to be brought up to the ureteral stump with a psoas hitch or Boari flap (Figs. 26.6 and 26.7). Standard principles of ureteroneocystostomy include a long, nontunneled, spatulated, stented anastomosis.

Ureteral injuries that occur during vascular graft surgery are a special case. Intraoperative management of these should be primary ureteroureterostomy with isolation of the repair with omentum to decrease the potential for urine leakage or infection of vascular grafts. Ureteral perforation during ureteroscopy can be treated by ureteral stenting, usually with no subsequent complications.

Injuries diagnosed postoperatively or in a delayed fashion can be considered for immediate repair if the injury is recognized

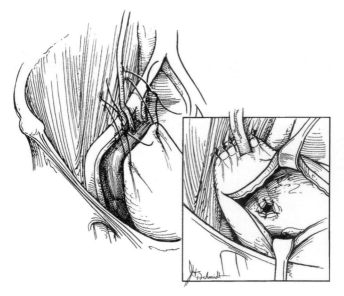

FIG. 26.6 Psoas hitch. Bladder is opened and secured to the psoas muscle to facilitate ureteral anastomosis. (From Hohenfellner M, Santucci RA. *Emergencies in urology,* Heidelberg, Germany, 2007, Springer. Copyright 2007, Dr. Markus Hohenfellner, with permission.)

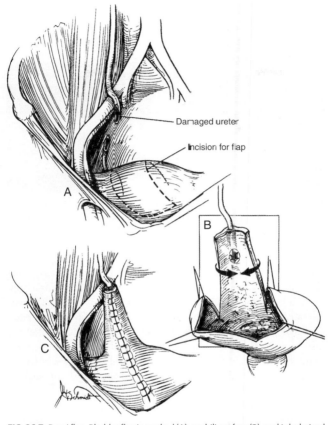

FIG. 26.7 Boari flap. Bladder flap is marked (A), mobilized free (B), and tubularized (C). (From Hohenfellner M, Santucci RA: *Emergencies in urology*, Heidelberg, Germany, 2007, Springer. Copyright 2007, Dr. Markus Hohenfellner, with permission.)

within 1 week (AUA urotrauma guideline). Injuries discovered after this 1 week period should be managed by retrograde ureteral imaging with ureteral stent placement, percutaneous nephrostomy, or both and definitive repair delayed until a minimum of 6 weeks after injury.

Intraoperative recognition of ureteral injuries occurs in as few as 34% of patients undergoing open operation and even more

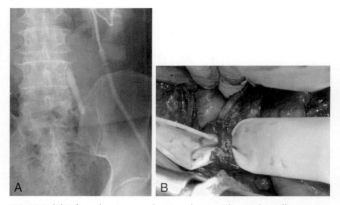

FIG. 26.8 (A) Left nephrostogram showing abrupt midureteral cutoff consistent with (inadvertent) suture ligation of the ureter. (B) Intraoperative view of left midureteral suture ligation.

rarely during laparoscopic surgery. Intraoperative injuries can include suture ligation, crush injury, partial or complete transection, devascularization, and injury from electrocautery (Fig. 26.8). Postoperatively, patients must be monitored for fever, abdominal pain, port site pain, and leukocytosis, which herald the potential for missed ureteral injury. Preoperative ureteral stenting can be used to improve identification of the ureter in high-risk cases; however, the gynecologic and colectomy literature is unclear about whether stents actually decrease ureteral injuries (Fig. 26.9).

Repair of delayed-recognition injuries is controversial. With an incomplete, delayed ureteral injury, retrograde ureteral imaging with stent placement is recommended (AUA urotrauma guideline). Failure to place a stent is due to complete obstruction of the ureter or complete ureteral transection with a long defect or gap. A majority of patients will eventually require definitive repair of significant ureteral injuries, whether or not stent placement is possible. If stents cannot be placed or the patient is unstable, then a percutaneous nephrostomy should be placed (Fig. 26.10). Endoscopic dilation and incision techniques in long, devascularized, postinjury or postoperative ureteral strictures have poor results.

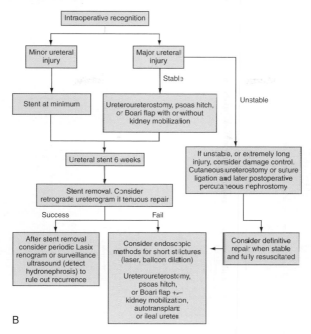

FIG. 26.9 Algorithm for the diagnosis and treatment of ureteral injuries discovered intraoperatively.

Follow-up imaging after any ureteral injury is recommended. After the ureteral stent is removed, renal ultrasonography is obtained in 4–6 weeks. If there is no hydronephrosis, we recommend at least yearly US examinations for 2–3 years.

GENITAL TRAUMA

Penile Fracture

Penile fracture is the disruption of the tunica albuginea with rupture of the corpus cavernosum. It is the result of blunt traumatic injury that typically occurs during vigorous sexual intercourse when the rigid penis strikes the perineum or pubic bone of the partner and results in a buckling injury.

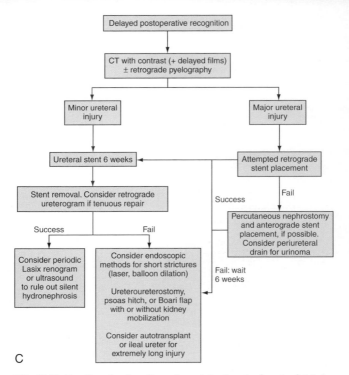

C

FIG. 26.10 Algorithm for the diagnosis and treatment of ureteral injuries discovered postoperatively.

The diagnosis of penile fracture is often straightforward and **can be made reliably by history and physical examination**. Patients usually describe a cracking or popping sound as the tunica tears followed by pain, rapid detumescence, discoloration, and swelling of the penile shaft (Fig. 26.11). **Penile US** can be used in situations of an **equivocal** evaluation.

Suspected penile fractures should be promptly explored and surgically repaired (Fig. 26.12). Surgical reconstruction results in faster recovery, decreased morbidity, lower complication rates, and lower incidence of long-term penile curvature.

If signs for urethral injury are present (hematuria or urinary retention), the urethra should be staged with a retrograde

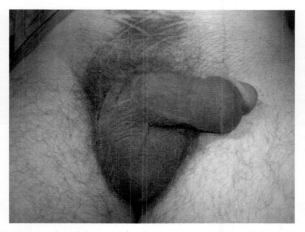

FIG. 26.11 Eggplant deformity—the classic appearance of a penile fracture sustained during intercourse, with hematoma of the penile shaft and ecchymosis extending into the scrotum.

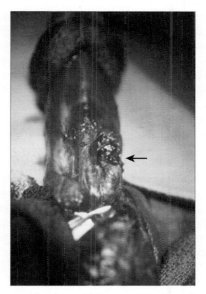

FIG. 26.12 Transverse laceration of left corpus cavernosum *(arrow)* associated with penile fracture, successfully repaired through a circumcision incision.

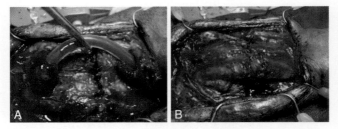

FIG. 26.13 (A) Completely transected urethra secondary to penile fracture. Repair of bilateral tunical rupture was performed previously. (B) Anastomotic repair of the urethra after urethral mobilization.

urethrogram or cystoscopy. Partial urethral injuries should be oversewn with fine absorbable suture over a urethral catheter. Complete urethral injuries should be debrided, mobilized, and repaired in a tension-free manner over a catheter (Fig. 26.13).

Penetrating Injuries

Gunshot injuries to the phallus are rarely isolated wounds. Treatment principles include **immediate exploration**, copious irrigation, excision of foreign matter, antibiotic prophylaxis, and surgical closure. Primary repair minimizes deformity and erectile dysfunction. **Retrograde urethrography should be strongly considered** in any patient with penetrating injury to the penis, especially with high-velocity missile injuries, blood at the meatus, or difficulty voiding and when the trajectory of the bullet was near the urethra. Urethral injuries resulting from penetrating trauma should be closed primarily by use of standard urethroplasty principles. Patients with urethral injury and extensive tissue loss may require staged repair and suprapubic urinary diversion. Penetrating scrotal lacerations should undergo surgical exploration to assess and repair deep tissues and remove contamination, regardless of US findings. Exploration can be managed simply with washout and closure given that the tunica vaginalis is not violated. Blunt scrotal injury can be evaluated by US for testicular rupture.

Bites

Animal bites should be irrigated, debrided, and closed primarily, whereas most human bites should be washed out and left open.

Vaginal Injury

Straddle injury the most common etiology of vaginal trauma, accounting for ~80% of all injuries. Straddle injuries typically result in minor trauma to the labia minora, with most not requiring surgical intervention. Larger injuries, particularly those involving the hymen, are more likely to require operative intervention, particularly if associated with perineal bleeding, hematoma, or swelling.

Any history or sign of penetrating vaginal injury must raise suspicion of abuse and should prompt careful assessment of the etiology of the trauma. **Perianal, hymen, and vaginal trauma are more suggestive of a penetrating mechanism.**

Pediatric Population

Although most genital injuries in children are accidental, it is critical to assess whether trauma to the penis or scrotum in boys or the vagina in girls is the result of abuse. About one in seven boys and one in three girls will be sexually abused in childhood. In most of these cases, the abuse is penetrative. When abuse is suspected, it is imperative to ensure that no other harm has been done. Often concomitant injuries go unnoticed, particularly to the anus and rectum. Hymenal injury has been strongly correlated with sexual abuse.

Penile injury in children happens inadvertently from a number of causes. These include circumcision, hair tourniquet strangulation, motor vehicle accidents, animal bites, zippers, toilet seat crush injuries, and burns or scalds. Newborn circumcision accounts for the majority of injuries.

TESTIS TRAUMA

Testicular injury results from blunt trauma in ~75% of cases, resulting in rupture of the tunica albuginea, contusion, hematoma, dislocation, or torsion of the testis. Most patients complain of severe scrotal pain and nausea. Swelling and ecchymosis are variable. Scrotal hemorrhage and hematocele along with tenderness to palpation often limit a complete physical examination. As a result, US should be performed to assess the integrity and vascularity of the testis in blunt trauma (AUA urotrauma guideline). US findings suggestive of testicular fracture include a heterogeneous echo pattern of the testicular parenchyma and disruption of the tunica albuginea (Fig. 26.14).

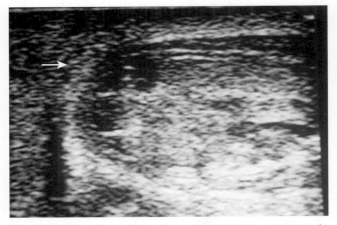

FIG. 26.14 Ultrasound examination demonstrates hypoechoic intratesticular areas *(arrow)* consistent with testicular rupture sustained by blunt trauma. Scrotal exploration revealed a large hematocele and exposed seminiferous tubules.

In contrast, exploration should not be delayed in penetrating scrotal trauma given the low sensitivity of US in these injuries. Likewise, significant hematoceles should also be explored, regardless of imaging studies, because up to 80% are caused by testicular rupture.

Early exploration and repair of testicular injury is associated with increased testicular salvage, reduced convalescence and disability, faster return to normal activities, and preservation of fertility and hormonal function. Orchiectomy rates are threefold to eightfold higher with conservative management and delayed surgery.

BLADDER INJURY

Most blunt bladder injuries are the result of rapid-deceleration motor vehicle collisions. Disruption of the bony pelvis tends to tear the bladder at its fascial attachments, but bone fragments also can directly lacerate the organ. Nearly half of all bladder injuries are iatrogenic. Obstetric and gynecologic complications are the most common causes of bladder injuries during open surgery.

Extraperitoneal bladder injury is usually associated with pelvic fracture (Fig. 26.15), but only 10% of patients with pelvic fracture

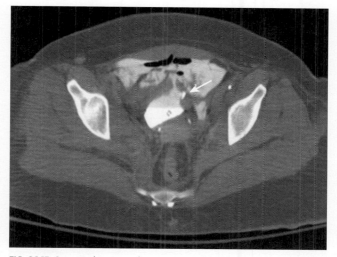

FIG. 26.15 Computed tomography cystogram of a patient with extraperitoneal bladder rupture after a motor vehicle–pedestrian collision and extensive pelvic fracture. *Arrow* indicates a fragment of bone in the bladder, removed at the time of laparotomy and repair of the bladder.

have bladder injuries. Intraperitoneal injuries can be associated with pelvic fracture but are more commonly caused by penetrating injuries or burst injuries at the dome by direct blow to a full bladder. Isolated bladder trauma is rare in children. This is possibly due, in part, to the fact that more of the bladder is intraperitoneal in children and that the bony pelvis in a child is more pliable, requiring more force to generate a pelvic fracture

After blunt external trauma, the absolute indication for immediate cystography is gross hematuria associated with pelvic fracture (29% of patients presenting with this combination have bladder rupture). Penetrating injuries of the buttocks, pelvis, or lower abdomen with any degree of hematuria warrant cystography. A dense, flame-shaped collection of contrast material in the pelvis is characteristic of extraperitoneal extravasation. Intraperitoneal extravasation is identified when contrast material outlines loops of bowel and/or the lower lateral portion of the peritoneal cavity (Fig. 26.16). If blood is noted at the meatus or the catheter does not pass easily, retrograde urethrography should be performed first

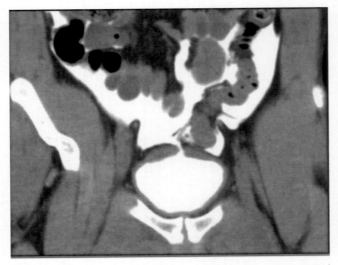

FIG. 26.16 Computed tomography cystogram demonstrates contrast material surrounding loops of bowel consistent with intraperitoneal bladder rupture.

because urethral injuries occur concomitantly in 10%–29% of patients with bladder rupture.

Any penetrating injury involving the ureteral orifice or intramural ureter warrants primary closure with stented reimplantation of the ureter and a perivesical drain. When **concurrent rectal or vaginal injuries exist**, the organ walls should be separated, overlapping suture lines should be avoided, and every attempt should be made to interpose viable tissue in between the repaired structures.

The treatment of uncomplicated extraperitoneal bladder ruptures is conservative, with urethral catheter drainage alone. Cystography in 2–3 weeks is necessary to verify complete healing before catheter removal. For patients undergoing **exploratory laparotomy for other associated injuries or internal fixation of pelvic fracture**, it is prudent to perform surgical repair of the extraperitoneal rupture at the same setting. When **internal fixation of pelvic fractures is performed**, concomitant bladder repair is recommended because urine leakage from the injured bladder onto the orthopedic fixative hardware is prevented, reducing the risk for hardware infection.

Penetrating or intraperitoneal injuries resulting from external trauma should be managed by immediate operative repair. Additional indications for immediate repair of bladder injury include **inadequate bladder drainage or clots in urine, bladder neck injury, and bone fragments projecting into the bladder.** Bladder neck injuries are more common in children and best served with early repair.

When bladder injuries are explored after penetrating trauma without preliminary imaging, the ureteral orifices should be inspected for clear efflux. Ureteral integrity also may be ensured by intravenous administration of indigo carmine, methylene blue, or fluorescein green or with retrograde passage of a ureteral catheter.

POSTERIOR URETHRAL INJURIES

Urethral disruption is heralded by the triad of a**n inability to urinate, blood at the meatus, and a palpably full bladder** When blood at the urethral meatus is discovered, an immediate retrograde urethrogram should be performed to rule out urethral injury (Fig. 26.17).

Immediate suprapubic tube placement remains the standard of care in men with severe posterior urethral injuries. Primary endoscopic realignment is associated with a prolonged clinical course because an overwhelming majority of patients, despite realignment, will develop posterior urethral stenosis. Close follow-up is essential in this population. Immediate urethroplasty is not recommended because it often requires further endoscopic treatment or open revision and has been shown to have higher incontinence and erectile dysfunction rates when compared to delayed repair. Posterior urethroplasty by excision and primary anastomosis is the treatment of choice for urethral distraction injuries.

Incomplete urethral tears are best treated by stenting with a urethral catheter. There is no evidence that a gentle attempt at urethral catheterization converts an incomplete transection into a complete transection.

ANTERIOR URETHRAL INJURIES

In contrast with posterior urethral distraction, anterior injuries are most often isolated. Most occur after straddle injury and involve the bulbar urethra, which is susceptible to compressive injury because of its fixed location beneath the pubis. A smaller percentage of injuries to the anterior urethra are the result of direct penetrating injury to the penis.

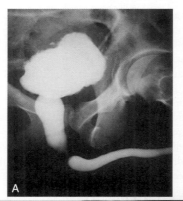

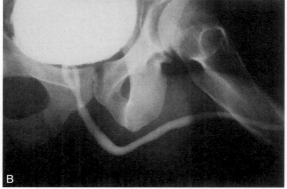

FIG. 26.17 (A) Combined cystogram and urethrogram 4 months after pelvic fracture shows complete posterior urethral disruption injury. (B) Postoperative appearance reveals normal urethral caliber.

Contusions and incomplete injuries can be treated with urethral catheter diversion alone. Initial suprapubic cystostomy is the standard of care for major straddle injuries involving the urethra. Delayed reconstruction with anastomotic urethroplasty is the procedure of choice in the totally obliterated bulbar urethra after a straddle injury.

Primary surgical repair is recommended for low-velocity urethral gunshot injuries. Initial suprapubic urinary diversion is recommended after high-velocity gunshot wounds to the urethra followed by delayed reconstruction.

Suggested Readings

Breyer BN, McAninch JW, Elliott SP, et al. Minimally invasive endovascular techniques to treat acute renal hemorrhage. *J Urol* 2008 179:2248-2253.

Buckley JC, McAninch JW. Pediatric renal injuries management guidelines from a 25-year experience. *J Urol* 2004;172:687-690.

Carroll PR, McAninch JW. Major bladder trauma: mechanism of injury and a unified method of diagnosis and repair. *J Urol* 1984;132:254-257.

Chung PH, Wessells H, Voelzke BB. Updated outcomes of early endoscopic realignment for pelvic fracture urethral injuries at a level 1 trauma center. *Urology* 2018;112:191-197.

Cooperberg MR, McAninch JW, Alsikafi NF, et al. Urethral reconstruction for traumatic posterior urethral disruption: outcomes of a 25-year experience. *J Urol* 2007;178:2006-2010.

Kozar, RA, Crandall M, Sharmuçanathan K, et al. Organ injury scaling 2018 update: spleen, liver, and kidney. *J Trauma* 2018;85:1119-1122.

Morey AF, Brandes SB, Dugi DD, et al. Urotrauma: AUA guideline. *J Urol* 2014 192:327-335.

27

Pathophysiology, Evaluation, and Management of Urinary Lithiasis

DAVID A. LEAVITT AND ROBERT M. SWEET

CONTRIBUTORS OF CAMPBELL-WALSH-WEIN, 12TH EDITION

Margaret S. Pearle, Jodi A. Antonelli, Yair Lotan, Nicole L. Miller, Michael S. Borofsky, David A. Leavitt, Jean Jmch De La Rosette, David Hoenig, Brian R. Matlaga, and Amy E. Krambeck

EPIDEMIOLOGY

The lifetime prevalence of kidney stones is 1%–15%, and it varies by age, gender, race, and geographic location. Globally, prevalence rates are increasing and vary from 7%–13% in North America, 5%–9% in Europe, and 1%–5% in Asia. The US prevalence is currently at 9%–10%. Stones are more common in hot, arid, and dry climates (mountains, deserts, tropics). Bladder stones and urethral stones account for about 5% and <1% of urolithiases, respectively.

Historically, nephrolithiasis was more common in men than women (2–3:1). However, now the rate is almost equal (1.3:1), driven by an increase in female stone disease. Men are more commonly affected in whites and Asians, and women are more commonly affected in African Americans and Hispanics.

Kidney stone incidence peaks in the fourth to sixth decades of life, with a rising incidence in children and an up to 50% risk of stone recurrence within 10 years. Kidney stone prevalence and incident risk directly corelate with weight and body mass index. Stone disease has been correlated with several systemic disorders, including diabetes, metabolic syndrome, hypertension, cardiovascular disease (heart disease, stroke), and chronic kidney disease

(CKD). Health-related quality of life appears worse in stone formers compared to nonstone formers.

PHYSIOCHEMISTRY AND PATHOGENESIS

Stone Pathogenesis

Stone formation requires supersaturated urine and begins with homogenous or heterogenous (more common) nucleation. Nuclei are the earliest crystal structures that will not dissolve. Heterogenous nucleation occurs as crystals adsorb onto existing epithelial cells, cell debris, and other crystals.

Stone promoters stabilize nuclei, while stone inhibitors destabilize nuclei (Table 27.1). Early crystal particle growth can progress as free crystal particle growth (crystals grow, aggregate and are retained within tubules) and fixed particle growth (crystals adhere onto anchoring sites within collecting system, or Randal's plaques). Randall's plaques are composed of calcium apatite (hydroxyapatite), originate from the basement membrane of the thin loop of Henle, extend into the collecting system, and act as a nidus for

Table 27.1 Urinary Promoters and Inhibitors of Stone Formation

PROMOTERS	INHIBITORS
Calcium	Inorganic
	Citrate
Oxalate	Magnesium
	Pyrophosphate
Sodium	Phosphate
	Organic
Urate	
	Urinary prothrombin fragment 1
Cystine	Glycosaminoglycans
	Heparin sulfate, chondroitin sulfate A and C, keratin sulfate, hyaluronan
Tamm-Horsfall protein (acidic urine)	Glycoproteins
	Tamm-Horsfall protein (uromodulin): inhibits calcium oxalate aggregation (basic urine)
	Nephrocalcin
	Osteopontin (uropontin)
Matrix[a]	

[a]Noncrystalline, mucoprotienaceous part of stones.

stone growth (especially, calcium oxalate). The cause of the plaques is unknown. Urinary stasis from any cause likely encourages stone formation and growth.

Calcium. From the (mainly small) intestines, 30%–40% of dietary calcium is absorbed depending on calcium intake and occurs via a saturable transcellular pathway and a nonsaturable, paracellular pathway. Many substances in the gut complex with calcium and reduce its availability for absorption: oxalate, fatty acids, citrate, phosphate, and sulfate.

Oxalate. Urinary oxalate is derived from endogenous liver production (50%) and dietary sources (50%). About 6%–14% ingested oxalate is absorbed transcellularly and paracellularly, though it varies widely among individuals (10%–70%) and occurs about equally between the small and large intestines. Many substances complex with oxalate, including calcium, magnesium, and oxalate-degrading bacteria *(Oxalobacter formigenes)*. Coingestion of calcium- and oxalate-containing foods leads to nonabsorbable calcium oxalate complexes and less free oxalate available for absorption. The contribution of *O. formigenes* to the overall risk of stone formation is not fully understood.

Citrate. From endogenous and dietary sources, citrate inhibits stone formation by many mechanisms.

1. **Complexes** with calcium, reducing urinary saturation of calcium salts
2. Directly **prevents** spontaneous nucleation of calcium oxalate crystals
3. **Inhibits** agglomeration and sedimentation of calcium oxalate crystals
4. **Inhibits** the growth of calcium oxalate and calcium phosphate crystals
5. **Enhances** the inhibitory effect of Tamm-Horsfall glycoproteins

Magnesium. Complexes with oxalate; synergistic with citrate; negated by uric acid.

Glycosaminoglycans. Inhibits calcium oxalate crystal nucleation and aggregation.

Glycoproteins. Inhibits calcium oxalate nucleation, growth, aggregation, and crystal-urothelial cell binding.

Matrix. The noncrystalline component of stones (mucoproteins, proteins, carbohydrates, urinary inhibitors), usually 2.5% by weight; can comprise >50% of infectious stones.

PATHOPHYSIOLOGY OF UPPER URINARY TRACT CALCULI

A number of pathophysiologic derangements contribute to calcium stone formation, with true idiopathic calcium stone formation uncommon (<3%). Uric acid (acidic urine), cystine (genetic defect), and infectious/struvite stones (alkaline urine, urease-producing bacteria) form in relatively unique settings.

Calcium Stones

Calcium-based stones are the most common stone type, and calcium is the major constituent of nearly 80% of stones (Table 27.2). Similarly, calcium stones have the largest number of potential metabolic abnormalities and therapies. Stone classification is often based on the dominant mineral subtype, and urinary calcium and oxalate contribute equally to calcium oxalate stone formation. Calcium phosphate stones tend to predominately affect women, present at a younger age, and are (especially brushite) often associated with metabolic abnormalities and nephrocalcinosis.

Hypercalciuria. The most common abnormality found in calcium stone formers, occurs in 35%–65% of patients, and defined as

Table 27.2 Stone Composition and Relative Occurrence

STONE COMPOSITION	CHEMICAL NAME	OCCURRENCE (%)
Calcium stones	Calcium oxalate (monohydrate and dihydrate)	60
	Calcium phosphate (apatite)	20
	Calcium hydrogen phosphate dihydrate (brushite)	2
Noncalcium stones	Uric acid	7
Infectious stones	Magnesium ammonium phosphate (Struvite)	7
	Carbonate apatite	<5
	Ammonium acid urate	<1
Genetic related stones	Cystine	1–2
	Xanthine	<1
	2,8-D hydroxyadenine	<1
Drug stones	Triamterene, indinavir, topiramate, etc.	<1

Table 27.3 Hypercalciuria Subtypes

HYPERCALCIURIA SUBTYPE	URINE CALCIUM		SERUM CHEMISTRY	
	Random diet	Restricted diet	Calcium	PTH
Dietary	↑	NL	NL	NL
Absorptive, type I	↑	↑	NL	NL or ↓
Absorptive, type II	↑	NL	NL	NL or ↓
Renal	↑	↑	NL	↑
Resorptive	↑	↑	↑	↑

NL, Normal; *PTH,* parathyroid hormone.
Adopted from AUA Core Curriculum.

>200 mg calcium/day on a calcium and sodium-controlled diet, or >4 mg/kg/day. Dysregulation of calcium metabolism and transport at the intestine, bone, or kidney can lead to hypercalciuria. Historically, hypercalciuria is classified as absorptive (20%–40%), renal (5%–8%) or resorptive (2%–8%; primary hyperparathyroidism) (Table 27.3). Clinically, the distinction between absorptive and renal hypercalciuria is not important because therapy does not change. Elevated serum parathyroid hormone (PTH) warrants evaluation for primary hyperparathyroidism.

Hyperoxaluria. Defined as urinary oxalate >40 mg/day. Increased urinary oxalate potentiates calcium oxalate stone formation and may trigger renal tubular cell injury, which can promote crystal deposition and growth. Up to half of urinary oxalate is derived from diet (24%–42%), and the rest is from liver metabolism. Causes of hyperoxaluria include primary (urine oxalate >80–100 mg/day, autosomal recessive, faulty glyoxylate metabolism), enteric (intestinal malabsorptive states), dietary (urinary oxalate <80 mg/day, excess dietary oxalate intake), and idiopathic.

Hypocitraturia. No exact cutoff defines hypocitraturia. Historically, urinary citrate <320 mg/day; more recently <450 mg/day (men) and <550 mg/day (women). An isolated abnormality in 10% and in combination with other abnormalities in 20%–60% of calcium stone formers. Systemic acidosis causes hypocitraturia secondary to enhanced renal tubular reabsorption and decreased synthesis of citrate in peritubular cells. Most hypocitraturia is idiopathic, though it is commonly seen in distal renal tubular acidosis (RTA) (type I), chronic diarrheal states (loss of intestinal bicarbonate/alkali), high animal protein diets, thiazides (hypokalemia and intracellular acidosis), and carbonic anhydrase inhibitors (e.g., topiramate, prevent bicarbonate reabsorption)

Hyperuricosuria. Defined as urinary uric acid >750 mg/day (women) or >800 mg/day (men) and seen in up to 40% of calcium stone formers. At a urine pH <5.5, undissociated uric acid predominates, while at urine pH >5.5, sodium urate predominates, mainly caused by increased dietary animal protein (purine) intake. Also acquired and hereditary causes (gout, myeloproliferative disorders). Exact mechanism unknown.

Hypercalcemic-Induced Hypercalciuria

1. *Sarcoidosis and granulomatous disease* – Sarcoid/granuloma macrophages produce excessive vitamin D_3, leading to increased intestinal calcium absorption and bone resorption. High serum and urinary calcium with low serum PTH are suggestive.
2. *Malignancy* – Tumors can produce PTH-related protein (PTHrP), which increases intestinal calcium absorption and bone resorption and stimulates vitamin D_3 synthesis.
3. *Glucocorticoids* – promote bone resorption (main effect) and stimulate PTH release.
4. Vitamin D toxicity
5. Thyrotoxicosis

Low Urine pH. At low urine pH (<5.5) the undissociated form of uric acid predominates and acts as a nidus for heterogenous nucleation with calcium oxalate. Idiopathic low urine pH was previously called "gouty diathesis."

Renal Tubular Acidosis (RTA). Clinical syndrome of metabolic acidosis caused by impaired renal tubular hydrogen ion secretion (distal or type 1) or bicarbonate reabsorption (proximal or type 2). Three types of RTA: 1, 2, and 4. Type 1 (distal) RTA is the most common and associated with stone formation (≤70% of individuals), usually calcium phosphate, and may be hereditary, acquired, or idiopathic (most common). Classic findings include low serum bicarbonate, hypokalemic, hyperchloremic, nonanion gap metabolic acidosis, bone demineralization, secondary hyperparathyroidism, elevated urine pH (>6.0), hypercalciuria, and profound hypocitraturia. Nephrocalcinosis is common.

Hypomagnesuria. Seen in up to 11% of stone formers. Magnesium inhibits stone formation by complexing with oxalate and calcium salts.

Noncalcium Stones

Uric Acid Stones. The three main determinants of uric acid stone formation are low pH (most important), low urine volume, and hyperuricosuria. Most uric acid stone formers have normal urinary uric acid excretion and persistently low urine pH. This differs from hyperuricosuric calcium stone formers with high urinary uric acid and normal pH. Uric acid is a weak acid, pKa 5.35 at 37°C. At low urine pH ($<$5.5), uric acid predominates and easily precipitates, while at higher urine pH ($>$6), sodium urate predominates (20 times more soluble than uric acid). Acquired causes of uric acid stones include metabolic syndrome, diabetes mellitus, and high animal protein intake.

Cystine Stones. Cystinuria is autosomal recessive disorder (rarely autosomal dominant with incomplete penetrance) whereby dibasic amino acids cystine ornithine, lysine, and arginine are not reabsorbed from the urine. Cystine, with the lowest solubility, readily precipitates to form stones. Cystine is a dimer composed of two cysteine molecules linked via a disulfide bond. Cystine solubility increases with elevating urinary pH. Classified based on the chromosomal mutation: type A (chromosome 2), type B (chromosome 19), and type AB (both chromosomes). Homozygotes (type AB) excrete much more cystine, have more active stone disease, and present at an earlier age. Type B heterozygotes have significantly higher urinary cystine than type A heterozygotes, though stone formation is similar between the two and is usually infrequent and much less common than in homozygotes.

Infectious Stones. These account for 5%–15% of all stones and are more common in women than men (2:1). Composed primarily of magnesium ammonium phosphate hexahydrate (struvite), carbonate apatite (calcium phosphate), and sometimes ammonium urate. Associated with urinary infection by urease-splitting bacteria, mainly *Proteus (most common), Klebsiella, Pseudomonas,* and *Staphylococcus* spp. (Table 27.4). Carbonate apatite precipitates at urine pH $>$6.8, and struvite precipitate at urine pH $>$7.2. Rapid stone growth can occur with recurrent or persistent urinary tract infections (UTIs). Urealysis produces alkaline urine and higher concentrations of ammonium, carbonate, and phosphate.

Table 27.4 Important Urease-Producing Bacteria

GRAM NEGATIVE	GRAM POSITIVE
Proteus spp. (most common)	Staphylococcus aureus
Klebsiella	Staphylococcus epidermidis
Pseudomonas spp. (≤5% strains)	Corynebacterium spp.
Escherichia coli (≤5% strains)	Enterococcus spp. (≤5% strains)
Serratia marcescens	
Providencia spp.	
Ureaplasma and Mycoplasma spp.	

Matrix Stones. Stones of pure matrix are rare, radiolucent, poorly visualized on noncontrast computed tomography (CT), and potentially mistaken for tumor or uric acid stones depending on the imaging study. They are more common in women, and associated with recurrent UTIs (*Proteus* spp., *E. coli*), alkaline urine, hemodialysis, and CKD (increased proteinuria). Matrix is composed of mucoproteins (two thirds) and mucopolysaccharides (one third). Pure matrix stones may contain >65% protein, while calcium-based stones usually contain ≤3% matrix. Matrix is thought to serve as a nidus for stone growth.

Medication-Related Stones. Drug-induced stones form either directly as crystallized drug or its metabolite or indirectly from unfavorable urine changes caused by the drug that promote stone formation (Table 27.5).

DIAGNOSIS AND EVALUATION

American Urological Association (AUA) guidelines on the medical management of kidney stones recommend

1. Screening (basic) evaluation for any patient who develops a kidney or ureteral stone
2. Metabolic evaluation in high-risk or interested first-time stone formers

Many risk factors predispose to stone disease, and those with risk factors from Table 27.6 are considered high risk.

Screening Evaluation

Includes medical and diet history, serum chemistries, urinalysis, stone analysis, imaging studies, and serum PTH if possible primary hyperparathyroidism (Box 27.1).

Table 27.5 Medication-Related Stones

MEDICATION	MECHANISM
Carbonic anhydrase Inhibitors	Metabolic acidosis, hypocitraturia
Acetazolamide	Zonisamide (can also crystallize)
Topiramate (Topamax)	
Zonisamide	
Vitamin C (ascorbic acid)	Hyperoxaluria
Calcium and vitamin D	Hypercalciuria
Loop diuretics (furosemide, bumetanide)	Hypercalciuria
Phosphate-binding antacids	Hypercalciuria
Chemotherapy agents	Hyperuricosuria
Probenecid (uricosuria)	Hyperuricosuria
Allopurinol	Xanthine stones from xanthine oxidoreductase inhibition
Laxatives	Ammonium acid urate stones (low urine volume, pH, sodium)
Triamterene	Triamterene stones
Protease inhibitors	Indinavir, ritonavir stones, others
Ephedrine	Ephedrine stones
Guaifenesin	Guaifenesin stones
Antibiotics (quinolones, amoxicillin, ampicillin, ceftriaxone)	Antibiotic stones
Silicate (certain antacids, e.g., magnesium trisilicate)	Silicate stones

Urinalysis. Crystal shapes on urine microscopy may provide clues to diagnosis (Table 27.7).

Stone Analysis. Usually done by x-ray diffraction or infrared spectroscopy and requires the stone to be pulverized into powder before analysis. May implicate underlying cause and guide medical therapy and prevention. Repeat stone analysis is recommended, when available. Most stones have mixed mineral composition.

Imaging. Necessary to diagnose stone disease and quantify stone burden, location, characteristics, urinary tract anatomy, and estimate metabolic activity. The optimal imaging usually depends on the clinical situation (Tables 27.8 and 27.9). Nephrocalcinosis suggests an underlying metabolic disorder.

Computed Tomography (CT). Noncontrast CT is considered the gold standard, with approximately 98% sensitivity and 97%

Table 27.6 Risk Factors Associated with Stone Formation

Past stone history
Family history of stone disease
Bowel disease, intestinal malabsorption, chronic diarrhea
History of bowel surgery (resection, gastric bypass)
Gout
Hyperparathyroidism, hyperthyroidism
Type 2 diabetes mellitus, metabolic syndrome
Obesity
Chronic kidney disease
Osteoporosis, pathologic skeletal fracture
Poor health: limited reserve to tolerate repeat stone episodes
Recurrent urinary tract infections
Neurogenic bladder, spinal cord injury
Stones composed of cystine, uric acid, struvite or infectious, brushite
Sarcoidosis
Anatomic abnormalities of urinary tract: solitary kidney, horseshoe
   kidney, urinary diversion, UPJO, medullary sponge kidney, ureterocele
Stone-provoking medications or excess supplements (probenecid,
   protease inhibitors, vitamin C, carbonic anhydrase inhibitors, calcium
   supplements)
Pediatric patients, early-onset stone formation
Solitary kidney (not necessarily higher risk of stone formation but
   prevention more important)
Environmental: high temperature, arid climates
Vocational: pilots, sailors, truck and bus drivers

UPJO, Ureteropelvic junction obstruction.

specificity. Contrast/urogram is helpful when detailed anatomy of the collecting system is necessary. CT is rapid, commonly available, highly accurate, provides excellent anatomic detail, and provides some insight into stone composition. Relatively higher cost and radiation exposure. Low-dose (<4 mSv) and ultra-low dose (<1 mSv) protocols available, often maintaining $>80\%$ and $>90\%$ sensitivity and specificity, respectively.

   Radiography: Plain Radiography (KUB) and Intravenous Pyelography (IVP). Kidney, ureter, and bladder (KUB) is the oldest imaging modality, with an estimated 57% sensitivity and 76% specificity. IVP has an estimated 70% sensitivity and 95% specificity. Up to 15%–20% of stones are radiolucent and missed. Overlying bones and bowel gas interfere with stone detection.

Box 27.1 Abbreviated Evaluation of Single Stone Formers

HISTORY

- Underlying predisposing conditions
- Medications (calcium, vitamin C, vitamin D, acetazolamide, steroids)
- Dietary excesses, inadequate fluid intake, excessive fluid loss

MULTICHANNEL BLOOD SCREEN

- Basic metabolic panel (sodium, potassium, chloride, carbon dioxide, blood urea nitrogen, creatinine)
- Calcium
- Intact parathyroid hormone
- Uric acid

URINE

- Urinalysis
  - pH >7.5: infection lithiasis
  - pH <5.5: uric acid lithiasis
  - Sediment for crystalluria
- Urine culture
  - Urea-splitting organisms: suggestive of infection lithiasis
- Qualitative cystine

RADIOGRAPHY

- Radiopaque stones: calcium oxalate, calcium phosphate, magnesium ammonium phosphate (struvite), cystine.
- Radiolucent stones: uric acid, xanthine, triamterene
- Intravenous pyelogram: radiolucent stones, anatomic abnormalities

STONE ANALYSIS

Ultrasound (US). US is widely available (many point-of-care options), cost effective, and avoids ionizing radiation. Operator variability, stone size, body habitus all influence accuracy. Relative low sensitivity (50%), better specificity (70%–90%). US has 90% sensitivity for detecting hydronephrosis. Doppler ultrasonography allows for evaluation of ureteral jets and twinkle artifact (mosaic of colors seen over a stone; distinguishes stone from other echogenic structures). Ureteral stones infrequently visible in adults.

Table 27.7 Urine Microscopic Appearance of Common Urinary Stone Crystals

STONE TYPE	CRYSTAL APPEARANCE
Calcium oxalate monohydrate	Hourglass, dumbbels, ovals
Calcium oxalate dihydrate	Envelopes, tetrahedral
Calcium phosphate: apatite	Amorphous, powder appearance
Calcium hydrogen phosphate: brushite	Needles, rosettes, pointing fingers
Magnesium ammonium phosphate: struvite	"Coffin lid." rectangular
Cystine	Hexagons
Uric acid	Amorphous shards, plates, parallelograms

Table 27.8 Imaging Studies and Effective Radiation Dose in Adults

IMAGING STUDY	EFFECTIVE DOSE (MSV)
Ultrasonography	0
Magnetic resonance imaging	0
Kidney, ureter, bladder (KUB)	0.7
KUB with tomograms	3.9
Intravenous pyelography (IVP)	3
Computed tomography (CT) urogram, with contrast (three-phase)	10–40
CT abdomen and pelvis, noncontrast	5–10
CT abdomen and pelvis, noncontrast, low dose	<4
CT abdomen and pelvis, noncontrast, ultra-low dose	<1

Digital Tomosynthesis. Similar to conventional KUB and obtains several low-dose images via a tomographic sweep of the x-ray emitter. Multiple coronal slice images are then digitally reconstructed. More sensitive than KUB, and significantly less radiation than standard CT.

Magnetic Resonance Imaging (MRI). Stone detections is variable and relies on inferring stone presence from a signal void rather than truly detecting the stone. MRI has 82% sensitivity and 98% specificity for renal stones. Considered in rare situations (pregnancy).

Table 27.9 Stone X-ray and Computed Tomography Characteristics

RADIOPAQUE	FAINTLY RADIOPAQUE	RADIOLUCENT	NOT VISIBLE ON NCCT
Calcium oxalate mono- and dihydrate	Struvite	Uric acid	
Calcium phosphate (brushite)	Calcium phosphate	Matrix	Protease inhibitor stones (indinavir, nelfinavir)
Calcium phosphate (apatite)	Matrix	Ammonium acid urate	
	cystine	Drug-stones	
		Xanthine	
		2,8-Dihydroxyadenine	

NCCT, Noncontrast comptued tomography.

Metabolic Evaluation

Metabolic evaluation is recommended in:
1. High-risk individuals (Table 27.6).
2. Interested first-time stone formers

This should include one or two 24-hour urine collections on a random diet, analyzed for, at least, total volume pH, calcium, oxalate, uric acid, citrate, sodium, potassium, and creatinine. Magnesium, sulfate, and urea nitrogen (estimates protein load from animal meat) may be included as well. Consider qualitative cystine screening test in children and at-risk adults. Fast and calcium load testing are not recommended to distinguish hypercalciuria type because treatment does not change. It is unclear whether an initial one or two 24-hour urine collections is better

Table 27.10 shows reference ranges for 24-hour urine parameters in adults. Normal ranges in children vary by gender, age, body weight, and surface area.

TREATMENT

The clinical management of nephrolithiasis depends on both patient- and stone-related factors. The prevention and medical management of kidney stones relies on dietary measures and medications. This can be done empirically but is enhanced by knowing stone composition, underlying risk factors, and 24-hour urine results (Fig. 27.1). Surgical management of stones includes shock wave lithotripsy (SWL), ureteroscopy (URS), percutaneous nephrolithotomy (PCNL), and rarely open, robotic, or laparoscopic surgery. For many clinical situations, more than one treatment option may be reasonable, with a common tradeoff between relative invasiveness and stone clearance.

Medical Management

General Diet Therapies. Several dietary prevention strategies should be followed by all stone formers, regardless of underlying risk (Table 27.11). Most of these measures are best studied in calcium stone formers.

Pharmacologic Therapies. Drug therapies are best utilized in high-risk stone formers, can reduce stone recurrences, and usually guided by stone type and metabolic abnormalities (Table 27.12 and Fig. 27.1).

Table 27.10 Normal Values for 24-hour Urine Analytes in Adults

URINARY ANALYTE	REFERENCE RANGES
Calcium	<200 mg/day (women), <250 mg/day (men)
Citrate	>550 mg/day (women), >450 mg/day (men)
Oxalate	<40 mg/day
Uric acid	<750 mg/day (women), <800 mg/day (men)
Sodium	<150 mg/day
Magnesium	30–120 mg/day
Potassium	20–100 mg/day
Cystine	<75 mg/day
pH	5.8–6.2
Creatinine/kg	15–20 (women), 18–24 (men)

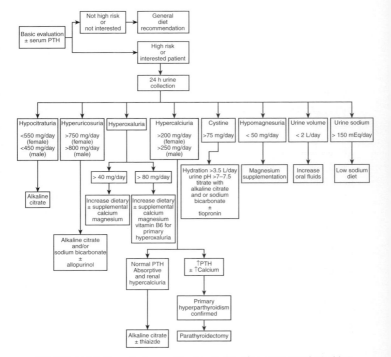

FIG. 27.1 Metabolic evaluation and treatment algorithm. *PTH*, Parathyroid hormone.

Table 27.11 General Dietary Therapies

Oral fluid intake to achieve urine volume ≥2.5 L/day
Circadian fluid intake
Dietary calcium intake of 1000–1200 mg calcium/day
Limit sodium intake to ≤2300 mg/day (≤ 100 mEq/day)
If urinary oxalate is elevated, limit high oxalate foods
Increase fruits and vegetables (increases dietary citrate) and fiber
Limit nondairy animal protein (0.8–1.0 g/kg/day; red meat, poultry, fish,
  pork, lamb)

• Calcium Oxalate and Calcium Phosphate Stones

Diet Therapies. General dietary measures (Table 27.11)

Pharmacologic Therapies

- **Thiazides** (hydrochlorothiazide, chlorthalidone, indapamide) – Recommended for recurrent calcium stone formers. Reduce stone recurrence in hypercalciuria and idiopathic calcium stone formers. Improve health-related quality of life. Reduce urinary calcium by directly stimulating calcium resorption at the distal tubule and indirectly at the proximal tubule through extracellular volume depletion. Inhibit sodium reabsorption at the distal tubule. Most studied medication for stone prevention. Long-term thiazide use can increase bone mineral density and decrease bony fractures. Hypercalciuria is potentiated by a low sodium diet.

  Adverse Effects. Hypokalemia, hypocitraturia, hyperglycemia, hyperuricemia, dyslipidemia, thirst, polyuria, gastrointestinal (GI) upset, fatigue, weakness. Often coadministered with potassium citrate to counter hypokalemia and hypocitraturia.

- **Alkaline Citrates** (potassium citrate, sodium citrate, calcium citrate) – Recommended for recurrent calcium stone formers and those with hypocitraturia. Reduce calcium stone recurrence and improve health-related quality of life. Citrate delivers an alkali load, corrects acidosis, and increases urinary citrate and urinary pH. Citrate is converted to bicarbonate in the liver, which increases urinary pH and citrate excretion (indirectly by reducing proximal tubular citrate reabsorption). Potassium citrate is preferred because it has the best supporting data, the potassium improves intracellular acidosis, and can offset hypokalemia induced by thiazides. Unclear

Table 27.12 Pharmacotherapies Used to Prevent Kidney Stones

MEDICATION	MECHANISM	EFFECT	STONE TYPE	TYPICAL DOSE
Thiazide/thiazide-like diuretics HCTZ Chlorthalidone Indapamide	↑ Calcium reabsorption	↓ Urinary calcium	Calcium oxalate Calcium phosphate	HCTZ 25 mg bid Chlorthalidone 25–50 mg/day Indapamide 1.25–2.5 mg/day
Alkaline citrates Potassium citrate Sodium citrate Calcium citrate	Binds calcium; inhibits calcium oxalate and calcium phosphate crystallization	↓ Urine calcium ↑ Urine citrate ↑ Urine pH	Calcium oxalate Uric acid Cystine	15–20 mEq bid–tid Dose varies by urine pH goal Alternative 1/2 mEq/kg/day in equally divided doses
Sodium bicarbonate	↑ Urine pH	↑ Urine pH ↑ Urine citrate	Uric acid Calcium oxalate Cystine	650 mg tid–qid
Allopurinol Febuxostat	Xanthine oxidase inhibitor	↓ Urine and serum uric acid	Calcium oxalate Uric acid Ammonium urate 2,8-Dihydroxyadenine	100–300 mg/day 80–120 mg/day
Thiols Tiopronin	Binds cystine via disulfide exchange	↓ Urine cystine ↑ Cystine solubility	Cystine	Titrate to effect Start: 100–300 mg/day Max: 2000 mg/day

Captopril	Binds cystine via disulfide exchange	↓ Urine cystine ↑ Cystine solubility	Cystine	25 mg tid
D-penicillamine	Binds cystine via disulfide exchange	↓ Urine cystine ↑ Cystine solubility	Cystine	Titrate to effect Start 250 mg/day
Acetohydroxamic acid	Inhibits urease	Urease inhibitor ↓ Urine urea ↓ Urine pH	Struvite	250 mg bid–tid
Calcium	Binds oxalate	↓ Urine oxalate	Calcium oxalate	1000–1200 mg/day
magnesium	Binds calcium and oxalate	May ↓ urine calcium, oxalate	Calcium oxalate	200–400 mg/day
Pyridoxine (vitamin B_6)	Cofactor AGT, ↓ liver oxalate production	↓ Urine oxalate	Calcium oxalate or primary hyperoxaluria	5–20 mg/kg/day

AGT, Alanine-glyoxylate aminotransferase
Modified from AUA Core Curriculum and EAU Guidelines on Urolithiasis.

if citrate supplementation benefits calcium phosphate stone formers because the potential benefits may be offset by the rise in urine pH. Formulations include wax tablet, liquid, and crystal/powder. Prescription and over the counter.

Adverse Effects. GI (nausea, heartburn, loose stools), 3%–17%; hyperkalemia in renal insufficiency.

- **Sodium Bicarbonate** (i.e., baking soda) – Delivers an alkali load, improves acidosis, and indirectly increase urinary citrate and pH. Sodium load can promote hypercalciuria, fluid retention, and edema. Alternative to potassium citrate in CKD or if hyperkalemia is a concern.

- **Allopurinol** – Xanthine oxidase inhibitor that reduces serum and urinary uric acid. Recommended for recurrent calcium oxalate stone formers with hyperuricosuria and normal urinary calcium. Febuxostat is another xanthine oxidase inhibitor.

Adverse Effects. Liver enzyme elevation, rash, Stevens-Johnson syndrome.

Special Situations with Calcium Stones

- **Thiazides and potassium citrate** reduce stone recurrence in recurrent calcium stone formers with no identifiable metabolic derangements and when the derangements have been fully corrected but stone recurrence continues.

- **Corticosteroids** are used in sarcoidosis and some granulomatous disease to suppress granuloma formation of 1,25-dihydroxy vitamin D, thereby reducing serum and urinary calcium.

- **Enteric Hyperoxaluria – Dietary and sometimes supplemental calcium** (taken with high oxalate meals) binds to and reduces available gut oxalate. In the setting of malabsorption, chronic diarrhea, or bowel disease or resection, liquid citrate formulation is preferred because extended-release tables may not dissolve and can be excreted whole.

- **Primary Hyperoxaluria – Potassium citrate and vitamin B_6 (pyridoxine).** Vitamin B_6 serves as a cofactor to the enzyme that converts oxalate to glyoxylate (AGT). No robust data showing a benefit to vitamin B_6 in other causes of hyperoxaluria.

- **Primary Hyperparathyroidism** (resorptive hypercalciuria) – If caused by an overactive parathyroid adenoma, **parathyroidectomy** is recommended.

• Uric Acid Stones

Diet Therapies. General dietary measures apply (Table 27.11). Correct metabolic syndrome and diabetes. Limit dietary animal protein if hyperuricosuria is found, though most uric acid stone formers have normal urinary uric acid.

Pharmacologic Therapies

- **Alkaline Citrates, Sodium Bicarbonate** – Acidic urine (pH <5.5) promotes uric acid precipitation, while increasing urine pH >6 coverts uric acid to the more soluble urate salt. Can dissolve pure uric acid stones but can take months and usually requires higher doses of alkali.
- **Allopurinol** (and febuxostat) – Not considered first-line therapy for most uric acid stone formers because most do not exhibit hyperuricosuria. A secondary measure if adequate urinary alkalization fails to prevent recurrent uric acid stones (common in chronic diarrhea, ileostomies, inflammatory bowel disease), if hyperuricosuria is present, and in rare situations of uric acid overproduction (myeloproliferative disorders, Lesch-Nyhan syndrome).

• Infectious Stones

Diet Therapies. General dietary measures (Table 27.11). Low calcium and low phosphorus diets have failed to show benefit.

Pharmacologic Therapies

- **Acetohydroxamic Acid** – Irreversible urease inhibitor; minimizes ammonium production, lowers urinary ammonia and pH, and increases struvite dissolution. Does not reduce struvite recurrence. Considered selectively in patients with recurrent or persistent struvite stones and no further reasonable surgical options. Poorly excreted with renal insufficiency.

  Adverse Effects. Common (22%–62%) and often interfere with long term compliance. Headache (30%), nausea and GI symptoms (25%–30%), hemolytic anemia (15%), tremor, hair loss, and deep vein thrombosis.

• Cystine Stones

Diet Therapies. General dietary measures (Table 27.11), with extra attention to high fluid intake (goal, >3 L urine output daily), limited sodium (reduces cystine urine excretion) and protein intake (reduces methionine, which is a cystine substrate).

Pharmacologic Therapies

- **Alkaline Citrates: Sodium Bicarbonate** – Cystine solubility greatly increases with urine pH >7–7.5; unknown if isolated citrate therapy can reduce cystine stone recurrence.
- **Cystine-Binding Thiol Drugs (tiopronin** [alpha mercaptopropionyl glycine]) – Recommended for cystine stone recurrence despite adequate fluid intake and urinary alkalization. Bind to cystine. Encourage a disulfide exchange, replacing relatively insoluble cystine-cystine dimers with the more soluble cystine-thiol complex. Titrated to reduce urinary cystine concentration while minimizing side effects.
  Adverse Effects. GI symptoms (17%), hematologic (5%, anemia, cytopenia), proteinuria (5%), rash, and loss of taste (4%)

Follow-Up

Periodic repeat stone imaging (KUB, renal US, or low-dose CT) and 24-hour urine specimens are important in patients initiated on stone treatment, with timing tailored to stone activity. Repeat 24-hour urine collection is encouraged within 6 months of dietary and medical therapy initiation or changes to assess treatment response. Blood testing to evaluate for adverse effects should be done periodically in patients taking pharmacologic stone therapy.

Surgical Management

The cornerstones of surgical treatment include SWL, URS, and PCNL. Observation is an option for asymptomatic, nonobstructing calyceal stones. In rare, select instances open, robotic, and laparoscopic approaches may be considered for stone clearance. For many clinical situations, more than one treatment option may be reasonable, with a tradeoff between relative invasiveness and stone clearance (Table 27.13). Careful attention to stone-, anatomic-, and patient clinical-related factors can guide optimal treatment recommendations.

Indications for Rapid Renal Decompression of an Obstructed Kidney

- UTI, sepsis
- Worsening renal function
- Bilateral obstruction
- Obstruction of solitary kidney
- Prolonged unilateral obstruction
- Intractable pain, nausea or vomiting

Table 27.13 Stone Clearance by Location, Size, and Treatment Modality

LOCATION	SIZE	STONE-FREE RATES (%)			
		SWL[a]	URS[a]	PCNL	Open
Renal	≤10 mm (nonstaghorn)	40–70	50–90	>80	
	>10 mm (nonstaghorn)	10–58	50–90	>80	
	Staghorn (and >2 cm)	19–57	50–80	70–78	71
Total Ureter	≤10 mm	64	93		
	>10 mm	62	83		
Proximal ureter	≤10 mm	66	85		
	>10 mm	74	79		
Mid Ureter	≤10 mm	75	91		
	>10 mm	67	82		
Distal Ureter	≤10 mm	74	94		
	>10 mm	71	92		

[a]stone-free rates are for single ureteroscopy procedure for ureteral stones. For shock wave lithotripsy (SWL) for ureteral stones, stone-free rates are for ≥1 procedure (mean number of SWL sessions: 1.34 [proximal ureter], 1.29 [mid ureter], 1.26 [distal ureter]).

Medical Expulsive Therapy (MET). The use of medication to facilitate ureteral stone passage. AUA guidelines recommend MET with alpha-blockers for distal ureteral stones ≤10 mm. Clear benefit for stones >5 mm. It is unclear if MET is beneficial for mid and proximal ureteral stones. Alpha-blocker use for MET is "off label." There is no benefit for MET in nonobstructing renal stones. Calcium-channel blockers (nifedipine) and steroids have been used for MET in the past, but contemporary efficacy data are lacking.

Shock Wave Lithotripsy. During SWL, weak shock waves (pressure waves) are generated externally, transmitted through the body, and focused onto the stone. Shock waves cause large pressure and shear stress changes at the wave front and have a positive-pressure (compressive phase) and negative-pressure (tensile phase) component. Stone fragmentation occurs by many mechanisms, including spallation, circumferential compression, shear stress, superfocusing, and cavitation. The three main types of shock wave generators include electrohydraulic (spark gap), electromagnetic, and piezoelectric. Fluoroscopy and ultrasound are used to target stones and guide treatment, with contemporary machines incorporating both modalities.

Indications and Contraindications. SWL success rates are influenced by many stone- and patient-related factors. SWL is most efficacious for smaller, less dense stones in favorable locations (not lower pole) and in patients with favorable anatomy (Box 27.2). SWL has the least morbidity and lowest complication rate but also lowest the stone clearance rate. The AUA guidelines considers SWL as an alternative to URS for mid and distal ureteral stones. The EAU guidelines recommend SWL or URS for ureteral stones <10 mm and URS as first line with SWL as an alternative for stones >10 mm. Per AUA guidelines, routine perioperative antibiotics are unnecessary in the absence of UTI. Routine ureteral stenting should not be performed during SWL, while postoperative alpha blocker use is encouraged to promote fragment passage. SWL should not be considered first line for lower pole stones >10 mm or staghorn stones. Box 27.3 shows contraindications to SWL.

Adverse Events

- Renal injury (contusion, hematoma): 1%–20%; 1% symptomatic
- Renal hemorrhage: ≤1%, some require transfusion

Box 27.2 Factors Negatively Affecting Shock Wave Lithotripsy Success

Stone composition (cystine, brushite, calcium oxalate monohydrate, matrix)
Stone attenuation ≥1000 HU
Skin-to-stone distance >10 cm (morbid obesity)
Renal anatomic anomalies (horseshoe kidney, calyceal diverticulum)
Unfavorable lower pole anatomy (narrow infundibulopelvic angle, narrow infundibulum, long lower pole calyx)
Relative or complete patient immobility

> **Box 27.3** Contraindications to Shock Wave Lithotripsy
>
> Pregnancy
> Uncorrected coagulopathy or bleeding diathesis
> Untreated urinary tract infection
> Arterial aneurysm near stone (renal or abdominal aortic aneurysms)
> Obstruction of urinary tract distal to stone
> Inability to target stone (skeletal malformation)

- Infection: rare, <1%
- Steinstrasse (street of stones): 2%–10%; more frequent with increasing stone burden
- Renal colic: 2%–4%
- Dysrhythmia: 10%–60%
- Liver and spleen hematoma; bowel perforation: case reports
- Hypertension: unclear if SWL increases hypertension risk in some patients
- Diabetes and renal impairment not seen in large population studies of SWL

Ureteroscopy. Ureteroscopes can be semirigid (distal or mid ureteral stones) or flexile (preferred for proximal ureteral and renal stones), fiberoptic or digital, and reusable or single use. URS is an option for almost any stone in almost any location within the upper urinary tract. However, certain patient and intrarenal anatomy can preclude successful retrograde access (steep lower pole angle, calyceal diverticuli, transplant ureters).

Indications and Contraindications. Besides untreated UTI, certain precluding anatomic abnormalities, and patients too unfit for any anesthesia or surgery, URS can be done in essentially any patient and for any stone. Recommended for suspected or known cystine or uric acid ureteral stones. Improved stone clearance compared with SWL for all stones at all upper urinary tract locations. Inferior stone clearance compared with PCNL, especially for larger lower pole and staghorn calculi. URS morbidity is more than SWL and less than PCNL. Can be done safely in patients on uninterrupted antiplatelets and or anticoagulants; however, longer postoperative hematuria is possible. Staged URS is an alternative for large burden renal stones in patients unfit or unwilling to undergo PCNL.

Adverse Events. Reports of overall adverse events vary widely from 9%–25%

- Failure to access the stone: 1%–8%
- Intraoperative bleeding severe enough to abort URS: <2%
- Delayed renal bleeding: <1%
- Renal hematoma: ≤1%
- Infection/sepsis: <5%/<2%
- Silent hydronephrosis: <1%–2%
- Stricture: 0.5%–4%. More common with long-term impacted ureteral stones, intraoperative ureteral injury
- Perforation: ≤4%. Occurs with excessive balloon and other ureteral dilation, misguided stone manipulation, over aggressive stone extraction, intracorporeal lithotripsy, and basket extraction devices
- Avulsion: <1%. Often overzealous attempts to extract large stones or fragments

Percutaneous Nephrolithotomy

Indications and Contraindications. AUA and EAU guidelines recommend PCNL as first-line treatment for total renal stone burdens >2 cm. Also indicated for certain complex renal anatomy, lower pole stone burdens >1 cm, staghorn stones, and ureteral and renal stones unsuccessfully managed by SWL or URS. Higher single-session stone clearance than SWL or URS and higher morbidity. PCNL is contraindicated in uncorrected coagulopathies, untreated UTI, pregnant women, potential malignant renal tumors, and when safe renal access is precluded by certain body habitus and anatomy. Preoperative noncontrast CT is recommended to best define stone burden and renal and perirenal anatomy.

Percutaneous access occurs via fluoroscopy, US, and rarely CT. Posterior calyceal access is preferred to theoretically reduce bleeding. Adjunctive flexible nephroscopy, if available, is recommended for all PCNLs. Tract dilation occurs with balloon or sequential dilators (plastic or metal). Smaller access tracts may correlate with less bleeding, similar stone clearance, and longer operative duration. Lithotripsy devices (ultrasonic, pneumatic/ballistic, combination, laser), suction, graspers and baskets are used for stone retrieval. Lasers are commonly employed during smaller-access (mini, micro) PCNL. Renal drainage by nephrostomy or ureteral stent is recommended, with optimal duration and type influenced by surgical and patient factors.

Adverse Events. Reports of overall adverse events vary widely, 4%–61%

- Fever: ≤11%
- Transfusion: 2%–10%
- Angioembolization: 1%–2%
- Infection
- Sepsis: <2%
- UTI: <5%
- Urinoma: <0.5%
- Thoracic complications: 2%–16% (subcostal (<2%) < below 11th < above 11th)
- Pneumothorax, hydrothorax, hemothorax
- Surround visceral injury <1%
- Liver or spleen <1%
- Bowel or intestine (duodenum) <1%

Laparoscopic, Robotic, and Open. In general, these should not be considered first-line therapy because almost all stones can be adequate treated with SWL, URS, and or PCNL. PCNL has almost completely supplanted anatrophic nephrolithotomy for staghorn stones. Open, laparascopic, and robotic approaches are considered in rare circumstances and often include anatomic abnormalities (large, anterior calyceal diverticuli with large stones), ectopic kidneys (e.g., pelvic kidneys), when additional reconstruction is planned (ureteropelvic junction obstruction [UPJO] with large stones), or for poorly functioning kidneys (nephrectomy indicated).

Treatment Selection

Figs. 27.2 and 27.3 show surgical treatment recommendations based on stone size and location.

LOWER URINARY TRACT STONES

Bladder Stones

Traditionally classified as migrant (3%–17%, nonexpelled kidney stones), primary idiopathic (children, nutritional deficiencies) and secondary (associated bladder pathology, e.g., bladder outlet obstruction, foreign body, long-term catheters). Usually presents with hematuria, lower urinary tract symptoms, and rarely urinary retention. More common in males. Treated with dissolution (slow,

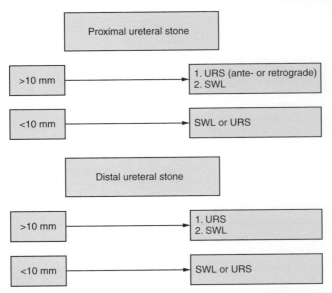

FIG. 27.2 Treatment algorithm: ureteral stones. *SWL,* Shock wave lithotripsy; *URS* ureteroscopy. (Modified from Turk et al. *EAU Guidelines on urolithiasis.* 2017.)

often incomplete), SWL, transurethral lithotripsy, suprapubic cystolithotomy or cystolithotripsy, or open removal.

Urethral Stones

Rare and most common in males; classified as primary (form secondary to urethral obstruction and or foreign body) or secondary (migratory, more common). Most patients present with acute painful urinary retention from sudden stone impaction.

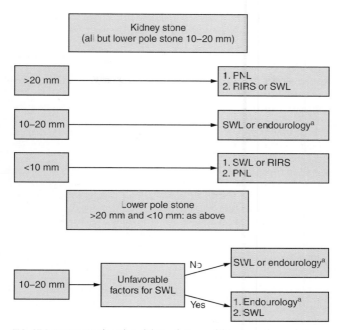

FIG. 27.3 Treatment algorithm. (A) Renal stones. (B) Lower pole renal stones. [a]The term "endourology" encompasses all PNL and ureteroscopy (URS) interventions. (Modified from Turk et al. *EAU Guidelines on urolithiasis.* 2017.).

Suggested Readings

Albala DM, Assimos DG, Clayman RV, et al. Lower pole I: a prospective randomized trial of extracorporeal shock wave lithotripsy and percutaneous nephrostolithotomy for lower pole nephrolithiasis-initial results. *J Urol* 2001;166 2072.

Assimos D, Krambeck A, Miller NL, et al. Surgical management of stones: American Urological Association/Endourological Society guideline, part I. *J Urol* 2016;196:1153-1160.

Assimos D, Krambeck A, Miller NL, et al. Surgical management of stones: American Urological Association/Endourological Society guideline, part II. *J Urol* 2016;196:1161-1169.

Borghi L, Meschi T, Amato F, et al. Urinary volume, water and recurrences in idiopathic calcium nephrolithiasis: a 5-year randomized prospective study. *J Urol* 1996;155(3): 839-843.

Borghi L, Schianchi T, Meschi T, et al. Comparison of two diets for the prevention of recurrent stones in idiopathic hypercalciuria. *N Engl J Med* 2002;346(2):77-84.

Escribano J, Balaguer A, Pagone F, et. al. Pharmacological interventions for preventing complications in idiopathic hypercalciuria. *Cochrane Database Syst Rev* 2009; CD004754

Ettinger B, Tang A, Citron JT, et al. Randomized trial of allopurinol in the prevention of calcium oxalate calculi. *N Engl J Med* 1986;315(22):1386-1389.

Pearle MS, Lingeman JE, Leveillee R, et al. Prospective, randomized trial comparing shock wave lithotripsy and ureteroscopy for lower pole caliceal calculi 1 cm or less. *J Urol* 2005;173:2005-2009.

Pearle MS, Roehrborn CG, Pak CY. Meta-analysis of randomized trials for medical prevention of calcium oxalate nephrolithiasis. *J Endourol* 1999;13(9):679-685.

Phillippou P, Moraitis K, Massod J, et. al. The management of bladder lithiasis in the modern era endourology. *Urology* 2012;79:980-986.

Phillips R, Hanchanale VS, Myatt A, et al. Citrate salts for preventing and treating calcium containing kidney stones in adults. *Cochrane Database Syst Rev* 2015;(10):CD010057.

Raffin EP, Penniston KL, Antonelli JA, et al. The effect of thiazide and potassium citrate use on the health-related quality of life of patients with urolithiasis. *J Urol* 2018;200(6):1290-1294.

Smith-Bindman R, Aubin C, Bailitz J, et al. Ultrasonography versus computed tomography for suspected nephrolithiaisis. *N Eng J Med* 2014;371:1100.

Surgical management of stones: American Urological Association/Endourological Society Guideline. https://www.auanet.org/educadtion/guiedlines/surgical-management-of-stones.cfm.

Urolithiasis: European Association of Urology Guideline. https://uroweb.org/guideline/urolithiasis/#1.

28

Evaluation and Management of Localized Renal Tumors

ATREYA DASH AND ROBERT M. SWEET

CONTRIBUTORS OF CAMPBELL-WALSH-WEIN, 12TH EDITION

William P. Parker, Matthew T. Gettman, Steven C. Campbell, Brian R. Lane, Phillip M. Pierorazio, Panagiotis Kallidonis, Evangelos Liatsikos, Thomas W. Jarrett, Surena F. Matin, Armine K. Smith, Ramaprasad Srinivasan, and W. Marston Linehan

CLASSIFICATION

Renal masses can be malignant, benign, or inflammatory (Table 28.1), or they can be classified based on radiographic appearance (simple cystic, complex cystic, solid) (Table 28.2).

BENIGN RENAL TUMORS

Renal Cysts

Epidemiology, Etiology, and Pathophysiology. Renal cyst disease is the most common benign renal tumor. Up to 10% of the population may harbor a renal cyst, with putative risk factors being age, male gender, hypertension, and worsening renal function.

Evaluation. To aid in the evaluation of renal cyst disease, the Bosniak classification (Table 28.3) is a commonly used method to characterize cysts and their risk of malignancy

Management Options. For most simple renal cysts, no additional follow-up is required, with the maximal intervention of serial imaging recommended for Bosniak IIF lesions.

Surgical resection or ablation is recommended for Bosniak III/IV lesions.

Table 28.1 Renal Masses Classified by Pathologic Features

MALIGNANT		BENIGN	
Renal Cell Carcinoma (RCC)	**Nephroblastic Tumors**[a]	**Cystic Lesions**	
• Clear cell RCC	• Nephrogenic rests	• Simple cyst	
• Multilocular cystic clear cell renal cell neoplasm of low malignant potential	• Nephroblastoma (Wilms tumor)	• Hemorrhagic cyst	
• Papillary RCC	• Cystic partially differentiated nephroblastoma	**Solid Lesions**	
• Chromophobe RCC		• Angiomyolipoma	
• Hybrid oncocytic chromophobe tumor	**Carcinoma Associated with Neuroblastoma**	• Oncocytoma	
• Carcinoma of the collecting ducts of Bellini	Neuroendocrine Tumors	• Papillary adenoma (renal adenoma)	
• Renal medullary carcinoma	• Carcinoid (low-grade neuroendocrine tumor)	• Metanephric tumors (adenoma, adenofibroma, stromal tumor)	
• MiT family translocation RCC[a]	• Neuroendocrine carcinoma (high-grade neuroendocrine tumor)	• Congenital mesoblastic nephroma[a]	
• Xpn translocation RCC	• Primitive neuroectodermal tumor	• Cystic nephroma/mixed epithelial stromal tumor	
• t(6;11) RCC	• Neuroblastoma	• Reninoma (juxtaglomerular cell tumor)	
• Mucinous tubular and spindle cell carcinoma	• Pheochromocytoma	• Renomedullary interstitial tumor	
• Tubulocystic RCC	**Hematopoietic and Lymphoid Tumors**	• Leiomyoma	
• Acquired cystic disease–associated RCC	• Lymphoma	• Fibroma	
• Clear cell (tubulo) papillary RCC	• Leukemia	• Hemangioma	
• Hereditary leiomyomatosis RCC syndrome–associated RCC	• Plasmacytoma	• Lymphangioma	
• RCC, unclassified	**Germ Cell Tumors**	• Schwannoma	
	• Teratoma	• Solitary fibrous tumor	
	• Choriocarcinoma		

Urothelium-Based Cancers	Metastasis	Vascular Lesions
	Invasion by Adjacent Neoplasm	• Renal artery aneurysm
• Urothelial carcinoma		• Arteriovenous malformation
• Squamous cell carcinoma		
• Adenocarcinoma		**Pseudotumor**
		Inflammatory
Sarcomas		• Abscess
		• Focal pyelonephritis
• Leiomyosarcoma		• Xanthogranulomatous pyelonephritis
• Liposarcoma		• Infected renal cyst
• Other sarcomas		• Tuberculosis
		• Rheumatic granuloma

aMore common in children and young adults.
Modified from Srigley JR, Delahunt B, Eble, et al. The International Society of Urological Pathology (ISUP) Vancouver Classification of Renal Neoplasia. Am J Surg Pathol 2013;37(10):1469-1489.

Table 28.2 Radiologic and Pathologic Correlates for Renal Masses

Simple Cystic	Strongly Enhancing Mass	Infiltrative Mass
Benign cyst	Clear cell RCC	Lymphoma
Parapelvic cyst	Angiomyolipoma	High-grade urothelial carcinoma
Hydronephrosis	Oncocytoma	Sarcomatoid differentiation
Caliceal diverticulum	Papillary RCC (occasionally)	Collecting duct carcinoma
	Chromophobe RCC (occasionally)	Renal medullary carcinoma
		Xanthogranulomatous pyelonephritis
		Metastasis (occasionally)

Complex Cystic	Moderately Enhancing Solid Mass	Calcified Mass
Cystic RCC	Papillary RCC	RCC
Hemorrhagic cyst	Chromophobe RCC	Urothelial carcinoma
Hyperdense cyst	Clear cell RCC (occasionally)	Benign complex cyst
Benign complex cyst	Oncocytoma	Xanthogranulomatous pyelonephritis
Cystic nephroma	Fat-poor angiomyolipoma	Renal artery aneurysm
Mixed epithelial-stromal tumor	Adenoma/metanephric adenoma	Concomitant nephrolithiasis
Cystic Wilms tumor	Unifocal lymphoma	
Infected cyst or abscess	Sarcoma	
Hydrocalix	Lobar nephronia	
Arteriovenous malformation	Pseudotumor	
Renal artery aneurysm	Infarct	
	Metastasis	

Fat-Containing Mass	Multifocal/Bilateral Masses
Angiomyolipoma	Familial RCC
Liposarcoma	Metastases
Lipoma	Sporadic, multifocal RCC (particularly papillary RCC or clear cell RCC)
	Angiomyolipomas (tuberous sclerosis)
	Lymphoma
	Cystic tumors (autosomal dominant polycystic kidney disease)

RCC, Renal cell carcinoma.
Modified from Simmons MN, Herts BR, Campbell SC. Image based approaches to the diagnosis of renal masses [lesson 39]. *AUA Update Series* 2007;26:382-391.

Table 28.3 Classification of Complex Renal Cysts

BOSNIAK CLASSIFICATION	RADIOGRAPHIC FEATURES	RISK OF MALIGNANCY	MANAGEMENT
I	Water density Homogeneous, hairline thin wall No septa No calcification No enhancement	None	Surveillance not necessary
II	Few hairline septa in which "perceived" enhancement may be present Fine calcification or short segment of slightly thickened calcification in wall or septa No unequivocal enhancement	Minimal	Surveillance not necessary
	Hyperdense lesion: ≤3 cm, well marginated, with no unequivocal enhancement	Minimal	Periodic surveillance
IIF	Multiple hairline thin septa Minimal smooth wall thickening "Perceived" enhancement of wall or septae may be present Calcification may be thick or nodular but must be without enhancement Generally well marginated No unequivocal enhancement	3%–5%	Periodic surveillance
	Hyperdense lesion: >3 cm or totally intrarenal with no enhancement	5%–10%	Periodic surveillance
III	"Indeterminate," thickened irregular or smooth walls or septa in which measurable enhancement is present	50%	Surgical excision[a]

Table 28.3 Classification of Complex Renal Cysts—cont'd

BOSNIAK CLASSIFICATION	RADIOGRAPHIC FEATURES	RISK OF MALIGNANCY	MANAGEMENT
IV	Clearly malignant lesions that can have all the criteria of category III but also contain enhancing soft-tissue components	75%–90%	Surgical excision[a]

[a]Surgical excision should be considered if the patient is in good health. Active surveillance is an option for select patients. Thermal ablation is probably best avoided for cystic lesions because of concern about tumor spillage.

Management can include aspiration, cyst decortication, cyst resection, sclerotherapy, arterial embolization, and even nephrectomy depending on the cause and symptom. Acquired cystic kidney disease (ACKD) is associated with a significant increase in malignancy risk and should be followed closely.

Oncocytoma

Epidemiology, Etiology, and Pathophysiology. Up to 25% of renal masses smaller than 3 cm represent oncocytomas. The most common benign enhancing renal mass. Associated with Birt-Hogg-Dube syndrome: pulmonary cysts, spontaneous pneumothoraces, and fibrofolliculomas.

Oncocytoma can be associated with perirenal fat invasion and renal vein invasion, findings that carry prognostic significance in renal cell carcinoma (RCC) but do not in oncocytoma and should not be interpreted as an aggressive pathology

Evaluation. Hypervascularity and a central scar on axial imaging, but these alone are insufficient for a definitive diagnosis. Histologically similar to chromophobe RCC, and immunohistochemical staining may be required to distinguish the two.

Management. When diagnosed by renal mass biopsy, the role of active surveillance (AS) has been explored with favorable results

Angiomyolipoma

Diagnosis. Contrary to other benign renal masses, the diagnosis of angiomyolipoma (AML) can be made on imaging. The presence of macroscopic fat on computed tomography (CT) or magnetic resonance imaging (MRI) is diagnostic of AML. On CT the presence of intralesional fat (-15 to -20 Hounsfield units [HU]) on nonenhanced series is diagnostic. Tuberous sclerosis is associated with the development of multifocal and bilateral renal AML and is associated with activation of the mTOR pathway.

Management. The management of patients with an AML should be individualized on the basis of sporadic versus syndromic AML, the presence of symptoms, the perceived risk of hemorrhage (Fig. 28.1), and with the goal of preserving renal function. The treatment of choice in patients with acute hemorrhage is selective renal angioembolization. Everolimus is indicated for the management of larger, multifocal AMLs in patients with tuberous sclerosis complex (TSC) and lymphangioleiomyomatosis (LAM).

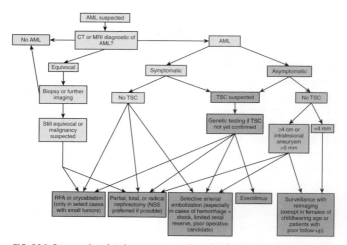

FIG. 28.1 Proposed updated management algorithm for renal angiomyolipoma (AML) by Flum et al. Algorithm represents suggested options. *CT,* Computed tomography; *MRI,* magnetic resonance imaging; *NSS,* nephron sparing surgery; *RFA,* radiofrequency ablation; *TSC,* tuberous sclerosis complex. (From Flum AS, Hamoui N, Said MA, et al. Update on the diagnosis and management of renal angiomyolipoma. *J Urol* 2016;195[4 Pt 1]:834-846.)

Other Benign Tumors

Other tumors include papillary adenoma, metanephric adenoma, cystic nephroma/mixed epithelial-stromal tumors, leiomyoma, and other rare tumors.

MALIGNANT RENAL TUMORS

Renal Cell Carcinoma

Incidence

- Up to 2%–3% of all adult malignant neoplasms, with a male-to-female predominance of 1.9 to 1. RCC typically is diagnosed between 55 and 75 years of age.
- The most lethal of the common urologic cancers.
- Usually sporadic; only 4%–6% are believed to be familial.
- The incidence has increased since the 1970s by an average of 3% per year, with more prevalent use of ultrasonography and CT for other nonspecific abdominal complaints, which increases the relative risk by 1.4 to 2.5-fold compared with control participants. Hypertension and obesity are also associated with increased prevalence of RCC.

Etiology. The strongest risk factor for RCC is tobacco exposure, which provides a relative risk of 1.4 to 2.5 compared with control participants.

Obesity provides a relative risk of 1.07 for each additional unit of body mass index.

Hypertension appears to be the third major causative factor for RCC. Approximately 4%–6% of RCC is familial in origin.

Familial Renal Cell Carcinoma and Molecular Genetics. The distinct nature of the various subtypes of RCC and advances in molecular genetics have contributed to a major revision in the histologic classification of this malignancy (Tables 28.4 and 28.5).

Pathology. All RCCs are, by definition, adenocarcinomas, derived from renal tubular epithelial cells (Table 28.6).

Most RCCs are round to ovoid and circumscribed by a pseudocapsule of compressed parenchyma and fibrous tissue rather than a true histologic capsule. Unlike upper tract urothelial carcinomas, most RCCs are not grossly infiltrative, with the notable exception of collecting duct carcinoma and sarcomatoid variants.

Table 28.4 Familial Renal Cell Carcinoma Subtypes

SYNDROME	PREDISPOSING GENE (CHROMOSOME)	RENAL TUMOR HISTOLOGY AND OTHER MAJOR CLINICAL MANIFESTATIONS	RECOMMENDED MANAGEMENT FOR RENAL TUMORS	POTENTIAL THERAPEUTIC TARGETS
von Hippel-Lindau disease (VHL)	*VHL* (3p25)	Clear cell RCC, often multifocal Retinal angiomas Central nervous system hemangioblastomas Pheochromocytoma Other tumors	Active surveillance <3 cm Surgical excision ≥3 cm, preference for nephron-sparing approaches	HIF-VEGF pathway
Hereditary papillary renal carcinoma (HPRC)	*MET* (7q31)	Multiple, bilateral type 1 papillary RCC	Active surveillance <3 cm Surgical excision ≥3 cm, preference for nephron-sparing approaches	MET kinase
Hereditary leiomyomatosis and renal cell carcinoma (HLRCC)	*Fumarate hydratase (FH)* (1q42-43)	Type 2 papillary RCC most common Collecting duct carcinoma Leiomyomas of skin or uterus Uterine leiomyosarcomas Low-grade variants of RCC also seen in children	Surgical excision, preference for PN but only when wide margins can be achieved	HIF-VEGF pathway; antioxidant response pathway; reductive carboxylation pathway
Succinate dehydrogenase-deficient RCC (SDH-RCC)	*SDHA SDHB* (1p36.13), *SDHC* (1q23.3), *SDHD* (11q23.1), *SDHAF2*	SDH-associated RCC (chromophobe, clear cell, type 2 papillary RCC; or oncocytoma), variable aggressiveness Paragangliomas (benign and malignant) Papillary thyroid carcinoma	Surgical excision, preference for PN but only when wide margins can be achieved	HIF-VEGF pathway; reductive carboxylation pathway

Syndrome	Gene (location)	Features	Management	Pathway
Birt-Hogg-Dube syndrome (BHD)	Folliculin (17p11.2)	Multiple chromophobe RCC, hybrid oncocytic tumors, oncocytomas; Clear cell RCC (occasionally); Papillary RCC (occasionally); Facial fibrofolliculomas; Lung cysts; Spontaneous pneumothorax	Active surveillance <3 cm; Surgical excision ≥3 cm, preference for nephron-sparing approaches	mTOR pathway
PTEN hamartoma tumor syndrome (Cowden syndrome)	PTEN (10q23)	Papillary RCC or other histology; Breast tumors (malignant and benign); Epithelial thyroid carcinoma	Active surveillance <3 cm; Surgical excision ≥3 cm, preference for nephron-sparing approaches	
Tuberous sclerosis complex (TSC)	TSC1 (9q34) or TSC2 (16p13.3)	Multiple renal angiomyolipomas; Clear cell RCC (2%–3% incidence); Renal cysts/polycystic kidney disease; Cardiac rhabdomyomas; Cutaneous angiofibromas; Pulmonary lymphangiomyomatosis; Neuropsychiatric disorders, including autism spectrum disorder and cognitive disability	AML: surveillance for <3 cm, everolimus for 3–5 cm, consideration for embolization or excision for ≥5 cm, preference for nephron-sparing approaches; RCC: surgical excision >3 cm, preference for nephron-sparing approaches	mTOR pathway
BAP1 tumor predisposition syndrome	BAP1 (3p21.2)	Clear cell RCC, can be high grade	Surgical excision, preference for nephron-sparing approaches	To be determined
MiTF-associated cancer syndrome	MiTF (3p14.1–p12.3)	Not defined	To be determined	To be determined

AML, Angiomyolipoma; CNS, central nervous system; MiTF, microphthalmia-associated transcription factor; PN, partial nephrectomy; PTEN, pentaerythritol tetranitrate; RCC, renal cell carcinoma.
Modified from Schmidt LS, Linehan WM. Genetic predisposition to kidney cancer. Semin Oncol 2016;43:566-574.

Table 28.5 Manifestations of von Hippel-Lindau Disease

TUMOR	AGE OF ONSET, MEAN (RANGE), YEARS	INCIDENCE (%)
Central Nervous System		
Retinal hemangioblastoma	25 (1–68)	25–60
Endolymphatic sac tumor	22 (12–50)	10–15
Craniospinal hemangioblastoma (overall)	30 (9–70)	60–80
Cerebellum	33 (9–78)	44–72
Brainstem	32 (12–46)	10–25
Spinal cord	33 (11–66)	13–50
Visceral		
Renal cell carcinoma	39 (13–70)	25–75
Renal cysts	39 (13–70)	20–60
Pheochromocytoma	27 (5–58)	10–25
Pancreatic neuroendocrine tumors (benign and malignant)	36 (5–70)	11–17
Pancreatic cysts	36 (5–70)	45–75
Epididymal cystadenoma	Unknown	25–60
Broad ligament cystadenoma	Unknown (16–46)	Unknown

Modified from Nielsen SM, Rhodes L, Blanco I, et al. von Hippel-Lindau disease: genetics and role of genetic counseling in a multiple neoplasia syndrome. *J Clin Oncol* 2016;34(18):2172-2181.

Nuclear features can be highly variable and are an independent prognostic factor for RCC generally and for clear cell and papillary RCC in particular.

A new four-tiered grading system developed by the World Health Organization and International Society of Urological Pathology has been validated for clear cell and papillary RCC (Table 28.7).

One unique feature of RCC is its predilection for involvement of the venous system (10% of cases).

Most sporadic RCCs are solitary. Bilateral involvement (2%–4%) can be synchronous or asynchronous and is more common in patients with familial forms of RCC, such as von Hippel-Lindau disease.

Multicentricity (10%–20%) is more common in association with papillary and familial RCC.

Table 28.6 Pathologic Subtypes of Renal Cell Carcinoma

HISTOLOGY[a]	FAMILIAL FORM AND GENETIC FACTORS	GROSS CHARACTERISTICS	MICROSCOPIC PATHOLOGIC CHARACTERISTICS	OTHER CHARACTERISTICS
Common Subtypes				
Clear cell RCC (70%–80%)	von Hippel-Lindau (VHL) disease	Typically well-circumscribed, lobulated, golden yellow tumor but can be infiltrative	Hypervascular tumor	Originates from proximal tubule
	VHL gene (3p25) mutation or hypermethylation		Nests or sheets of clear cells with delicate vascular network	Aggressive behavior more common
	Chromosome 3p deletions	Necrosis, hemorrhage, and cystic degeneration common	IHC[b]: LMWCKs[c], vimentin, EMA, CA IX	Often responds to targeted molecular therapy and immunotherapy
	Loss of chromosome 8p, 9p, 14q; gain of chromosome 5q	Venous involvement also common		
Papillary RCC Type 1 (5%–10%)	HPRC	Fleshy tumor with fibrous pseudocapsule	Hypovascular tumor	Originates from proximal tubule
	Altered MET proto-oncogene status present in 81% of sporadic cases	Necrosis and hemorrhage are common	Papillary structures with single layer of cells around fibrovascular cores	Good prognosis
	Trisomy of chromosome 7 and 17		Basophilic cells with low-grade nuclei	Often multicentric
			IHC[b]: LMWCKs[c], CK7 (type 1 > type 2), AMACR	Common in ARCD

Table 28.6 Pathologic Subtypes of Renal Cell Carcinoma—cont'd

HISTOLOGY[a]	FAMILIAL FORM AND GENETIC FACTORS	GROSS CHARACTERISTICS	MICROSCOPIC PATHOLOGIC CHARACTERISTICS	OTHER CHARACTERISTICS
Common Subtypes				
Papillary RCC type 2 (5%–10%)	HLRCC Fumarate hydratase (FH) gene (1q42-43) mutation in HLRCC	Fleshy tumor with fibrous pseudocapsule Necrosis and hemorrhage are common	Hypovascular tumor Papillary structures with single layer of cells around fibrovascular cores Eosinophilic cells with high-grade nuclei IHC[b]: LMWCKs[c], AMACR	Originates from proximal tubule Worse prognosis then type 1 papillary RCC; similar or worse prognosis when compared with clear cell RCC
Chromophobe RCC (3%–5%)	Birt-Hogg-Dube (BHD) syndrome Folliculin (FLCN) gene mutation (17pn) Loss of multiple chromosomes (1, 2, 6, 10, 13, 17, 21, Y) TP53 and PTEN mutations	Well-circumscribed, homogeneous Tan or light brown cut surface	"Plant cells" with pale cytoplasm, perinuclear clearing or "halo," nuclear "raisins," and prominent cell borders (classic subtype) Positive Hale's colloidal iron staining IHC[b]: diffuse CK7 Eosinophilic subtype has dense pink cytoplasm and mitochondrial gene mutations	Originates from intercalated cells of collecting duct Generally good prognosis, although sarcomatoid variant associated with poor prognosis

Clear cell papillary RCC (~5%)	VHL disease	Well-circumscribed, well-developed capsule	Low-grade clear epithelial cells organized in linear papillae and tubules; IHC[b]: diffuse CK7; cuplike CA-IX distribution	Arise in ESRD and VHL; Good prognosis, indolent tumor behavior
Unclassified RCC (1%-3%)	Unknown	Varied	Varied	Origin not defined; Generally poor prognosis
Rare Subtypes (Each Represents <1%)				
Carcinoma of the collecting ducts of Bellini (collecting duct carcinoma)	Unknown; Multiple chromosomal losses	Firm, centrally located tumor with infiltrative borders; Light gray to tan white	Complex, highly infiltrative cords within inflamed (desmoplastic) stroma; High grade nuclei, mitoses	Originates from collecting duct; Poor prognosis; May respond to cytotoxic chemotherapy
Renal medullary carcinoma	Associated with sickle cell trait	Infiltrative, gray-white; Extensive hemorrhage and necrosis	Poorly differentiated cells with lacelike appearance; Inflammatory infiltrate; Hypovascular tumor	Originates from collecting duct; Dismal prognosis; Tendency to metastasize early with extremely poor prognosis
Hereditary leiomyomatosis and renal cell carcinoma (HLRCC)-associated RCC	HLRCC; Fumarate hydratase (FH) gene (1q42-43) mutation	Fleshy tumor with fibrous pseudocapsule; Necrosis and hemorrhage are common	Papillary structures with single layer of cells around fibrovascular cores; Eosinophilic cells with high grade nuclei; IHC[b]: LMWCKs[c], AMACR	Low grade variant recently described in children

Table 28.6 Pathologic Subtypes of Renal Cell Carcinoma—cont'd

HISTOLOGY[a]	FAMILIAL FORM AND GENETIC FACTORS	GROSS CHARACTERISTICS	MICROSCOPIC PATHOLOGIC CHARACTERISTICS	OTHER CHARACTERISTICS
Rare Subtypes (Each Represents <1%)				
Succinate dehydrogenase-deficient renal carcinoma	*SDH-RCC* SDHA, SDHB (1p36:13), SDHC (1q23.3), SDHD (1q23.1), SHDAF2	Solitary lesion	Vacuolated eosinophilic or clear cells Shares features with chromophobe RCC, oncocytoma, clear cell RCC, type 2 papillary RCC IHC[b]: loss of SDHB	Presents in young adults, most often in those with a germline mutation in an SDH gene HIF-VEGF pathway; reductive carboxylation pathway High- and low-grade variants have been described
MiT family translocation RCC (includes Xp11 translocation RCC and t(6;11) RCC)	Various mutations involving chromosome Xp11.2 resulting in TFE3 gene fusion	Well-circumscribed, tan-yellow tumor	Variable; often clear cells with papillary architecture IHC[b]: nuclear TFE3	Occurs in children and young adults; accounts for 40% of pediatric RCC t(X;17) presents with advanced stage and often follows indolent course t(X;1) can recur with late lymph node metastases

Acquired cystic disease-associated RCC	VHL gene alterations Chromosome 3p deletion	Cystic degeneration	Cribriform, microcystic or sieve-like architecture. Cysts lined with single layer of clear cells. IHC[b]: absent CK7	Occurs in patients with ESRD and acquired cystic kidney disease. Excellent prognosis
Multilocular cystic clear cell renal neoplasm of low malignant potential	Identical to clear cell RCC	Well-circumscribed mass of small and large cysts	Cysts lined by single layer of low grade clear cells. No expansive nodules of tumor cells	Almost uniformly benign clinical behavior
Tubulocystic RCC	Unknown	Multiple small to medium renal cysts with spongy appearance	Enlarged nucleoli (grade 3). Eosinophilic and oncocytoma like cytoplasm	Favorable prognosis
Mucinous tubular and spindle cell carcinoma	Unknown	Well-circumscribed, tan-white-pink tumors centered in medulla	Mixture of tubules and spindle-shaped epithelial cells; mucin background	Favorable prognosis
Hybrid oncocytic chromophobe tumor	Birt-Hogg-Dube (BHD) syndrome Folliculin (FLCN) gene mutation (17p11)	Well-circumscribed, homogeneous appearance tan or light brown cut surface	Shares features with chromophobe RCC and oncocytoma; often coexists with these tumors in BHD patients	Generally good prognosis

[a]Sarcomatoid variants of all of these subtypes have been described and are associated with compromised prognosis.

[b]Immunohistochemistry (IHC) using these markers can help to differentiate between renal cell carcinoma (RCC) subtypes.

[c]Cytokeratin (CK): low-molecular-weight cytokeratins (LMWCKs).

AMACR, Alpha-methylacyl-coenzyme A racemase; *CA-IX,* carbonic anhydrase IX; *CK7,* cytokeratin 7; *EMA,* epithelial membrane antigen; *ESRD,* end-stage renal disease; *HI RCC,* hereditary leiomyomatosis and RCC; *HPRC,* hereditary papillary RCC; *IHC,* immunohistochemistry; *VHL,* von Hippel-Lindau.

Modified from Eble JN, Sauter G, Epstein JI, et al. *WHO classification of tumours: pathology and genetics of tumours of the urinary system and male genital organs.* Lyon, France: IARC Press, 2004; Srigley JR, Delahunt B, Eble J N, et al. The International Society of Urological Pathology (ISUP) Vancouver classification of renal neoplasia. *Am J Surg Pathol* 2014;37(10):1469-1489; Moch H, Cubilla AL, Humphrey PA, et al. The 2016 WHO classification of tumours of the urinary system and male genital organs—part A: renal, penile, and testicular tumours. *Eur Urol* 2016;70(1):93-105.

Table 28.7 World Health Organization/International Society of Urological Pathology Grading System for Clear Cell and Papillary Renal Cell Carcinoma

GRADE	DESCRIPTION
1	Nucleoli are absent or inconspicuous and basophilic at 400× magnification
2	Nucleoli are conspicuous and eosinophilic at 400× magnification and visible but not prominent at 100× magnification
3	Nucleoli are conspicuous and eosinophilic at 100× magnification
4	There is extreme nuclear pleomorphism, multinucleated giant cells, and/or rhabdoid and/or sarcomatoid differentiation

Modified from Delahunt B, Srigley JR, Egevad L, et al. International Society of Urological Pathology grading and other prognostic factors for renal neoplasia. *Eur Urol* 2014;66(5):795-798.

Histologic Subtypes. Clear cell renal cell carcinoma accounts for 70%–80% of all RCCs. Origin is the proximal tubule, and hypervascularity and necrosis are frequently present. Typically, these are more aggressive than the other common subtypes of RCC but also more likely to respond to immunotherapy and other targeted molecular therapies. Papillary renal cell carcinoma is the second most common histologic subtype (10%–15%). There is a tendency toward multicentricity (40%).

Papillary RCC (10%–15% of RCC) is divided into type 1, an indolent form associated with MET mutations and frequently multifocal, and type 2, which is associated with poorer prognosis.

Chromophobe renal cell carcinoma represents 3%–5% of all RCCs and is typically an indolent type of RCC that shares some histopathologic features with benign oncocytomas.

Collecting duct carcinoma is a relatively rare subtype of RCC, with a predictably poor prognosis. Most reported cases of collecting duct carcinoma have been high grade, advanced stage, and unresponsive to conventional therapies.

Renal medullary carcinoma represents an uncommon subtype of RCC that occurs almost exclusively in patients with sickle cell trait. It is typically diagnosed in young African Americans, often in the third decade of life, and many cases are locally advanced and metastatic at the time of diagnosis.

Sarcomatoid and rhabdoid differentiation is no longer recognized as a distinct histologic subtype of RCC and is found in 1%–5% of RCCs, most commonly in association with clear cell RCC or chromophobe RCC.

Unclassified renal cell carcinoma represent a minority of cases (1%–5%) of presumed RCC with features that remain indeterminate even after careful analysis. Many are poorly differentiated and are associated with a highly aggressive biologic behavior and a particularly poor prognosis.

Clinical Presentation. Because of the sequestered location of the kidney within the retroperitoneum, many renal masses remain asymptomatic and nonpalpable until they are locally advanced. With the more pervasive use of noninvasive imaging for the evaluation of a variety of nonspecific symptom complexes, more than 60% of RCCs are now detected incidentally.

Symptoms associated with RCC can be due to local tumor growth, hemorrhage, paraneoplastic syndromes, or metastatic disease (Table 28.8).

The classic triad of flank pain, gross hematuria, and palpable abdominal mass is now rarely seen.

Table 28.8 Clinical Presentation of Renal Cell Carcinoma

Incidental presentation
Symptoms of localized or locally advanced disease
    Hematuria
    Flank pain
    Abdominal mass
    Perinephric hematoma
Obstruction of the inferior vena cava
    Bilateral lower extremity edema
    Nonreducing or right-sided varicocele
Symptoms of systemic disease
    Persistent cough
    Bone pain
    Cervical lymphadenopathy
    Constitutional symptoms
    Weight loss, fever, or malaise
    Paraneoplastic syndromes

A less common but important presentation of RCC is that of spontaneous perirenal hemorrhage, in which the underlying mass may be obscured. More than 50% of patients with perirenal hematoma of unclear cause have an occult renal tumor, most often AML or RCC.

Paraneoplastic syndromes are found in 10%–20% of patients with RCC.

Hypercalcemia has been reported in up to 13% of patients and can be due to either paraneoplastic phenomena or osteolytic metastatic involvement of the bone.

Hypertension and polycythemia are other important paraneoplastic syndromes commonly found in patients with RCC.

Nonmetastatic hepatic dysfunction, or Stauffer syndrome has been reported in 3%–20% of cases.

In general, treatment of paraneoplastic syndromes associated with RCC has required surgical excision or systemic antineoplastic therapy to reduce the burden of disease, and except for hypercalcemia, medical therapies alone have not proved helpful.

Screening is focused on patients with end-stage renal disease and acquired renal cystic disease, tuberous sclerosis, and familial RCC (Table 28.9). Overall, the relative risk of RCC in patients with end-stage renal disease has been estimated to be 5- to 20-fold higher than the general population.

Staging. The recommended staging system for RCC is the eighth edition of the American Joint Committee on Cancer tumor-lymph node-metastasis (AJCC TNM) classification, which was released in 2016 (Tables 28.10 and 28.11).

The clinical staging of renal malignant disease begins with a thorough history, physical examination, and judicious use of laboratory tests.

The radiographic staging of RCC can be accomplished in most cases with a high-quality abdominal CT scan and a routine chest radiograph. Tumor (T) stage is based on size and extension of the cancer into renal or extrarenal structures.

Patients with an enlarged or indistinct adrenal gland on CT, extensive malignant replacement of the kidney, or a palpably abnormal adrenal gland are at risk for malignant adrenal involvement and should be managed accordingly.

Table 28.9 Screening for Renal Cell Carcinoma: Target Populations

Patients with End-Stage Renal Disease

Screen only patients with long life expectancy and minimal major comorbidities

Periodic ultrasound examination or CT scan beginning during third year on dialysis

Patients with Known von Hippel-Lindau Disease

Obtain biannual abdominal CT or ultrasound beginning at the age of 15–20 years

Periodic clinical and radiographic screening for nonrenal manifestations

Relatives of Patients with von Hippel-Lindau Disease

Obtain genetic analysis
  If positive, follow screening recommendations for patients with known von Hippel-Lindau disease
  If negative, less stringent follow-up is required

Relatives of Patients with Other Familial Forms of Renal Cell Carcinoma

Obtain periodic ultrasound or CT and consider genetic analysis

Patients with Tuberous Sclerosis

Periodic screening with ultrasound examination or CT scan

Patients with Autosomal Dominant Polycystic Kidney Disease

Routine screening not justified

General Population

Routine screening not justified

CT, Computed tomography.

Contiguous extension of tumor into the ipsilateral adrenal gland is classified as T4 and noncontiguous involvement of either adrenal as M1, reflecting likely patterns of dissemination.

Enlarged hilar or retroperitoneal lymph nodes (≥ 2 cm in diameter) on CT almost always harbor malignant change, but this should be confirmed by surgical exploration or percutaneous biopsy if the patient is not a surgical candidate. Many smaller lymph nodes prove to be inflammatory rather than neoplastic and should not preclude surgical therapy.

Table 28.10 International Tumor, Node, Metastasis (TNM) Staging System for Renal Cell Carcinoma

T: Primary Tumor			
TX	Primary tumor cannot be assessed		
T0	No evidence of primary tumor		
T1a	Tumor ≤4.0 cm and confined to the kidney		
T1b	Tumor >4.0 cm and ≤7.0 cm and confined to the kidney		
T2a	Tumor >7.0 cm and ≤10.0 cm and confined to the kidney		
T2b	Tumor >10.0 cm and confined to the kidney		
T3a	Tumor extends into the renal vein or its segmental branches, invades the pelvicalyceal system, or invades perirenal and/or renal sinus fat but not beyond Gerota fascia		
T3b	Tumor grossly extends into the vena cava below the diaphragm		
T3c	Tumor grossly extends into the vena cava above the diaphragm or invades the wall of the vena cava		
T4	Tumor invades beyond Gerota fascia (including contiguous extension into the ipsilateral adrenal gland)		

N: Regional Lymph Nodes			
NX	Regional lymph nodes cannot be assessed		
N0	No regional lymph nodes metastasis		
N1	Metastasis in regional lymph node(s)		

M: Distant Metastases			
MX	Distant metastasis cannot be assessed		
M0	No distant metastasis		
M1	Distant metastasis present		

Stage Grouping			
Stage I	T1	N0	M0
Stage II	T2	N0	M0
Stage III	T1 or T2	N1	M0
	T3	Any N	M0
Stage IV	T4	Any N	M0
	Any T	Any N	M1

Modified from Edge SB, Byrd DR, Compton CC. *AJCC cancer staging manual*, 8th ed. New York: Springer-Verlag, 2016.

Table 28.11 Tumor, Node, Metastasis (TNM) Stage and 5-Year Cancer-Specific Survival for Renal Cell Carcinoma

FINDINGS	ROBSON STAGE	TNM (6th ed. 2002)	TNM (7th ed. 2009)	TNM (8th ed. 2016)	5-YEAR SURVIVAL RATE (%)
Organ-confined (overall)		T1-2N0M0	T1-2N0M0	T1-2N0M0	70–90
≤4.0 cm	I	T1aN0M0	T1aN0M0	T1aN0M0	90–100
>4.0 cm to 7.0 cm	I	T1bN0M0	T1bN0M0	T1bN0M0	80–90
>7.0 to 10.0 cm	I	T2N0M0	T2aN0M0	T2aN0M0	65–80
>10.0 cm	I	T2N0M0	T2bN0M0	T2bN0M0	50–70
Invasion of pelvicalyceal system	I	T1-2N0M0	T1-2N0M0	T3aN0M0	50–70
Invasion of perinephric or renal sinus fat	II	T3aN0M0	T3aN0M0	T3aN0M0	50–70
Extension into renal vein or branches	IIIA	T3bN0M0	T3aN0M0	T3aN0M0	40–60
Extension into IVC below diaphragm	IIIA	T3cN0M0	T3bN0M0	T3bN0M0	30–50
Extension into IVC above diaphragm or invasion of IVC wall	IIIA	T3cN0M0	T3cN0M0	T3cN0M0	20–40
Direct adrenal involvement	II	T3aN0M0	T4N0M0	T4N0M0	0–30
Locally advanced (invasion beyond Gerota fascia)	IVA	T4N0M0	T4N0M0	T4N0M0	0–20
Lymph node involvement	IIIB	T(Any)N1-2M0	T(Any)N1M0	T(Any)N1M0	0–20
Systemic metastasis	IVB	T(Any)N1-2M1	T(Any)N1M1	T(Any)N1M1	0–10

IVC, Inferior vena cava.

Data from Amin MB, Edge SB, Greene FL, et al. *AJCC cancer staging manual*, 8th ed. New York: Springer; 2017; Bailey GC, Boorjian SA, Ziegelmann MJ, et al. Urinary collecting system invasion is associated with poor survival in patients with clear-cell renal cell carcinoma. *BJU Int* 2017;119(4):585-590; Campbell SC, Novick AC, Belldegrun A, et al. Guideline for management of the clinical T1 renal mass. *J Urol* 2009;182(4):1271-1279; Haddad H, Rini BI. Current treatment considerations in metastatic renal cell carcinoma. *Curr Treat Options Oncol* 2012;13(2):212-229; Hafez KS, Fergany AF, Novick AC. Nephron sparing surgery for localized renal cell carcinoma: impact of tumor size on patient survival, tumor recurrence and TNM staging. *J Urol* 1999;162(6):1930-1933; Kim SP, Alt AL, Weight CJ, et al. Independent validation of the 2010 American Joint Committee on Cancer TNM classification for renal cell carcinoma: Results from a large, single institution cohort. *J Urol* 2011;185(6):2035-2039; Lane BR, Kattan MW. Prognostic models and algorithms in renal cell carcinoma. *Urol Clin North Am* 2008;35(4):613-625; Leibovich BC, Cheville JC, Lohse CM, et al. Cancer specific survival for patients with pT3 renal cell carcinoma–can the 2002 primary tumor classification be improved? *J Urol* 2005;173(3):716-719; Martinez-Salamanca JI, Huang WC, Millan I, et al. Prognostic impact of the 2009 UICC/AJCC TNM staging system for renal cell carcinoma with venous extension. *Eur Urol* 2011;59(1):120-127; Thompson RH, Cheville JC, Lohse CM, et al. Reclassification of patients with pT3 and pT4 renal cell carcinoma improves prognostic accuracy. *Cancer* 2005;104(1):53-60.

MRI is still the premier study for evaluation of invasion of tumor into adjacent structures and for surgical planning in these challenging cases.

The sensitivities of CT for detection of renal venous tumor thrombus and inferior vena cava (IVC) involvement are 78% and 96%, respectively.

MRI is well established as the premier study for the evaluation and staging of inferior vena cava (IVC) tumor thrombus, although several studies suggest that multiplanar CT is likely equivalent in many patients.

Metastatic evaluation in all cases should include a routine chest radiograph, systematic review of the abdominal and pelvic CT or MRI, and liver function tests. Pathologic stage is the most important prognostic factor for RCC. Invasion of neighboring organs (T4), involvement of retroperitoneal lymph nodes (N1), and the presence of metastatic disease (M1) confer a poor outcome for patients with RCC. Other important pathologic features include nuclear grade, tumor size, and histologic subtype. Important prognostic factors for cancer-specific survival in patients with RCC include specific clinical signs or symptoms, tumor-related factors, and various laboratory findings. Integrated systems, such as nomograms, often outperform other prediction methods.

Prognosis. Important prognostic factors for cancer-specific survival in patients with nonmetastatic RCC include specific clinical signs or symptoms, tumor-related factors, and various laboratory findings (Table 28.12).

Overall, tumor-related factors such as pathologic stage (most important), tumor size, nuclear grade, and histologic subtype have the greatest individual predictive ability. However, an integrative approach, combining a variety of factors that have independent value on multivariate analysis, appears to be most powerful. Clinical findings that suggest a compromised prognosis in patients with presumed localized RCC include symptomatic presentation, unintended weight loss of >10% of body weight, and poor performance status.

Venous involvement was once thought to be a very poor prognostic finding for RCC, but several reports demonstrate that many patients with tumor thrombi can be salvaged with an aggressive surgical approach. These studies document 45%–69% 5-year survival rates for patients with venous tumor thrombi as long as the cancer is otherwise confined to the kidney.

Table 28.12 Adverse Prognostic Factors for Renal Cell Carcinoma

CLINICAL	ANATOMIC	HISTOLOGIC
Poor performance status	Larger tumor size	High nuclear grade
Systemic symptoms	Venous involvement	Certain histologic subtypes
Anemia	Extension into contiguous organs, including adrenal gland	Sarcomatoid features
Hypercalcemia		Presence of histologic tumor necrosis
Elevated lactate dehydrogenase		Vascular invasion
Elevated erythrocyte sedimentation rate	Lymph node metastases	Invasion of perinephric or renal sinus fat
Elevated C-reactive protein	Distant metastases and greater metastatic burden	Collecting system invasion
Thrombocytosis		Positive surgical margin
Elevated alkaline phosphatase		

Data from Lane BR, Kattan MW. Prognostic models and algorithms in renal cell carcinoma. *Urol Clin North Am* 2008;35(4):613-625; Sun M, Vetterlein M, Harshman LC, et al. Risk assessment in small renal masses: a review article. *Urol Clin North Am* 2017;44(2) 189-202.

Direct invasion of the wall of the vein appears to be a more important prognostic factor than level of tumor thrombus and is now classified as pT3c independent of the level of tumor thrombus.

The major drop in prognosis comes in patients whose tumor extends beyond Gerota's fascia involving contiguous organs (stage T4) and in patients with lymph node or systemic metastases.

Lymph node involvement is associated with 5- and 10-year survival rates of 5%–30% and 0%–5%, respectively.

Systemic metastases have a 1-year survival of <50%, 5-year survival of 5%–30%, and 10-year survival of 0%–5%, although these numbers have improved modestly in the era of VEGF-targeted treatments and checkpoint inhibitors.

For patients with asynchronous metastases the metastasis-free interval can be a useful prognosticator because it often reflects the tempo of disease progression.

Other important prognostic factors for patients with systemic metastases include performance status, number and sites of metastases, anemia, hypercalcemia, elevated alkaline phosphatase or lactate dehydrogenase levels, thrombocytosis, and sarcomatoid histology.

TREATMENT OF LOCALIZED RENAL CELL CARCINOMA

We now recognize great heterogeneity in the tumor biology of these lesions, and multiple management strategies are available, including radical nephrectomy (RN), partial nephrectomy (PN), thermal ablation (TA), and AS.

American Urological Association Guidelines for Renal Mass and Localized Renal Cancer

The 2017 AUA Guidelines for Renal Mass and Localized Renal Cancer (Fig. 28.2) provide an evidence-based review of this topic, along with comprehensive recommendations for evaluation, counseling, and management.

An increased focus on functional issues, preoperatively and postoperatively, recognizing their importance for cancer survivorship for many patients with localized RCC.

Risk Stratification and Renal Mass Biopsy

Overall, about 20% of solid, enhancing, clinical T1 renal masses are benign, most often oncocytomas or atypical AMLs, although

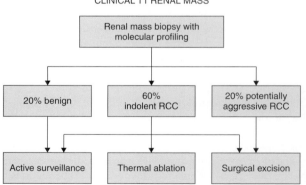

FIG. 28.2 The American Urological Association guideline panel for the management of renal mass and localized renal cancer strongly advocates research priority for renal mass biopsy with molecular profiling to facilitate more rational management. The distribution of benign, indolent, and potentially aggressive RCC can vary based on tumor size, gender, and other patient and tumor characteristics. *RCC,* Renal cell carcinoma.

the incidence of benign pathology can vary greatly in different populations.

An even more important determinant of benign pathology is tumor size.

Tumor size also correlates strongly with biologic aggressiveness for clinical T1 renal masses, as reflected by high tumor grade, locally invasive phenotype, or unfavorable histology.

Current algorithms incorporating clinical and radiographic factors to predict tumor aggressiveness for small renal tumors are very limited in their accuracy.

Renal mass biopsy (RMB) can substantially improve on this and should be considered for further risk stratification when it may influence management (Fig. 28.2). RMB is not indicated for young, healthy patients who are unwilling to accept the limitations of RMB or for older, frail patients who will be managed conservatively even if RMB suggests a potentially aggressive tumor. RMB is safe with relatively low rates of hematoma (4.9%), clinically significant pain (1.2%), gross hematuria (1.0%), pneumothorax (0.6%), and hemorrhage requiring transfusion (0.4%). There have been no reported cases of RCC tumor seeding in the contemporary literature. A positive biopsy is reliable with high specificity (96%) and positive predictive value (99.8%). The nondiagnostic rate for RMB is approximately 14%, which can be substantially reduced with repeat biopsy. Histologic evaluation of RCC subtype is dependable (>90%), but accuracy for grade is variable (60%–80%). A nonmalignant biopsy result may not truly indicate that a benign entity is present.

Renal Function After Partial or Radical Nephrectomy: Survival Implications

Surgery remains the mainstay for curative treatment of this disease.

RN has fallen out of favor for small renal tumors because of concerns about cystic kidney disease (CKD) and should only be performed when necessary in this population.

The main downside of RN is that it predisposes to CKD, which can be associated with morbid cardiovascular events and increased mortality rates.

Several studies illustrate the potential negative implications of CKD, including a population-based analysis that reported increased rates of cardiovascular events and death as the degree of CKD worsened. These data highlight the potential need to optimize renal function and underscore nephron sparing as an important principle in the management of clinical T1 renal masses, particularly small renal masses. Subsequent studies have suggested that there may be a difference between CKD resulting from medical causes (CKD-M) and CKD primarily related to surgical removal of nephrons (CKD-S). PN is preferred for small renal masses (stage T1a, <4.0 cm) whenever feasible. RN represents gross overtreatment for most such lesions, which often have limited biologic potential.

PN is also strongly preferred whenever preservation of renal function is potentially important, such as patients with preexisting CKD or proteinuria, an abnormal contralateral kidney, or multifocal or familial RCC.

Larger tumors (clinical stages T1b/T2) have increased oncologic potential and have often already replaced a substantial portion of the parenchyma, leaving less to be saved by PN. In this setting, if a normal contralateral kidney is present, the relative merits of PN versus RN can be debated.

The AUA guidelines provide well-defined oncologic and functional criteria for consideration for RN (Fig. 28.3). If these criteria are not satisfied, PN should be considered, if feasible.

Well-designed randomized, prospective trials are required to provide higher quality data and allow for more rational management of patients with localized renal tumors.

Radical Nephrectomy

Prototypical RN encompasses the basic principles of early ligation of the renal artery and vein, removal of the kidney with primary dissection external to Gerota fascia, excision of the ipsilateral adrenal gland, and performance of an extended lymph node dissection (LND).

Performance of a perifascial nephrectomy is of undoubted importance during RN for preventing postoperative local tumor recurrence because approximately 25% of clinical T1b/T2 RCCs manifest perinephric fat involvement.

Preliminary renal arterial ligation remains an accepted practice; however, in large tumors with abundant collateral vascular supply, it is not always possible to obtain complete preliminary control of the arterial circulation.

Renal mass and localized renal cancer[a]

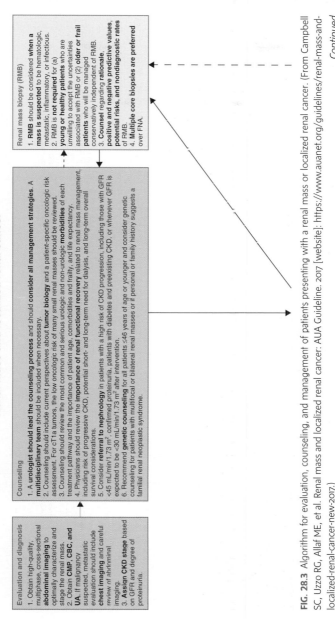

Evaluation and diagnosis

1. Obtain high-quality, multiphase, cross-sectional **abdominal imaging** to optimally characterize and stage the renal mass.
2. Obtain **CMP, CBC, and UA.** If malignancy suspected, metastatic evaluation should include **chest imaging** and careful review of abdominal imaging.
3. **Assign CKD stage** based on GFR and degree of proteinuria.

Counseling

1. A **urologist should lead the counseling process** and should **consider all management strategies.** A **multidisciplinary team** should be included when necessary.
2. Counseling should include current perspectives about **tumor biology** and a patient-specific oncologic risk assessment. For cT1a tumors, the low oncologic risk of many small renal masses should be reviewed.
3. Counseling should review the most common and serious urologic and non-urologic **morbidities** of each treatment pathway and the importance of patient age, comorbidities and frailty, and life expectancy.
4. Physicians should review the **importance of renal functional recovery** related to renal mass management, including risk of progressive CKD, potential short- and long-term need for dialysis, and long-term overall survival considerations.
5. Consider **referral to nephrology** in patients with a high risk of CKD progression, including those with GFR <45 mL/min/1.73 m² confirmed proteinuria, patients with diabetes and preexisting CKD, or whenever GFR is expected to be <30 mL/min/1.73 m² after intervention.
6. Recommend **genetic counseling** for all patients ≤46 years of age or younger and consider genetic counseling for patients with multifocal or bilateral renal masses or if personal or family history suggests a familial renal neoplastic syndrome.

Renal mass biopsy (RMB)

1. **RMB** should be considered **when a mass is suspected** to be hematologic, metastatic, inflammatory, or infectious.
2. RMB **is not required** for (a) **young or healthy patients** who are unwilling to accept the uncertainties associated with RMB or (2) **older or frail patients** who will be managed conservatively independent of RMB.
3. **Counsel** regarding rationale, **positive and negative predictive values, potential risks, and nondiagnostic rates** of RMB.
4. **Multiple core biopsies are preferred** over FNA.

FIG. 28.3 Algorithm for evaluation, counseling, and management of patients presenting with a renal mass or localized renal cancer. (From Campbell SC, Uzzo RG, Allaf ME, et al. Renal mass and localized renal cancer: AUA Guideline. 2017 [website]: https://www.auanet.org/guidelines/renal-mass-and-localized-renal-cancer-new-2017.)

Continued

Management

Partial nephrectomy (PN) and nephron-sparing approaches

1. **Prioritize PN for the management of the cT1a renal mass when intervention is indicated.**
2. Prioritize nephron-sparing approaches for patients with an anatomic or functionally solitary kidney, bilateral tumors, known familial RCC, preexisting CKD, or proteinuria.
3. Consider nephron-sparing approaches for patients who are young, have multifocal masses, or have comorbidities that are likely to impact renal function in the future.

Radical nephrectomy (RN)

Physicians should consider **RN** for patients **in whom increased oncologic potential is suggested** by tumor size, RMB, and/or imaging characteristics. In this setting, RN is preferred if all of the following criteria are met:
1. High tumor complexity and PN would be challenging even in experienced hands
2. No preexisting CKD or proteinuria
3. Normal contralateral kidney and new baseline eGFR will likely be >45 mL/min/1.73 m².

Thermal ablation (TA)

1. **Consider TA an alternate approach for management of cT1a renal masses <3 cm in size.** A percutaneous approach is preferred.
2. Both radiofrequency ablation and cryoablation are options.
3. A RMB should be performed prior to TA.
4. **Counseling about TA** should include information regarding increased likelihood of tumor persistence or recurrence after primary TA, which may be addressed with repeat TA if further intervention is elected.

Active surveillance (AS)

1. For patients with renal masses suspicious for cancer, especially those <2 cm, AS is an option for initial management.
2. **Prioritize AS and expectant management when the anticipated risk of intervention or competing risks of death outweigh the potential oncologic benefits of active treatment.**
3. When the risk-benefit analysis for treatment is equivocal and the patient prefers AS, physicians should repeat imaging in 3–6 months to assess for interval growth and may consider RMB for additional risk stratification.
4. When the oncologic benefits of intervention outweigh the risks of treatment and competing risks of death, physicians should recommend active treatment. In this setting, AS may be pursued only if the patient understands and is willing to accept the associated oncologic risk

Factors favoring AS or expectant management

Patient related	Tumor related
Older adult	Tumor size <3 cm
Life expectancy <5 years	Tumor growth <5 mm/year
High comorbidities	Noninfiltrative
Excessive perioperative risk	Low complexity
Frailty (poor functional status)	Favorable histology
Patient preference for AS	
Marginal renal function	

Principles related to PN

1. **Prioritize preservation of renal function** through efforts to optimize nephron mass preservation and avoidance of prolonged warm ischemia.
2. **Negative surgical margins should be a priority.** The extent of normal parenchyma removed should be determined by surgeon discretion taking into account the clinical situation; tumor characteristics, including growth pattern; and interface with normal tissue. Enucleation should be considered in patients with familial RCC, multifocal disease, or severe CKD to optimize parenchymal mass preservation.

Surgical principles

1. In the presence of clinically concerning regional lymphadenopathy, **lymph node dissection** should be performed for staging purposes.
2. **Adrenalectomy** should be performed if imaging and/or intraoperative findings suggest metastasis or direct invasion.
3. A **minimally invasive approach** should be considered when it would not compromise oncologic, functional, and perioperative outcomes.
4. **Pathologic evaluation of the adjacent renal parenchyma** should be performed after PN or RN to assess for possible nephrologic disease, particularly for patients with CKD or risk factors for developing CKD.

[a]The focus is on clinically localized renal masses suspicious for renal cell carcinoma (RCC) in adults, including solid enhanced tumors and Bosniak 3 and 4 complex cystic lesions. *CBC,* Complete blood count; *CKD,* chronic kidney disease; *CMP,* complete metabolic profile; *FNA,* fine-needle aspiration; *GFR,* glomerular filtration rate; *UA,* urinalysis.

FIG. 28.3—cont'd

Removal of the ipsilateral adrenal gland is not routinely necessary.

There is strong consensus that LND need not be performed for most patients with localized kidney cancer and clinically negative nodes.

The surgical approach for RN is determined by the size and location of the tumor as well as the body habitus of the patient.

Laparoscopic RN is now established as a less-morbid alternative to open surgery in the management of low- to moderate-volume RCCs with no local invasion, limited or no venous involvement, and manageable lymphadenopathy.

Several studies on outcomes after RN for localized RCC have demonstrated that the risk of postoperative recurrence is stage dependent, and surveillance protocols should reflect this (Tables 28.13 and 28.14).

Table 28.13 Surveillance for Clinically Localized Renal Neoplasms: General Considerations

FOLLOW-UP MEASURE	RECOMMENDATION
Physical examination and history	History and physical examination directed at detecting signs and symptoms of metastatic spread or local progression
Laboratory testing	Basic laboratory testing, including BUN/creatinine, urinalysis, and eGFR, for all patients
	Progressive renal insufficiency or proteinuria should prompt nephrology referral
	CBC, LDH, LFTs, alkaline phosphatase, and serum calcium per discretion of the physician
CNS imaging	Acute neurologic signs should lead to prompt neurologic cross-sectional imaging of the head or spine based on localized symptoms
Bone scan	Elevated alkaline phosphatase, clinical symptoms such as bone pain, and/or radiographic findings suggestive of a bony neoplasm should prompt a bone scan
	Bone scan should not be performed in the absence of these signs and symptoms

BUN, Blood urea nitrogen; *CBC*, complete blood count; *CNS*, central nervous system; *eGFR*, estimated glomerular filtration rate; *LDH*, lactate dehydrogenase; *LFTs*, liver function tests
Modified from Donat SM, Diaz M, Bishoff JT, et al. Follow-up for clinically localized renal neoplasms: AUA guideline. *J Urol* 2013;190:407-416.

Table 28.14 Surveillance After Radical or Partial Nephrectomy[a]

FOLLOW-UP MEASURE	RECOMMENDATION
Low-Risk Patients	
Abdominal imaging	**Partial nephrectomy:** Obtain a baseline abdominal scan (CT or MRI) within 3–12 months after surgery.
	If the initial postoperative scan is negative, abdominal imaging (US, CT, or MRI) may be performed yearly for 3 years based on individual risk factors.
	Radical nephrectomy: Patients should undergo abdominal imaging (US, CT, or MRI) within 3–12 months after surgery.
	If the initial postoperative imaging is negative, abdominal imaging beyond 12 months may be performed at the discretion of the clinician.
Chest imaging	**Partial and radical nephrectomy:** Obtain a yearly CXR for 3 years and only as clinically indicated beyond that time period.
Moderate- to High-Risk Patients (Pt2-4Nomx or Pt[Any]N1mx): Partial or Radical Nephrectomy	
Abdominal imaging	A baseline abdominal scan (CT or MRI) within 3–6 months after surgery with continued imaging (US, CT, or MRI) every 6 months for at least 3 years and annually thereafter to year 5.
	Imaging beyond 5 years may be performed at the discretion of the clinician.
	Perform site-specific imaging as symptoms warrant.
Chest imaging	Obtain a baseline chest scan (CT) within 3–6 months after surgery with continued imaging (CXR or CT) every 6 months for at least 3 years and annually thereafter to year 5.
	Imaging beyond 5 years is optional and should be based on individual patient characteristics and tumor risk factors.

[a]Please also refer to Table 28.13 for general considerations related to surveillance.
CT, Computed tomography; *CXR*, chest x-ray; *MRI*, magnetic resonance imaging; *US*, ultrasound.
Modified from Donat SM, Diaz M, Bishoff JT, et al. Follow-up for clinically localized renal neoplasms: AUA guideline. *J Urol* 2013;190:407-416.

Partial Nephrectomy

Interest in PN for RCC has been stimulated by advances in renal imaging, experience with renal vascular surgery for other conditions, improved methods of preventing ischemic damage, growing numbers of incidentally discovered renal tumors, greater appreciation of the potentially deleterious effects of CKD, and encouraging long-term survival in patients undergoing this form of treatment.

Accepted indications for PN traditionally included situations in which RN would render the patient anephric or at high risk for ultimate need of dialysis.

In patients with bilateral synchronous RCC, the general approach has been to perform bilateral PNs whenever feasible, usually as staged procedures, particularly if the tumors are relatively large.

Margin width appears to be immaterial as long as the final margins are negative; this is particularly relevant when the tumor is located within the hilum and preservation of renal function is at a premium.

Patients with RCC involving a functionally or anatomically solitary kidney must be advised about the potential need for temporary or permanent dialysis. A functioning renal remnant of at least 20%–30% of one kidney is necessary to avoid end-stage renal failure, although this presumes good functional status of the remaining parenchyma.

PN is now standard of care for the management of small renal masses (clinical T1a) in the presence of a normal contralateral kidney, presuming that the mass is amenable to this approach.

The literature demonstrates equivalent oncologic outcomes for PN compared with RN in appropriately selected patients, and the functional outcomes tilt the balance in favor of PN whenever feasible.

Prior experience with "elective" PN for T1a RCC demonstrated local recurrence rates of 1%–2% and overall cancer-free survival well over 90%.

The AUA guidelines now provide evidence-based recommendations for use of PN (Fig. 28.3) relative to RN with emphasis on well-defined selection criteria for RN.

Tumors that demonstrate features suggesting increased oncologic potential (e.g., large tumor size, aggressive histology on RMB, or concerning imaging characteristics, such as infiltrative appearance) should be considered for RN, and RN is generally preferred in this setting only if all of the following criteria are met: (1) high tumor complexity and PN would be challenging even in experienced hands; (2) no preexisting CKD or proteinuria; and (3) normal contralateral kidney and new baseline glomerular filtration rate (GFR) will likely be >45 mL/min/1.73 m².

Evaluation of patients with RCC for PN should include preoperative testing to exclude locally extensive or metastatic disease and additional specific renal imaging to delineate the relationship of the tumor to the intrarenal vascular supply and collecting system.

Urologic complications, such as urine leak or postoperative bleed, are more common after PN than other management strategies.

The quality of the parenchyma is for the most part nonmodifiable, essentially setting the ceiling for functional recovery after any intervention (Fig. 28.4). Most studies that have incorporated the other two factors into multivariable analysis suggest that the number of preserved nephrons is the primary factor determining functional outcomes after PN, while irreversible ischemic injury plays a secondary role.

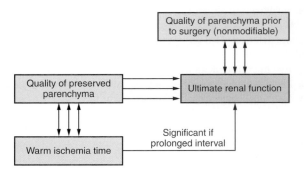

FIG. 28.4 Determinants of renal function after partial nephrectomy. The quality and quantity of preserved parenchyma are the main determinants of renal function after partial nephrectomy, with ischemic injury playing a secondary role as long as limited warm ischemia or hypothermia is used. Prolonged warm ischemia, however, can lead to irreversible loss of nephron function.

Hypothermia should be considered for more complex cases or whenever a prolonged ischemic interval (>25–30 minutes) is anticipated, particularly for patients with a solitary kidney or preexisting CKD.

Surveillance of patients after PN, similar to RN, can be tailored to pathologic tumor stage.

Patients who undergo nephron-sparing surgery for RCC may be left with a remnant kidney and are at risk for development of long-term functional impairment from hyperfiltration

Tumor Enucleation

Tumor enucleation (TE) is well-established for patients with familial kidney cancer, although its role for sporadic RCC remains controversial.

TE entails blunt dissection along the pseudocapsule, thereby reducing the amount of normal parenchyma removed with the tumor.

In summary, review of the TE literature suggests that this approach is reasonable for many patients, but selection criteria are not well defined.

The AUA guidelines emphasize that negative surgical margins should always be a top priority with PN.

Thermal Ablative (TA) Therapies

TA, including renal cryosurgery, microwave and radiofrequency ablation (RFA), are now established as alternate nephron-sparing treatments for patients with localized RCC.

Both can be administered percutaneously and thus offer the potential for reduced morbidity.

Long-term efficacy of TA is still not as well established as surgical excision, and local recurrence rates with primary TA are somewhat higher than those reported for traditional surgical approaches.

Most local recurrences after TA can be salvaged with repeat ablation, and cancer-specific survival rates for clinical T1a tumors are generally high across all management strategies.

Overall survival is primarily determined by age and general health status, not approach to management.

The traditional candidates for TA have been patients with reason-able life expectancy despite advanced age or significant comorbidities, who prefer a proactive approach but are not optimal candidates for conventional surgery. Although TA is still a reasonable choice for such patients, AS is now more commonly used in this setting.

Other candidates for TA include patients with local recurrence after previous nephron-sparing surgery, and those with hereditary renal cancer who present with multifocal lesions for whom multiple PNs may be cumbersome.

The 2017 AUA guidelines advocate for TA as an alternate approach for the management of clinical T1a renal masses smaller than 3.0 cm in diameter.

Clinical experience after primary renal cryoablative therapy suggests successful local control in about 80%–90% of patients (Fig. 28.5), although many studies provide only limited follow-up.

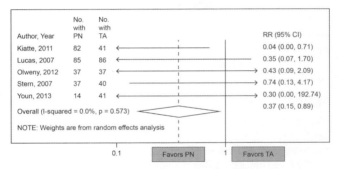

Author, Year	No. with PN	No. with TA		RR (95% CI)
Kiatte, 2011	82	41		0.04 (0.00, 0.71)
Lucas, 2007	85	86		0.35 (0.07, 1.70)
Olweny, 2012	37	37		0.43 (0.09, 2.09)
Stern, 2007	37	40		0.74 (0.13, 4.17)
Youn, 2013	14	41		0.30 (0.00, 192.74)
Overall (I-squared = 0.0%, p = 0.573)				0.37 (0.15, 0.89)
NOTE: Weights are from random effects analysis				

0.1 Favors PN 1 Favors TA

Risk Ratio and 95% Confidence Intervals of Local Recurrence

CI = confidence interval; No = numbers; PN = partial nephrectomy; RR = risk ratio for local recurrence; TA = thermal ablation
Note: The width of the horizontal lines represents the 95 percent confidence intervals for each study. The diamond at the bottom of the graph indicates the 95 percent confidence interval.

FIG. 28.5 Meta-analysis of local recurrence rates after partial nephrectomy (PN) versus primary tumor ablation (TA) incorporating studies with 48 ± 12 months of follow-up. Risk ratios with 95% confidence intervals are shown for each study and for the overall analysis. Most such recurrences can be salvaged with repeat TA and the observed differences in local recurrence rates were no longer present when secondary ablations were taken into account. (Modified from Campbell SC, Uzzo RG, Allaf ME, et al. Renal mass and localized renal cancer: AUA Guideline. https://www.auanet.org/guidelines/renal-mass-and-localized-renal-cancer-new-(2017).)

Active Surveillance

The incidental discovery of many small RCCs in asymptomatic older adult patients or those of poor surgical risk provided the opportunity to observe the growth rate of these tumors in patients who were unable or unwilling to undergo surgery.

Subsequent series from several institutions confirmed that many small renal masses will grow slowly (median growth rate, 0.09–0.34 cm/year) and with a relatively low rate of metastasis (<2.0% during 2–5 years of follow-up).

Studies suggest that patients with small, solid renal lesions, who are older, or who have increased surgical risk can safely be managed with observation and serial renal imaging at 6-month or 1-year intervals.

The AUA guidelines now provide specific recommendations about AS or expectant management and well-defined criteria for monitoring patients on surveillance (Table 28.15).

For small, solid or Bosniak 3–4 complex cystic masses, AS should be considered on option for initial management, and for tumors with reduced malignant potential, such as those smaller than 2.0 cm diameter, this applies to healthy patients, too.

Table 28.15 Active Surveillance: Imaging Recommendations[a]

FOLLOW-UP MEASURE	RECOMMENDATION
Percutaneous biopsy	Percutaneous biopsy may be considered before active surveillance.
Abdominal imaging	Cross-sectional scanning (CT or MRI) within 3–6 months of active surveillance initiation to establish a growth rate, with continued imaging (US, CT, or MRI) at least annually thereafter.
Chest imaging	Patients with biopsy-proven renal cell carcinoma or a tumor with oncocytic features on active surveillance should undergo annual CXR. Continued surveillance should also be considered by oncocytoma.

[a]Please also refer to Table 28.13 for general considerations related to surveillance.
CT, Computed tomography; *CXR*, chest x-ray; *MRI*, magnetic resonance imaging; *US*, ultrasound.
Modified from Donat SM, Diaz M, Bishoff JT, et al. Follow-up for clinically localized renal neoplasms: AUA guideline. *J Urol* 2013;190:407-416.

Shared decision making about AS versus intervention can be complex, and patient- and tumor-related factors that favor conservative management are detailed (Fig. 28.3).

Suggested Readings

Blom JH, van Poppel H, Maréchal JM, et al. Radical nephrectomy with and without lymph-node dissection: final results of European Organization for Research and Treatment of Cancer (EORTC) randomized phase 3 trial 30881. *Eur Urol* 2009;55: 28-34.

Borregales LD, Kim DY, Staller AL, et al. Prognosticators and outcomes of patients with renal cell carcinoma and adjacent organ invasion treated with radical nephrectomy. *Urol Oncol* 2016;34:e219-e226.

Campbell S, Uzzo RG, Allaf ME, et al. Renal mass and localized renal cancer: AUA guideline. *J Urol* 2017;198:520-529.

Cancer Genome Atlas Research Network: Comprehensive molecular characterization of clear cell renal cell carcinoma. *Nature* 2013;499:43-49.

Capitanio U, Montorsi F. Renal cancer. *Lancet* 2016;387:894-906.

Curatolo P, Bombardieri R, Jozwiak S. Tuberous sclerosis. *Lancet* 2008;372:657-668.

Delahunt B, Cheville JC, Martignoni G, et al. International Society of Urological Pathology (ISUP) grading system for renal cell carcinoma and other prognostic parameters. *Am J Surg Pathol* 2013;37:1490-1504.

Donat SM, Diaz M, Bishoff JT, et al. Follow-up for clinically localized renal neoplasms: AUA guideline. *J Urol* 2013;190:407-416.

Eknoyan G. A clinical view of simple and complex renal cysts. *J Am Soc Nephrol* 2009;20:1874-1876.

Flum AS, Hamoui N, Said MA, et al. Update on the diagnosis and management of renal angiomyolipoma. *J Urol* 2016;195:834-846.

Gershman B, Thompson RH, Moreira DM, et al. Radical nephrectomy with or without lymph node dissection for nonmetastatic renal cell carcinoma: a propensity score-based analysis. *Eur Urol* 2017;71:560-567.

Grantham JJ. Clinical practice. Autosomal dominant polycystic kidney disease. *N Engl J Med* 2008;359:1477-1485.

Halpenny D, Snow A, McNeill G, et al. The radiological diagnosis and treatment of renal angiomyolipoma-current status. *Clin Radiol* 2010;65:99-108.

Helenon O, Crosnier A, Verkarre V, et al. Simple and complex renal cysts in adults: classification system for renal cystic masses. *Diagn Interv Imaging* 2018;99:189-218.

Kim SP, Campbell SC, Gill I, et al. Collaborative review of risk benefit trade-offs between partial and radical nephrectomy in the management of anatomically complex renal masses. *Eur Urol* 2017;72:64-75.

Ljungberg B, Bensalah K, Canfield S, et al. EAU guidelines on renal cell carcinoma: 2014 update. *Eur Urol* 2015;67:913-924.

Moch H, Cubilla AL, Humphrey PA, et al. The 2016 WHO classification of tumours of the urinary system and male genital organs—part A: renal, penile, and testicular tumours. *Eur Urol* 2016;70:93-105.

Ristau BT, Correa AF, Uzzo RG, et al. Active surveillance for the small renal mass: growth kinetics and oncologic outcomes. *Urol Clin North Am* 2017;44:213-222.

Scosyrev E, Messing EM, Sylvester R, et al. Renal function after nephron-sparing surgery versus radical nephrectomy: results from EORTC randomized trial 30904. *Eur Urol* 2014;65:372-377.

Silverman SG, Pedrosa I, Ellis JH, et al. Bosniak classification of cystic renal masses, version 2019: an update proposal and needs assessment. *Radiology* 2019;292(2):475-488.

Van Poppel H, Da Pozzo L, Albrecht W, et al. A prospective, randomised EORTC intergroup phase 3 study comparing the oncologic outcome of elective nephron-sparing surgery and radical nephrectomy for low-stage renal cell carcinoma. *Eur Urol* 2011;59:543-552.

29

Evaluation and Management of Advanced Renal Cell Carcinoma and Upper Tract Urothelial Tumors

ATREYA DASH AND ROBERT M. SWEET

CONTRIBUTORS OF CAMPBELL-WALSH-WEIN, 12TH EDITION

William P. Parker, Matthew T. Gettman, Steven C. Campbell, Brian R. Lane, Phillip M. Pierorazio, Panagiotis Kallidonis, Evangelos Liatsikos, Thomas W. Jarrett, Surena F. Matin, Armine K. Smith, Ramaprasad Srinivasan, and W. Marston Linehan

TREATMENT OF LOCALLY ADVANCED RENAL CELL CARCINOMA

Inferior Vena Cava Involvement

One of the unique features of renal cell carcinoma (RCC) is its frequent pattern of growth intraluminally into the renal venous circulation, also known as venous tumor thrombus.

About 45%–70% of patients with RCC and inferior vena cava (IVC) thrombus can be cured with an aggressive surgical approach, including radical nephrectomy (RN) and IVC thrombectomy.

Staging of the level of IVC thrombus is as follows: I, adjacent to the ostium of the renal vein; II, extending up to the lower aspect of the liver and below the hepatic veins; III, involving the intrahepatic portion of the IVC but below the diaphragm; and IV, extending above the diaphragm.

In all series, a significant proportion of patients with level IV IVC thrombi are cured with surgical resection, typically in the absence of metastases and other adverse features.

Magnetic resonance imaging (MRI) is the preferred diagnostic study at many centers; however, recent literature indicates that an appropriately performed computed tomography (CT) can provide essentially equivalent information.

The surgical approach is tailored to the level of IVC thrombus but uniformly begins with early ligation of the arterial blood supply and in the process the kidney is gently mobilized, leaving it only attached via the renal vein.

Vascular control for level III and level IV IVC thrombi requires more extensive dissection, venovenous bypass, or cardiopulmonary bypass and hypothermic circulatory arrest. For level III thrombi, mobilization of the liver and exposure of the intrahepatic IVC often allows the thrombus to be mobilized caudad to the hepatic veins, and venous isolation can then proceed as for a level II thrombus (Fig. 29.1). Patient selection is critical because many patients, especially those with metastatic disease, will have a limited life expectancy.

However, surgery can impart a significant palliative benefit by preventing pulmonary emboli and minimizing disability from intractable edema, ascites, cardiac dysfunction, or associated local symptoms such as abdominal pain and hematuria.

Locally Invasive Renal Cell Carcinoma

In evaluation of patients with large, invasive retroperitoneal masses, a broad differential diagnosis should be considered, including adrenocortical carcinoma, urothelial carcinoma, sarcoma, and lymphoma, in addition to locally invasive RCC.

Because surgical therapy is the only potentially curative management for RCC, extended operations with en bloc resection of adjacent organs are occasionally indicated.

However, even with an aggressive surgical approach, the prognosis remains poor. Despite a significant likelihood of recurrence of RCC with poor-risk features, there is no established evidence of a benefit for adjuvant therapy in patients who appear to be cancer free after surgical resection, and observation remains the standard of care. Ongoing adjuvant clinical trials investigating targeted molecular agents, checkpoint inhibitors, and other novel systemic approaches should be supported in an effort to identify an efficacious adjuvant strategy.

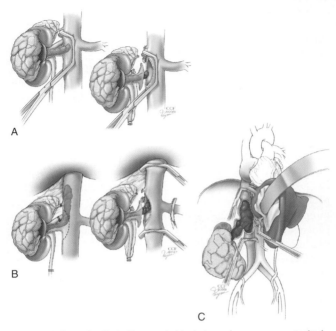

FIG. 29.1 Schematics illustrating surgical techniques for management of inferior vena cava (IVC) thrombi according to level. (A) Level I IVC thrombus managed with a Satinsky clamp to achieve vascular isolation. (B) Level II IVC thrombus managed by sequential clamping of the lower IVC, contralateral renal vein, and cephalad IVC, along with mobilization of the IVC and occlusion of lumbar veins, allowing for vascular isolation. (C) Level III IVC thrombus managed by mobilization of the liver, providing exposure of the intrahepatic IVC and retraction of the thrombus to facilitate placement of the upper IVC clamp just below the level of the hepatic veins. Through this approach, vascular isolation is achieved in a manner similar to that in B. If the cephalad clamp must be placed above the level of the hepatic veins, a Pringle maneuver should be performed to temporarily occlude the hepatic blood flow. (Reprinted with permission, Cleveland Clinic Center for Medical Art and Photography, Copyright 2007-2009. All rights reserved.)

Lymph Node Dissection for Renal Cell Carcinoma

The presence of lymph node metastasis is an important prognostic factor and defines a high-risk subset of patients with advanced RCC.

Although lymphadenectomy for RCC provides accurate staging (Table 29.1, Fig. 29.2), the therapeutic benefits of routine lymphadenectomy are controversial.

Most important, the European Organization for Research and Treatment of Cancer (EORTC) 30881 randomized trial of lymphadenectomy at RN failed to show a survival advantage for most patients undergoing lymphadenectomy.

Lymphadenectomy may be performed in patients with clinically suspicious (radiographic or intraoperative) lymphadenopathy for staging purposes and, because of lack of data indicating a reliable therapeutic benefit, need not be performed routinely in patients with localized kidney cancer and clinically negative nodes.

Local Recurrence After Radical Nephrectomy or Nephron-Sparing Surgery

Local recurrence of RCC after RN, which includes recurrence in the renal fossa, ipsilateral adrenal gland, renal vein stump or adjacent

Table 29.1 Risk of Regional Lymph Node Metastases in Renal Cell Carcinoma Based on Pathologic Risk Factors

NO. OF RISK FACTORS[a]	PERCENTAGE OF PATIENTS IN THIS RISK GROUP	PERCENTAGE WITH POSITIVE LYMPH NODES IN RETROSPECTIVE SERIES[b]	PERCENTAGE WITH POSITIVE LYMPH NODES IN PROSPECTIVE SERIES[c]
0	4		
	4% (729/1652)	0.4% (3/729)	—
1	18% (302/1652)	1.0% (3/302)	—
2	17% (276/1652)	4.4% (12/276)	20% (7/35)
3	13% (209/1652)	12% (26/209)	37% (26/71)
4	7.3% (121/1652)	13% (16/121)	49% (26/53)
5	0.9% (15/1652)	53% (8/15)	50% (5/10)

[a]Risk factors for regional lymph node metastases include (1) large primary tumor (>10 cm); (2) clinical stage T3/T4; (3) high tumor grade (Fuhrman grade 3 or 4); (4) sarcomatoid features; or (5) histologic tumor necrosis.
[b]Data from (Blute et al., 2004b); lymph node dissection performed in 58% of 1652 patients overall.
[c]Data from (Crispen et al., 2011); lymph node dissection performed in 41% of 415 patients with 2– risk factors.

SIDE OF PRIMARY TUMOR

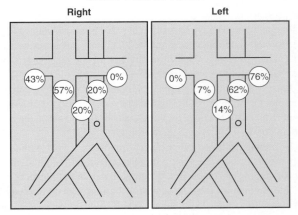

FIG. 29.2 Frequency of lymph node positivity detected at extended lymph-adenectomy in patients with lymph node positive renal cancer at nephrectomy. (From Crispen PL, Breau RH, Allmer C, et al. Lymph node dissection at the time of radical nephrectomy for high-risk clear cell renal cell carcinoma: indications and recommendations for surgical templates. *Eur Urol* 2011;59:18-23.)

IVC, or ipsilateral retroperitoneal lymph nodes, is an uncommon event, occurring in 2%–4% of cases.

Risk factors include locally advanced or node-positive disease and adverse histopathologic features.

Only about 20%–40% of local recurrences are isolated; the majority of patients with local recurrence also have systemic disease, and a thorough metastatic evaluation should be pursued.

Surgical resection of isolated local recurrence of RCC after RN should be considered because it can provide long-term cancer-free status for 30%–40% of patients.

Local recurrence in the remnant kidney after PN for RCC has been reported in 1.4%–10% of patients, and the main risk factors are advanced T stage or high tumor grade.

Patients with isolated local recurrence after PN can be considered for repeat PN, completion nephrectomy, TA, or AS.

TREATMENT OF ADVANCED RENAL CELL CARCINOMA

Approximately one-third of all patients with newly diagnosed RCC are seen initially with synchronous metastatic disease, and an additional 20%–40% of patients with clinically localized disease at diagnosis eventually develop metastases.

Prognostic Factors

Several clinical features, such as a long time interval between initial diagnosis and appearance of metastatic disease and presence of fewer sites of metastatic disease, have been associated with better outcome.

Poor performance status and the presence of lymph node and/or liver metastases have long been recognized to be associated with shorter survival.

A multivariate analysis showed a poor performance status (Karnofsky score <80), an elevated serum lactate dehydrogenase level (>1.5 times upper limit of normal), a low hemoglobin (less than the lower limit of normal), an elevated corrected calcium concentration (>10 g/dL), and lack of prior nephrectomy were independent predictors of a poor outcome (Table 29.2).

Patients could be stratified into three distinct prognostic groups based on these five poor prognostic factors (Table 29.3). The overall survival (OS) times in patients with no adverse factors (favorable-risk group), one to two risk factors (intermediate-risk group), and more than three risk factors (poor-risk group) were 20 months, 10 months, and 4 months, respectively.

The International Metastatic Renal Cell Carcinoma Database Consortium (IMDC) investigators confirmed the prognostic relevance of several components of the Memorial Sloan Kettering Cancer Center (MSKCC) model (performance status, hypercalcemia, anemia, and time from diagnosis to treatment); in addition, neutrophilia and thrombocytosis were identified as additional, independent predictors of poor outcome. Patients were divided into three risk categories (Tables 29.4 and 29.5).

Table 29.2 Adverse Prognostic Factors in 670 Patients Treated With Chemotherapy or Immunotherapy at the Memorial Sloan Kettering Cancer Center

- Karnofsky performance score <80%
- Elevated lactate dehydrogenase (>1.5 times upper limit of normal)
- Low hemoglobin (<lower limit of normal)
- Elevated corrected calcium (>10 mg/dL)
- Absence of prior nephrectomy

Table 29.3 Risk Stratification Based on Adverse Prognostic Factors in 670 Patients Treated with Chemotherapy or Immunotherapy at the Memorial Sloan Kettering Cancer Center

RISK GROUP	NO. OF ADVERSE PROGNOSTIC FACTORS	MEDIAN OVERALL SURVIVAL (months)
Good	0	20
Intermediate	1–2	10
Poor	3–5	4

Data from Motzer RJ, Mazumdar M, Bacik J, et al. Survival and prognostic stratification of 670 patients with advanced renal cell carcinoma. *J Clin Oncol* 1999;17:2530-2540.

Table 29.4 Adverse Prognostic Factors in 849 Patients Treated with First-Line Vascular Endothelial Growth Factor (VEGF)–Targeted Therapy

- Karnofsky performance score <80%
- Neutrophilia (>upper limit of normal)
- Low hemoglobin (<lower limit of normal)
- Elevated corrected calcium (>upper limit of normal)
- Thrombocytosis (>upper limit of normal)
- <1 yr from diagnosis to VEGF-targeted therapy

Table 29.5 Risk Stratification Based on Adverse Prognostic Factors in 849 Patients Treated with First-Line Vascular Endothelial Growth Factor–Targeted Therapy

RISK GROUP	NO. OF ADVERSE PROGNOSTIC FACTORS	MEDIAN OVERALL SURVIVAL (months)
Good	0	43.2
Intermediate	1–2	22.5
Poor	3–6	7.8

Data from Heng DY, Xie W, Regan MM, et al. External validation and comparison with other models of the International Metastatic Renal-Cell Carcinoma Database Consortium prognostic model: a population-based study. *Lancet Oncol* 2013;14(2):141-148.

SURGICAL MANAGEMENT OF METASTATIC RENAL CELL CARCINOMA

Debulking or Cytoreductive Nephrectomy in Patients with Metastatic Renal Cell Carcinoma

Nephrectomy as the sole therapeutic intervention in the context of metastatic disease is unlikely to alter outcome.

The most compelling evidence in support of cytoreductive nephrectomy is provided by two randomized phase III studies conducted by the Southwest Oncology Group (SWOG) and the EORTC.

Although there were no significant differences in the response rates to interferon observed in the two study arms, OS was improved in the surgery plus interferon arm (median, 11.1 vs 8.1 months for interferon alone; $P = .05$) (Fig. 29.3).

These data supported the use of cytoreductive nephrectomy in carefully selected patients with metastatic RCC who are likely candidates for subsequent cytokine therapy (Table 29.6).

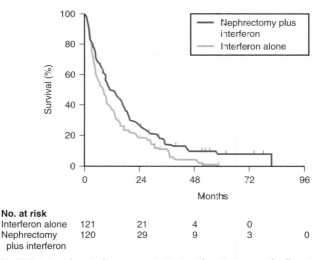

No. at risk				
Interferon alone	121	21	4	0	
Nephrectomy plus interferon	120	29	9	3	0

FIG. 29.3 Actuarial survival among 241 patients with metastatic renal cell carcinoma randomized to either interferon-α alone or interferon-α after cytoreductive nephrectomy. (Modified from Flanigan RC, Salmon SE, Blumenstein BA, et al. Nephrectomy followed by interferon alfa-2b compared with interferon alfa-2b alone for metastatic renal-cell cancer. *N Engl J Med* 2001;345:1655-1659.)

Table 29.6 Summary of Outcome in Randomized Studies of Interferon-α Alone or Interferon-α After Cytoreductive Nephrectomy in Patients with Metastatic Kidney Cancer

STUDY	NO. OF ELIGIBLE PATIENTS			RESPONSE RATE AFTER IFN (%)			MEDIAN OVERALL SURVIVAL (MO)		
	TOTAL	IFN	Nx Plus IFN	IFN	Nx Plus IFN	P	IFN	Nx Plus IFN	P
Flanigan et al., 2001	241	121	120	3.6	3.3	NS	8.1	11.1	.05
Mickisch et al., 2001	83	42	41	12	19	.38	7	17	.03
Flanigan et al., 2004	331	163	161	5.7	6.9	.60	7.8	13.6	.002

IFN, Interferon-α; *Nx,* cytoreductive nephrectomy.

Since the advent of vascular endothelial growth factor receptor–targeted therapy, cytoreductive nephrectomy had remained the practice, based largely on data generated in the era of cytokine therapy and supported by retrospective series and outcome analysis from a national cancer database.

The CARMENA (Cancer du Rein Metastatique Nephrectomie et Antiangiogéniques) study was a prospective study designed to address the issue of cytoreductive nephrectomy in the vascular endothelial growth factor era.

Although findings from this study reiterate that patients with poor prognosis are not likely to benefit from cytoreductive nephrectomy, the impact of these data on current clinical practice (i.e., the use of cytoreductive surgery in appropriately selected patients with low metastatic burden and other favorable features) remains uncertain.

Resection of Metastases

Resection of limited metastatic disease has been reported by several groups to be associated with long disease-free intervals and OS in some patients.

Metastasectomy has not been evaluated systematically in a prospective, randomized fashion, and the favorable outcome ascribed to resection in patients with solitary metastatic disease may reflect patient selection bias, inherent differences in tumor biology, and natural history or other confounding factors.

In a series from MSKCC, complete or "curative" resection was associated with a longer OS (44% 5-year survival vs 14% in patients undergoing incomplete resection); multivariate analysis also identified the presence of a solitary metastatic lesion, age younger than 60 years, and a disease-free interval of >1 year as favorable prognostic indicators.

In addition, some studies have suggested that pulmonary metastases, smaller tumor size (<4 cm in one series), and metachronous lesions are predictors of better outcome after metastasectomy.

Although not supported by convincing evidence of survival benefit from prospective studies, resection of isolated metastatic lesions is a reasonable and widely employed practice in well-selected patients with RCC.

Palliative Surgery

Cytoreductive nephrectomy can be performed with palliative intent in patients with intractable pain, hematuria, constitutional symptoms, or a variety of paraneoplastic manifestations such as hypercalcemia, erythrocytosis, secondary thrombocytosis, or hypertension.

Resection of the primary renal tumor does not always result in clinical benefit.

Cytoreductive nephrectomy with palliative intent is therefore performed relatively infrequently but is appropriate in some patients.

UROTHELIAL TUMORS OF THE UPPER URINARY TRACT AND URETER

Epidemiology
Incidence. Upper urinary tract carcinomas (UTUCs) make up only 5%–10% of urothelial tumors.

The majority of UTUCs are presented in a single renal unit, although up to 5% of patients have bilateral disease.

The involvement of the pelvicalyceal system is twice as common as with ureteral tumors.

Multifocal presence of UTUC is diagnosed in 10%–20% of cases.

Concurrent bladder cancer is diagnosed in 17% of cases.

Up to 41% of American men with UTUC have a history of bladder cancer.

Disease recurrence after treatment involves the bladder in 22%–47% of cases and the contralateral upper tract in 2%–6%.

Metachronous UTUC after treated bladder cancer could reach 80% of cases, and most of these occurrences take place in the renal pelvis rather than the ureter.

Approximately 60% of the UTUCs are invasive, and 7% have metastasized at diagnosis.

UTUCs are twice more frequent in men than in women.

Familial or hereditary upper tract tumors should be considered when the patient is younger than 60 years.

Mortality Rate. Disease mortality has been related to increasing age, male gender, black non-Hispanic race, and advanced tumor stage.

Risk Factors
Genetic Predisposition. Familial or hereditary UTUCs are linked to hereditary nonpolyposis colorectal carcinoma (HNPCC) syndrome (or Lynch syndrome).

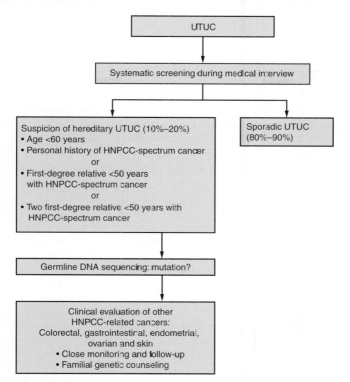

FIG. 29.4 Selection of patients with upper tract urothelial cancer (UTUC) for hereditary screening during the first medical interview. *HNPCC,* Hereditary nonpolyposis colorectal carcinoma. (From Rouprêt M, Babjuk M, Compérat E, et al. European Association of Urology Guidelines on Upper Urinary Tract Urothelial Carcinoma: 2017 Update. *Eur Urol* 2018;73[1]:111-122.)

Patients with HNPCC and UTUC are younger than 60 years (mean age, 55 years).

Suspicion for genetic predisposition should be raised in young patients with UTUC, personal history, or having two first-degree relatives with a cancer related to HNPCC (especially colon or endometrial tumors) (Fig. 29.4).

Environmental Factors. The routine use of tobacco increases the relative risk for UTUC from 2.5 to 7 times.

Histopathology

Urothelial carcinomas represent >90% of the upper urinary tract tumors. Pure nonurothelial upper urinary tract cancers are rare conditions. Variants of urothelial cancer are encountered in approximately 25% of UTUCs. Papillomas, inverted papillomas, and von Brunn nests are usually benign lesions. UTUC develops through a gradual progression of hyperplasia to dysplasia and eventually carcinoma in situ (CIS) in a significant proportion of UTUC cases. CIS is difficult to diagnose with significant morphologic variations. The muscle invasion or invasion to the renal parenchyma or the surrounding adventitia is more likely to take place on the upper tract.

Diagnosis

Localized disease is characterized by hematuria, dysuria, and flank pain. Advanced disease is characterized by flank or abdominal mass, weight loss, anorexia, and bone pain.

Cystoscopy should always be performed.

Flexible ureteroscopy with biopsy is a key approach for diagnosis.

Computed tomography urography has the highest diagnostic accuracy.

Urine collection or washing of the ureter with a ureteral catheter could provide the most accurate cytologic results.

Staging and Classification

Ureteral tumors are in the distal ureter (70% of cases), mid-ureter (25% of cases), and upper ureter (5% of cases). Bilateral disease is found in in 3% to 5% of cases. The prognosis for recurrence after radical nephroureterectomy is related to the location of the tumor and stage. The recurrence rate is 2%–4% with an interval of 17–170 months. Bladder recurrence is 15%–75% within 5 years. CIS involves a higher incidence of bilateral and multifocal disease. Disease spread is typically direct expansion of the tumor to lymphatics and bloodstream.

Prognosis

TNM Classification. The tumor, node, metastasis (TNM) classification and staging system is the most commonly used (Table 29.7).

The regional lymph nodes (LNs) for pelvic and upper ureteral tumors are the hilar and retroperitoneal LNs.

Table 29.7 Tumor, Node, Metastasis (TNM) Classification for Upper Urinary Tract Carcinoma

T: Primary Tumor	
TX	Primary tumor cannot be assessed
To	No evidence if primary tumor
Ta	Noninvasive papillary carcinoma
Tis	Carcinoma in situ
T1	Tumor invades subepithelial connective tissue
T2	Tumor invades muscularis
T3	Renal pelvis: tumor invades beyond muscularis into peripelvic fat or renal parenchyma Ureter: tumor invades beyond muscularis into perinephric fat
T4	Tumor invades adjacent organs or through the kidney into perinephric fat

N: Regional Lymph Nodes	
NX	Regional lymph nodes cannot be assessed
No	No regional lymph nodes metastasis
N1	Metastasis in a single lymph node ≤2 cm in the greatest diameter
N2	Metastasis in a single lymph node >2 cm in the greatest diameter

M: Distant Metastasis	
Mo	No distant metastasis
M1	Distant metastasis

For the mid and distal ureteral tumors the respective LNs are the intrapelvic LNs. The laterality of the LNs does not affect N classification.

The renal pelvic subclassification (pT3) provides discrimination between the microscopic infiltration of the renal parenchyma, which is represented as pT3a, and the macroscopic infiltration or invasion of the peripelvic adipose tissue, which is represented as pT3b.

The American Joint Committee on Cancer staging system could also be used (Table 29.8).

Histologic Grading. The 2004/2016 World Health Organization classification distinguishes between noninvasive tumors: papillary urothelial neoplasia of low malignant potential and low- and high-grade carcinomas based on histologic characteristics (low grade vs high grade).

Table 29.8 American Joint Committee on Cancer Staging System in Conjunction With the Tumor, Node, Metastasis (TNM) System

AJCC STAGING SYSTEM	TNM CLASSIFICATION SYSTEM
0	T0
I	Ta, Tis, T1, N0, M0
II	T2, N0, M0
III	T3, N0, M0
IV	T4 or T, N+, M+

Prognostic Factors

Tumor Stage and Grade – The primary recognized prognostic factors are tumor stage and grade (Fig. 29.5). UTUCs that invade the muscle wall usually have a very poor prognosis. The 5-year specific survival is less than 50% for pT2/pT3 stage and <10% for pT4 stage.

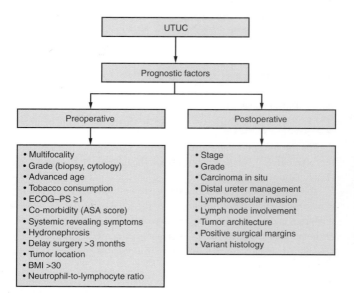

FIG. 29.5 Upper urinary tract urothelial carcinoma (UTUC): prognostic factors. *ASA,* American Society of Anesthesiologists; *BMI,* body mass index; *ECOG–PS,* Eastern Cooperative Oncology Group Performance Status. (Modified from Rouprêt M, Babjuk M, Compérat E, et al. European Association of Urology Guidelines on Upper Urinary Tract Urothelial Carcinoma: 2017 update. *Eur Urol* 2018;73[1]:111-122.)

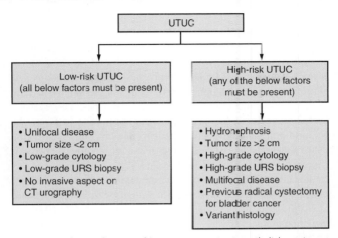

FIG. 29.6 Risk stratification of upper urinary tract urothelial carcinoma (UTUC). *CT,* Computed tomography; *URS,* ureteroscopy. (Modified from Rouprêt M, Babjuk M, Compérat E, et al. European Association of Urology Guidelines on Upper Urinary Tract Urothelial Carcinoma: 2017 update. *Eur Urol* 2018;73[1]:111-122.)

Tumor stage is difficult to assert based on the clinical criteria. The UTUC cases could be stratified between low- and high-risk tumors to distinguish the cases that are more appropriate for kidney-sparing treatment rather than radical surgery (Fig. 29.6).

SURGICAL MANAGEMENT UPPER TRACT UROTHELIAL CARCINOMA

Diagnosis

Ureteroscopic Evaluation and Biopsy. Preoperative ureteroscopy has clear benefits when there is a question of diagnosis and/or if conservative management is being considered. Because of the small size and shallow depth of ureteroscopic biopsy specimens, a precise correlation with eventual tumor stage is difficult. In predicting the tumor stage, a combination of the radiographic studies, the visualized appearance of the tumor, and the tumor grade provides the surgeon with the best estimation for risk stratification.

Treatment

Radical Nephroureterectomy. Radical nephroureterectomy with excision of a bladder cuff is the gold standard for large, high-grade, suspected invasive tumors of the renal pelvis and proximal ureter. Open, laparoscopic, and robotic techniques are surgical options. The entire distal ureter, including the intramural portion and the ureteral orifice, must be removed. Many approaches have been described.

Lymphadenectomy. Prospective studies are needed to assess the role and optimal extent of lymphadenectomy in UTUC, emerging data validate its importance in the treatment of patients with this cancer.

It is safe and beneficial for accurate staging and appears to have prognostic and therapeutic value in patients with invasive disease (T2–T4), especially in the setting of tumors of renal pelvis and proximal ureter.

Results. Multiple series reported on strong correlation of outcome with tumor stage and grade (Table 29.9). Complete ureterectomy with bladder cuff excision should accompany nephroureterectomy for UTUC.

Nondefinitive management of the distal ureter was associated with a higher rate of local and distal recurrence and inferior disease-specific and overall survival.

Table 29.9 Literature Review of Overall Survival of Patients with Upper Tract Urothelial Tumors (Renal Pelvis or Ureter) by Stage and Grade

	5-YEAR SURVIVAL (%)
Tumor Grade	
1–2	40–87
3–4	0–33
TMN Stage	
Ta, T1, Tcis	60–90
T2	43–75
T3	16–33
T4	0–5
N+	0–4
M+	0

TNM, Tumor, node, metastasis.

Endourologic Management

Basic Attributes. Tumors of the upper urinary tract can be approached in a retrograde or antegrade fashion. The approach chosen depends largely on the tumor location and size. In general, a retrograde ureteroscopic approach is used for low-volume ureteral and renal tumors (Fig. 29.7).

An antegrade percutaneous approach is preferred for larger tumors of the upper ureter or kidney and for those that cannot be adequately manipulated in a retrograde approach because of location (e.g., lower pole calyx) or previous urinary diversion.

Results. The literature shows the long-term feasibility of the ureteroscopic approach (Table 29.10), but concerns over the high rate of ipsilateral recurrences remain.

Management of Positive Upper Tract Urinary Cytology and Carcinoma In Situ. An unequivocal positive voiding urinary cytology

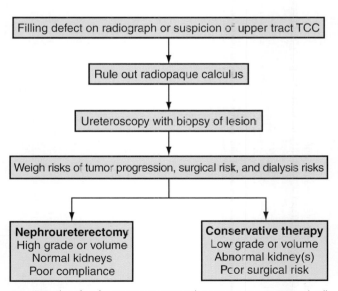

FIG. 29.7 Algorithm for endoscopic approach to upper tract transitional cell carcinoma (TCC).

Table 29.10 Ureteroscopic Management

STUDY	PATIENTS (n)	FOLLOW-UP (mo)	UPPER TRACT RECURRENCE (%)	BLADDER RECURRENCE (%)	NEPHROURETERECTOMY RATE (%)	DISEASE PROGRESSION (%)	FAILED MANAGEMENT (%)	COMPLICATIONS (%)
Martínez-Piñeiro et al., 1996	54	31	23	ND	10	ND	28	23
Daneshmand et al., 2003	30	31	90	23	13	20	47	17
Johnson et al., 2005	35	52	68	ND	3	0	3	9
Gadzinski et al., 2010	34	18	31	15	ND	15	ND	9
Pak et al., 2009	57	53	90	ND	19	7	19	ND
Thompson et al., 2008	83	55	55	45	33	14	33	
Cutress et al., 2012	73	54	69	43	19	19	30	16

ND, Not disclosed.
Modified from Cutress ML, Stewart GD, Zakikhani P, et al. Ureteroscopic and percutaneous management of upper tract urothelial carcinoma (UTUC): systematic review. *BJU Int* 2012;110:614-628.

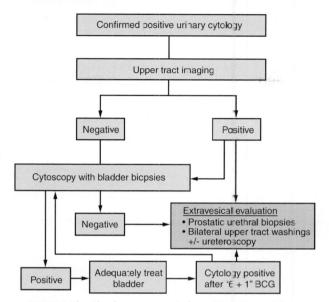

FIG. 29.8 Algorithm for management of a positive urinary cytology.

usually indicates the presence of urothelial carcinoma. Most cases are from a bladder source; however, extravesical sites may be involved, including the upper urinary tracts and the prostatic urethra in men (Fig. 29.8).

Suggested Readings

Atkins MB, Dutcher J, Weiss G, et. al. Kidney cancer: the Cytokine Working Group experience (1986-2001): part I. IL-2-based clinical trials. *Med Oncol* 2001;18:197-207.

Choueiri TK, Escudier B, Powles T, et. al. Cabozantinib versus everolimus in advanced renal-cell carcinoma. *N Engl J Med* 2015;373:1814-1823.

Choueiri TK, Escudier B, Powles T, et. al. Cabozantinib versus everolimus in advanced renal cell carcinoma (METEOR): final results from a randomised, open-label, phase 3 trial. *Lancet Oncol* 2016;17:917-927.

Choueiri TK, Halabi S, Sanford BL et. al. Cabozantinib versus sunitinib as initial targeted therapy for patients with metastatic renal cell carcinoma of poor or intermediate risk: the Alliance A031203 CABOSUN Trial. *J Clin Oncol* 2017;35:591-597.

Flanigan RC, Salmon SE, Blumenstein BA, et. al. Nephrectomy followed by interferon alfa-2b compared with interferon alfa-2b alone for metastatic renal-cell cancer. *N Engl J Med* 2001;345:1655-1659.

Fyfe GA, Fisher RI, Rosenberg SA, et. al. Long-term response data for 255 patients with metastatic renal cell carcinoma treated with high-dose recombinant interleukin-2 therapy. *J Clin Oncol* 1996;14:2410-2411.

Heng DY, Xie W, Regan MM, et. al. External validation and comparison with other models of the International Metastatic Renal-Cell Carcinoma Database Consortium prognostic model: a population-based study. *Lancet Oncol* 2013;14:141-148.

Hudes G, Carducci M, Tomczak P, et al. Temsirolimus, interferon alfa, or both for advanced renal-cell carcinoma. *N Engl J Med* 2007;356:2271-2281.

Mejean A, Ravaud A, Thezenas S, et al. Sunitinib alone or after nephrectomy in metastatic renal-cell carcinoma. *N Engl J Med* 2018;379:417-427.

Motzer RJ, Hutson TE, Tomczak P, et. al. Sunitinib versus interferon alfa in metastatic renal-cell carcinoma. *N Engl J Med* 2007;356:115-124.

Motzer RJ, Mazumdar M, Bacik J, et. al. Survival and prognostic stratification of 670 patients with advanced renal cell carcinoma. *J Clin Oncol* 1999;17:2530-2540.

Motzer RJ, Escudier B, McDermott DF, et. al. Nivolumab versus everolimus in advanced renal-cell carcinoma. *N Engl J Med* 2015;373:1803-1813.

Motzer RJ, Tannir NM, McDermott DF, et. al. Nivolumab plus ipilimumab versus sunitinib in advanced renal-cell carcinoma. *N Engl J Med* 2018;378:1277-1290.

30

Pathophysiology, Evaluation, and Management of Adrenal Disorders

BRADLEY F. SCHWARTZ AND ROBERT M. SWEET

CONTRIBUTORS OF CAMPBELL-WALSH-WEIN, 12TH EDITION

Simpa S. Salami, David Mikhail, Simon J. Hall, Manish A. Vira, Christopher J. Hartman, Casey A. Dauw, Stuart I. Wolf, and Melissa R. Kaufman

Also known as suprarenal glands, the adrenal glands are paired, retroperitoneal organs that lie immediately above the kidneys within Gerota's fascia. They are known to have significant hormonal activity and are central to homeostasis. Because of their location and physiology, the diseases and surgical procedures are well within the urologic surgeon's realm of management.

ADRENAL ANATOMY AND PHYSIOLOGY

Embryology

The gland is made of two embryologically and functionally distinct units: the cortex (outer layer and endocrine) and medulla (inner layer and neurocrine). The cortex is derived from the intermediate mesoderm of the urogenital ridge in the fifth week of gestation as mesenchymal cells proliferate to form the outer layer of the fetal adrenal. These cells become encapsulated at the end of the eighth week by cells from the peritoneal mesothelium. The medulla is derived from neural crest cells located in the sympathetic ganglia, which become enveloped by the cortex by the ninth week and ends by week 18. At birth the gland is twice the weight of the adult gland and continues to develop until 12 months of age.

Unilateral agenesis is rare, and bilateral agenesis is incompatible with life. However, because of the differences in embryologic development of the kidney and adrenal glands, in cases of renal agenesis, malrotation, or malascent, the adrenal glands will be in their normal anatomic location but more discoid in shape. Other embryologic anomalies include heterotopia (adrenal rests), which can be found anywhere along the path of gonadal descent in the retroperitoneum. These rests can be found in up to 50% of neonates but because of atrophy, only 1% of adults. In cases of congenital adrenal hyperplasia (CAH), rests may lie in the testis, manifesting as a testis mass. This needs to be considered prior to orchiectomy in patients with CAH.

Anatomy

The glands weigh 4–5 g each, are 4–6 cm in length and are 2–3 cm wide and lie at the level of the 11th and 12th ribs. The right gland is triangular and is bordered medially by the inferior vena cava (IVC), superiorly and anteriorly by the liver, inferiorly by the kidney and renal vein, posteriorly by the psoas muscle, and laterally by the body wall. The left is crescent shaped and is bordered medially by the aorta; superiorly and anteriorly by the spleen, stomach, and splenic vessels; inferiorly by the kidney and renal vein, posteriorly by the psoas muscle; and laterally by the body wall. The blood supply is variable but arises from three arteries: superior adrenal (inferior phrenic artery), middle adrenal (aorta), and inferior (ipsilateral renal artery). The short right adrenal vein drains directly into the IVC; the left vein is longer and drains into the renal vein. Extensive collateral vasculature allows for partial adrenalectomy when indicated. Right lymphatic drainage is via the paracaval chain, and the left is drained by the paraaortic chain. Autonomic innervation is by preganglionic sympathetic fibers off the sympathetic trunk directly to the chromaffin cells of the medulla, whereas postganglionic fibers from the splanchnic ganglia supply the cortex (Figs. 30.1 and 30.2).

Adrenal Cortex Physiology

Much of the hormone synthesis in the adrenal gland arises from the common precursor, cholesterol. Low-density lipoprotein

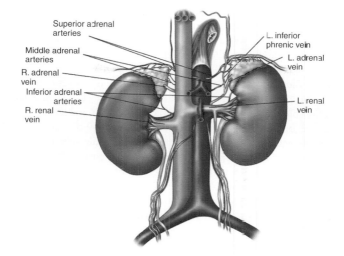

FIG. 30.1 Adrenal vascular supply demonstrating inflow from the superior, middle, and inferior adrenal arteries bilaterally. Whereas the right (R.) adrenal vein drains directly into the posterior inferior vena cava, the left (L.) adrenal vein often communicates with the inferior phrenic vein before draining into the left renal vein. (Courtesy of the University of Kentucky.)

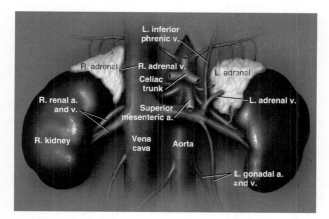

FIG. 30.2 Vascular supply of adrenal glands. *a,* Artery; *L,* left; *R,* right; *v,* vein.

(LDL) serves as the primary source of cholesterol for the adrenals. The cortex is composed of three major zones: the zona glomerulosa (mineralocorticoid), zona fasciculate (glucocorticoid) and reticularis (androgen). The zone layers can best be remembered as "salt, sugar, sex" (Fig. 30.3).

Zona Glomerulosa. The outermost region of the adrenal gland and the only source of aldosterone synthase (CYP11B2), making it the sole source of aldosterone (the primary mineralocorticoid) in the body. Aldosterone stimulates distal nephron epithelial cells to reabsorb sodium and chloride ions while secreting hydrogen and potassium ions. Aldosterone primarily affects total body volume and not sodium concentration. Its levels are regulated by angiotensin II through the renin-angiotensin-aldosterone system (RAAS) and by serum potassium levels. The main inhibitor of aldosterone secretion is atrial natriuretic peptide (ANP), suggesting strong relationships between cardiac, adrenal, and renal function.

Zona Fasciculata. The site of production of glucocorticoids from expression of 17α-hydroxylase, 21-hydroxylase, and 11β-hydroxylase enzymes. Cortisol is the primary product, and its secretion is under tight control of adrenocorticotrophic hormone (ACTH). Production of cortisol follows a strict circadian rhythm with the majority being produced in the early morning.

Zona Reticularis. This innermost zone contains large amounts of 17α-hydroxylase and 17,20-lyase, resulting in the production of dehydroepiandrosterone (DHEA), sulfated DHEA (DHEA-S), and androstenedione, which may have roles in the treatment of advanced prostate cancer. Aberrations in the production of these hormones result in CAH.

Adrenal Medulla

The medulla composes 10% of adrenal mass but is integral to the autonomic nervous system. Chromaffin cells in the medulla are innervated by preganglionic sympathetic fibers of T11 to L2 similar to the sympathetic ganglia. The systemic stress response is modulated by catecholamines that are produced from the amino acid tyrosine and consist of epinephrine (E) (80%), norepinephrine (NE) (19%), and dopamine (1%).

The majority of catecholamine metabolism occurs in the adrenal medulla. The metabolites metanephrine, normetanephrine,

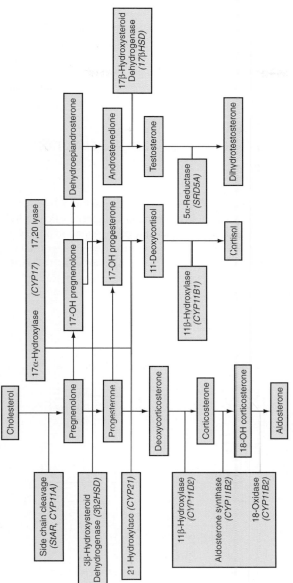

FIG. 30.3 Steroid hormone synthesis beginning with cholesterol and resulting in mineralocorticoid, glucocorticoid, and androgen production in the adrenal cortex. Enzymes are listed in boxes and genes in parentheses. (From Hyun G, Kolon TF. A practical approach to intersex in the newborn period. *Urol Clin North Am* 2004;31:435-443.)

and vanillylmandelic acid (VMA) and the enzymes catechol-O-methyltransferase (COMT) and monoamine oxidase (MAO) are the most important. More than 90% of metanephrine and 20% of normetanephrine in the bloodstream are produced in the medulla. These can be important in the diagnosis of pheochromocytoma. These metabolites are also excreted in the urine in a sulfonated form, making them measurable in urine collections.

ADRENAL DISORDERS
DISORDERS OF INCREASED ADRENAL FUNCTION
Cushing Syndrome
Pathophysiology

Cushing syndrome (CS) is rare and is defined as hypercortisolism secondary to excessive production of glucocorticoids by the adrenal cortex. Corticotropic cells of the anterior pituitary gland secrete ACTH, also known as corticotropin, under the influence of the hypothalamus (Fig. 30.4). Physiologically, the most

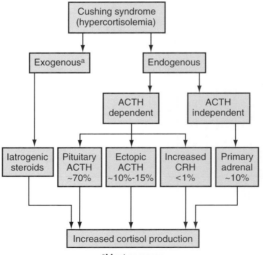

FIG. 30.4 Clinically relevant causes of excess cortisol production. *ACTH*, Adrenocorticotropic hormone; *CRH*, corticotropin-releasing hormone.

important promoter of ACTH release is corticotropin-releasing hormone (CRH), but oxytocin and vasopressin also play a role. Stress is the most important variable in modulating the hypothalamus-pituitary-adrenal (HPA) axis. Glucocorticoids bind receptors in the hypothalamus and the pituitary gland and complete the negative feedback loop by inhibiting production of CRH and ACTH by these structures, respectively. Given the sophistication of the HPA axis, hypercortisolism can result from a number of different pathologies that result in oversecretion of cortisol by the adrenal glands. Causes of CS can be divided into three main groups: (1) exogenous, (2) ACTH dependent, and (3) ACTH independent.

Exogenous Cushing Syndrome. Exogenous CS is the most common cause of hypercortisolism in patients of the Western world. Synthetic glucocorticoids are used for a multitude of conditions, and CS may result from administration of even low doses taken orally, topically, or inhaled. CS can also be seen in patients not realizing they are getting exogenous preparations or in people using them for performance enhancement.

ACTH-Dependent Cushing Syndrome. ACTH-dependent hypercortisolism accounts for 80%–85% of cases of endogenous CS. Approximately 80% of ACTH-dependent disease results from primary pituitary pathology and is known as Cushing disease (CD). Ectopic ACTH production is the other main cause of ACTH-dependent hypercortisolism. CD is caused by excessive secretion of ACTH by the pituitary gland. This also accounts for 70% of cases of CS. Microadenomas and small tumors of the pituitary are the most common causes of CD.

Ectopic ACTH Syndrome. Production of ACTH by nonpituitary tumors can also result in hypercortisolism. These tumors are frequently malignant and account for approximately 10% of cases of CS. The hypercortisolism of ectopic ACTH syndrome can precede a cancer diagnosis by many years and include lung, thyroid, gastrointestinal (GI), and neuroendocrine cancers and pheochromocytoma.

Adrenal Tumors. Cortisol-secreting tumors of the adrenal represent 10% of cases of CS. They are usually small, unilateral hyperplastic nodules. Roughly 8% of CS cases have overproduction of cortisol from adrenocortical carcinoma (ACC) and represents a poor prognosis.

Rare Causes. Rare causes include ACTH-independent macronodular adrenal hyperplasia and primary pigmented nodular adrenocortical disease.

Clinical Characteristics

Clinical characteristics of CS vary considerably. The classic symptoms of hypercortisolism, such as central obesity, moon facies, buffalo hump, proximal muscle weakness, easy bruisability, and abdominal striae, are nonspecific. CS also results in systemic symptomatology that is identical to the common metabolic syndrome, such as central obesity, dyslipidemia, insulin resistance, and hypertension (HTN). Many men with CS have erectile dysfunction and may present with decreased libido and hypogonadism. Up to 50% of CS patients have urolithiasis. Patients who exhibit cushingoid features should be worked up for hypercortisolism.

Diagnostic Tests

The two most frequently used tests to diagnose CS are the 24-hour urinary free cortisol (UFC) test and the overnight low-dose dexamethasone suppression test (LD-DST). When evaluating incidentalomas, the UFC test may be inadequate because of its low sensitivity. In normal patients, dexamethasone stimulates the corticotropic cells of the anterior pituitary, which in turn suppresses ACTH production and results in lower serum cortisol levels. A patient's failure to suppress cortisol after dexamethasone administration is indicative of CS.

The UFC test is a 24-hour direct measurement of bioavailable cortisol. Late-night salivary cortisol and midnight plasma cortisol measurements take advantage of a common feature of all causes of CS—a perturbation and in some cases complete disruption in the diurnal variation of cortisol levels. The abnormality is the inability to suppress cortisol levels at night. Peak morning cortisol levels in patients with CS are often within the normal range; however, persistent elevation at night may signal the loss of diurnal variance associated with CS. Although midnight plasma cortisol measurements are clinically impractical in an outpatient setting, late-night salivary cortisol measurements are becoming a popular diagnostic tool for identification of hypercortisolism.

Identifying the Cause of Cushing Syndrome. First, measure serum ACTH. Low levels indicate an ACTH-independent cause, and abdominal imaging should be performed. If the adrenals are normal, then an exogenous source of steroids should be considered. If the levels are high, one must decipher between CD and ectopic ACTH syndrome. Identifying pituitary microadenomas as extra-adrenal ACTH-producing tumors with modern imaging techniques can be challenging. Also, incidental lesions found in the lung, pancreas, and pituitary gland confuse the issue greatly. Direct measurements of ACTH in a downstream venous plexus that drains the pituitary gland—the inferior petrosal sinus—after CRH stimulation has become the gold standard approach for distinguishing ectopic ACTH production from CD. High levels of ACTH in the inferior petrosal sinus, when compared with those in peripheral blood, indicate CD, whereas levels similar to peripheral plasma suggest an ectopic ACTH source. The high-dose dexamethasone test is not routinely used currently.

Treatment

Exogenous CS. Cessation of glucocorticoid administration must be gradual so that the HPA axis has ample time to recover. The process can take weeks to months and varies greatly among patients. Be aware of steroid withdrawal syndrome, wherein the patient cannot tolerate steroid dose reduction despite apparent normalization in HPA axis testing.

Cushing Disease. The current standard of care for ACTH-secreting pituitary adenomas is trans-sphenoidal surgical resection. Only 60%–80% of patients are cured, and up to 25% of individuals relapse. Macroadenomas are resistant to neurosurgical treatment, and fewer than 15% are cured after excision of tumors 1 cm or larger. After resection, a severe addisonian state is common, and careful glucocorticoid replacement is necessary in the year after surgery. Hypopituitarism after resection of a pituitary adenoma is a known complication, with rates varying from 5% to 50%. Currently, bilateral adrenalectomy is recommended when at least one attempt to treat the primary tumor has failed. It is also necessary when hypercortisolism is life threatening, and swift definitive treatment is mandatory. The advantages of the procedure include a lack of postoperative hypopituitarism and an extremely high success rate with rapid resolution of hypercortisolism. Lifelong mineralocorticoid and glucocorticoid replacement is required in all patients. Moreover, the patients are at risk for progressive growth of their pituitary adenoma, which can result in ocular chiasm compression, oculomotor deficiencies, and, rarely, a rise in intracranial pressure. This is known as the Nelson-Salassa syndrome, or just Nelson syndrome, which is found in 8%–29% of patients who have undergone bilateral adrenalectomy.

Ectopic ACTH Syndrome. Excision of the ACTH-producing tumor is ideal but possible in only 10% of patients. In unresectable or unidentifiable ACTH-producing tumors, bilateral adrenalectomy is an excellent option.

ACTH-Independent Disease. Cortisol-producing adrenal masses should be treated with either partial or total adrenalectomy.

Medical Treatment of Hypercortisolism. Medications that block enzymes of steroid synthesis such as metyrapone, aminoglutethimide, ketoconazole and etomidate can be used to bridge the patient waiting for surgery or when surgical intervention is not possible.

PRIMARY ALDOSTERONISM

Pathophysiology

The release of renin from the JG cells is the rate-limiting step in the RAAS cascade. Normally, renin release is stimulated by low renal perfusion pressure, increased renal sympathetic nervous activity, and low sodium concentration sensed by the macula densa. Renin then cleaves angiotensinogen to angiotensin I, which in turn is cleaved by angiotensin-converting enzyme (ACE) to angiotensin II. Angiotensin II functions as a potent vasoconstrictor and triggers the release of aldosterone from the zona glomerulosa. Additional regulators of aldosterone release include potassium and ACTH. In Conn syndrome, aldosterone secretion is independent of the RAAS, and plasma renin levels will be suppressed. This finding is in contrast with patients who have secondary hyperaldosteronism, in whom elevated renin levels are the cause of elevations in aldosterone secretion. There are subtypes of primary aldosteronism that differ in their therapy. Idiopathic hyperplasia and aldosterone-producing adenomas account for >95% of cases. Clinically, patients with idiopathic hyperplasia have less severe HTN and are less likely to be hypokalemic compared with patients with aldosterone-producing adenomas. Whereas both adrenal glands are responsible for increased aldosterone production in idiopathic hyperplasia, unilateral adrenalectomy is not therapeutic. Unilateral adrenal hyperplasia is distinctly uncommon but, when appropriately diagnosed, is potentially curable

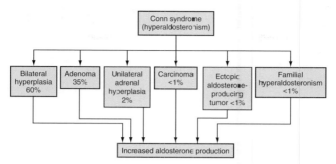

FIG. 30.5 Subtypes of primary aldosteronism. (Modified from Young WF. Primary aldosteronism: renaissance of a syndrome. *Clin Endocrinol [Oxf]* 2007;66:607-618.)

with adrenalectomy. In comparison with idiopathic hyperplasia, aldosterone-producing adenomas are associated with more profound HTN and hypokalemia (Fig. 30.5).

Familial hyperaldosteronism (FH) type I, also called glucocorticoid-remediable aldosteronism, is autosomal dominant and is manifested by aldosterone being secreted to the circadian rhythm of ACTH instead of the RAAS. Patients often have early-onset severe HTN or cerebral vascular accidents and/or a family history of HTN.

Type II is autosomal dominant and presents with either hyperplasia or adenomas indistinct from the sporadic type of hyperaldosteronism. FH type III is characterized by bilateral adrenal hyperplasia, refractory HTN, severe hypokalemia, and the overproduction of hybrid steroids. Genetic testing for types I and III is recommended (Box 30.1).

Clinical Characteristics

Virtually all patients present with refractory HTN. Hypokalemia is classically a hallmark of the disease but may only be present 10%–50% of the time. Cardiac and renal disease may be present because of the HTN. Stroke, atrial fibrillation, cardiac events, proteinuria, and renal failure are all increased in hyperaldosteronism.

Screening

Hypokalemia needs correction and significant medications discontinued prior to screening the patient (Fig. 30.6) Alpha or calcium

---

Box 30.1 Subtypes of Primary Aldosteronism

SURGICALLY CORRECTABLE

Aldosterone-producing adenoma
Primary unilateral adrenal hyperplasia
Ovarian aldosterone-secreting tumor
Aldosterone-producing carcinoma

NOT CORRECTABLE BY SURGERY

Bilateral adrenal hyperplasia
Familial hyperaldosteronism type I
Familial hyperaldosteronism type II
Familial hyperaldosteronism type III

---

channel blockers should be employed as first line to treat HTN. Patients should be encouraged to take sodium and avoid licorice and chewing tobacco. Obtain a morning (between 8–10 AM) plasma aldosterone concentration (PAC) and PRA. From these, the PAC and aldosterone-to-renin ratio (ARR) can determine autonomous aldosterone secretion. PAC >20 ng/dL and PRA below the detection level are abnormal. All patients suspected of primary hyperaldosteronism should get cross-sectional imaging. Hyperaldosteronomas are typically unilateral, low-density, nonenhancing lesion <10 Hounsfield units (HU), with an average size of 1.6–1.8 cm and a normal-appearing contralateral adrenal gland.

Confirmatory Testing

If there is HTN, hypokalemia, PRA below detection and PAC >20 ng/dL, no confirmatory testing is needed. The flurocortisone suppression test involves 0.1 mg every 6 hours in addition to NaCl 2 g every 8 hours, both for 4 days. PAC is measured in the upright position. Failure to suppress PAC to less than 6 ng/dL is diagnostic of primary aldosteronism.

The oral sodium loading test is conducted by administering a high-sodium diet and NaCl for 3 days followed by 24-hour urine measurements of aldosterone, sodium, and creatinine. The diagnosis of primary aldosteronism is made when the 24-hour aldosterone is >12 μg/day.

The intravenous (IV) saline infusion test spares the patient from several days of sodium loading by the administration of 2 L of

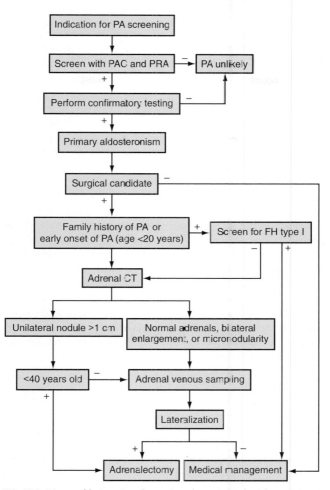

FIG. 30.6 Primary aldosteronism diagnosis and treatment algorithm. *CT*, Computed tomography; *FH*, familial hyperaldosteronism; *PA*, primary aldosteronism; *PAC*, plasma aldosterone concentration; *PRA*, plasma renin activity.

0.9% sodium chloride intravenously over 4 hours. The infusion is performed in the morning after an overnight fast while the patient is in a recumbent position. After the IV infusion of saline, PAC is measured; a level >5 ng/dL is diagnostic of primary aldosteronism, and levels >10 ng/dL are suggestive of aldosterone-producing adenomas.

Adrenal vein sampling (AVS) can be useful. Proper patient preparation is essential and includes 1 hour of recumbency, correction of hypokalemia, and discontinuation of antihypertensive agents. AVS is performed in the morning after an overnight fast. Percutaneous samples are collected from three sites: right adrenal vein, left adrenal vein, and IVC. Aldosterone and the cortisol concentrations are determined. Appropriate specimen collection from the adrenal vein is determined by comparing the cortisol concentrations from the adrenal vein with the cortisol concentration from the IVC. The ratio of adrenal vein to IVC cortisol should be >1.1−5 : 1, depending on the use of cosyntropin stimulation. If cosyntropin stimulation is used, a higher ratio is expected in properly collected samples. AVS that demonstrates adrenal vein–to–IVC ratios below the cutoff, on either side, should be considered "nonselective" and discarded. An adrenal vein–to–IVC ratio above the cutoff, bilaterally, is considered "selective," and comparisons between aldosterone concentrations can be made to determine the presence of lateralization.

Treatment And Prognosis

When total or partial adrenalectomy is feasible, this is the procedure of choice. The majority undergoing adrenalectomy will have improvement in HTN, and most will discontinue some or all medications, a significant portion will have no change in blood pressure. Potassium is corrected in the vast majority of patients.

Medical therapy is successful at normalizing both HTN and potassium and consists of aldosterone receptor agonists spironolactone and eplerenone. Spironolactone is initiated at doses of 25–50 mg/day and can be titrated up to 400 mg/day, depending on blood pressure, serum potassium levels, and side effects. Side effects include gynecomastia, impotence, and menstrual disturbances. Eplerenone is better tolerated because of increased selectivity for the aldosterone receptor. Treatment should be initiated with 25 mg/day and titrated up to 100 mg/day (Table 30.1).

Table 30.1 Perioperative Glucocorticoid Administration in Patients on Chronic Steroid Therapy

DEGREE OF SURGICAL STRESS	DEFINITION	GLUCOCORTICOID DOSE
Minor	Procedure under local anesthesia and >1 hour in duration (e.g., inguinal hernia repair)	Hydrocortisone 25 mg or equivalent
Moderate	Procedure such as vascular surgery of a lower extremity or a total joint replacement	Hydrocortisone 50–75 mg or equivalent This could be continuation of usual daily steroid dose (e.g., prednisone 10 mg/day) and hydrocortisone 50 mg intravenously during surgery
Major	Procedure such as esophagogastrectomy or operation on cardiopulmonary bypass	Usual glucocorticoid (e.g., prednisone 40 mg or the parenteral equivalent within 2 hours before surgery) and hydrocortisone 50 mg intravenously every 8 hours after the initial dose for the first 48–72 hours of postoperative period

Data from Salem M, Tainsh RE Jr, Bromberg J, et al. Perioperative glucocorticoid coverage. A reassessment 42 years after emergence of a problem Ann Surg 1994;219(4):416-425; and Axelrod L. Perioperative management of patients treated with glucocorticoids. Endocrinol Metab Clin North Am 2003;32(2):367-383.

FH type I can be treated with oral glucocorticoids, which will reduce ACTH release, leading to decreased aldosterone production. In FH type I patients whose blood pressure is not controlled with glucocorticoids alone or in those who develop iatrogenic CS, the addition of an aldosterone receptor antagonist should be considered.

PHEOCHROMOCYTOMA

A tumor of medullary catecholamine-producing cells, it is a rare tumor responsible for 0.5% of HTN cases and 5% of incidental adrenal masses. Extra-adrenal pheochromocytomas (paragangliomas) and can occur in the head, neck, thorax, abdomen, pelvis, and bladder. Chromaffin bodies called the organ of Zuckerkandl lie between the aortic bifurcation and the root of the inferior mesenteric artery (IMA) are common locations of paragangliomas.

Pathophysiology

Medullary cells possess the enzyme phenylethanolamine-N-methyltransferase (PNMT), which synthesizes E from NE. The variability of this enzyme causes the variability of clinical manifestations of this tumor depending upon the amounts of E, NE, and dopamine that are produced.

Familial cases account for 33% of pheochromocytomas. Genes such as Von Hippel-Lindau (VHL) and neurofibromatosis are examples of hereditary pheochromocytomas.

Malignant pheochromocytomas is defined by the presence of clinical metastases. Histopathologic information of the primary tumor is of limited value in determining metastatic potential. Metastasis in patients with VHL and MEN-2 syndromes is rare.

Clinical Characteristics

Pheochromocytoma is often referred to as the 10% tumor: extra-adrenal, familial, pediatric, bilateral, and malignant. Tumors in the right gland are more common, are larger, and have higher recurrence rates.

Paroxysmal HTN is classic; however, such episodic spikes in blood pressure are documented in only approximately 30%–50% of patients and can occur in essential hypertension. The remainder of patients demonstrate persistently elevated blood pressure, and a minority are normotensive. The triad of headache, episodic sudden perspiration, and tachycardia is a classic hallmark of pheochromocytoma. More than 20% of patients can be asymptomatic. Depending on the catecholamine milieu of each tumor, symptomatology can vary greatly.

Hereditary pheochromocytomas occurs at a younger age and is more often multifocal and bilateral.

Metastatic disease is more common in extra-adrenal lesions and in the SDHB mutation. Common sites include bone, lung, liver, and lymph nodes. Most discovered within 5 years of the original diagnosis.

Diagnostic Tests

Cross-Sectional Imaging. On computed tomography (CT) or magnetic resonance imaging (MRI), adrenal pheochromocytomas appear as well-circumscribed lesions. Given their rich vascularity and low lipid content, pheochromocytomas typically measure an attenuation of >10 HU on unenhanced CT. Bright signal intensity on T2-weighted images (light-bulb sign) may help in the diagnosis of pheochromocytoma but not pathognomonic.

Functional Imaging. When CT or MRI reveals an adrenal mass and biochemical testing suggests a pheochromocytoma, surgery is indicted. In the vast majority of cases, functional imaging is not required.

Positron Emission Tomography. Fluorine-18 fluorodeoxyglucose positron emission tomography is the gold standard for imaging pheochromocytoma.

Metaiodobenzylguanidine Scintigraphy. MIBG is the most sensitive and specific agent for diagnosing pheochromocytoma. It is used for recurrences or extra-adrenal disease.

Biochemical Evaluation. Metanephrine conversion is an uninterrupted process allowing plasma measurements that are much more accurate than paroxysmal catecholamine production (Table 30.2).

VMA is end metabolite of catecholamine production, and urine VMA has 99% specificity in nonfamilial cases (Table 30.3).

Table 30.2 Test Characteristics for Diagnosis of Pheochromocytoma From a Large Multicenter Cohort Study[a]

| | SENSITIVITY (%) | | SPECIFICITY (%) | |
	HEREDITARY	SPORADIC	HEREDITARY	SPORADIC
Plasma-free metanephrines	97 (74/76)	99 (137/138)	96 (326/339)	82 (249/305)
Catecholamines	69 (52/75)	92 (126/137)	89 (305/339)	72 (220/304)
Urinary fractionated metanephrines	96 (26/27)	97 (76/78)	82 (237/288)	45 (73/164)
Catecholamines	79 (54/68)	91 (97/107)	96 (312/324)	75 (159/211)
Total metanephrines	60 (27/45)	88 (61/69)	97 (91/94)	89 (79/89)
Vanillylmandelic acid	46 (30/65)	77 (66/86)	99 (310/312)	86 (132/153)

[a]n = 858: 214 patients with pheochromocytoma and 644 control participants.
Data from Lenders J, Pacak K, Walther M, et al. Biochemical diagnosis of pheochromocytoma which test is best? *JAMA* 2002;287(11):1427-1434.

Table 30.3 Relative Merits for and Against Use of Plasma-Free Metanephrines and Urinary Fractionated Metanephrines in the Diagnosis of Pheochromocytoma

URINARY FRACTIONATED METANEPHRINES	PLASMA-FREE METANEPHRINES
Well-established, widely available test	Relatively new test with limited availability
Urinary concentrations (200–2000 nmol) make analysis relatively easy	Plasma concentrations (0.1–0.5 nmol) can make analysis difficult
Easy for clinicians to implement with minimal expenditure of time and effort	Blood collections require some time and effort by medical staff
24-hour collections can be inconvenient for patients	Blood sampling relatively more convenient for patients
Problems with reliability of incomplete timed urine collections	Collection and handling of blood samples can be better regulated
Difficult to control dietary and daily life influences on sympathoadrenal function	Influences of diet and sympathoadrenal function more easily controlled
In children, 24-hour collections are difficult to interpret without age-appropriate reference intervals	In children, blood sampling may be stressful, but results are more easily interpreted without age-appropriate reference intervals
Urine collections may be inappropriate in patients with renal failure	Test is applicable in patients with renal failure

From Grossman A, Pacak K, Sawka A, et al. Biochemical diagnosis and localization of pheochromocytoma: can we reach a consensus? *Ann N Y Acad Sci* 2006;1073:332-347.

All patients younger than 50 years of age should receive genetic testing for the RET, VHL, SDHB, and SDHD gene mutations. Routine testing for the NF1 gene is not recommended in patients who do not meet clinical criteria for neurofibromatosis.

Treatment

Preoperative Management. Surgical excision via minimally invasive surgery is the gold standard. Preoperative evaluation by a cardiologist is recommended (Fig. 30.7).

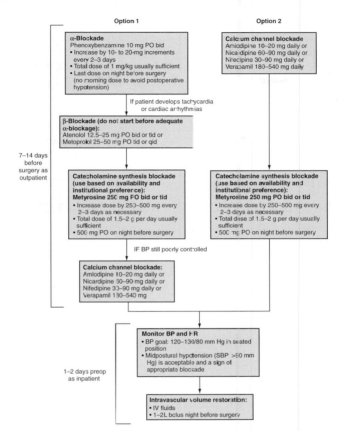

FIG. 30.7 Preoperative medical management in patients with pheochromocytoma. *bid*, Twice a day; *BP*, blood pressure; *HR*, heart rate; *IV*, intravenous; *PO*, by mouth; *SBP*, systolic blood pressure; *tid*, three times a day. (Modified from Pacak K. Preoperative management of the pheochromocytoma patient. *J Clin Endocrinol Metab* 2007;92:4069-4079.)

Alpha blockers are the mainstay of preoperative treatment. The irreversible agent phenoxybenzamine is the drug of choice started 14 days prior to surgery and titrated to blood pressure (BP) 120–130/80 mm Hg in a seated position. Selective reversible alpha blockers such as terazosin, doxazosin, or prazosin may be used but data are not as compelling.

Beta blockers should never be used before alpha blockers. Can be used for reflex tachycardia and arrhythmias. Atenolol and metoprolol are preferred.

Calcium blockers may be useful for patients with mild symptomology prior to surgery.

Intravascular volume crucial to successful outcome. Once alpha blockade initiated, encourage salt and fluid intake prior to surgery. IV fluid resuscitation can be utilized day prior to surgery.

Postoperative Management. Postoperatively, the following can occur and need to be monitored: hypotension from the lasting effects of alpha blockade or hypoglycemia from the increase in insulin after tumor excision.

DISORDERS OF DECREASED ADRENAL FUNCTION

Causes of Addison's disease include autoimmune adrenalitis, infections, and surgical excision. Caution should be exercised when performing a nephrectomy in a patient with a prior history of contralateral renal surgery.

Clinical Characteristics

Patients may have fatigue, anorexia, and hyperpigmentation, the hallmark of Addison's crisis. Acute crisis is life threatening and may include acute abdomen, nausea, vomiting, fever, and hypovolemia.

Diagnostic Tests

A low morning serum cortisol and elevated ACTH can help confirm adrenal crisis.

Treatment

Adrenal hormones need to be replaced. Cortisol is replaced with hydrocortisone two-thirds in the morning and one-third in the evening. Mineralocorticoid is replaced with fludrocortisone.

DISORDERS OF ABNORMAL ADRENAL FUNCTION

Congenital Adrenal Hyperplasia

CAH is autosomal recessive characterized by low cortisol caused by a deficiency in 21-hydroxylase 95% of the time. ACTH is increased causing adrenal hyperplasia.

ADRENAL LESIONS

Malignant

Adrenocortical Carcinoma (ACC). Rare and universally poor prognosis. May be associated with a number of syndromes but mostly sporadic.

Incidental detection has increased, but >50% of patients have symptoms at time of diagnosis. Abdominal pain or fullness and symptoms related to increased adrenal hormone production are the most common symptoms. The most common is cortisol resulting in CS. The second most common is increased androgens mainly 17-ketosteroids, resulting in virilization: male-pattern baldness, hirsutism, and oligmenorrhea.

Diagnostic Tests. Cross sectional imaging is the best test to identify an adrenal tumor. ACC presents large with 90% >5 cm and the majority greater than 10–12 cm. MRI may be useful for identification of adjacent soft tissue involvement or venous invasion. Other scans may be useful but adrenal lesions this large should be removed.

Staging. Classic tumor, node, metastasis staging applies.

Management. ACCs >8 cm should be considered for open surgery. Smaller tumors should be considered for laparoscopic or robotically assisted proedures.

Neuroblastoma. Neuroblastoma, a malignancy derived from the neural crest cells, which give rise to the adrenal medulla and sympathetic ganglia, is the most common solid extracranial tumor of childhood.

Metastases. Melanoma, lung, RCC, breast, medullary thyroid, ACC, GI, prostate, cervical and others can metastasize to the adrenal. The majority are found on cross sectional imaging. Excision of the involved adrenal is recommended in the vast majority of cases.

Benign

Adenoma. Adenoma is the common mass in the adrenal found on 6% of autopsies. It is the common "incidentaloma" found on cross-sectional imaging. The majority are nonfunctional. Once inert always inert.

Noncontrast CT is the most valuable diagnostic tool. Adenomas are usually <4 cm, well rounded, and homogeneous. High lipid content leads to an attenuation of <10 HU on unenhanced CT. When IV

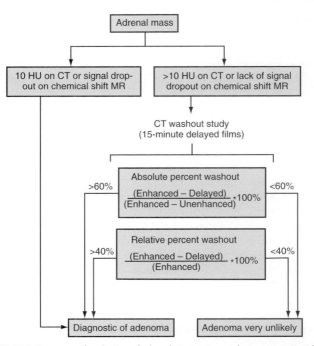

FIG. 30.8 Summary of evaluation of adrenal mass using modern cross-sectional imaging. *CT,* Computed tomography; *HU,* Hounsfield units; *MR,* magnetic resonance.

contrast is used, lesions that wash out >50% of gained enhancement on delayed films are usually benign adenomas. There is no need for intervention unless they are large or functional (Fig. 30.8).

Myelolipoma. These are nonfunctional fat-containing tumors of the adrenal glands. Usually no intervention is necessary unless they are larger than 4–5 cm.

Evaluation of Adrenal Lesions in Urologic Practice

Tumors <4 cm warrant no intervention unless they are functional. Tumors >4 cm should be strongly considered for excision whether functional or not. In contemplating extirpation, a functional study is recommended. Growth rates of >5 mm/yr warrant excision (Table 30.4, Fig. 30.9).

Table 30.4 Characteristics of Incidental Adrenal Masses as Described in a Systematic Review of Published Series of Adrenal Incidentalomas That Include 20 or More Patients

ADRENAL LESION	PERCENT OF TOTAL (n = 2005)
Metabolically active	11.2
Cortisol-producing adenoma	5.3
Aldosterone-producing adenoma	1.0
Pheochromocytoma	5.1
Malignant	7.2
Adrenocortical carcinoma	4.7
Metastasis	2.5
Total potentially surgical lesions	18.4

Data from Young WF Jr. Management approaches to adrenal incidentalomas. A view from Rochester, Minnesota. *Endocrinol Metab Clin North Am* 2000;29(1):159-185; and Young WF Jr. The incidentally discovered adrenal mass. *N Engl J Med* 2007;356(6):601-610.

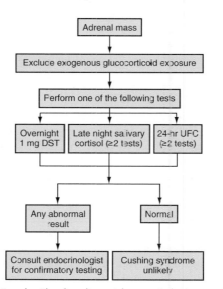

FIG. 30.9 Testing algorithm for ruling out hypercortisolemia secondary to an adrenal mass. In case of a positive result during late-night salivary cortisol or 24-hour urinary free cortisol evaluations, repeat testing is often prudent. *DST,* Dexamethasone suppression test; *UFC,* urinary free cortisol.

Biopsy is of limited value unless differentiating between malignant and benign process.

Functional Assessment of Adrenal Masses

Need to test for cortisol, catecholamine, and in HTN patients, aldosterone.

Test for hypercortisolism with LD-DST, late-night salivary cortisol test, a 24-hour UFC test.

Failure to suppress cortisol levels after steroid administration is indicative of CS. The patient should take 1 mg of dexamethasone between 11 PM and midnight. Serum cortisol should then be obtained between 8–9 AM.

The late-night salivary cortisol test collects the saliva between 11 PM and midnight. A persistently elevated cortisol represents hypercortisolism.

Conn syndrome is diagnosed from an ARR of ≥20 along with serum aldosterone >15 ng/mL. Adrenal vein sampling may be needed to localize a micro-adenoma.

Pheochromocytoma can be diagnosed by using free fractionated plasma metanephrines and the 24-hour urinary fractionated metanephrines.

Surgery of the Adrenals

Indications include functional tumors that fail medial therapy, suspicion of malignancy, tumors >6 cm, and tumors between 4–6 cm that are equivocal or that are symptomatic (Fig. 30.10).

Contraindications include uncorrected coagulopathy, widespread metastatic disease, and severe cardiopulmonary morbidity precluding anesthesia.

ACC. The debate continues as to the optimal approach to ACC: laparoscopic or robotic versus open. Tumors >6 cm that are most certainly ACC might want to be addressed with open surgery. Smaller tumors or tumors that are equivocal can be removed with minimally invasive surgery, ideally transperitoneal. Either method should include a lymph node dissection and avoid tumor spillage.

Open Adrenalectomy

Transperitoneal – These include anterior transabdominal and thoracoabdominal. The advantages are excellent surgical exposure and better vascular access and control but at the expense of ileus and major organ injury.

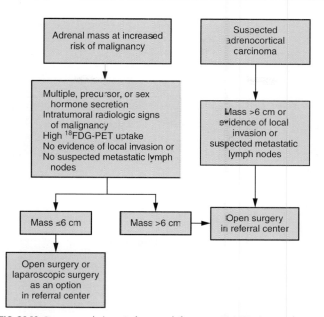

FIG. 30.10 Recommended surgical approach for nonmetastatic primary adrenocortical carcinoma. *18FDG*, [18F]fluoroceoxyglucose. (From Gaujoux S, Mihai R; Joint Working Group of ESES and ENSAT: European Society of Endocrine Surgeons (ESES) and European Network for the Study of Adrenal Tumours (ENSAT) recommendations for the surgical management of adrenocortical carcinoma. *Br J Surg* 2017;104(4):358-376.)

Retroperitoneal – These include the flank and lumbodorsal approaches, which have smaller operative fields but have less ileus and shorter hospitalizations. This approach may be better for the obese patient.

Flank Retroperitoneal. The patient is placed in lateral decubitus position with the table flexed and the kidney rest elevated. An axillary roll is placed, and the ipsilateral arm is placed over the opposite arm with the elbow slightly flexed. The lower leg is flexed, and the upper leg is overlapped with adequate padding or all pressure points, between the legs and arms. The patient is secured to the table at the shoulders, hips, and knees.

The incision is made along the course of the 11th rib (Figs. 30.11–30.14). Overlying muscles are incised, and the rib is

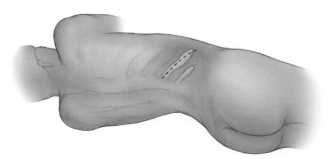

FIG. 30.11 Surgical incision over 11th rib for flank adrenalectomy. The patient is in flexion, with the kidney rest deployed to maximally expose the right retroperitoneum.

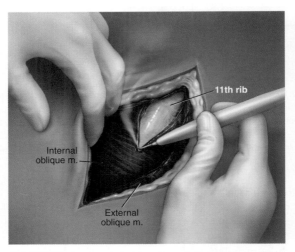

FIG. 30.12 Flank approach. Incision of muscle (m.) overlying 11th rib.

exposed and removed. The lumbodorsal fascia is entered, and anterior dissection identifies the peritoneal fold. This is dissected off until the great vessels are seen. Cephalad exposure identifies the adrenal gland and the renal vein. Retractors aid in exposure. The gland is then systematically excised. On the right, the vein is short and is found superiorly entering the IVC. One must use extreme

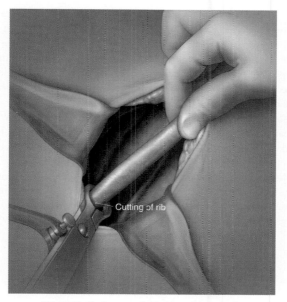

FIG. 30.13 Flank approach. Excision of the 11th rib.

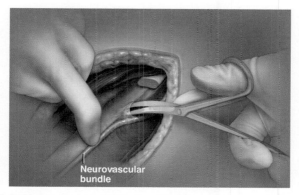

FIG. 30.14 Flank approach. Mobilization of the intercostal neurovascular bundle from the 11th rib. This is performed with a combination of blunt dissection with a Kittner dissector and sharp dissection with Metzenbaum scissors.

caution not to avulse the vein and not damage the gland or mass. Adrenal arteries are seldom seen. On the left, the longer vein enters the superior portion of the left renal vein. The veins are divided. For functional tumors, early ligation of the vein is optimal to prevent traumatic handling of the gland, which can release catecholamines into the circulation causing hypertensive crisis. The incision is closed in two layers, and the skin is closed.

Posterior Lumbodorsal Approach. The adrenals are directly approached through this incision, though exposure is severely limited. This approach is not to be used for large tumors or ACC. It can be used for bilateral hyperplasia (Figs. 30.15 and 30.16).

Anterior Transabdominal Approach. Indicated for large tumors requiring adequate exposure, caval involvement, or extensive nodal dissection. Approaches are subcostal, chevron, or midline (Figs. 30.17–30.20). On the left, the colon is reflected medially, the

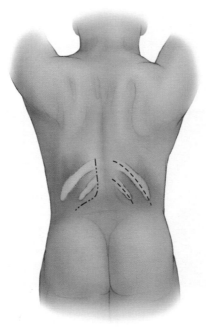

FIG. 30.15 Posterior approach—possible locations for lumbodorsal incisions.

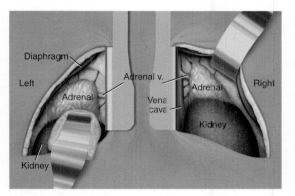

FIG. 30.16 Bilateral posterior approach—anatomic relations to the adrenal gland as seen from behind. *v*, Vein.

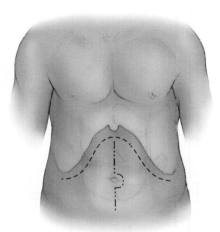

FIG. 30.17 Anterior approach. The transperitoneal approach may be attempted through a midline incision or subcostal incision. The subcostal incision can be extended into a full chevron for bilateral adrenalectomy or if a large unilateral tumor is encountered.

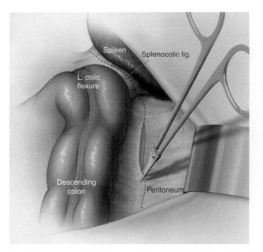

FIG. 30.18 Anterior approach. Peritoneum lateral to the left colon is incised at the line of Toldt and extended cephalad to the splenocolic ligament and inferiorly. *L,* Left; *lig.,* ligament.

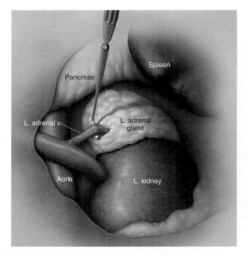

FIG. 30.19 Anterior approach. The left adrenal vein is dissected out and ligated. *L,* Left; *v,* vein.

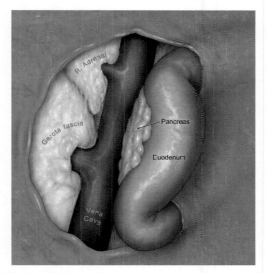

FIG. 30.20 Kocher maneuver. The peritoneum is incised, and sharp dissection and blunt dissection are used to mobilize the second stage of the duodenum away from the renal hilum. *R*, Right.

spleen is elevated, and the adrenal can be seen just posterior and inferior to the splenic artery and lateral to the pancreas. The adrenal vein should be divided close to the insertion of the renal vein. The gland is then dissected out in its entirety having caution of the spleen, pancreas, and kidney. The incision is closed in two layers.

The right adrenal is approached by retracting the liver, releasing the hepatic flexure of the colon, Kocherizing the duodenum, and identifying the gland just lateral to the IVC and just superior to the right renal vein.

Minimally Invasive Surgery. Laparoscopic (trans-and retroperitoneal approaches) (Figs. 30.21–30.27), robotic (Figs. 30.28– 30.31), single-site (LESS), and natural orifice (NOTES) techniques have all been applied to surgery of the adrenal gland and are emerging as the gold standard for adrenal surgery. The principles are the same and the approaches are very similar.

Partial Adrenalectomy. Partial adrenalectomy should be considered in patients with bilateral adrenal tumors, solitary adrenal

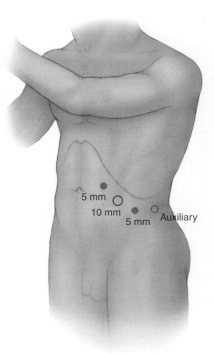

FIG. 30.21 Four-trocar configuration for left transperitoneal laparoscopic adrenalectomy.

gland, or familial syndromes such as von Hippel-Lindau disease, familial pheochromocytoma, and multiple endocrine neoplasia type IIA (Box 30.2). All approaches can be used. Intraoperative ultrasound is important to localize the tumor for accurate incision.

Ablative Therapy. Microwave, radiofrequency, and cryoablation techniques have been performed for adrenal disease. These are not recommended for tumors >4 cm or pheochromocytoma.

Complications

Complications of adrenal surgery are no different than those of other major abdominal procedures (Box 30.3). Right adrenalectomies can have injuries to the liver, gallbladder, large and small

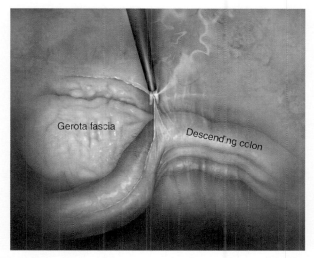

FIG. 30.22 Transperitoneal laparoscopic adrenalectomy. Incision of the line of Toldt and medial dissection of the left colon with cautery endoscopic scissors.

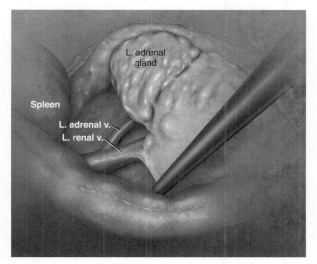

FIG. 30.23 Transperitoneal laparoscopic adrenalectomy. Exposure and dissection of the renal vein and left adrenal vein. *L,* Left; *v,* vein.

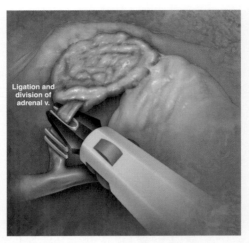

FIG. 30.24 Transperitoneal laparoscopic adrenalectomy. Ligation and division of left adrenal vein. *v,* Vein.

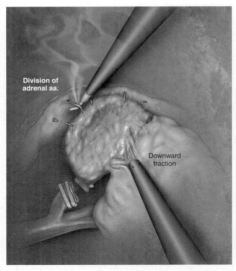

FIG. 30.25 Transperitoneal laparoscopic adrenalectomy. Division of adrenal arterial supply and superomedial dissection with downward traction on the kidney. *aa,* Arteries.

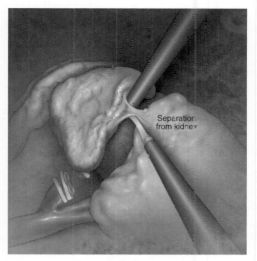

FIG. 30.26 Transperitoneal laparoscopic adrenalectomy. The adrenal gland is mobilized off the medial aspect of the kidney.

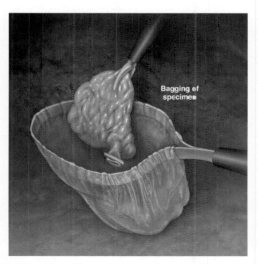

FIG. 30.27 Transperitoneal laparoscopic adrenalectomy. Placement of specimen in an endoscopic extraction sac.

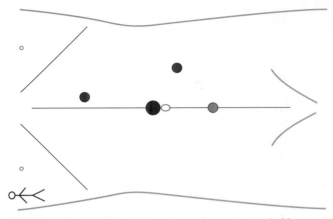

FIG. 30.28 Left robotic adrenalectomy trocar placement. A total of four ports are placed: one 12-mm camera port (●), one 12-mm assistant port (●), and two 8-mm robotic arm ports (●). The distance between each port should be at least 8 cm.

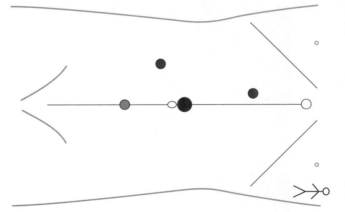

FIG. 30.29 Right robotic adrenalectomy trocar placement. A total of five ports are used: one 12-mm camera port (●), one 12-mm assistant port (●), two 8-mm robotic arm ports (●) are established, and to retract the liver, a 5-mm trocar (○) is placed with a retraction device.

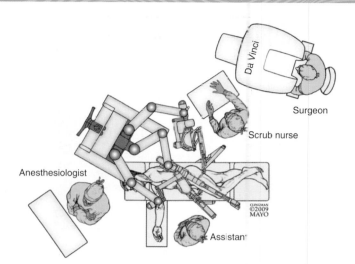

FIG. 30.30 Surgical room setup for left robotic adrenalectomy. The slave unit of the robot is brought in over the patient's left shoulder as indicated in the diagram. (By permission of Mayo Foundation for Medical Education and Research. All rights reserved.)

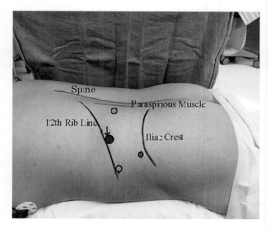

FIG. 30.31 Robot-assisted posterior retroperitoneal adrenalectomy. ● Camera port; ● 8-mm robotic ports; ● assistant port. (From Feng Z, Feng MP, Levine JW, et al. Robotic retroperitoneoscopic adrenalectomy: useful modifications of the described posterior approach. *J Robot Surg* 2017;11(4):409-414.)

Continued

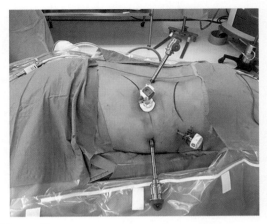

FIG. 30.31—cont'd

intestine, kidney, renal vasculature, pleura, and IVC. Left-sided surgery can injure the spleen, pancreas, large and small intestine, and kidney and its vasculature and pleura. Profound hyper- or hypotension can occur as well as electrolyte disturbances intra- or postoperatively (Box 30.4).

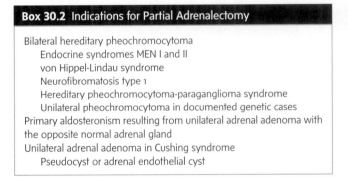

Box 30.2 Indications for Partial Adrenalectomy

Bilateral hereditary pheochromocytoma
    Endocrine syndromes MEN I and II
    von Hippel-Lindau syndrome
    Neurofibromatosis type 1
    Hereditary pheochromocytoma-paraganglioma syndrome
    Unilateral pheochromocytoma in documented genetic cases
Primary aldosteronism resulting from unilateral adrenal adenoma with the opposite normal adrenal gland
Unilateral adrenal adenoma in Cushing syndrome
    Pseudocyst or adrenal endothelial cyst

Box 30.3 Intraoperative Complications of Adrenal Surgery

Access related
    Abdominal wall hemorrhage
    Cutaneous nerve injury
    Visceral injury by Veress needle or trocar
Hemorrhage
    Inferior vena cava or aorta
    Adrenal vein
    Lumbar vein
    Hepatic vein
    Remnant adrenal gland after partial adrenalectomy
Ischemia
    Ligation of renal artery or vein
    Ligation of superior mesenteric artery and vein
Injury to neighboring organs as a result of thermal energy or incorrect plane of dissection
    Lung—pneumothorax
    Pancreas
    Liver
    Spleen
    Stomach and bowel, especially duodenum
    Kidney
Hemodynamic instability
    Pheochromocytoma

Modified from Vaughn ED. Complications of adrenal surgery. In Taneja SS, Smith RB, Ehrlich RM, eds. *Complications of urologic surgery: prevention and management,* 3rd ed. Philadelphia: 2001:366.

Box 30.4 Postoperative Complications of Adrenal Surgery

Primary aldosteronism
    Hypokalemia: secondary to continued potassium loss immediately postoperative
    Hyperkalemia: secondary to failure of contralateral adrenal to secrete aldosterone
Cushing syndrome
    Inadequate steroid replacement leading to hypocorticism
    Fracture secondary to osteoporosis
    Hyperglycemia
    Poor wound healing
    Increased risk of infections

Continued

Box 30.4 Postoperative Complications of Adrenal Surgery—cont'd

Pheochromocytoma
  Hypotension secondary to α-adrenergic blockade after tumor removal
Generic complications
  Hemorrhage
  Pneumothorax
  Pancreatitis
  Pneumonia
  Prolonged ileus
  Intraabdominal collections

Modified from Vaughn ED. Complications of adrenal surgery. In: Taneja SS, Smith RB, Ehrlich RM, eds. *Complications of urologic surgery: prevention and management,* 3rd ed. Philadelphia: Saunders, 2001:368.

Suggested Readings

Ball MW, Hemal AK, Allaf ME. International Consultation on Urological Diseases and European Association of Urology International Consultation on Minimally Invasive Surgery in Urology: laparoscopic and robotic adrenalectomy. *BJU Int* 2017;119:13-21.

El-Maouche D, Arlt W, Merke DP. Congenital adrenal hyperplasia. *Lancet* 2017;390(10108): 2194-2210.

Lam AK. Update on adrenal tumours in 2017 World Health Organization (WHO) of endocrine tumours. *Endocr Pathol* 2017;28(3):213-227.

Lee FT, Elaraj D. Evaluation and management of primary hyperaldosteronism. *Surg Clin North Am.* 2019;99(4):731-745.

Neumann HPH, Young WF Jr, Eng C. Pheochromocytoma and paraganglioma. *N Engl J Med* 2019;8;381(6):552-565.

Rossi GP. Primary aldosteronism: JACC state-of-the-art review. *J Am Coll Cardiol* 2019;3;74(22):2799-2811.

Schreiner F, Anand G, Beuschlein F. Perioperative management of endocrine active adrenal tumors. *Exp Clin Endocrinol Diabetes* 2019;127(2-03):137-146.

Vaidya A, Nehs M, Kilbridge K. Treatment of adrenocortical carcinoma. *Surg Pathol Clin* 2019;12(4):997-1006.

Young WF Jr. Clinical practice. The incidentally discovered adrenal mass. *N Engl J Med* 2007;356(6):601-610.

31

Complications of Urologic Surgery

JESSICA C. DAI, PETER SUNARYO, CRAIG A. PETERS, AND ROBERT M. SWEET

CONTRIBUTORS OF CAMPBELL-WALSH-WEIN, 12TH EDITION

Reza Ghavamian, Charbel Chalouhy, Michael J. Schwartz, Jessica E. Kreshover, Brian Duty, Michael Joseph Conlin, Mcr, Roshan M. Patel, Kamaljot S. Kaler, and Jaime Landman

ADULT COMPLICATIONS

A wide array of physiologic, medical, and surgical complications may occur following urologic surgery. Although the growth of endourology and minimally invasive surgery has helped to minimize surgical morbidity, unique periprocedural complications have also emerged from these techniques.

Classification

Postoperative complications may be quantified based on standardized classification systems. The Clavien-Dindo Scale (Table 31.1) is validated for urologic surgery and captures complication severity by the required management and the relative invasiveness of the management intervention.

Neuromuscular Complications

Positioning Injuries. Neuromuscular complications occur following 1%–3% of urologic surgeries. Positioning-related injuries typically result from prolonged nerve compression, excessive stretch, or ischemia. This may be exacerbated by extended operative time and inadequate pressure point padding. Obese patients are particularly vulnerable, given their increased weight and longer operative times. Specific patient positioning for various urologic

Table 31.1 Clavien-Dindo Scale for Postoperative Complications

GRADE	DEFINITION
1	Any deviation from the normal postoperative course without the need for pharmacologic treatment or surgical, endoscopic, or radiologic intervention
	Allowed therapeutic regimens are drugs as antiemetics, antipyretics, analgesics, diuretics, and electrolytes and physiotherapy. This grade also includes wound infections opened at the bedside
2	Requiring pharmacologic treatment with drugs other than those allowed for grade 1 complications
	Blood transfusions and total parenteral nutrition are also included
3	Requiring surgical, endoscopic, or radiologic intervention
3A	Intervention not under general anesthesia
3B	Intervention under general anesthesia
4	Life-threatening complication (including central nervous system complications) requiring intensive care or intensive care unit management
4A	Single-organ dysfunction (including dialysis)
4B	Multi-organ dysfunction
5	Death of a patient
Suffix "d"	If the patient has a complication at the time of discharge, the suffix "d" (for "disability") is added to the respective grade of complication. This label indicates the need for a follow-up to fully evaluate the complication

surgeries may result in characteristic nerve compression injury patterns (Table 31.2). Strategies for prevention of perioperative peripheral neuropathies are outlined by the American Society of Anesthesiologists (Box 31.1).

Direct Nerve Injury. Specific urologic procedures are associated with direct intraoperative nerve injury (Table 31.3). Careful attention to patient and retractor positioning, as well as deliberate identification and avoidance of the nerves at risk may help avoid injury. Clips inadvertently placed on nerves must be removed, and transected nerves should be repaired in a tension-free manner with nonabsorbable suture. Postoperative physical therapy may optimize recovery of any resulting functional deficits.

Compartment Syndrome. Compartment syndrome of the gluteal or lower extremity compartments results from prolonged time in

Table 31.2 Positioning-Related Nerve Injuries

POSITION	NERVE AFFECTED	MECHANISM	DEFICIT	PREVENTION
Supine	Sciatic nerve	• Inadequate cushioning or padding	• Calf, foot numbness	• Avoid excessive upper extremity abduction >90 degrees
	Radial nerve	• Arm dislodged off armrest in supination; inadequate securement	• Wrist drop	• Pad arm board to avoid excessive pressure on ulnar + spiral groove of humerus
	Median nerve	• Arm dislodged off armrest in pronation; inadequate securement	• Weak hand grip • Diminished palmar sensation	
	Ulnar nerve	• Excess hyperextension of forearm in pronation • Elbow flexed at 90 degrees with arm folded across chest	• Weakened grip • Claw hand: extended metacarpophalangeal joint and flexed interphalangeal joint at the third and fourth fingers	
Lithotomy	Posterior tibial nerve	• Compression of posterior knee against stirrups	• Weak plantarflexion • Sensory loss in sole, lateral aspect of foot • Posterior calf paresthesia	• Manipulate both legs simultaneously • Flex hips 80–100 degrees • Hip abduction 30–45 degrees
	Peroneal nerve	• Compression of stirrups laterally around fibular neck	• Foot drop • Weak dorsiflexion • Weakened foot eversion	
	Pudendal nerve	• Excess traction and compression against stirrups	• Variable perineal sensory loss • Incontinence (rare)	
	Obturator	• Hyperflexion of thigh at hip joint (exaggerated lithotomy position)	• Motor weakness with thigh adduction	

Continued

Table 31.2 Positioning-Related Nerve Injuries—cont'd

POSITION	NERVE AFFECTED	MECHANISM	DEFICIT	PREVENTION
	Peroneal nerve	Inadequate padding of dependent leg	• Foot drop • Weak dorsiflexion • Weakened foot eversion	• Adequate padding of dependent leg
	Brachial plexus	• Excessive arm abduction >90 degrees • External arm rotation • Posterior shoulder displacement	• Shoulder pain • Variable arm and hand weakness	• Avoid ipsilateral arm abduction >90 degrees • Careful ulnar padding of contralateral hand • Placement of axillary roll just caudal to axilla
Prone	Anterior tibial nerve	Extended period of plantarflexion	Foot drop	• Careful padding and positioning of ankles, foot, leg
	Lateral femoral cutaneous nerve	Excessive pressure on lateral thigh	Numbness of anterolateral thigh	
	Brachial plexus	• Excessive shoulder abduction >90 degrees	• Shoulder pain • Variable arm and hand weakness	• Avoid shoulder and elbow abduction >90 degrees

Box 31.1 American Society of Anesthesiologists Task Force Recommendations on the Prevention of Perioperative Peripheral Neuropathies

PREOPERATIVE ASSESSMENT

- When judged appropriately, it is helpful to ascertain that patients can comfortably tolerate the anticipated operative position.

UPPER EXTREMITY POSITIONING

- Arm abduction should be limited to 90 degrees in supine patients; patients who are positioned prone may comfortably tolerate arm abduction greater than 90 degrees.
- Arms should be positioned to decrease pressure on the postcondylar groove of the humerus (ulnar groove). When arms are tucked at the side, a neutral forearm position is recommended. When arms are abducted on arm boards, either supination or a neutral forearm position is acceptable.
- Prolonged pressure on the radial nerve in the spiral groove of the humerus should be avoided.
- Extension of the elbow beyond a comfortable range may stretch the median nerve.

LOWER EXTREMITY POSITIONING

- Lithotomy positions that stretch the hamstring muscle group beyond a comfortable range may stretch the sciatic nerve.
- Prolonged pressure on the peroneal nerve at the fibular head should be avoided.
- Neither extension nor flexion of the hip increases the risk for femoral neuropathy.

PROTECTIVE PADDING

- Padded arm boards may decrease the risk for upper extremity neuropathy.
- The use of chest rolls in laterally positioned patients may decrease the risk for upper extremity neuropathies.
- Padding at the elbow and at the fibular head may decrease the risk for upper and lower extremity neuropathies, respectively.

EQUIPMENT

- Properly functioning automated blood pressure cuffs on the upper arms do not affect the risk for upper extremity neuropathies.
- Shoulder braces in steep head-down positions may increase the risk for brachial plexus neuropathies.

Continued

> **Box 31.1** American Society of Anesthesiologists Task Force Recommendations on the Prevention of Perioperative Peripheral Neuropathies—cont'd
>
> **POSTOPERATIVE ASSESSMENT**
> - A simple postoperative assessment of extremity nerve function may lead to early recognition of peripheral neuropathies.
>
> **DOCUMENTATION**
> - Charting specific positioning actions during the care of patients may result in improvements of care by (1) helping practitioners focus attention on relevant aspects of patient positioning and (2) providing information that continuous improvement processes can use to effect refinements in patient care.
>
> ---
>
> Modified from American Society of Anesthesiologists Task Force on Prevention of Perioperative Peripheral Neuropathies. Practice advisory for the prevention of perioperative peripheral neuropathies: a report by the American Society of Anesthesiologists Task Force on Prevention of Perioperative Peripheral Neuropathies. *Anesthesiology* 2000;92(4):1168-1182.

lithotomy position. Impaired tissue perfusion, tissue ischemia, and increased compartment pressures result. Risk factors include obesity, peripheral vascular disease, muscular build, and intraoperative blood loss or hypotension. Typical presenting symptoms include pain out of proportion to exam, swelling, and loss of lower extremity sensation. Management includes urgent orthopedic consult, compartment pressure monitoring, and urgent fasciotomy for compartment pressures >30 mm Hg. Irreversible damage may occur with prolonged pressures >50 mm Hg. Prevention includes intermittently relieving the legs from lithotomy position and minimizing operative time.

Rhabdomyolysis. Prolonged operative time in lithotomy or flank position may result in rhabdomyolysis, resulting in release of intracellular myoglobin, creatine kinase, and lactate dehydrogenase into the bloodstream. Obese patients are at particularly high risk. Patients may present with myalgias, limb weakness, and myoglobinuria ("tea-colored urine"). Acute kidney injury, oliguria, or anuria may result. This should be managed expectantly with intravenous hydration and urinary alkalinization as needed.

Table 31.3 Common Nerve Injuries Associated with Specific Urologic Procedures

PROCEDURE	NERVES AT RISK	DEFICITS	AVOIDANCE
Psoas hitch	Genitofemoral nerve	Paresthesias or pain distributed along base of scrotum and penis, upper/medial thigh	Longitudinal placement of anchoring sutures parallel to psoas tendon
	Femoral nerve	Weakness in knee extension, paresthesias or pain over anteromedial thigh	Careful placement of retractors, avoidance of compression on psoas muscle
Inguinal orchiectomy; hernia repair	Ilioinguinal nerve	Paresthesias or pain of lateral hemiscrotum, groin	Careful identification, isolation, and preservation of nerve within inguinal canal
Pelvic lymph node dissection	Obturator nerve	Paresthesias or pain of medial thigh; weak thigh adduction	Complete visualization of nerve prior to clip placement

Intraoperative Complications

Trocar and Veress Needle-Related Injuries. Similar rates of injury have been described for open Hassan technique and blind Veress needle placement. Careful attention to the angle of entry, sufficient skin incision, and rotational movement during trocar placement may all minimize risk of injury during trocar placement.

Subcutaneous Emphysema, Pneumothorax. Subcutaneous emphysema develops owing to improper placement of the Veress needle or, more commonly, to leakage of carbon dioxide (CO_2) around ports. The pathognomonic sign is crepitus over the abdomen and thorax; in male patients, a pneumoscrotum may also develop. It is important to place each port so that it is pointing toward the surgical field, to avoid the continued forceful redirection of the port during the procedure that results in widening of the tissue tract around the port. The earliest signs of pneumothorax may be the development of subcutaneous emphysema, especially in the neck and chest area. More ominous signs, such as hypotension and decreased breath sounds with an increase in ventilatory pressure, are indicative of a tension pneumothorax.

Major Vascular Injury. Access-related vascular injury is rare (0.04%–0.1% incidence). The left common iliac vessels are at greatest risk. Immediate recognition and expeditious management of vascular injury is critical. This includes direct pressure on the area of injury, increasing pneumoperitoneum pressure (to 25 mm Hg), and gaining proximal and distal control/exposure. Vascular surgery consultation should be done if the injury is significant. The trocar should be left in place because this may help tamponade bleeding and help identify the location of injury. Small Veress needle punctures may be self-limited and is simply managed by choosing a different site. However, trocar-related injuries are typically more extensive and nearly always require rapid conversion to open surgery for immediate repair.

Injury to Epigastric Vessels. Delayed presentation of epigastric vessel injury is common after minimally invasive surgery because trocars may initially tamponade these vessels. Transillumination of the abdominal wall prior to trocar placement and careful inspection of lateral ports following trocar removal may help avoid or identify any potential injury. Minor bleeding may be managed with electrocautery; more significant bleeding may require direct suturing by laparoscopic approaches or the Carter-Thomason CloseSure system.

Gas Embolus. Gas embolus is a rare complication that may occur following Veress placement and accidental carbon dioxide insufflation into the vascular system. This manifests as sudden hypoxia, hypercarbia, and hypotension and a characteristic "mill wheel murmur." Management includes immediate desufflation, administration of 100% FiO_2, and repositioning of the patient in Trendelenberg and left lateral decubitus position (i.e., right side up), to trap the air bubble in the right atrium. The patient is hyperventilated with 100% oxygen. A central line should be placed to aspirate out the air embolus.

Bowel Injury. The initial signs of visceral injury consist of aspiration of blood, urine, or bowel contents through the Veress needle or, in the case of a solid organ, high pressures on initial insufflation.

Bowel or bladder entry by the Veress needle needs no further treatment other than needle withdrawal. The first sign of this bowel insufflation is asymmetrical abdominal distention followed by flatus and insufflation of only a small amount of CO_2 (<2 L) before high pressures are reached. If this complication is suspected, then the insufflation line should be disconnected; the outflow of gas will immediately confirm bowel entry. The surgeon should routinely pass the laparoscope through the secondary port to inspect the puncture site of the initial port to identify possible through and through bowel injury.

Barotrauma. Prolonged elevated pressures (>15 mm Hg) may result in barotrauma. Prolonged high pressures may be caused by insufficient and infrequent monitoring of CO_2 pressure, malfunction of the insufflator, or additional pressures produced by auxiliary devices. Furthermore, barotrauma may be caused by using positive end-expiratory pressure resulting in rupture of a pulmonary bleb or bulla. The initial sign of barotrauma may be hypotension caused by decreased cardiac output secondary to an acute drop in venous return caused by compression of the vena cava. Also, a pneumothorax or pneumomediastinum may develop because of the high ventilation pressures. The surgeon should desufflate the abdomen and, after the hemodynamic changes have been reversed, reinitiate the pneumoperitoneum.

Stapler Malfunction. The reported incidence of stapler malfunction is about 1%. The most common cause of malfunction is excessive thickness of the stapled tissue; thus, adequate dissection of vascular pedicles is critical to ensure proper stapler application. Clip placement should be avoided in the area of the staple line, and both stapler jaws should be visualized prior to staple firing. A jammed stapler may be rescued by a second staple fire if adequate room is maintained proximal to the initial staple line.

Vascular Injury. Most major vascular injuries occur intraoperatively and are immediately recognized and addressed. Risk factors include prior abdominal surgery, aberrant vascular anatomy, and concomitant abdominal pathology. Adequate exposure and identification of the injured vessel is critical. Controlled injuries may be managed laparoscopically or robotically by primary repair with selective use of vascular clamps or careful application of surgical clips or staplers (Fig. 31.1). Conversion to hand-assist or laparotomy should be performed without delay. A Satinsky

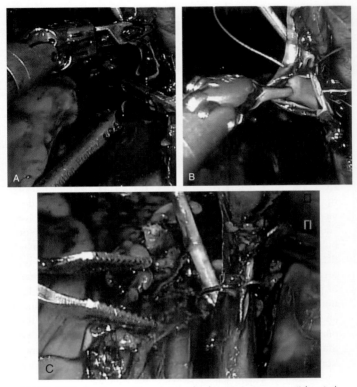

FIG. 31.1 (A) The fourth arm of the robot is utilized to gain temporary partial control. (B) The defect is repaired with a 5.0 running suture with excellent visualization and control. (C) Final repair with some luminal narrowing but proximal and distal filling of the vein with the sequential pneumatic device confirming flow. (From Tare D, Maria P, Ghavamian R. Vascular complications in laparoscopic and robotic urologic surgery. In: Ghavamian R, ed. *Complications of laparoscopic and robotic urologic surgery.* 1st ed. New York: Springer, 2010:45–58.)

clamp can be used for larger injuries. Ligation may be performed without significant consequences if the injured vessel has adequate collateral circulation (e.g., internal iliac artery, inferior mesenteric artery). In contrast, injury to the superior mesenteric artery universally warrants immediate repair. There should be a low threshold for open conversion and vascular surgery consult, particularly for major injuries. Blood transfusion should be administered as needed. When suspected, it is important to immediately communicate the situation to anesthesia and nursing staff so they can prepare for resuscitation measures.

Bowel Injury. Bowel injury may also result from forceful tissue handling or thermal injury due to inappropriate direct activation, coupling to another instrument, capacitive coupling, and insulation failure (Fig. 31.2). For small perforations or serosal injury, primary suture repair is appropriate. Bowel resection should be performed if viability is in question. Limited colonic injury may be managed through open, laparoscopic, or robotic approaches if there is no fecal spillage. Extensive colonic injuries with obvious fecal spillage may require diverting colostomy, and general surgery consultation is prudent.

> **Delayed Presentation** – Unrecognized bowel injury may present within 24–48 hours of injury with trocar site pain disproportionate to exam, abdominal distension, ileus, or diarrhea. Patients may lack typical signs of peritonitis, acute abdomen, or leukocytosis. Computed tomography (CT) with oral and intravenous contrast is diagnostic. Abdominal radiographs are notoriously inaccurate because the CO_2 may remain as free air for up to 9 days after the procedure. Minor postoperative thermal injuries of the bowel discovered late in the postoperative period (i.e., >5–7 days) may be managed conservatively with antibiotics and an elemental diet. A closed fistula may develop that will heal with this approach. However, if the patient does not respond rapidly or develops worsening peritonitis, open surgical exploration is mandatory.

Rectal Injury. Rectal injury may occur during radical prostatectomy. The overall incidence is low (<0.5%) for both open and robotic approaches but >10-fold higher for salvage prostatectomy. A rectal end to end anastomosis (EEA) dilator may aid intraoperative identification of the rectum during challenging cases, and electrocautery should be avoided during dissection of the posterior prostatic plane. For minor lacerations in the absence of gross fecal spillage, multilayer primary closure with omental overlay and drainage may be performed; the integrity of the repair should be tested with air injection. More extensive injury is best

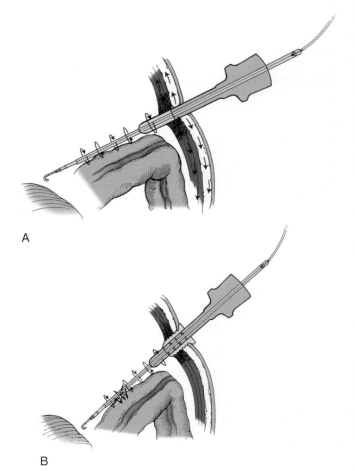

A

B

FIG. 31.2 Capacitive coupling. (A) Charge surrounding the activated monopolar electrode is conducted back to the all-metal cannula and dispersed by the abdominal wall. (B) The electrosurgical instrument is being used through a metal cannula that has been anchored to the skin with a nonconductive plastic grip; accordingly, the electrical field cannot be conducted to the abdominal wall because the plastic retainer acts as an insulator; a stronger electrical charge is thus conducted to any other tissue in contact with the cannula.

managed with diverting colostomy. General surgery consultation should be considered.

> **Delayed Presentation** – Unrecognized rectal injuries may present with nausea, vomiting, ileus, focal pelvic pain, or peritonitis. CT with rectal contrast or gastrograffin enema is typically diagnostic. Surgical exploration and diverting colostomy should be performed to minimize risk of sepsis and rectourethral fistula formation.

Pancreatic Injury. The tail of the pancreas is at risk of injury during left renal or adrenal surgery often caused by mechanical retraction. The typical presentation is abdominal discomfort, elevated serum lipase and amylase levels, and leukocytosis. Pancreatic injury may progress to pancreatic fistula, pseudocyst, or intraabdominal abscess if not managed appropriately. Obvious intraoperative injury should be managed with distal pancreatectomy.

> **Delayed Presentation** – Postoperative manifestations include increased drainage from intraabdominal drains and elevated drain amylase and lipase. Cross-sectional imaging should be performed to assess for undrained fluid collections. Management includes bowel rest, total parenteral nutrition (TPN), and percutaneous drainage of large fluid collections. Octreotide and somatostatin analogues may further minimize pancreatic injury-related morbidity. Distal pancreatectomy may be needed for refractory cases.

Duodenal Injury. The duodenum is at risk of injury during right renal procedures because kocherization of the duodenum is necessary to expose the right renal hilum. Even minor shear or puncture injuries may lead to perforation, with patients presenting with postoperative fever, abdominal pain, and sepsis. Duodenal wall hematomas secondary to compression injury may lead to prolonged ileus, requiring bowel rest and total parenteral nutrition for management.

Injury to Genitourinary Structures

Intraoperative injury to genitourinary structures may occur during both urologic and nonurologic surgeries. Injuries recognized postoperatively are associated with more severe patient morbidity and more complex management; thus, timely recognition and work-up of suspected intraoperative injuries is critical.

Urethral Injuries. Urethral injury may commonly occur following traumatic attempts at Foley catheterization, in the setting of female urethral reconstructive surgery, or during colorectal surgery. Risk factors for traumatic catheterization in particular include history of known urethral stricture, prior urethral surgery or pelvic radiation, known prostatic enlargement, and inexperienced operators.

>   **Diagnosis** – Cystoscopy and intraoperative retrograde urethrogram is diagnostic in cases of suspected urethral injury. During female pelvic reconstructive surgery, direct visualization of trocars or mesh within the urethra may occur, though signs of urethral injury may also be more subtle (ex: tethering of the urethra or bladder neck). Obvious transection injury may also be identified by visualization of the urethral catheter through a urethrotomy.

>   **Management** – Urethral injury should be managed with indwelling Foley catheter placement and drainage; this may require use of special catheters (e.g., coudé) or cystoscopic guidance. Transection injuries may be repaired using absorbable monofilament suture. In women, peritoneal, omental, or labial fat interposition should also be considered between the anterior vaginal wall and urethra to minimize risk of fistula formation. If the injury is too extensive, suprapubic catheter placement may be considered, with delayed definitive repair.

Bladder Injury. The bladder is the most commonly injured organ during pelvic surgery. Injury most commonly results from inadvertent laceration, though devascularization injury may also occur. Occasionally, intentional cystotomy may be made, such as in cases of tumor excision or placenta accreta. Classification of injury is determined by depth, location, and size of injury (Table 31.4). Risk factors include anatomic distortion (e.g., from mass effect, prolapse), previous pelvic surgery, and pelvic radiation.

>   **Diagnosis** – Immediate diagnosis requires a high index of suspicion. Visualization of the Foley catheter, urinary extravasation, and presence of blood (or gas in laparoscopic cases) may be indicators of injury. Intraoperative instillation of contrast, fluid, or dye may help localize the injury when an obvious defect is not visible. Cystoscopy may also be used

Table 31.4 Grading System for Classifying Bladder Injury

GRADE	INJURY	DESCRIPTION
1	Hematoma	Contusion, intramural hematoma
1	Laceration	Partial thickness
2	Laceration	Extraperitoneal bladder wall laceration <2 cm
3	Laceration	Extraperitoneal (>2 cm) or intraperitoneal (<2 cm) bladder wall laceration
4	Laceration	Intraperitoneal (>2 cm) bladder wall laceration
5	Laceration	Laceration extending into trigone (bladder neck or ureteral orifice)
6		Not salvageable

Data from Moore EE, Cogbill TH, Jurkovich GJ, et al. Organ injury scaling. III: chest wall, abdominal vascular, ureter, bladder, and urethra. *J Trauma* 1992:33(3):337-339.

to directly visualize the bladder. Patients with unrecognized bladder injury may present in a delayed fashion with abdominal distension, ileus, fevers, chills, and leukocytosis. CT cystogram provides definitive diagnosis in these cases. In either case, concomitant injury to the ureters, trigone, bladder neck, vagina, and rectum must also be ruled out.

Management – Recognized bladder lacerations should be closed in two layers with absorbable suture. When the area of injury is not immediately visible, cystotomy may be performed to facilitate identification of the area of injury. Cystotomy closure should be tested intraoperatively to ensure it is watertight. Bladder drainage for 7–14 days is recommended.

Ureteral Injury. Ureteral injury may occur through inadvertent ligation, thermal injury, transection, crush injury, devascularization, or avulsion, with varying degrees of injury severity (Table 31.5). The distal ureter is the most common site of injury. Risk factors include prior pelvic radiation, malignancy, and significant adhesions. Prophylactic ureteral catheter placement does not decrease the rate of intraoperative ureteral injury, though this may facilitate ureteral identification. However, these may also cause ureteral edema, leading to postoperative acute kidney injury (AKI).

Diagnosis – Ureteral efflux alone is an inadequate indicator of ureteral integrity, and cystoscopy and retrograde pyelogram remain the gold standard to assess for ureteral injury. Intraoperative urogram may also be performed. Postoperatively,

Table 31.5 Grading System for Classifying Ureteral Injury

GRADE	INJURY	DESCRIPTION
1	Hematoma	Contusion or hematoma without devascularization
2	Laceration	<50% transection
3	Laceration	>50% transection
4	Laceration	Complete transection with ≤2 cm devascularization
5	Laceration	Complete transection with >2 cm devascularization
6		Not salvageable

From Best CD, Petrone P, Buscarini M, et al. Traumatic ureteral injuries: a single institution experience validating the American Association for the Surgery of Trauma-Organ Injury Scale grading scale. *J Urol* 2005;173(4):1202-1205.

elevated drain creatinine may indicate unrecognized injury. Definitive postoperative diagnosis is made through cross-sectional imaging such as CT with intravenous contrast and delayed phase imaging.

Management – When recognized acutely, management of ureteral injury is dictated by the location and severity of injury (Table 31.6). When appropriate, endoscopic management is preferred. Repair of ureteral transection should be performed with absorbable suture in a tension-free, watertight manner

Table 31.6 Management of Ureteral Injuries

LOCATION	SEVERITY	MANAGEMENT
Distal	Grade 1–2	Ureteral stent or nephrostomy tube × 2–6 weeks (stent preferred)
	Grade 3–5	Ureteroneocystotomy ± psoas hitch or Boari flap
Mid or proximal	Grade 1–2	Ureteral stent or nephrostomy tube × 2–6 weeks (stent preferred)
	Grade 3–5	Uretero-ureterostomy over ureteral stent
Proximal	Grade 5	Temporization with percutaneous nephrostomy tube
		Delayed repair
		• Ureterocalicostomy
		• Transureteroureterostomy
		• Ileal ureter interposition
		• Autotransplantation
		• Appendiceal on lay or buccal mucosal graft

over an indwelling stent. Omental or peritoneal interposition should be considered in these cases.

For highly complex injuries or those diagnosed in a delayed fashion, temporary drainage with a stent or percutaneous nephrostomy tube should be performed, and delayed repair is preferred. After definitive management, patients should be monitored for delayed complications such as stricture or fistula formation.

Renal Injury. Most renal injuries result from trauma rather than iatrogenic causes. Hemorrhage from renal vascular or parenchymal injuries is most common and may typically be managed conservatively with close monitoring and transfusion. In refractory or severe cases, selective embolization may be used. This is preferred over open exploration because of lower rates of renal parenchymal loss and patient morbidity.

Postoperative Complications

Urine Leak. Urine leak may occur following any urinary anastomoses (e.g., urethrovesical junction anastomosis, uretero-enteric anastomosis) or following partial nephrectomy with collecting system entry.

Diagnosis – Small leaks may be relatively asymptomatic, but larger leaks may present with fever, ileus, or abdominal pain related to chemical peritonitis. Drainage may increase from surgical drains, and drain fluid creatinine will be elevated. Imaging with delayed phase CT or cystogram defines the location and extent of the leak.

Management – In the absence of complicating factors (e.g., infection, distal obstruction, foreign bodies), some urinary leaks will heal over time with adequate drainage. When bladder injury is diagnosed postoperatively, the key factor is whether the drainage is extraperitoneal or intraperitoneal. Extraperitoneal extravasation may be treated by placing a Foley catheter. Intraperitoneal drainage is an indication for laparoscopic or open repair.

Renal Vascular Complications. Delayed postoperative bleeding may occur following partial nephrectomy in ~1%–3% of patients, resulting from arterio venous fistula or pseudoaneurysm formation. Greater risk is associated with deeper tumors and increasing tumor complexity.

Diagnosis – Patients typically present 2–3 weeks postoperatively with significant hematuria, flank pain, hypotension, and decline in hematocrit. Up to 10% of patients may be asymptomatic and diagnosed on CT angiography alone. Imaging may demonstrate a blush of contrast corresponding to active extravasation (Fig. 31.3).

Management – Small asymptomatic aneurysms may resolve spontaneously with conservative management and close monitoring. However, symptomatic pseudoaneurysms (e.g., acute blood loss anemia, hypotension) should be addressed with arterial angiography and selective embolization (Fig. 31.4).

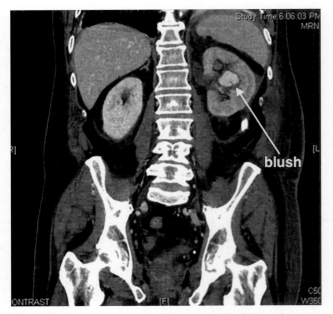

FIG. 31.3 Segmental renal arterial pseudoaneurysm. Arterial phase of a contrast computed tomography image revealing an arterial blush in a patient 2 days after a left laparoscopic partial nephrectomy. (From Tare D, Maria P, Ghavamian R. Vascular complications in laparoscopic and robotic urologic surgery. In: Ghavamian R, ed. *Complications of laparoscopic and robotic urologic surgery.* 1st ed. New York: Springer, 2010:45-58.)

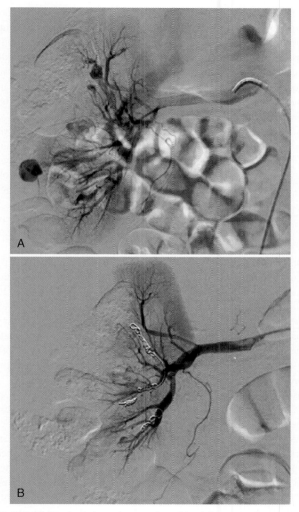

FIG. 31.4 (A) Renal arteriography revealing at least three pseudoaneurysms 2 days after a right robotic partial nephrectomy for a 6-cm midpole renal mass. (B) Selective coil embolization revealing resolution of the bleeding pseudoaneurysms.

Lymphocele. Lymphoceles are the most common complication resulting from lymph node dissection. These are caused by disruption in lymphatic drainage and may occur as early as 48–72 hours postoperatively. Risk increases with greater extent of lymphadenectomy. There are no robust data to support a single optimal approach to management of lymphatics (e.g., clips versus bipolar). Use of adjunctive hemostatic agents such as fibrin sealants has been described to optimize lymphostasis.

> **Diagnosis** – Most small lymphoceles are asymptomatic. However, large lymphoceles may cause symptoms due to mass effect, such as lower urinary tract symptoms or lower extremity edema.

> **Management** – Small, asymptomatic lymphoceles may be observed. Drainage with marsupialization and a peritoneal window should be considered if the lymphocele is large or symptomatic. Simple drainage alone may increase the risk of superinfection and may not be sufficient to prevent reaccumulation of lymphatic fluid.

Port Site Hernias. Port site hernias may occur in up to 5% of patients following minimally invasive surgeries. Risk factors include older age, previous hernia, operating time, and trocar size (10-fold greater for 12-mm vs 10-mm trocars). Single-port surgery also carries greater hernia risk. Cross-sectional imaging is diagnostic, and most port-site hernias can be repaired in a minimally invasive fashion. Closure of large fascial defects with figure-of-8 absorbable suture at the time of initial surgery may prevent this complication.

Fascial Dehiscence. The incidence of fascial dehiscence is ~1%–2%. Risk factors include advanced age, malnutrition, corticosteroid use, obesity, radiotherapy, surgical site infection (SSI), and technical errors at the time of wound closure (e.g., knot slippage, excessive suture tension, sutures placed too close to the fascial edge). There appears to be no difference in fascial dehiscence or incisional hernia risk between running or interrupted closure with slowly absorbable suture. Retention sutures have become less frequently used because of greater patient morbidity and discomfort, and inconsistent efficacy in reducing rates of evisceration, wound infection, and incisional hernia.

> **Diagnosis** – Dehiscence typically occurs about 1 week postoperatively and may be heralded by a gush of serosanguinous fluid. Nausea and vomiting, obstipation, abdominal

bulge, or frank evisceration of bowel contents are other presenting symptoms. Cross-sectional imaging is diagnostic and provides information regarding the location and extent of the dehiscence.

Management – Small fascial disruptions may be managed with wound packing and close observation. However, most dehiscences require urgent return to the operating room, particularly if evisceration has occurred. In the interim, bowel contents should be protected with saline-moistened towels. Intraoperatively, the fascial edges should be carefully inspected; primary closure may be appropriate if these are healthy and may be brought back together without tension. Otherwise, wound debridement and closure with absorbable mesh or biologic grafts is indicated.

Stomal Complications. In the immediate postoperative period, stomal necrosis or mucocutaneous separation may occur. Over the longer term, stomal retraction, stenosis, or fistula formation may develop. Peristomal skin complications such as candidiasis, skin trauma, contact dermatitis, folliculitis, or hyperplastic growth may also affect nearly half of all patients undergoing urinary diversion. Attention to stomal perfusion and configuration intraoperatively, as well as perioperative education and engagement of stomal therapists, may help minimize these complications.

Venous Thromboembolism (VTE). The reported incidence of VTE is 0.7% following renal surgery, 1.1% following radical prostatectomy, and 5%–8% following cystectomy. Most events occur following discharge. Risk factors include pelvic surgery, malignancy, obesity, and longer surgical times. Risk-adapted approaches to thromboprophylaxis are based on procedure type and patient factors (Table 31.7). Level I evidence exists to support the use of extended thromboprophylaxis for 1 month following major abdominal or pelvic surgery for urologic malignancy.

PEDIATRIC COMPLICATIONS

Complications in pediatric urologic surgery are similar to those in adult practice. A child's response, however, can be quite unique. Children can physiologically compensate for blood loss, respiratory insufficiency, and electrolyte abnormalities until they rapidly decline clinically. Management approaches are generally similar; however, children often require sedation

Table 31.7 Recommendations for Thromboprophylaxis in Various Risk Groups

| RISK FOR SYMPTOMATIC VTE | RISK AND CONSEQUENCES OF MAJOR BLEEDING | |
	AVERAGE RISK (~1%)	HIGH RISK (~2%) OR SEVERE CONSEQUENCES
Very low (<0.5%)	No specific prophylaxis	No specific prophylaxis
Low (~1.5%)	IPC	IPC
Moderate (~3.0%)	LDUH, LMWH, or IPC	IPC
High (~6.0%)	LDUH or LMWH plus IPC	IPC until risk for bleeding diminishes and pharmacologic prophylaxis can be added
High-risk cancer surgery	LDUH or LMWH plus IPC and extended duration prophylaxis with LMWH postdischarge	IPC until risk for bleeding diminishes and pharmacologic prophylaxis can be added
High risk, LDUH an LMWH contraindicated or not available	Fondaparinux or low-dose aspirin (160 mg), IPC, or both	IPC until risk for bleeding diminishes and pharmacologic prophylaxis can be added

IPC, Intermittent pneumatic compression; *LDUH*, low-dose unfractionated heparin; *LMWH*, low–molecular-weight heparin; *VTE*, venous thromboembolism.
From Gould MK, Garcia DA, Wren SM, et al. American College of Chest Physicians: Prevention of VTE in nonorthopedic surgical patients: Antithombotic therapy and prevention of thrombosis, 9th ed: American College of Chest Physician Evidence-Based Clinical Practice Guidelines. *Chest* 2012;141(2 suppl):e227S-e277S.

or anesthesia for even minor drainage procedures. Conventional predictors of perioperative morbidity are of less value in children. Unfortunately, the standard Clavien system for grading complications is not very suitable to children because of their need for sedation for even minor procedures.

PATTERNS OF COMPLICATIONS

Hemorrhage

Surgical hemorrhage in children is relatively uncommon and typically occurs with pelvic or renal surgery, yet it can occur with hypospadias and even circumcision. The child may compensate for significant blood loss, but the usual clinical signs of pallor, tachycardia, labile blood pressure, and abdominal pain are all indicators of possible bleeding.

Management is directed at identifying the source in determining whether direct or indirect measures such as pressure may be adequate. Retrovesical hemorrhage after ureteral reimplantation can be a significant source of blood loss and is often overlooked. Its presence may be indicated by persistent bladder symptoms despite catheter removal even in the absence of significant hematuria.

Obstruction

Urinary obstruction following reconstructive procedures, in particular, ureteral reimplantation, pyeloplasty, and ureteroureterostomy, is a significant risk that must be identified early. Acute indications include nausea and vomiting, flank pain, and obviously oliguria if this represents bilateral obstruction. A high index of suspicion is important. Ultrasound imaging can usually identify the problem, but functional imaging may be necessary for confirmation. In the setting of oliguria, careful attention to concomitant electrolyte disorders is important.

Subacute obstruction can develop in the weeks to months after surgery, and routine ultrasound or renal scan monitoring is important to identify this. In the setting of preoperative hydronephrosis, judging the clinical significance of postoperative dilation may be challenging. In general, if the degree of dilation in the first 3–4 months after surgery is worse than preoperative, functional assessment and possible decompression is needed. Otherwise continued monitoring is reasonable.

Management in the acute setting requires prompt decompression, and the options of percutaneous nephrostomy or ureteral stenting are both useful depending on the clinical context. Maintaining a percutaneous nephrostomy tube can be difficult in small children but does provide the opportunity of assessing whether obstruction has resolved without losing access to the kidney. Many of these obstructions are transient, but if clinical symptoms are significant enough, intervention is required. Nonresolving obstruction can respond to balloon dilation with stenting, but this is unpredictable. Formal reconstruction may be necessary.

Urine Leak

As with adult patients, urine leak is common following reconstructive surgeries. Identification and management principles are similar. In children, voiding dysfunction and withholding of urination can produce urine leak in the setting of a ureteral stent with retrograde flow.

Management of urine leak requires identification of the location and usually proximal drainage or stenting are sufficient. In the setting of an augmentation cystoplasty, bladder leakage can be difficult to control and may require multiple drainage sites or even proximal diversion.

Infection

Infection in pediatric surgical wounds is uncommon but present with the usual signs of swelling, erythema, tenderness, drainage, and fever. Prophylactic antibiotics are rarely needed or indicated. The risk factors for infections include urinary contamination, prior infections, and even colonized parents.

Urinary tract infections following surgery, particularly with indwelling drainage tubes such as stents, can be difficult to prevent and there is controversy whether prophylactic antibiotics after perioperative antibiotics are useful. In the setting of a prior history of recurrent infections, continued prophylaxis while drainage tubes are in place is probably appropriate.

Management of infections is similar to adults with drainage of any surgical wound infection, although preemptive treatment can sometimes prevent the need for drainage. Urinary infection is usually treatable with parenteral or oral antibiotics based on cultures. Preoperative cultures can be useful in patients considered at high risk.

Tissue Breakdown

In hypospadias repair and genital reconstructive surgeries, tissue breakdown is a frustrating complication that often necessitates secondary repairs. The more extensive the surgery, the greater the likelihood of impaired healing. Prevention is directed at basic concepts of delicate tissue handling, drainage, avoidance of foreign materials, and maintaining a healthy blood supply. Reported enthusiasm for hyperbaric treatment has little objective support.

Management is directed at maintaining as much healthy tissue as possible, draining any hematoma, and keeping the tissues clean. It is essential to be patient and defer any secondary surgery for at least 4 months. Only in the case of a urethral fistula with distal urethral stenosis is early intervention justified. Temporary drainage may facilitate fistula healing.

Bowel Injury

Bowel injury in laparoscopic and robotic procedures or open reconstructive surgeries can be devastating but will usually follow the adult patterns of presentation and management.

Suggested Readings

Abdel-Meguid T, Gomella L. Prevention and management of complications. St. Louis: Quality Medical Publishing, 1996

Alberts BD, Woldu SL, Weinberg AC, et al. Venous thromboembolism after major urologic oncology surgery: a focus on the incidence and timing of thromboembolic events after 27,455 operations. *Urology* 2014;84:799-806.

American Society of Anesthesiologists Task Force on Prevention of Perioperative Peripheral Neuropathies: Practice advisory for the prevention of perioperative peripheral neuropathies: an updated report by the American Society of Anesthesiologists Task Force on Prevention of Perioperative Peripheral Neuropathies. *Anesthesiology* 2018;128:11-26.

Bishoff JT, Allaf ME, Kirkels W, et al. Laparoscopic bowel injury: incidence and clinical presentation. *J Urol* 1999;161:887-890

Chuang KW, Zaretz W, Gordon S. Complications of surgical positioning AUA Update Series. 2011. Vol 30, Lesson 17. Dindo classification of surgical complications is not a statistically reliable system for grading morbidity in pediatric urology. *J Urol* 2016;195(2):460-464.

Clavien PA, Barkun J, de Oliveira ML, et al. The Clavien-dindo classification of surgical complications: five-year experience. *Ann Surg* 2009;250:187-196.

Dwyer ME, Dwyer JT, Cannon GM Jr, et al. The Clavien-dissection at the time of robot-assisted radical prostatectomy. *Eur Urol* 2017;71(2):155-158.

Felder S, Rasmussen MS, King R, et al. Prolonged thromboprophylaxis with low molecular weight heparin for abdominal or pelvic surgery. *Cochrane Database Syst Rev* 2019;8(8):CD004318.

Grande P, Di Pierro GB, Mordasini L, et al. Prospective randomized trial comparing titanium clips to b polar coagulation in sealing lymphatic vessels during pelvic lymph node dissection at the time of robot-assisted radical prostatectomy. *Eur Urol* 2017;71(2):155-158.

Hefermehl LJ, Largo RA, Hermanns T, et. al. Lateral temperature spread of monopolar, bipolar and ultrasonic instruments for robot assisted laparoscopic surgery. *BJU Int* 2013;114:245-252.

Hershlag A, Loy R, et al. Femoral neuropathy after laparoscopy. *J Reprod Med* 1990;35:575-576.

Hyams ES, Pierorazio P, Proteek O, et al. Iatrogenic vascular lesions after minimally invasive partial nephrectomy: a multi-institutional study of clinical and renal functional outcomes. *Urology* 2011;78:820-826.

Jiang R, Wolf S, Alkazemi MH, et al. The evaluation of three comorbidity indices in predicting postoperative complications and readmissions in pediatric urology. *J Pediatr Urol.* 2018;14(3):244, e1-e7.

Liss M, Skarecky D, Morales B, et al. Preventing perioperative complications of robotic-assisted radical prostatectomy. *Urology* 2013;81:319-323.

Morey AF, Brandes S, Dugi DD, et al. Urotrauma: AUA guideline. *J Urol* 2014;192:327-335.

Mumtaz FH, Chew H, Gelister JS. Lower limb compartment syndrome associated with the lithotomy position: concepts and perspectives for the urologist. *BJU Int* 2002;90:792-799

Smith A, Anders M, Auffenberg G, et al. *Optimizing outcomes in urologic surgery: postoperative.* American Urological Association White Paper, 2018.

Index

Page numbers followed by "*f*" indicate figures, "*t*" indicate tables, and "*b*" indicate boxes